Heart Failure: Clinical Assessment

Heart Failure: Clinical Assessment

Editor: Bernard Tyler

FOSTER ACADEMICS

www.fosteracademics.com

www.fosteracademics.com

FOSTER ACADEMICS

Cataloging-in-Publication Data

Heart failure : clinical assessment / edited by Bernard Tyler.
p. cm.
Includes bibliographical references and index.
ISBN 978-1-63242-547-8
1. Heart failure. 2. Cardiac arrest. 3. Heart--Diseases. 4. Outcome assessment (Medical care).
I. Tyler, Bernard.
RC685.C53 H43 2018
616.129--dc23

Foster Academics,
118-35 Queens Blvd., Suite 400,
Forest Hills, NY 11375, USA

ISBN 978-1-63242-547-8 (Hardback)

Printed and bound in China.

Contents

Preface

This book has been a concerted effort by a group of academicians, researchers and scientists, who have contributed their research works for the realization of the book. This book has materialized in the wake of emerging advancements and innovations in this field. Therefore, the need of the hour was to compile all the required researches and disseminate the knowledge to a broad spectrum of people comprising of students, researchers and specialists of the field.

The inability of the heart to function properly and its incapability to pump blood is known as heart failure. The common causes of heart failure are high blood pressure, valvular heart disease, cardiomyopathy and excessive intake of alcohol. Excessive tiredness, shortness of breath and leg swelling are some of the most common symptoms of heart failure. The topics included in this book on heart failure are of utmost significance and are bound to provide incredible insights to readers. It will serve as a valuable source of reference for graduate and postgraduate students.

At the end of the preface, I would like to thank the authors for their brilliant chapters and the publisher for guiding us all-through the making of the book till its final stage. Also, I would like to thank my family for providing the support and encouragement throughout my academic career and research projects.

Editor

Allopurinol Therapy in Gout Patients Does Not Associate with Beneficial Cardiovascular Outcomes: A Population-Based Matched-Cohort Study

Victor C. Kok[1,2*], Jorng-Tzong Horng[1,3*], Wan-Shan Chang[3], Ya-Fang Hong[4], Tzu-Hao Chang[5]

1 Public Health and Clinical Informatics Research Group, Department of Biomedical Informatics, Asia University, Wufeng, Taichung, Taiwan, **2** Department of Internal Medicine, Kuang Tien General Hospital, Shalu, Taichung, Taiwan, **3** Department of Computer Science and Information Engineering, National Central University, Jhongli, Taoyuan, Taiwan, **4** Institute of Molecular Biology, Academia Sinica, Nankang, Taipei, Taiwan, **5** Graduate Institute of Biomedical Informatics, Taipei Medical University, Taipei, Taiwan

Abstract

Introduction: Previous studies have shown an association between gout and/or hyperuricemia and a subsequent increase in cardiovascular disease (CVD) outcomes. Allopurinol reduces vascular oxidative stress, ameliorates inflammatory state, improves endothelial function, and prevents atherosclerosis progression. Accordingly, we tested the hypothesis that a positive association between allopurinol therapy in gout patients and future cardiovascular outcomes is present using a population-based matched-cohort study design.

Methods: Patients aged ≥40 years with newly diagnosed gout having no pre-existing severe form of CVD were separated into allopurinol (n = 2483) and non-allopurinol (n = 2483) groups after matching for age, gender, index date, diabetes mellitus, hypertension, hyperlipidemia, and atrial fibrillation. The two groups were also balanced in terms of uric acid nephrolithiasis, acute kidney injury, hepatitis, and Charlson comorbidity index.

Results: With a median follow-up time of 5.25 years, the allopurinol group had a modest increase in cardiovascular risk [relative risk, 1.20; 95% confidence interval (CI), 1.08–1.34]. A Cox proportional hazard model adjusted for chronic kidney disease, uremia, and gastric ulcer gave a hazard ratio (HR) for cardiovascular outcomes of 1.25 (95% CI, 1.10–1.41) in gout patients receiving allopurinol compared with the non-allopurinol group. In further analysis of patients receiving urate-lowering therapy, the uricosuric agent group (n = 1713) had an adjusted HR of 0.83 (0.73–0.95) for cardiovascular events compared with the allopurinol group.

Conclusions: The current population-based matched-cohort study did not support the association between allopurinol therapy in gout patients with normal risk for cardiovascular sequels and beneficial future cardiovascular outcomes. Several important risk factors for cardiovascular disease, such as smoking, alcohol consumption, body mass index, blood pressure were not obtainable in the current retrospective cohort study, thus could potentially bias the effect estimate.

Editor: Guoying Wang, Johns Hopkins Bloomberg School of Public Health, United States of America

Funding: This work was partially supported by the National Science Council of the Republic of China under contract no. NSC 101-2221-E-008-125-MY3. There are no other funders to support the work. The funders had no role in study design, data collection and analysis, decision to publish, or preparation of the manuscript.

Competing Interests: The authors have declared that no competing interests exist.

* E-mail: doctorkok@hotmail.com (VCK); horng@db.csie.ncu.edu.tw (J-TH)

Introduction

Gout is a common disease resulting from urate crystal deposition in joints, connective tissues, and parenchymal organs including the kidneys, which may present clinically as gouty arthropathy, accumulation of urate crystals in the form of tophaceous deposits in numerous tissues, gouty nephropathy, or uric acid nephrolithiasis.[1] The prevalence of gout among the general United States population in 2007–2008 was 3.9% (8.3 million individuals).[2] All gout patients have hyperuricemia, defined as extracellular fluid urate supersaturation, at some point during the course of their illness. The prevalence of hyperuricemia is 10%–20% in the Western population.[1] Over the past two decades, a number of studies have shown that hyperuricemia portends an increased risk for subsequent cardiovascular outcomes, including mortality.[3–7]

In a population-based cohort study, we showed that among non-diabetic individuals aged ≥50 years who had no pre-existing serious cardiovascular disease (CVD), those with gout were 1.1 times more likely than those without gout to die from CVD in the next 5 years.[8]

The causative role of elevated serum uric acid concentrations (hyperuricemia) in CVD is suggested by studies showing its deleterious effect on endothelial function, inducing production of pro-inflammatory and pro-oxidative substances and platelet adhesiveness.[6]

There are three main types of urate-lowering therapy in clinical practice: reduction of urate production by use of a xanthine oxidase inhibitor such as allopurinol; enhancement of urinary excretion of uric acid with uricosuric agents; or conversion of uric acid to the more soluble purine end product allantoin using exogenous urate oxidase, also known as uricase. Allopurinol, as an antihyperuricemic agent, has been demonstrated to protect the cardiovascular system by reducing vascular oxidative stress, ameliorating inflammatory state, improving endothelial function, and preventing atherosclerosis progression.[4,9–14] At higher doses (≥300 mg a day), allopurinol was even able to regress the left ventricular mass in patients with ischemic heart disease.[15]

The positive effect of allopurinol treatment on future cardiovascular risk among patients with chronic kidney disease (CKD) was shown in a small prospective randomized trial of 113 patients with estimated glomerular filtration rates of <60 milliliter/min. In this open label study conducted by Spanish investigators, patients were randomly assigned to treatment with allopurinol at 100 mg/day (n = 57) or to continue their usual therapy (n = 56). Allopurinol treatment slowed renal disease progression independently of age, gender, diabetes, C-reactive protein, albuminuria, or renin–angiotensin system blockers use. After a mean follow-up time of 23.4±7.8 months, allopurinol treatment reduced the risk of cardiovascular events by 71% [hazard ratio (HR), 0.29; 95% confidence interval (CI), 0.09–0.86] compared with the usual therapy.[16]

A cohort study using a record linkage database to study the impact of allopurinol treatment on cardiovascular and mortality outcomes showed that higher doses of allopurinol were associated with better control of urate and lower risks of both cardiovascular events and mortality. In this study, there was no significant increase in the risk of cardiovascular events for allopurinol users (n = 1035) when compared with non-urate-lowering therapy users [adjusted hazard ratio (aHR), 1.10; 95% CI, 0.95–1.26]. Compared with low-dose (100 mg) allopurinol users, high-dose (≥300 mg) users showed a significant reduction in the risk of cardiovascular events (aHR, 0.69; 95% CI, 0.50–0.94) and mortality (aHR, 0.75; 95% CI, 0.59–0.94).[17]

An observational study using data from a Health Maintenance Organization evaluated the effect of uric acid and allopurinol use on clinical outcomes in 6204 patients with heart failure. This study demonstrated that high uric acid levels (>7.7 mg/dL or > 458 μmol/L) were a predictor of increased mortality (aHR, 1.37; 95% CI, 1.17–1.60) and an increase in cardiac hospitalizations (aHR, 1.10; 95% CI, 1.01–1.22). An increase in uric acid levels during follow-up was also an independent predictor of mortality (aHR, 1.46; 95% CI, 1.25–1.71) and cardiac hospitalizations (aHR, 1.15; 95% CI 1.06–1.23). With a median follow-up time of 498 days, treatment with allopurinol was independently associated with improved survival (aHR, 0.79; 95% CI, 0.64–0.98).[18] Another large, time-matched, nested case-control analysis using health care databases in Quebec, Canada, was designed to determine whether gout and allopurinol use are associated with heart failure outcomes. This study, which targeted a cohort of elderly patients aged ≥66 years with heart failure (n = 25,090), showed that >30 days of continuous allopurinol use is associated with reduced heart failure readmissions or death (HR, 0.69; 95% CI, 0.60–0.79; P<0.001) and all-cause mortality (HR, 0.74; (95% CI, 0.61–0.90; P<0.001) among patients with a history of gout.[19]

Therefore, it would be of great interest and academic appeal to examine the hypothesis that among different urate-lowering therapies for gout patients, allopurinol therapy would have better cardiovascular outcomes than non-allopurinol treatments, including a uricosuric agent in matched patients with gout. We thus designed a large-scale population-based retrospective matched-cohort study to answer this question.

Methods

Data Sources

We conducted a population-based retrospective matched-cohort study using the Taiwan National Health Insurance Research Database (NHIRD). The Taiwan National Health Insurance (NHI) program commenced on March 1, 1995. As of 2007, 98.4% of Taiwan's population of 22.96 million individuals was enrolled in this program. The NHIRD contains a number of computerized databases that incorporate files and original data on claims reimbursements derived from the insurance system held by the NHI Administration. These data have been provided to researchers for academic research purposes. The NHIRD comprises four main database files: ambulatory expenditures by visit, inpatient expenditures by admission, details of ambulatory care orders, and details of inpatient orders. These data files were de-identified by scrambling the identification codes of both individuals and medical facilities. The NHIRD is widely regarded as very accurate and complete and has become one of the largest and most comprehensive population-based databases in the world.[8,20–22]

This study used a dataset of one million randomly selected enrollees representing 4.5% of the Taiwanese population in the entire NHI enrollee profile. There was no significant difference in age or gender between the patients in the dataset used in this study and the population in the mother NHIRD, as verified by the National Health Research Institute (NHRI), Taiwan.

Ethics Statement

Because this study used only NHIRD data files that were de-identified by scrambling the identification codes of both individuals and medical facilities, this research fits the criteria for exemption from review by the Institution Review Board contained within the legal statements promulgated by the Ministry of Health and Welfare of Taiwan pursuant to Paragraph 1, Article 5 of the *Human Subjects Research Act* enacted on December 28, 2011. This study adhered to strict confidentiality guidelines that are in accordance with the regulations set forth by the *Personal Information Protection Act* of Taiwan, amended on May 26, 2010. The research was conducted in accordance with the *Declaration of Helsinki* as revised in 1989.

Study Population and Study Cohorts

We limited our study population to every individual diagnosed with gout in the years 1999 to 2008 (n = 46,586). We defined individuals with gout as those with gout-related diagnoses according to code 274 of the International Classification of Diseases, 9th Revision, Clinical Modification (ICD-9-CM). Under ICD-9-CM code 274, subjects with gouty arthropathy (code 274.0), gouty nephropathy (274.1), gouty iritis (274.89), gouty tophi (274.8), gouty tophi of ear (274.81), gouty tophi of heart (274.82), gout with other manifestations (274.89), and uric acid nephrolithiasis (274.11) were included. Gout and gout-related diagnoses are used interchangeably in this paper.

From this pool of 46,586 subjects with gout, we excluded 7200 subjects who were <40 years old or whose gender was unknown; 10,420 who visited the clinic less than 2 times during the defined study period; 2904 who had a pre-existing severe form of hypertensive, cerebrovascular, or CVD; and 2033 who had pre-existing gout in the preceding 2 years. This process resulted in a target population of 24,029 patients aged ≥40 years, with newly

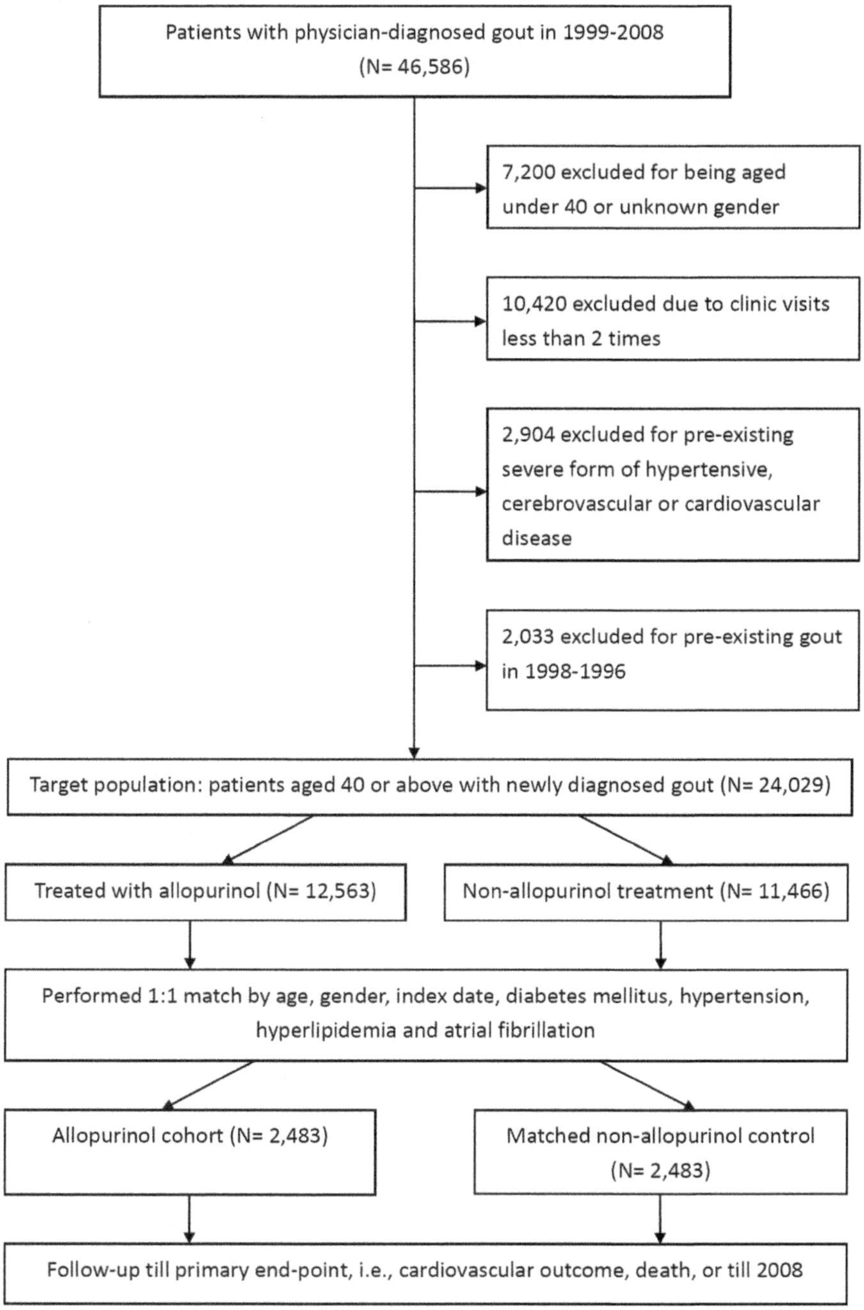

Figure 1. Study flowchart showing target population, exclusion reasons, matching and follow-up details in this retrospective matched-cohort population-based study using Taiwan National Health Research Institute Database.

diagnosed gout, having no history of pre-existing severe form of hypertension, cardiovascular, or cerebrovascular disease (Figure 1).

The severe CVDs included malignant hypertension, hypertensive nephropathy, myocardial infarction, or any form of congestive heart failure, as well as a coronary artery bypass surgery or percutaneous transluminal coronary angioplasty. In addition, subjects with intracerebral hemorrhage, intracranial hemorrhage, occlusion/stenosis of pre-cerebral arteries, and occlusion of cerebral arteries were also excluded. The detailed list of the corresponding ICD-9-CM codes can be found in our previously published article.[8] By excluding this group of patients, we ensured that the study would not contain patients with pre-existing severe cardiovascular and/or cerebrovascular comorbidities and, therefore, with a high pre-existing risk of a cardiovascular outcome.

The study population was divided into two groups: those who received allopurinol treatment and those who did not. The allopurinol group consisted of 12,563 patients and the non-allopurinol group consisted of 11,466 patients. We then performed one-to-one matching by age at accrual, gender, index date of subjects in the allopurinol group, diabetes mellitus, hypertension, hyperlipidemia, and atrial fibrillation. After matching, we finalized two matched study group, an allopurinol group and a non-allopurinol group, each containing 2483 patients. Follow-up continued until the occurrence of a primary cardiovascular outcome, death, or the end of 2008 (Figure 1).

Main Outcome Measures

A cardiovascular outcome is defined as an event requiring hospitalization during follow-up that is given a primary final diagnosis among several CVD-related diagnoses. These diagnoses included a spectrum of diseases from coronary heart disease (CHD) (ICD-9-CM codes 410–414) to hypertensive heart disease (401–405), heart failure (428), cerebrovascular disease (stroke) (430–438), and other CVDs (390–400, 406–409, 415–427, 429, and 439–459).[8,23] Cases with fatal CVD event ended up in the Emergency Room that did not require hospitalization were very rare in Taiwan due to practice culture and fairly easy access to hospitals.

Demographic data such as age and gender, as well as medical comorbidities including hypertension, diabetes mellitus, hyperlipidemia, atrial fibrillation, uric acid nephrolithiasis, acute kidney injury, hepatitis, contact dermatitis and other eczema, CKD, uremia, and gastric ulcer were collected for baseline evaluation. The Charlson comorbidity index (CCI) was also calculated for each case in the two groups. Comorbid medical conditions, identified using their standard ICD-9-CM codes, were used to calculate cumulatively the CCI score for each individual. The established CCI, adapted from the Charlson index for use with ICD-9-CM coded administrative databases, contains 17 weighted categories related to chronic concomitant diseases and is able to predict the subsequent 1-year mortality among inpatients. Each category has a score between 1 and 6 points (1 point each for myocardial infarction, congestive heart failure, peripheral vascular disease, cerebrovascular disease, dementia, chronic lung disease, rheumatologic disease, peptic ulcer disease, mild liver disease, and diabetes without organ damage; 2 points each for diabetes with organ damage, hemiplegia or paraplegia, severe renal disease, and any malignancy including leukemia and lymphoma; 3 points for severe liver disease; and 6 points each for metastatic solid tumor and HIV infection), and the sum of these scores is regarded as a measure of the burden of medical comorbidity.[24,25]

We assessed the use of uricosuric agents for urate-lowering therapy in the comparator cohort not receiving allopurinol. In Taiwan, three kinds of uricosuric agent are reimbursed: benzbromarone, probenecid, and sulfinpyrazone. The daily dose and duration of allopurinol use were also evaluated in this matched-cohort study.

Statistical Analysis

Pre-analysis data file merging and other data management operations before statistical analysis were performed using the SAS statistical package (SAS System for Windows, version 8.2, SAS Institute, Cary, NC, USA). Statistical analyses were performed using SPSS software (version 17.0, SPSS Inc., Chicago, Illinois, USA). All statistical tests were two-sided. Values of $P<0.05$ were considered statistically significant. The risk of cardiovascular outcomes associated with gout was evaluated using Cox proportional hazards analysis. All Cox regression models included the following covariates: CKD, uremia, and gastric ulcer. Adjusted hazard ratios (aHR) with a 95% CI were calculated. The relative risks of cardiovascular outcomes were calculated and analyzed using the Chi-square test (2×2). The distribution of comorbidity characteristics were compared between the two groups, and the differences were examined using the Chi-squared test and t test, as well as the Mann–Whitney U test (also called the Wilcoxon rank-sum test), which is a non-parametric statistical hypothesis test for assessing whether one of two samples of independent observations tends to have larger values than the other. Variables such as age, sex, underlying comorbidity, daily dose of allopurinol, use of uricosuric agents, duration of allopurinol use, and follow-up in years are reported as percentages. StatsDirect statistical software (StatsDirect Ltd, England, 2008) was used to provide relative risk values and Yate's corrected 2×2 test computations. The cardiovascular event-free cumulative survival probabilities were estimated in each group using the Kaplan–Meier method. The log-rank test was used to compare the significance of inequalities with respect to the cardiovascular event-free survival curves of each group.

Results

Two matched groups, allopurinol and non-allopurinol, each consisting of 2483 patients, were followed-up throughout the defined study period, or until a cardiovascular event, with neither drop-out nor cross-over. Because the allopurinol and non-allopurinol groups were already matched with respect to seven pre-defined conditions (age at diagnosis of gout, gender, index date of the allopurinol group subjects, diabetes mellitus, hypertension, hyperlipidemia, and atrial fibrillation), there was no statistically significant difference between these two groups in terms of these seven variables. Furthermore, there was no statistically significant difference in the frequency of uric acid nephrolithiasis, acute kidney injury, hepatitis, contact dermatitis and other eczema, as well as overall Charlson–Deyo comorbidity index (Table 1). However, there was a statistically significant higher percentage of CKD and uremia in the allopurinol group compared with the non-allopurinol group (4.75% and 1.09% versus 2.38% and 0.52%, respectively). The allopurinol group also had a higher percentage of CKD, including uremia, although the percentage was considered low at approximately 7%. The allopurinol group had a slightly higher rate of gastric ulcer (2.34% versus 1.49%; $P=0.0296$) (Table 1). These minor inequalities were later adjusted in the Cox proportional hazard model to calculate the HR.

The mean age (± standard deviation) of the study group was 61.84 (±12.13) years. Men accounted for 62.22% of the total cases. Slightly more than half of the patients in both groups had hypertension at accrual. Twenty three percent of the patients had been diagnosed with diabetes and approximately 31% had hyperlipidemia (Table 1).

In the allopurinol group, 85.54% of gout patients took allopurinol at a dose of >100 mg/day. Of these, 16% were treated with a dose of ≥300 mg/day. Among patients receiving allopurinol, 59% took allopurinol for >6 months. Of these, 9% took allopurinol for 0.5–1 year; 13% for 1–2 years; 9% for 2–3 years; 5% for 3–4 years and 23% for >4 years.

In the non-allopurinol group, nearly 69% of the patients received a uricosuric agent. The most common uricosuric agent used was benzbromarone (66%), followed by sulfinpyrazone (3%), and probenecid (0.4%).

Follow-up of the patients in the two groups was complete; there was no drop-out or loss to follow-up. The median follow-up time for the allopurinol group was 5.25 years [interquartile range (IQR), 4.88 years], whereas it was 5.04 years (IQR, 4.98 years) for the non-allopurinol group. There was no statistically significant difference in the follow-up time between these two groups (Table 2). There were 566 cardiovascular events (22.8%) in the allopurinol group during the entire follow-up period and 470 events (18.9%) in the non-allopurinol group. The relative risk for cardiovascular outcomes of the allopurinol group was 1.2 times higher than that of the non-allopurinol group (95% CI, 1.08–1.34) (Table 2). In another words, the allopurinol group was 1.2 times

Table 1. Baseline characteristics of the two matched cohorts of patients with newly diagnosed gout either treated with or without allopurinol.

Characteristics		Allopurinol cohort (n = 2483)		Non-allopurinol cohort (n = 2483)		P-value
		N	%	N	%	
Age at gout diagnosis						1.0000
	40–49	481	19.37	481	19.37	
	50–59	621	25.01	621	25.01	
	60–69	628	25.29	628	25.29	
	70–79	561	22.59	561	22.59	
	≥80	192	7.73	192	7.73	
	Mean ±SD	61.84±12.13		61.84±12.13		
Gender						1.0000
	Men	1545	62.22	1545	62.22	
	Women	938	37.78	938	37.78	
Co-morbidities						
	Hypertension	1257	50.62	1257	50.62	1.0000
	Diabetes mellitus	573	23.08	573	23.08	1.0000
	Hyperlipidemia	766	30.85	766	30.85	1.0000
	Atrial fibrillation	1	0.04	1	0.04	1.0000
	Uric acid nephrolithiasis	1	0.04	0	0.00	1.0000
	Acute kidney injury	9	0.36	3	0.12	0.0829
	Hepatitis	53	2.13	49	1.97	0.6890
	Contact dermatitis and other eczema	424	17.08	431	17.36	0.7925
	Chronic kidney disease	118	4.75	59	2.38	<.0001
	Uremia	27	1.09	13	0.52	0.0262
	Gastric ulcer	58	2.34	37	1.49	0.0296
	Charlson's Comorbidities Index (CCI)					0.3013*
	0	793	31.94	887	35.72	
	1	515	20.74	633	25.49	
	2	381	15.34	321	12.93	
	3	282	11.36	236	9.50	
	4	204	8.22	147	5.92	
	5	122	4.91	106	4.27	
	6	81	3.26	70	2.82	
	7	43	1.73	45	1.81	
	8	29	1.17	15	0.60	
	9	18	0.72	13	0.52	
	10	8	0.32	4	0.16	
	>10	7	0.28	6	0.24	

*Wilcoxon's signed rank test (2-sided P value).
The 2 cohorts were matched for age at gout diagnosis, gender, diabetes mellitus, hypertension, hyperlipidemia, atrial fibrillation and index date. In addition, both cohorts were balanced in terms of Charlson's comorbidities index (CCI), acute kidney injury and hepatitis etc.

more likely to experience a cardiovascular outcome compared with the non-allopurinol group.

A Cox proportional hazards regression model established to calculate the effect of allopurinol therapy on future cardiovascular outcomes for gout patients aged ≥40 years, after adjusting for CKD, uremia, and gastric ulcer gave an aHR of 1.25 (95% CI, 1.10–1.41) compared with the non-allopurinol therapy (Table 3 and Figure 2).

With respect to the different forms of cardiovascular events, we further examined the effect of allopurinol therapy on subsequent hospitalizations due to CHD, cerebrovascular disease (stroke), hypertensive heart disease, heart failure, or other cardiovascular disorders. The HR and aHR for hospitalization due to each form of CVD are reported in Table 4. Compared with non-allopurinol therapy, allopurinol therapy for patients aged >40 years with gout was significantly associated with an increased aHR for hospitalization due to CHD (aHR, 1.41; 95% CI, 1.10–1.79), hypertensive

Table 2. Treatment with allopurinol by total daily dose, duration of use, duration of follow-up, and cardiovascular outcomes.

Treatment, follow-up, and outcomes		Allopurinol cohort (n = 2483)		Non-allopurinol cohort (n = 2483)		*P*-value
		N	%	N	%	
Allopurinol	daily dose	2483	100	-	-	
	<100 mg	359	14.46	-	-	
	100 mg	1262	50.83	-	-	
	200 mg	467	18.81	-	-	
	≥300 mg	395	15.90	-	-	
Uricosuric agent		-	-	1713	68.99	
	benzbromarone	-	-	1628	65.57	
	probenecid	-	-	11	0.44	
	sulfinpyrazone	-	-	74	2.98	
Duration of allopurinol use						
	<0.5 year	1011	40.72	NA	NA	
	0.5–1 year	233	9.38	NA	NA	
	1–2 years	325	13.09	NA	NA	
	2–3 years	215	8.66	NA	NA	
	3–4 years	134	5.40	NA	NA	
	>4 years	565	22.75	NA	NA	
Follow-up in years	Median, (IQR)	5.25, (4.88)		5.04, (4.98)		0.6971
Cardiovascular outcome	***Events***	566	22.80	470	18.93	
	Relative Risk (RR)	1.20 (95% CI = 1.08–1.34)				

With a median follow-up of 5.25 years, the allopurinol cohort has harbored a modestly increased risk of cardiovascular events.
CI: confidence interval; IQR: interquartile range; NA: not applicable; RR: relative risk; yr: year.

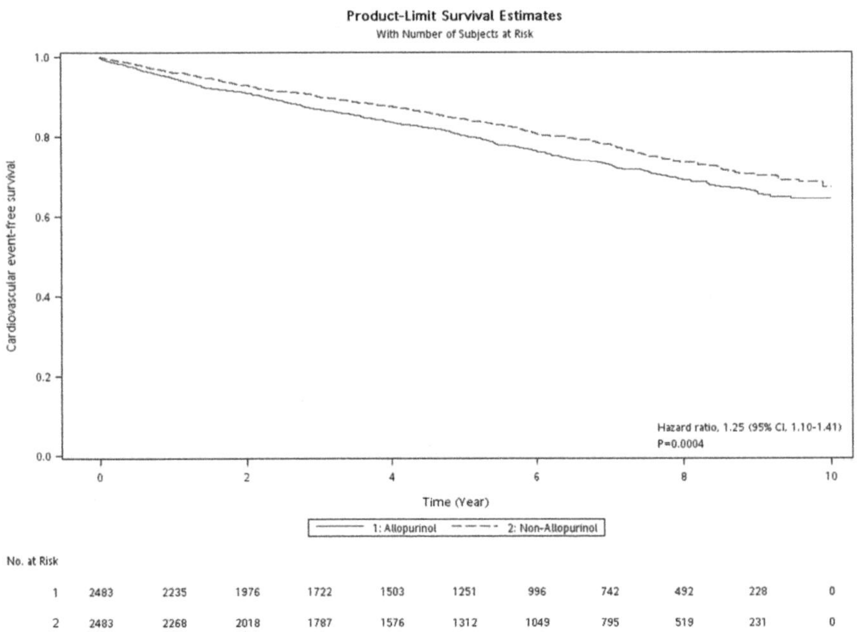

Figure 2. Kaplan-Meier cardiovascular event-free survival curves of gout patients treated with allopurinol and matched comparators of gout patients receiving no allopurinol. At a median follow up of 5.25 years, the allopurinol therapy group harbored an increased hazard ratio of 1.25 (95% confidence interval, 1.10–1.41).

Table 3. Univariate and multivariate hazard ratios (HR) for cardiovascular outcome in patient with essentially newly diagnosed gout receiving allopurinol as compared with non-allopurinol medications.

Cardiovascular Outcome	N (%)	Univariate		Multivariate	
		HR	95% CI	HR	95% CI
Non-allopurinol	470 (18.93)	Ref	-	Ref	-
Allopurinol	566 (22.80)	1.24*	1.10–1.41	1.25**	1.10–1.41

Multivariate HR was obtained after adjusting for chronic kidney disease, uremia, and gastric ulcer.
*P<0.05;
**P<0.001.
CI: confidence interval; HR: hazard ratio; Ref: reference.

heart disease (aHR, 1.34; 95% CI, 1.18–1.53), and heart failure (aHR, 1.52; 95% CI, 1.17–1.98) after adjusting for uremia, CKD, and gastric ulcer.

We fit a Cox model for gout patients receiving urate-lowering therapy to determine if allopurinol provided protection against cardiovascular outcomes compared with uricosuric therapy consisting of benzbromarone, sulfinpyrazone, and probenecid. The results showed that when allopurinol therapy was regarded as a reference, uricosuric therapy was shown to have cardiovascular protection (aHR, 0.83; 95% CI, 0.73–0.95) (Table 5).

Taking all these results into account, allopurinol therapy did not provide cardiovascular protection and also led to adverse outcomes in patients with gout. With a median follow-up time of 5.25 years, the allopurinol group had a modest increase in cardiovascular risk (relative risk, 1.20; 95% CI, 1.08–1.34). A Cox proportional hazard model adjusted for CKD, uremia, and gastric ulcer gave an HR for cardiovascular outcomes of 1.25 (1.10–1.41) in gout patients receiving allopurinol compared with those not receiving allopurinol. In a subgroup analysis of patients receiving urate-lowering therapy, the uricosuric agent group (n = 1713) had an aHR of 0.83 (0.73–0.95) compared with the allopurinol group.

We also fit a Cox model examining the associations of low- and high-dose allopurinol therapy with subsequent cardiovascular risk. The model used a daily allopurinol dose of <100 mg, which had an incidence of cardiovascular events of 23.68%, as its reference for comparison (Table 6). Using this model, the incidence of cardiovascular events was 25.67%, 19.70%, and 11.48% in the 100-mg group, 200-mg group, and ≥300-mg group, respectively. The univariate HRs were statistically significant at the higher doses of 200 mg (HR, 0.73; 95% CI, 0.55–0.98) and 300 mg (HR, 0.67; 95% CI, 0.48–0.92), demonstrating the beneficial effect of a higher daily dose of allopurinol therapy. Although the 200-mg and ≥300-mg groups retain their beneficial HRs (both HR were 0.91) after adjustment for CKD, uremia, and gastric ulcer, the differences lose statistically significance (Table 6). Nevertheless, because of the comparatively lower numbers of cases in the higher dosage groups, a true benefit from a higher daily dose of allopurinol cannot be completely ruled out.

Discussion

To the best of our knowledge, this is the first population-based study accruing a large number of patients with gout and including well-matched references that was designed to uncover an association between allopurinol therapy and subsequent cardiovascular risk. The quasi-experimental design of the study, with clear exclusion criteria and extensive matching, allowed profound control of variance by exclusion of subjects with pre-existing severe CVDs and control of known confounding variables. Excluding subjects with pre-existing severe CVD results in the exclusion of high-risk to very-high risk patients who are prone to experience a cardiovascular outcome during subsequent follow-up. The extensive matching process also allowed, in the early phase of the study, elimination of confounding variables other than age, gender, and index date only; thus, post-hoc statistical adjustments could be omitted.

Table 4. Hazard ratio and adjusted hazard ratio for hospitalization due to cardiovascular events in patients aged more than 40 having their gout treated with allopurinol as compared those matched control receiving no allopurinol.

	Allopurinol cohort (%) (n = 2,483)	Non-allopurinol control (%) (n = 2,483)	HR (95% CI)	Adjusted HR (95% CI)
Cardiovascular Events	566 (22.80)	470 (18.93)	1.24*** (1.10–1.41)	1.25*** (1.10–1.41)
Coronary heart disease	158 (6.36)	111 (4.47)	1.44** (1.13–1.84)	1.41** (1.10–1.79)
Cerebrovascular disease (Stroke)	176 (7.09)	150 (6.04)	1.18 (0.95–1.47)	1.18 (0.95–1.47)
Hypertensive heart disease	538 (21.67)	419 (16.87)	1.34*** (1.18–1.52)	1.34*** (1.18–1.53)
Heart failure	141 (5.68)	92 (3.71)	1.55** (1.19–2.02)	1.52** (1.17–1.98)
Other	233 (9.38)	208 (8.38)	1.13 (0.94–1.36)	1.12 (0.93–1.35)

Adjustment was made for uremia, chronic kidney disease and gastric ulcer.
**P*<0.05,
**<0.01,
***<0.001.
CI: confidence interval; HR: hazard ratio.

Table 5. Hazard ratio and adjusted hazard ratio for hospitalization due to cardiovascular events in patients or matched subjects aged more than 40 with gout and hyperuricemia receiving urate-lowering therapy, either allopurinol or uricosuric agent.

Urate-lowering therapy	Cardiovascular Events	Univariate Cox model		Adjusted Cox model	
	N (%)	HR	95% CI	HR	95% CI
Allopurinol (n = 2483)	566 (22.80)	ref	ref	ref	ref
Uricosuric agents (n = 1713)	334 (13.45)	0.83**	0.72–0.95	0.83**	0.73–0.95

Adjustment was made for uremia, chronic kidney disease and gastric ulcer.
*$P<0.05$,
**<0.01,
***<0.001.
CI: confidence interval; HR: hazard ratio

Selection bias was obviously avoided. The vast majority (84.5%) of the entire cohort received urate-lowering therapy (including allopurinol or uricosuric agents), indicating that selection methodology for the gout patients was adequate. Allocation bias was also avoided, because positive or negative exposure to allopurinol was unambiguous in the database. Furthermore, our use of administrative-based data enabled us to study allopurinol exposure and cardiovascular outcomes without the influence of recall bias in both groups. There was no drop-out or loss to follow-up because complete tracking of study subjects was feasible, even when a patient relocated or received treatment in different hospitals. The follow-up time was considered long enough to allow a cardiovascular event to be observed.

Using this study design, the results showed an association between allopurinol therapy for gout patients and increased CVD events. Allopurinol may have a harmful effect, with an increase in the risk of CVD even after adjustment for CKD and uremia. This means that a Taiwanese patient aged ≥40 years with newly diagnosed gout and hyperuricemia who is prescribed allopurinol therapy to lower urate levels is associated with a 25% increase in cardiovascular risk over the next 10 years of follow-up. This data is considered robust, with a narrow 95% confidence interval.

It is noteworthy that a published cohort study, using a United Kingdom record linkage database, conducted in a population of patients aged ≥60 years who underwent urate measurements either at a hospital or a community clinic, demonstrated that there was a statistically insignificant increase in the risk of cardiovascular events for allopurinol users compared with subjects not receiving urate-lowering therapy (aHR, 1.10; 95% CI 0.95–1.26) and with subjects not receiving urate-lowering therapy that had urate > 6 mg/dL (aHR, 1.07; 95% CI, 0.89–1.28). Nevertheless, the study showed that compared with subjects receiving low-dose (100 mg) allopurinol, those receiving high-dose (≥300 mg) allopurinol showed a significant reduction in the risk of cardiovascular events (aHR, 0.69; 95% CI, 0.50–0.94).[17] Our analysis of HRs by different daily dosages of allopurinol (Table 6) also suggested that a higher daily dose may benefit patients with gout in terms of cardiovascular risk.

Another retrospective cohort study of patients with chronic heart failure that investigated the association between different durations (short-term versus long-term) and daily dosages [low-dose versus high-dose (≥300 mg)] of allopurinol therapy and cardiovascular mortality merits mention here.[26] The results of this study disclosed that long-term low-dose allopurinol worsened cardiovascular mortality, with HR of 2.04 (95% CI, 1.48–2.81); whereas, long-term high-dose allopurinol provided benefit, with a relative risk of 0.59 (95% CI, 0.37–0.95).

Thus, we believe that it is the dosage of allopurinol may make a difference when reduction of cardiovascular risk is the main therapeutic aim. Further prospective studies are needed to test this hypothesis.

The mechanisms underlying the beneficial effect of higher daily dosage of allopurinol have been reported in recent years. Erdogan et al. published a single arm clinical trial of allopurinol at 300 mg/day for 3 months in patients diagnosed with dilated cardiomyopathy with concomitant hyperuricemia. Their results showed that this high dose of allopurinol can improve coronary microvascular and left ventricular function.[9] Rajendra et al. reported a double-

Table 6. Univariate and multivariate hazard ratios (HR) for cardiovascular outcome in patient with gout receiving higher dosage of allopurinol as compared with low-dose allopurinol.

Allopurinol therapy	Cardiovascular events	Univariate		Multivariate	
Daily dosage	Number (%)	HR	95% CI	HR	95% CI
<100 mg	85 (23.68)	Ref	-	Ref	-
100 mg	324 (25.67)	0.988	0.778–1.255	1.191	0.931–1.523
200 mg	92 (19.70)	0.731*	0.545–0.982	0.906	0.671–1.224
≥300 mg	65 (11.48)	0.669*	0.484–0.924	0.907	0.650–1.266

Multivariate HR was obtained after adjusting for chronic kidney disease, uremia, and gastric ulcer.
*$P<0.05$.
CI: confidence interval; HR: hazard ratio; Ref: reference.

blind, randomized, placebo-controlled trial of very high-dose allopurinol therapy (600 mg/day) with cross-over in patients with coronary artery disease. Their results showed that at this very high dose, allopurinol profoundly reduces vascular tissue oxidative stress and improves three different measures of vascular/endothelial dysfunction.[27] Recently, Noman et al. conducted a double-blind, randomized, placebo-controlled trial of allopurinol at 600 mg/day for 6 weeks before cross-over in patients with at least 2 months of angiographically documented stable chronic angina pectoris with positive exercise tolerance test. They found that this very high-dose allopurinol could increase the median time to ST depression, median total exercise time, and time to chest pain.[28]

There is also a possibility that our result, that allopurinol fared worse than the matched reference cohort consisting of uricosuric agent users (69%) and patients having no urate lowering therapy (31%), may have resulted just because of the capability of allopurinol therapy to serve as a prognostic factor suggesting a poorer cardiovascular outcome. However, this suggestion is only hypothetical.

There are some potential limitations to this study. We did not have access to the relevant biochemical datasets incorporating urate measurements and personal lifestyle histories such as cigarette smoking and alcohol consumption history, abdominal obesity, consumption of fruits and vegetables, and records of physical activity. This is because individual identities are not available because of de-identification of the cases within the NHI databases. The lack of such information could potentially bias the effect estimate. Another potential limitation is that data for medication other than urate-lowering medications and the compliance and adherence to treatment were too complex to incorporate in the covariate analyses.

In conclusion, allopurinol therapy as a urate-lowering treatment has previously been found to reduce cardiovascular risk, particularly in patients with coronary artery disease, heart failure, or CKD having concomitant hyperuricemia. Our large-scale study using population-based matched-cohort design in patients with gout and "normal risk" for cardiovascular events did not observe any beneficial effect of allopurinol, whereas the association with a modest increase in cardiovascular risk was detected. Several important risk factors for cardiovascular disease, such as smoking, alcohol consumption, body mass index, blood pressure were not obtainable in the current study, thus could potentially bias the effect estimate. A hypothesis-generating finding was suggested from a subgroup analysis of low- versus high-dose allopurinol therapy, showing a possible beneficial effect from high-dose therapy. Further prospective large-scale cohort studies or randomized controlled trials are needed.

Acknowledgments

We are immensely thankful to the National Health Insurance Administration, Ministry of Health and Welfare, Taiwan, and the National Health Research Institute, Taiwan, for kindly providing the research data for analysis. The interpretation and conclusions contained herein do not represent those of the aforementioned institutions.

Author Contributions

Conceived and designed the experiments: VCK JTH. Performed the experiments: VCK WSC. Analyzed the data: VCK JTH WSC YFH THC. Contributed reagents/materials/analysis tools: YFH THC. Wrote the paper: VCK. Obtained grants for research: JTH. Organized research meetings: JTH.

References

1. Bhansing KJ, van Bon L, Janssen M, Radstake TR (2010) Gout: a clinical syndrome illustrated and discussed. Neth J Med 68: 352-359.
2. Zhu Y, Pandya BJ, Choi HK (2011) Prevalence of gout and hyperuricemia in the US general population: the National Health and Nutrition Examination Survey 2007-2008. Arthritis Rheum 63: 3136–3141.
3. Krishnan E, Pandya BJ, Chung L, Dabbous O (2011) Hyperuricemia and the risk for subclinical coronary atherosclerosis—data from a prospective observational cohort study. Arthritis Res Ther 13: R66.
4. Kanbay M, Sanchez-Lozada LG, Franco M, Madero M, Solak Y, et al. (2011) Microvascular disease and its role in the brain and cardiovascular system: a potential role for uric acid as a cardiorenal toxin. Nephrol Dial Transplant 26: 430–437.
5. Puddu P, Puddu GM, Cravero E, Vizioli L, Muscari A (2012) Relationships among hyperuricemia, endothelial dysfunction and cardiovascular disease: molecular mechanisms and clinical implications. J Cardiol 59: 235–242.
6. Feig DI, Kang DH, Johnson RJ (2008) Uric acid and cardiovascular risk. N Engl J Med 359: 1811–1821.
7. Ford ES (2011) Uric acid and mortality from all-causes and cardiovascular disease among adults with and without diagnosed diabetes: findings from the National Health and Nutrition Examination Survey III Linked Mortality Study. Diabetes Res Clin Pract 93: e84–86.
8. Kok VC, Horng JT, Lin HL, Chen YC, Chen YJ, et al. (2012) Gout and subsequent increased risk of cardiovascular mortality in non-diabetics aged 50 and above: a population-based cohort study in Taiwan. BMC Cardiovasc Disord 12: 108.
9. Erdogan D, Tayyar S, Uysal BA, Icli A, Karabacak M, et al. (2012) Effects of allopurinol on coronary microvascular and left ventricular function in patients with idiopathic dilated cardiomyopathy. Can J Cardiol 28: 721–727.
10. George J, Carr E, Davies J, Belch JJ, Struthers A (2006) High-dose allopurinol improves endothelial function by profoundly reducing vascular oxidative stress and not by lowering uric acid. Circulation 114: 2508–2516.
11. Muir SW, Harrow C, Dawson J, Lees KR, Weir CJ, et al. (2008) Allopurinol use yields potentially beneficial effects on inflammatory indices in those with recent ischemic stroke: a randomized, double-blind, placebo-controlled trial. Stroke 39: 3303–3307.
12. Siu YP, Leung KT, Tong MK, Kwan TH (2006) Use of allopurinol in slowing the progression of renal disease through its ability to lower serum uric acid level. Am J Kidney Dis 47: 51–59.
13. Stone PH (2011) Allopurinol a new anti-ischemic role for an old drug. J Am Coll Cardiol 58: 829–830.
14. Yiginer O, Ozcelik F, Inanc T, Aparci M, Ozmen N, et al. (2008) Allopurinol improves endothelial function and reduces oxidant-inflammatory enzyme of myeloperoxidase in metabolic syndrome. Clin Res Cardiol 97: 334–340.
15. Rekhraj S, Gandy SJ, Szwejkowski BR, Nadir MA, Noman A, et al. (2013) High-dose allopurinol reduces left ventricular mass in patients with ischemic heart disease. J Am Coll Cardiol 61: 926–932.
16. Goicoechea M, de Vinuesa SG, Verdalles U, Ruiz-Caro C, Ampuero J, et al. (2010) Effect of allopurinol in chronic kidney disease progression and cardiovascular risk. Clin J Am Soc Nephrol 5: 1388–1393.
17. Wei L, Mackenzie IS, Chen Y, Struthers AD, MacDonald TM (2011) Impact of allopurinol use on urate concentration and cardiovascular outcome. Br J Clin Pharmacol 71: 600–607.
18. Gotsman I, Keren A, Lotan C, Zwas DR (2012) Changes in uric acid levels and allopurinol use in chronic heart failure: association with improved survival. J Card Fail 18: 694–701.
19. Thanassoulis G, Brophy JM, Richard H, Pilote L (2010) Gout, allopurinol use, and heart failure outcomes. Arch Intern Med 170: 1358–1364.
20. Wu CY, Chen YJ, Ho HJ, Hsu YC, Kuo KN, et al. (2012) Association between nucleoside analogues and risk of hepatitis B virus-related hepatocellular carcinoma recurrence following liver resection. JAMA 308: 1906–1914.
21. Wang YP, Liu CJ, Hu YW, Chen TJ, Lin YT, et al. (2012) Risk of cancer among patients with herpes zoster infection: a population-based study. CMAJ 184: E804–809.
22. Chang CW, Kok VC, Tseng TC, Horng JT, Liu CE (2012) Diabetic patients with severe sepsis admitted to intensive care unit do not fare worse than non-diabetic patients: a nationwide population-based cohort study. PLoS One 7: e50729.
23. Kuo CF, See LC, Luo SF, Ko YS, Lin YS, et al. (2010) Gout: an independent risk factor for all-cause and cardiovascular mortality. Rheumatology (Oxford) 49: 141–146.
24. Needham DM, Scales DC, Laupacis A, Pronovost PJ (2005) A systematic review of the Charlson comorbidity index using Canadian administrative databases: a perspective on risk adjustment in critical care research. J Crit Care 20: 12–19.
25. Schneeweiss S, Maclure M (2000) Use of comorbidity scores for control of confounding in studies using administrative databases. Int J Epidemiol 29: 891–898.

26. Struthers AD, Donnan PT, Lindsay P, McNaughton D, Broomhall J, et al. (2002) Effect of allopurinol on mortality and hospitalisations in chronic heart failure: a retrospective cohort study. Heart 87: 229–234.
27. Rajendra NS, Ireland S, George J, Belch JJ, Lang CC, et al. (2011) Mechanistic insights into the therapeutic use of high-dose allopurinol in angina pectoris. J Am Coll Cardiol 58: 820–828.
28. Noman A, Ang DS, Ogston S, Lang CC, Struthers AD (2010) Effect of high-dose allopurinol on exercise in patients with chronic stable angina: a randomised, placebo controlled crossover trial. Lancet 375: 2161–2167.

2

Phosphoproteomic Profiling of Human Myocardial Tissues Distinguishes Ischemic from Non-Ischemic End Stage Heart Failure

Matthew A. Schechter[1,9], Michael K. H. Hsieh[1,9], Linda W. Njoroge[1], J. Will Thompson[2], Erik J. Soderblom[2], Bryan J. Feger[1], Constantine D. Troupes[1], Kathleen A. Hershberger[3,4], Olga R. Ilkayeva[3], Whitney L. Nagel[1], Gina P. Landinez[1], Kishan M. Shah[1], Virginia A. Burns[5], Lucia Santacruz[1], Matthew D. Hirschey[3,4], Matthew W. Foster[6], Carmelo A. Milano[1], M. Arthur Moseley[2], Valentino Piacentino III[1], Dawn E. Bowles[1]*

1 Department of Surgery, Duke University Medical Center, Durham, North Carolina, United States of America, **2** Duke Proteomics Core, Duke University Medical Center, Durham, North Carolina, United States of America, **3** Sarah W. Stedman Nutrition and Metabolism Center, Duke University Medical Center, Durham, North Carolina, United States of America, **4** Department of Medicine, Duke University Medical Center, Durham, North Carolina, United States of America, **5** Duke Translational Research Institute, Duke University Medical Center, Durham, North Carolina, United States of America, **6** Division of Pulmonary, Allergy and Critical Care, Medicine, Duke University Medical Center, Durham, North Carolina, United States of America

Abstract

The molecular differences between ischemic (IF) and non-ischemic (NIF) heart failure are poorly defined. A better understanding of the molecular differences between these two heart failure etiologies may lead to the development of more effective heart failure therapeutics. In this study extensive proteomic and phosphoproteomic profiles of myocardial tissue from patients diagnosed with IF or NIF were assembled and compared. Proteins extracted from left ventricular sections were proteolyzed and phosphopeptides were enriched using titanium dioxide resin. Gel- and label-free nanoscale capillary liquid chromatography coupled to high resolution accuracy mass tandem mass spectrometry allowed for the quantification of 4,436 peptides (corresponding to 450 proteins) and 823 phosphopeptides (corresponding to 400 proteins) from the unenriched and phospho-enriched fractions, respectively. Protein abundance did not distinguish NIF from IF. In contrast, 37 peptides (corresponding to 26 proteins) exhibited a ≥2-fold alteration in phosphorylation state ($p<0.05$) when comparing IF and NIF. The degree of protein phosphorylation at these 37 sites was specifically dependent upon the heart failure etiology examined. Proteins exhibiting phosphorylation alterations were grouped into functional categories: transcriptional activation/RNA processing; cytoskeleton structure/function; molecular chaperones; cell adhesion/signaling; apoptosis; and energetic/metabolism. Phosphoproteomic analysis demonstrated profound post-translational differences in proteins that are involved in multiple cellular processes between different heart failure phenotypes. Understanding the roles these phosphorylation alterations play in the development of NIF and IF has the potential to generate etiology-specific heart failure therapeutics, which could be more effective than current therapeutics in addressing the growing concern of heart failure.

Editor: Toru Hosoda, Tokai University, Japan

Funding: This work was supported by Duke Department of Surgery funding (Bolognesi Award to DEB). We thank the Duke Proteomics Core Facility (http://www.genome.duke.edu/cores/proteomics/), which provided mass spectrometry proteomics service. The Duke Proteomics Core is funded in part by the Duke School of Medicine, the Duke Translational Medicine Institute (CTSA grant UL1RR024128), and the Duke Cancer Institute. The funders had no role in study design, data collection and analysis, decision to publish, or preparation of the manuscript.

Competing Interests: The authors have declared no competing interests exist.

* Email: dawn.bowles@duke.edu

9 These authors contributed equally to this work.

Introduction

Despite earlier diagnosis and improved therapy, heart failure (HF) continues to be a major health concern. In 2012, 5.7 million Americans were diagnosed with HF [1]. The lifetime risk of developing HF after age 40 is 20%, with the annual incidence approaching 10 per 1000 people after age 65 [2]. More than half of all HF patients will die within a 5-year period of being diagnosed [3,4]. These statistics are complicated by the fact that HF is a complex, multi-faceted disease that presents in two major forms: ischemic and non-ischemic.

Ischemic HF describes significantly impaired left ventricular function resulting from reduced blood supply to the heart muscle. In contrast, the reduced left ventricular function seen in non-ischemic HF has a range of etiologies, including congenital, infectious agents, autoimmune, and idiopathic. However, the current standard of care treats all cases of HF similarly, regardless of etiology. The treatment options for advanced heart failure are limited to implantation of a ventricular assist device to mechanically unload the heart, heart transplantation, or palliation with continuous intravenous inotropic support. These options, however, are associated with high morbidity and mortality, highlighting the continued need for improving HF treatment.

One such avenue of exploration is etiology-specific treatment. Such precise therapy would require an enhanced understanding of the molecular differences between heart failure phenotypes. Uncovering these molecular differences in a systematic and comprehensive way is made possible by utilizing high throughput 'omics profiling [5,6]. Genomics, proteomics, metabolomics, etc. have primarily focused on comparing the differences between one HF etiology and non-failing samples (reviewed by Gonzalez *et al* [7]). Recently, using two dimensional gel-based proteomics on tissue from diseased human hearts, Klawitter *et al* were able to demonstrate differences in the relative abundance of proteins in signaling pathways between ischemic or idiopathic cardiomyopathies [8]. However, differences in protein quantity represent only one aspect of the molecular picture; many of the key proteins involved in signal transduction pathways are highly regulated by post translational modification, such as phosphorylation. Whether protein phosphorylation patterns differ between heart failure etiologies is unknown. Such knowledge may enable the development of better and more precise heart failure therapeutics and diagnostics.

In the current investigation, cardiac tissues from a well-characterized and well-preserved human heart tissue bank were subjected to titanium dioxide resin to enrich for phosphopeptides, and then analyzed by a bottom-up LC/MS/MS global proteomics approach. This approach revealed amino acid residue-specific phosphorylation patterns on 400 cardiac proteins, which were compared between the IF and NIF etiologies. This revealed, for the first time, cardiac disease-specific phosphorylation pattern variations on key proteins involved in various aspects of cardiac physiology. Understanding how distinct protein phosphorylation patterns impact specific heart failure etiologies will support the development of therapeutics that better treat heart failure.

Materials and Methods

Human Cardiac Tissue Acquisition and Tissue Repository

The study protocol was approved by the Duke University Health System Institutional Review Board (DUHS IRB). The DUHS IRB, FWA #00009025, is duly constituted and complies with all U.S. regulatory requirements related to the protection of human research participants and the Guidelines of the International Conference on Harmonization (ICH) as adopted by the U.S. Food and Drug Administration. Tissue samples used for this study were procured from the Duke Human Heart Repository (DHHR), which is a DUHS IRB approved tissue repository. Samples were procured by the DHHR in accordance under an approved DUHS IRB protocol using written informed consent or a waiver of consent for discarded tissues. Some samples procured had been anonymized with all HIPAA identifiers removed, others were de-identified. Only DHHR personnel were privy to a key that could link the samples to patient information. No HIPAA information was provided with any of the samples used in this study. Human myocardium was acquired from the left ventricular free wall of explanted IF or NIF hearts following cardiac transplantation. Non-failing (NF) left ventricular tissue was acquired from donors whose hearts were not utilized for transplant, thus becoming available for research. After explantation, transmural tissue samples were processed and stored as described in the Methods S1.

Sample Preparation for Mass Spectrometry

Heart tissue samples were homogenized and subjected to phase separation by addition of chloroform. Protein was precipitated from the organic layer, washed, sonicated, recovered by centrifugation, and re-suspended in mass spectrometry-compatible detergent (RapiGest, Waters Corp., Milford, MA). Cardiac tissue homogenates used for mass spectrometry were subjected to Bradford Assay for protein quantification. A 625 µg aliquot of protein (per sample) was subjected to reduction, alkylation, followed by overnight proteolysis with sequencing grade trypsin (Promega, Madison, WI). A 25 µg aliquot from each sample was used for unenriched proteomic analysis of protein expression in the heart tissue. This 25 µg was spiked with 1.25 pmol ADH1_YEAST digest (Massprep standard, Waters Corporation) as a surrogate standard prior to analysis.

The remaining 600 µg of protein were then enriched for phosphopeptides using in-house packed TiO_2 spin columns as previously described [9].

LC/MS/MS Data collection

The sample cohort was randomized prior to LC/MS/MS analysis. Peptide digests obtained from each of the samples were analyzed in a label-free quantitative fashion using a nanoAcquity UPLC system coupled to a Synapt HDMS mass spectrometer (Waters Corp, Milford, MA) for unenriched peptide analyses and an LTQ Orbitrap XL (Thermo Fisher Scientific, Waltham, MA) for phosphopeptide analyses.

LC-MS Data Processing

Robust peak detection and label-free alignment of individual peptides across all sample injections was performed using the commercial package Rosetta Elucidator v3.3 (Rosetta Biosoftware, Inc., Seattle, WA) with PeakTeller algorithm [10]. Details are described in supporting methods. The raw data in the form of a flat file (excel) Excel File S1 is provided via this link: https://discovery.genome.duke.edu/express/resources/3772/Schechter_PLOSone_Supplemental_Data_June2014.xlsx.

Statistical Analysis

Basic statistical analysis was performed on both the unenriched (protein-level) and phosphopeptide (peptide-level) datasets in order to obtain candidate (phospho) proteins that were differentially expressed. Fold-changes were calculated for each failing group versus non-failing control, as the ratio of the average intensity between the groups; directionality of the ratio was established that positive fold-changes mean up-regulated in failing versus nonfailing control, and negative fold-changes mean down-regulated in failing versus nonfailing. P-values were calculated using an error-weighted ANOVA with Benjamini-Hochberg FDR correction for multiple hypotheses testing (Rosetta Elucidator v3.3). The input for this test was the protein-level data for unenriched analysis (intensity for all peptides summed per sample), or the peptide-level data for phosphopeptides, and the raw intensities were scaled to a normal distribution using the Error Model in Elucidator software prior to ANOVA. Fold-changes and p-values are shown for all proteins (Table S1) and phosphopeptides (Table S2). Statistical cutoffs for fold-change were established for proteins based on a power calculation using the average biological variation within each group. Using the protein average %CV (23%) and 4 reps per group at a 95% confidence, minimum cutoffs were set to 2-fold

(98% powering) for proteins. ANOVA p-value of 0.05 or less was required.

Western Blot Analysis

Cryopreserved heart tissue was mechanically disrupted by mortar and pestle in liquid nitrogen and suspended in lysis buffer (1% IGEPAL CA-630, 0.5% Deoxycholate, 2% SDS, 5 mM EDTA in 1X PBS) with protease and phosphatase inhibitor cocktail tablets (Roche Diagnostics, Indianapolis, IN). Samples were then pulse homogenized on ice via mechanical homogenization.

Cardiac tissue homogenates were subjected to Bicinchoninic acid (BCA) assay (Pierce Biotechnology/Thermo Fisher Scientific, Rockford, IL) for protein quantification. Western Blot for protein immunodetection was performed as described previously [11].

Metabolomics

Organic acids were quantified using methods described previously [12] employing Trace Ultra GC coupled to ISQ MS operating under Xcalibur 2.2 (Thermo Fisher Scientific, Austin, TX).

Bioinformatics Analysis of Protein Data Sets

Ingenuity Pathway Analysis (IPA, Winter 2012 Release) (Ingenuity Systems, Redwood City, CA) was used to classify the proteins according to primary function as well as for pathway analysis. KinasePhose 2.0 (http://kinasephos2.mbc.nctu.edu.tw/index.html) [13] was used to identify protein-kinase specific phosphorylation sites among the differentially phosphorylated proteins with a specificity threshold of at least 80%.

Supporting Materials and Methods

Detailed sample preparation, LC-MS processing, and western blot methodology is described in Methods S1.

Results

Patient Samples

Left ventricular tissue from 12 male patients matched for age and race was used in this study, with 4 patients in each of the following groups: ischemic failing (IF); non-ischemic failing (NIF); or non-failing (NF) hearts not used for transplantation. Groups were closely matched for cardiac function and treatment history (Table 1). All patients with HF exhibited significantly lower ejection fractions compared to NF controls, which had normal left ventricular function. All HF patients received intravenous inotropic agents and intra-aortic balloon pump support, whereas only patients from the IF subset received prior coronary artery bypass surgery. In the NIF group, two patients were diagnosed with non-ischemic cardiomyopathy of unknown etiology, one patient had a viral cardiomyopathy, and the fourth patient developed HF secondary to valvular disease.

Quantitative Analysis of Proteins in Human Left Ventricles

Following the workflow in Figure 1A, all heart tissue samples were subjected to quantitative analyses of the phospho-enriched and unenriched proteome. The reproducibility of the unenriched analytical approach was validated with a spike-in of the internal standard yeast ADH1 digest at a known concentration. Consistent ADH1 abundance (7% coefficient of variation (CV)) across all 12 samples was observed (Figure 1B).

Table 1. Demographic and clinical information.

Group	Sample Size (n)	Age (y±m)	Sex (% Male)	Race (% Caucasian)	% Prior Bypass Surgery	Ejection Fraction (%)	% Inotropic Agent	% Intra-aortic Balloon Pump
Non Failing (NF)	4	57.0±3.4	100	50	0	>55%	0	0
Ischemic Failing (IF)	4	58.0±7.0	100	75	100	<15%	100	100
Non Ischemic Failing (NIF)	4	51.5±7.6	100	50	0	<15%	100	100

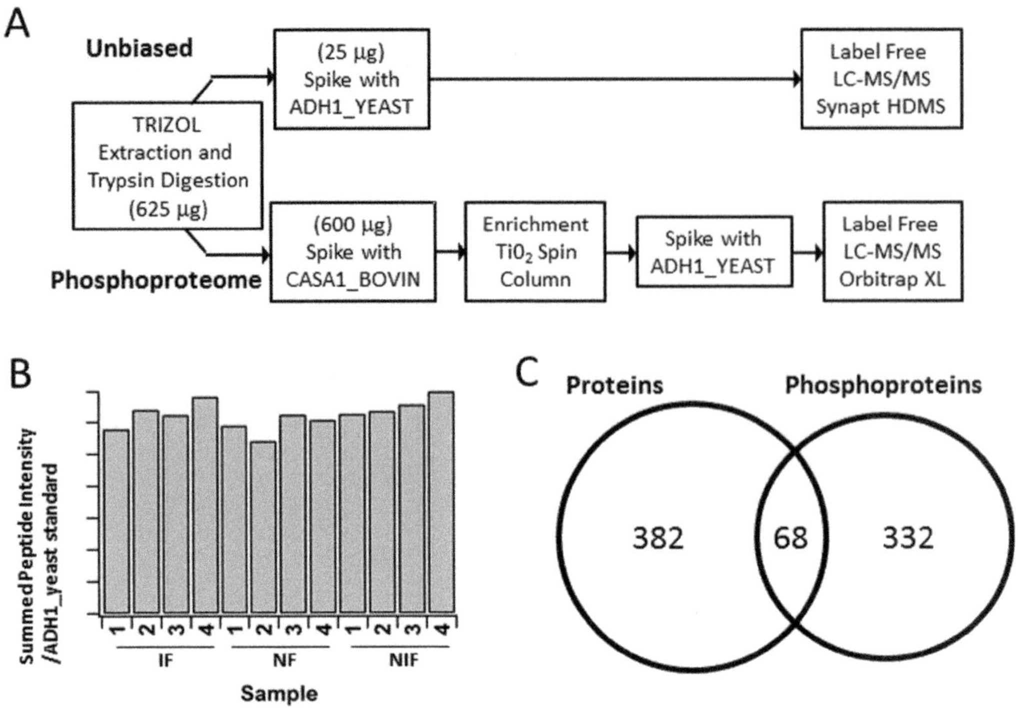

Figure 1. Experimental Approach. A: Illustration of the sample preparation and MS work flow. B: Reproducibility/Internal Control. Relative levels of the ADH1 protein spiked into each heart lysate as determined by chromatographic peak intensity. C: Venn Diagram demonstrating the protein and phosphoprotein yield and overlap.

Peptide/protein identification and quantification by Rosetta Elucidator with Mascot and IdentityE search algorithms yielded expression data for a total of 850 proteins: 4,436 peptide annotations representing 450 proteins in the unenriched samples, for which relative quantitation between samples was performed (Figure 1C; Table S1 for the complete list), and site-specific quantitation for 823 phosphopeptides corresponding to 400 phosphorylated proteins in the phospho-enriched samples were determined (Figure 1C; Table S2 for the complete list). Between the observed unenriched proteome and the phosphoproteome, 68 proteins overlapped (Figure 1C). These 68 proteins and their respective fold changes and p-values are listed in Table S3.

Differential Expression Analysis

Principal components analysis (PCA) was performed in order to observe any high-level differences between sample groups and to screen for outlier samples using the unenriched and phospho-enriched proteome expression data. Expression data was z-score transformed across all samples at the protein-level for unenriched samples (Figure 2A) or at the peptide level for phospho-enriched samples (Figure 2B), and Rosetta Elucidator v3.3 was used to calculate principal components. The two most prominent components (PC1 versus PC2) are plotted in Figures 2A and 2B, and no significant outliers are observed for either unenriched or phosphoproteomes. Interestingly, in unenriched proteomes (Figure 2A), the four NF samples separate from the failing samples along PC1; however, in the phosphoproteome, at least three of the four NIF appear unique along PC1 compared to the IF or NF groups (Figure 2B). This global observation of group classification suggests that the unenriched proteome may best separate failing from NF hearts, whereas phosphorylation status may play a larger role in distinguishing IF versus NIF.

Using the abundance levels of significantly different proteins and phosphopeptides, an unbiased 2D hierarchical clustering analysis was performed at the protein-level (Figure 2C) or phosphopeptide level (Figure 2D) in order to observe the overall expression pattern of these molecules in each individual sample and to determine how these candidates segregate the failing and NF hearts. Figure 2C shows clear differentiation between failing and NF hearts, but none between the two failing etiologies was observed. In contrast, the phosphopeptide analyses (Figure 2D) show a more robust differentiation between all three groups.

Comparison of the unenriched NIF and IF proteomes revealed no differential protein expression, except for carbonic anhydrase 3. The data from the unenriched proteome was filtered to exclude blood proteins and antibodies from consideration. 18 proteins represented by at least two high-confidence peptides and a significant (ANOVA, $p < 0.05$) fold change of at least two were identified between unenriched failing and NF proteomes (Table 2 and 3). Three proteins in the IF (Table 2) and 15 proteins in NIF (Table 3) differed in abundance from the NF. Moreover, four proteins were decreased in abundance, while the remaining proteins were increased in abundance in the failing hearts (Table 2 and 3). Among the proteins whose abundance was significantly changed in the failing human myocardial tissue were secreted glycoproteins, ceruloplasmin, carbonic anhydrase 1 and 3, serum amyloid A, and extracellular matrix proteins. Peptides from the fibulin family of extracellular matrix proteins (fibulin 1, fibulin2, and latent transforming growth factor beta binding protein 2 (fibulin 3)) were consistently up-regulated across the NIF samples.

Our primary goal was to determine etiology-specific changes in site-specific phosphorylation for the phosphopeptides. A phosphopeptide was considered of interest if it fulfilled the following criteria: 1) a ≥2-fold alteration in phosphorylation state (ANOVA

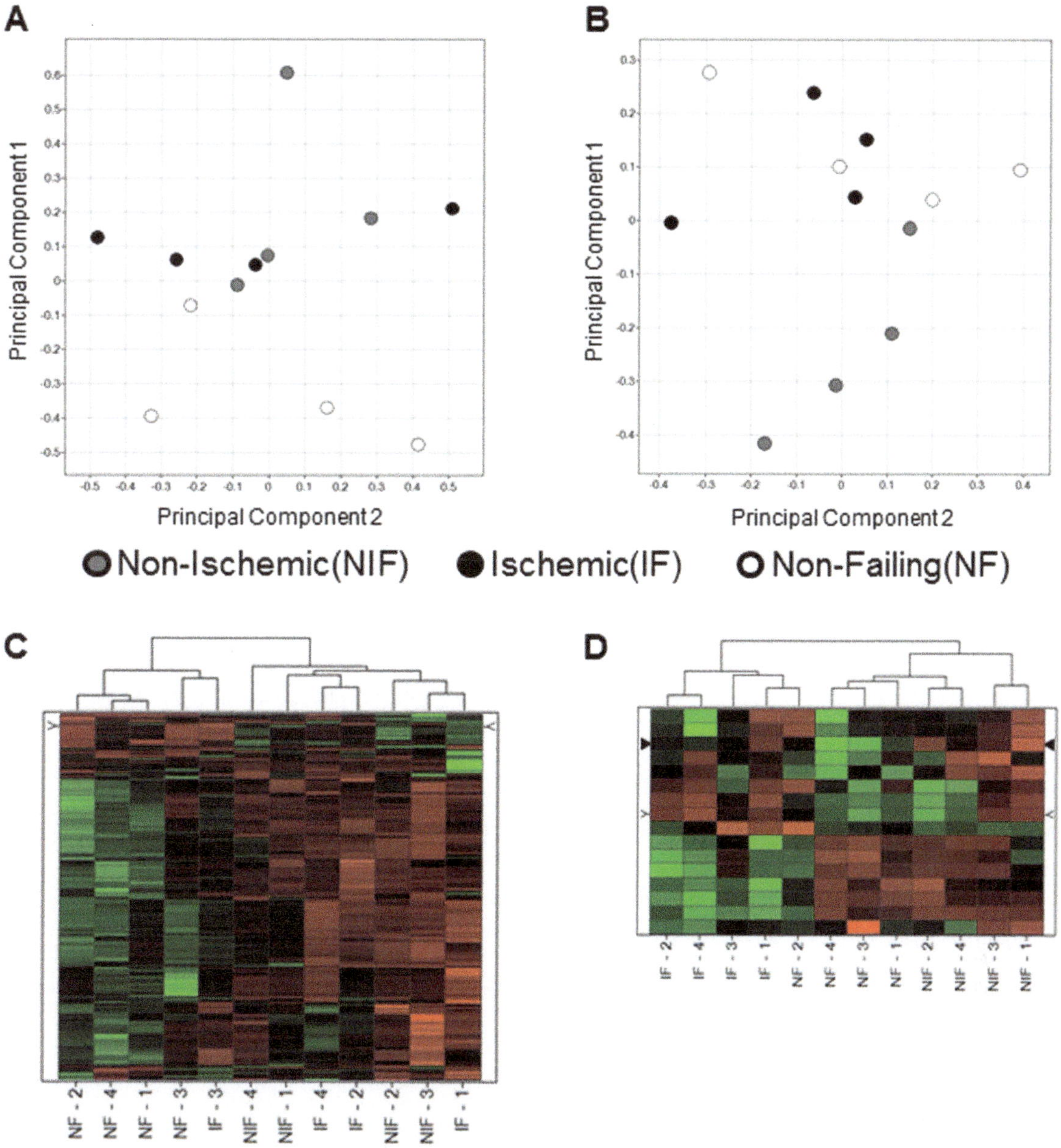

Figure 2. Principal Components Analysis and Hierarchical Clustering. The expression data for all peptides from the unenriched (A) and phosphopeptide enriched (B) samples were used to perform Principal Components Analysis (PCA) after z-score transformation of the peptide intensities. The top two principal components are plotted in each figure, showing no extreme outlier samples among the twelve individual patients tested, either among the unenriched samples or phosphopeptide-enriched. The statistically-significant differentially expressed peptides for each experiment were used to calculate 2D hierarchical clusters in order to view sample-to-sample relationships within these differentially expressed signals, at the unenriched proteome level from Tables 2 and 3 (C) and from the phosphoproteome in Table 4 (D).

p-value≤0.05) between NIF and IF; 2) significantly different phosphorylation levels between at least one etiology of failing hearts and NF hearts; and 3) phosphorylation level differences observed were unlikely to be due to protein level differences. The last criteria was fulfilled by using either the unenriched protein levels (if available; Table S3 for the 68 overlapping proteins) or the comparative levels of other phosphopeptides from the protein of interest (Table S4) and demonstrating that the levels of these other phosphopeptides are not significantly different between the three heart tissue groups nor do they trend in the same direction as the phosphopeptide under consideration.

From this analysis, 26 proteins were identified to contain at least one differently phosphorylated site between NIF and IF tissue that met our criteria (Table 4). Some of these proteins, such as lyric and leiomodin 1, were differentially phosphorylated in the two types of heart failure. Other phosphoproteins demonstrated either a significant hyper-phosphorylation or dephosphorylation in one or more amino acid sites, while phosphorylation levels at the corresponding amino acid sites were unchanged in the other etiology compared to NF tissue.

Table 2. Proteins with statistical significant differential expression between IF and NF heart tissue.

Entry Name	Protein Name	Peptide Count	Fold Change	p-value (ANOVA)	Protein Function
CAH1_HUMAN	**Carbonic anhydrase 1**	2	7.24	1.6×10^{-3}	Acid-Base balance
A2MG_HUMAN	**Alpha-2-macroglobulin**	33	2.31	1.0×10^{-4}	Protease Inhibitor
SAA_HUMAN	**Serum amyloid A protein**	2	−7.32	1.0×10^{-4}	Acute Phase Protein

Data was filtered to eliminate blood proteins and antibodies and to show only proteins with Protein Prophet probability >0.8, FDR-corrected p-value <0.05, absolute fold-change >2. Proteins in bold were validated by western blot analysis.

Validation Western Blot Analysis

The unenriched proteomic mass spec data were validated by Western Blot analysis of independently prepared tissue homogenates from the same 12 patients (Figure 3). Western blot quantitative data is shown in Figure 4. These Western blots confirmed the altered changes in IF and NIF compared to NF that were revealed by the mass spec data: an increase in carbonic anhydrase, ceruloplasmin, Fibulin1, Fibulin2 and Alpha 2-HS glycoprotein (FETUA); a decrease in serum amyloid A; and an increase in α2-Macroglobulin (α2M). Interestingly, a cleaved version of α2M was the prevalent form of α2M in both NIF and IF hearts, whereas the full-length α2M was the prevalent species in NF heart tissue (Figures 3 and 4).

Metabolomic analysis

Pyruvate dehydrogenase E1 component subunit alpha (ODPA or PDH) catalyzes the overall conversion of pyruvate to acetyl-CoA and CO_2, and provides the primary link between glycolysis and the tricarboxylic acid cycle. A significant decrease in phosphorylation of PDH at Ser 300 was observed in IF heart compared to both NIF and NF samples (Table 4) suggestive that PDH is more active in IF hearts than NIF or NF hearts. Mass spectrometry methods were used to examine pyruvate content in the same 12 human myocardial samples (Figure 5). The IF tissue had the lowest levels of pyruvate, supportive of our hypothesis that of the three groups of patients, PDH is most active in IF. Another enzyme that influences pyruvate levels in the myocardium is lactate dehydrogenase (LDH). LDH catalyzes the conversion of pyruvate to lactate and back. Lactate levels were the highest in IF (Figure 5) suggestive that in IF tissues both PDH and LDH are more active than in NIF.

Bioinformatics Analysis

Focusing on differential protein or phosphoprotein levels between NIF and NF samples, Ingenuity Pathway Analysis (IPA) was used to construct an interaction network of proteins (Figure 6). Many of the proteins that were significantly different (>2-fold change, $p<0.05$) were glycoproteins, proteoglycans, and structural

Table 3. Proteins with statistically significant differential expression between NIF and NF heart tissue.

Entry Name	Protein Name	Peptide Count	Fold Change	*p*-value (ANOVA)	Protein Function
CAH3_HUMAN	Carbonic anhydrase 3	2	7.02	1.2×10^{-02}	Acid-Base balance
LTBP2_HUMAN	Latent-transforming growth factor â-binding protein 2	6	4.12	9.8×10^{-03}	Elastic Fiber Structure
CAH1_HUMAN	**Carbonic anhydrase 1**	2	4.06	3.1×10^{-04}	Acid-Base balance
ASPN_HUMAN	Asporin	9	3.03	1.5×10^{-02}	Cartilage Homeostasis
CO6A3_HUMAN	Collagen alpha-3(VI) chain	6	2.93	5.6×10^{-03}	ECM Fibrillar Protein
FBLN2_HUMAN	**Fibulin-2**	4	2.52	7.1×10^{-03}	ECM Remodeling Protein
MFAP4_HUMAN	Microfibril-associated glycoprotein 4	5	2.50	1.4×10^{-02}	Elastic Fiber Formation
FIBG_HUMAN	Fibrinogen gamma chain	13	2.29	1.4×10^{02}	Primary Platelet Receptor Binding Site
FBLN3_HUMAN	EGF-containing fibulin-like extracellular matrix protein 1	2	2.25	1.7×10^{-02}	Elastic Fiber Formation
FBLN1_HUMAN	**Fibulin-1**	2	2.16	4.7×10^{-02}	ECM Organization
CERU_HUMAN	**Ceruloplasmin**	15	2.09	4.0×10^{-03}	Copper Homeostasis
DERM_HUMAN	Dermatopontin	5	2.08	2.8×10^{-02}	Fibroblast Cell Adhesion
MYH2_HUMAN	Myosin-2	2	−2.08	4.5×10^{-03}	Skeletal Muscle Contraction
ATPD_HUMAN	ATP synthase subunit delta, mitochondrial	2	−2.22	6.2×10^{-04}	ATP Synthase Core Subunit
SAA_HUMAN	**Serum amyloid A protein**	2	−6.41	1.7×10^{-04}	Acute Phase Protein

Data was filtered to eliminate blood proteins and antibodies and to show only proteins with Protein Prophet probability >0.8, FDR-corrected p-value <0.05 and absolute fold-change >2. Proteins in bold were validated by western blot analysis.

Table 4. Phosphopeptides with statistically significant differences between IF and NIF human heart tissue.

Primary Protein Name	Protein Description	Modified Peptide Sequence	NIF v IF Fold Change	NIF v IF p-value (ANOVA)	IF v NF Fold Change	IF v NF p-value (ANOVA)	NIF v NF Fold Change	NIF v NF p-value (ANOVA)	Function
LYRIC_HUMAN	Protein LYRIC	LSSQI**S**AGEEK	−7.29	<0.0001	3.31	0.0002	−2.21	0.0080	Transcription co-activator; regulator of apoptosis
LMOD1_HUMAN	Leiomodin-1	GSPKPSPQP**S**PKPSPK	9.66	<0.0001	−1.92	0.0001	5.04	0.0080	Poorly characterized (muscle contraction?)
LMOD1_HUMAN	Leiomodin-1	NSL**S**PATQR	9.18	<0.0001	−4.93	0.0030	1.86	0.7820	
LMOD1_HUMAN	Leiomodin-1	G**S**PKP**S**PQPSPKP**S**PK	4.40	0.0400	−6.84	0.0020	−1.56	0.7110	
BASI_HUMAN	Basigin precursor	KPEDVLDDDDAGSAPLKS**S**GQHQNDK	−7.27	<0.0001	4.62	0.0005	−1.57	0.6750	Tissue remodeling; cell shape & tensile properties
LARP7_HUMAN	La-related protein 7	KRS**SS**EDAESLAPR	−4.46	0.0100	3.48	0.0070	−1.28	0.8900	RNA processing; tumorgenesis
MLRV_HUMAN	Myosin regulatory light chain 2, ventricular/cardiac muscle isoform	AGGAN**S**NVFSMFEQTQIQEFK	−3.53	0.0060	1.70	0.7800	−2.08	0.0880	Cardiac muscle contraction, morphogenesis
HS90A_HUMAN	Heat shock protein HSP 90-alpha	E**S**EDKPEIEDVGSDEEEEKK	−3.42	0.0002	3.74	0.0000	1.09	0.9040	Molecular chaperone; cardiac muscle cell apoptosis
ACINU_HUMAN	Apoptotic chromatin condensation inducer in the nucleus	KSS**S**ISEEKGD**S**DDEKPR	−2.15	0.0000	2.50	0.0000	1.16	0.8960	Apoptosis
POPD1_HUMAN	Blood vessel epicardial substance	N**S**IASSSDSDDGLHQFLR	−10.06	<0.0001	1.30	0.9980	−7.72	<0.0001	Cell adhesion & signaling
POPD1_HUMAN	Blood vessel epicardial substance	GTS**S**M**S**SLHVSSPHQR	−8.02	0.0120	2.03	0.9410	−3.96	0.1710	Cell adhesion & signaling
FHL2_HUMAN	Four and a half LIM domains protein 2	YI**S**FEER	−3.34	0.0130	−1.04	0.9210	−3.49	0.0350	Transcription co-activator; ECM assembly
HSPB1_HUMAN	Heat shock protein beta-1	GP**S**WDPFRDWYPHSR	−3.32	<0.0001	−1.07	0.8020	−3.56	0.0001	Molecular chaperone
KAPO_HUMAN	cAMP-dependent protein kinase type I-alpha regulatory subunit	TD**S**REDEI**S**PPPPNPVVK	−2.81	0.0040	−1.77	0.3500	−4.98	<0.0001	Regulation of cAMP activity; cardiac muscle cell proliferation
MPRI_HUMAN	Cation-independent mannose-6-phosphate receptor	LV**S**FHDD**S**DEDLLHI	−2.64	0.0120	1.03	0.9350	−2.58	0.0360	Insulin-like growth factor 2 and mannose 6-phosphate signaling

Table 4. Cont.

Primary Protein Name	Protein Description	Modified Peptide Sequence	NIF v IF Fold Change	NIF v IF p-value (ANOVA)	IF v NF Fold Change	IF v NF p-value (ANOVA)	NIF v NF Fold Change	NIF v NF p-value (ANOVA)	Function
SRCH_HUMAN	Sarcoplasmic reticulum histidine-rich calcium-binding protein	GHDGEDDEGEE-EEEEEEEEEEA**S**TEYGHQAHR	−2.57	0.0280	−1.36	0.6690	−3.50	0.0040	Calcium homeostasis; regulation of heart contraction
KCRM_HUMAN	Creatine kinase M-type	GTGGVDTAAVG**S**VFDVSNADR	−2.11	0.0370	−1.79	0.5830	−3.77	0.0001	Energy homeostasis; biomarker for myocardial infarction
SRBS2_HUMAN	Sorbin and SH3 domain-containing protein 2	SFTSS**S**P**S**SPSR	5.55	<0.0001	−1.69	0.2940	3.28	0.0350	Z-band signaling; cytoskeleton regulation
AKA12_HUMAN	A-kinase anchor protein 12	EGVTPWA**S**FKK	4.43	0.0030	−1.02	0.9800	4.33	0.0080	Cell growth; signal transduction
SRBS2_HUMAN	Sorbin and SH3 domain-containing protein 2	TSPGRVDLPG**S**STTLTK	3.70	<0.0001	1.04	0.9970	3.85	0.0004	Z-band signaling; cytoskeleton regulation
MAP4_HUMAN	Microtubule-associated protein 4	VG**S**LDNVGHLPAGGAVK	3.32	0.0190	1.37	0.5590	4.55	<0.0001	Cell cycle progression
SRBS2_HUMAN	Sorbin and SH3 domain-containing protein 2	**T**SPGRVDLPGSSTTLTK	3.15	0.0010	-1.07	0.8410	2.95	0.0060	Z-band signaling; cytoskeleton regulation
TITIN_HUMAN	Titin	SR**S**TPPSIAAK	3.10	0.0300	1.73	0.5250	5.36	0.0001	Cardiac muscle development & contraction; tissue elasticity
LMO7_HUMAN	LIM domain only protein 7	RGE**S**LDNLDSPR	2.79	0.0340	1.32	0.7820	3.67	0.0040	Cell adhesion
SRBS2_HUMAN	Sorbin and SH3 domain-containing protein 2	DAS**S**PVPPPHVPPPVPPLRPR	2.64	0.0140	2.64	0.2380	6.98	0.0007	Z-band signaling; cytoskeleton regulation
MATR3_HUMAN	Matrin-3	SY**S**PDGKESPSDKK	2.61	0.0060	−1.11	0.0003	2.36	0.0750	Cell growth & proliferation; DNA damage response
SRBS2_HUMAN	Sorbin and SH3 domain-containing protein 2	DA**S**SPVPPPHVPPPVPPLRPR	2.26	0.0040	1.52	0.3420	3.44	<0.0001	Z-band signaling; cytoskeleton regulation
ODPA_HUMAN	Pyruvate dehydrogenase E1 component subunit alpha, somatic form, mitochondrial	YGMG**T**SVER	123.00	<0.0001	−61.57	<0.0001	2.00	0.7030	Glycolysis; cellular metabolism

Table 4. Cont.

Primary Protein Name	Protein Description	Modified Peptide Sequence	NIF v IF Fold Change	NIF v IF p-value (ANOVA)	IF v NF Fold Change	IF v NF p-value (ANOVA)	NIF v NF Fold Change	NIF v NF p-value (ANOVA)	Function
ODPA_HUMAN	Pyruvate dehydrogenase E1 component subunit alpha, somatic form, mitochondrial	YHGH**S**MSDPGV**S**YR	32.46	<0.0001	−32.49	<0.0001	−1.00	0.9390	
ODPA_HUMAN	Pyruvate dehydrogenase E1 component subunit alpha, somatic form, mitochondrial	YHGH**S**MSDPGVS**Y**R	25.87	<0.0001	−27.30	<0.0001	−1.06	0.9110	
NEXN_HUMAN	Nexilin	EMLA**S**DDEEDVSSKVEK	13.46	0.0005	−16.05	0.0003	−1.19	0.6860	Z-disc protein; cytoskeleton organization
PTRFL_HUMAN	PTRF/SDPR family protein	EIP**T**PEPLK	9.33	<0.0001	−2.60	0.0120	3.59	0.1390	Cardiac myofibril assembly
LMOD1_HUMAN	Leiomodin-1	NSL**S**PATQR	9.18	<0.0001	−4.93	0.0030	1.86	0.7820	Poorly characterized (? Muscle contraction)
HSPB8_HUMAN	Heat shock protein beta-8	DPFRD**S**PLSSR	5.28	<0.0001	−5.87	<0.0001	−1.11	0.8580	Molecular chaperone
TITIN_HUMAN	Titin	RVK**S**PEPSHPK	3.76	<0.0001	−2.18	0.0001	1.72	0.6440	Cardiac muscle development & contraction; tissue elasticity
TITIN_HUMAN	Titin	AV**S**PTETKPTPTEK	2.56	0.0370	−2.64	0.0450	−1.03	0.9640	
FA54B_HUMAN	Protein FAM54B	NA**S**VPNLR	2.51	0.0010	−4.67	<0.0001	−1.86	0.0320	Mitochondrial fission regulator

Phosphorylation sites are underlined.

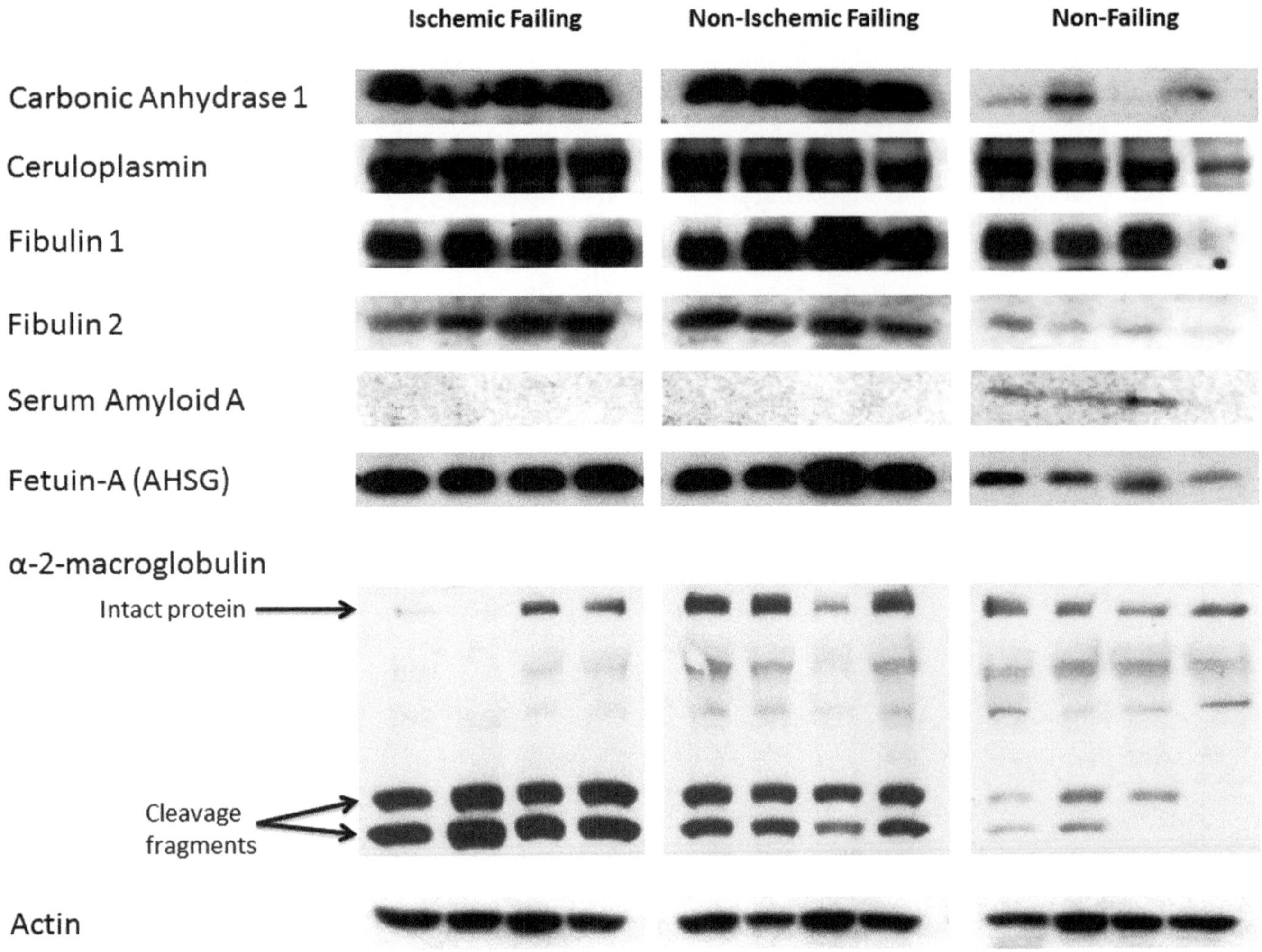

Figure 3. Western blot validations of selected statistically significant proteins identified by proteomics analysis. Protein extracts from IF, NIF, or NF samples (40 μg) were subjected to polyacrylamide gel electrophoresis. Replica nitrocellulose blots were incubated with anti- carbonic anhydrase, -ceruloplasmin, -fibulin 1, -fibulin 2, -serum amyloid A, -fetuin A, -alpha 2 macroglobulin, -PDH Serine 300, or -sarcomeric actin.

proteins, all components of the extracellular matrix (ECM). More ECM proteins were discovered when the inclusion criteria were expanded to significantly different proteins between NIF and NF with <2-fold change (min fold change 1.46) using the IPA analysis (Figure 6, light green). Pathway analysis also suggested that Akt, SMAD3, MMP14, and aryl hydrocarbon receptor (AHR), all of which have been implicated in cardiac remodeling [14–17], may be central regulators controlling the expression levels of many of the proteins included in the IPA analysis. IPA analysis validation was performed by Western blot analysis, which established that several of these more central proteins (AKT, SMAD3, and AHR) were also differentially expressed in NIF (Figures 7 and 8).

Further bioinformatics analysis of the phosphorylation data demonstrated that nine of the differentially phosphorylated proteins are possible targets of casein kinase 2 (Ck2, Figure 9). The four differentially phosphorylated proteins in NIF (LYRIC, SHRC, FHL2, KAP0 and MPRI) were all dephosphorylated in this disease state, while four of the six differentially phosphorylated proteins in IF (LYRIC, LARP7, HSP90A, ACINU) were increasingly phosphorylated.

Discussion

Heart failure remains a progressive disease with limited treatment options. Current standard of care does not differentiate between ischemic and non-ischemic etiologies, treating them similarly. However, as this study suggests, there are important protein phosphorylation differences between the two HF etiologies. Given the variety of cellular processes these proteins are involved in, these differences may be important in the design of therapies for heart failure.

Our analysis revealed the following general differences between the two main types of heart failure: 1) Protein abundances were similar between both types of heart failure compared to NF controls, with one exception; and 2) Site-specific phosphorylation differences on many proteins clearly distinguished non-ischemic and ischemic HF.

Protein abundance differences between non-ischemic and ischemic heart tissue

The only protein that displayed statistically significant differential expression between NIF and IF was carbonic anhydrase 3 (CAH3). CAH3 levels were 2.83-fold higher in the NIF than in the

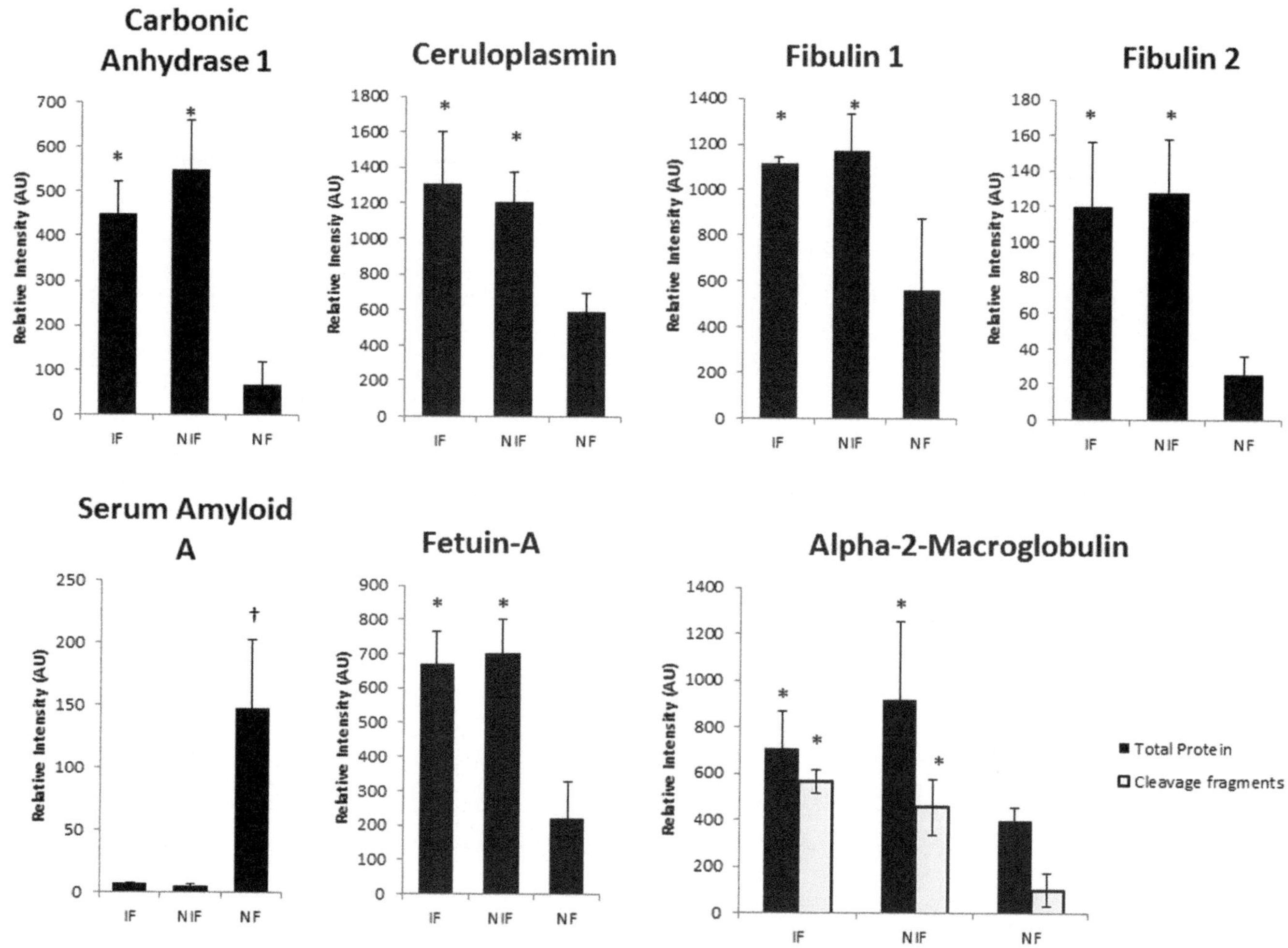

Figure 4. Quantitation of carbonic anhydrase 1, ceruloplasmin, fibulin 1, fibulin 2, serum amyloid A, fetuin A, and total and cleavage products of alpha 2 macroglobulin as determined by densitometry analysis and expressed as relative intensity (arbitrary units (AU)) normalized to actin levels. *: significantly elevated relative to NF samples, †: significantly elevated relative to both NIF and IF.

IF samples. Why the levels of CAH3 increase in HF, especially in NIF, is unclear. In general, many tissues contain carbonic anhydrases, which interconvert carbon dioxide and bicarbonate to maintain acid-base balance and help transport carbon dioxide out of tissues, especially metabolically active tissues like heart and brain. Therefore, the increase of CAH3 could be a sign that these hearts are increasingly metabolically active in an attempt to compensate for the decrease in function.

Protein abundance differences between failing and non-failing human tissue

Extracellular matrix remodeling in the context of NIF. The involvement of ECM remodeling in NIF was our most robust finding from evaluation of protein level differences between failing and non-failing tissues (Figure 6). This finding is not only consistent with other studies that have used proteomic analysis to investigate protein expression variation in cardiac disease, but it complements their findings as well [18,19]. The Barallobre-Barreiro *et al* study, which focused on the ECM remodeling in ischemia/reperfusion injury using a pig model, found an interaction network centered on transforming growth factor-β1 (TGFB1), a known profibrotic molecule[19]. TGFB1 was also heavily involved in our network (Figure 6). Additionally, our network demonstrated what the Barallobre-Barreiro *et al* study suggested, that fibulin 1, 2, and 3 (components of elastic fibers) were significantly up regulated in NIF and trended toward up regulation in IF. These revelations were confirmed by western blot analysis of fibulin 1 and 2 (Figures 3 and 4). Up regulation of fibulin-1 is associated with cardiac disease, [20–22] while up regulation of fibulin-2 and fibulin-3, although not implicated in cardiac disease, is associated with a variety of other fibrotic disorders [23]. Down regulating fibulins may be a therapeutic target in future treatments of heart failure.

Oxidative stress, cellular damage, and inflammation. NIF and IF samples had similarly modulated proteins involved in the oxidative stress and inflammatory pathways, including ceruloplasmin, heat shock protein 90, serum amyloid A, and α2-macroglobulin (α2M). These proteins had comparative abundances in human heart tissue that were confirmed by Western blot analyses (Figures 3 and 4).

When exposed to activated proteases, α2M exposes a "bait region" within its structure that traps the protease. Following protease binding, α2M promotes clearance and degradation of the bound protease while undergoing limited proteolysis [24]. This limited proteolysis, however, does result in α2M cleavage, and our findings reveal an increase in α2M cleavage products. Therefore,

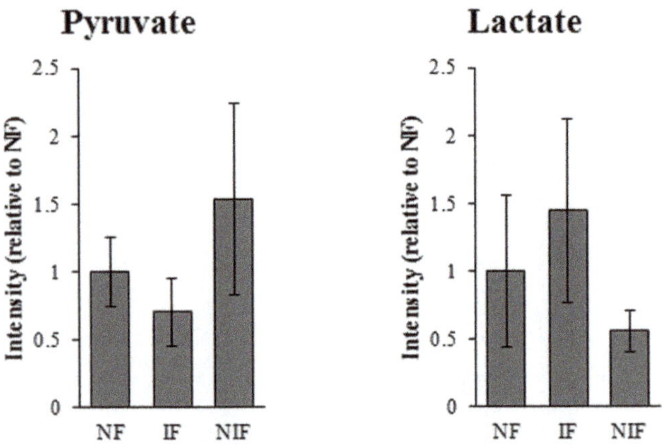

Figure 5. Evaluation of lactate and pyruvate levels in NF, non-failing; IF, ischemic failing; NIF, non-ischemic failing human myocardial tissues. Data is reported as fluorescent intensity relative to NF tissue.

the increased levels of cleaved α2M in HF tissue could be protective attempts to limit the effects of harmful proteases. In addition to binding proteases, the native form of α2M can bind to damaged proteins in order to limit cellular damage and abnormal protein deposition [25]. However this broader protective function of α2M is lost upon exposure to proteases [25] and this decreased ability of α2M to clear damaging protein deposits could be contributing to HF progression. Whether a cause of or response to cellular damage, the cleaved form of α-2M could be a useful biomarker for the progression of HF.

NIF and IF etiologies have different phosphorylation signatures

While the unenriched data set demonstrates the common pathways underlying both types of heart failure, the phosphorylation analysis indicates differences between the two disease etiologies. These differences can be grouped as: 1) etiology-specific differences in phosphorylation at a particular site; and 2) significantly different single- or multiple-site phosphorylation in only one type of HF (compared to NF control). Another notable finding was that over one-third of the differentially phosphorylated protein sequences (9/26) were potential targets of casein kinase 2 (Ck2) (Figure 9). Common functional themes of the significant phosphoproteins include cell growth/death, cardiac muscle development and/or function, and stress response, suggesting etiology-specific regulation of these functions contribute to the development or progression of heart failure.

Etiology-specific differences in phosphorylation. Lyric, also known as metadherin, is a transcription co-factor. Increased Lyric content and phosphorylation play a major role in cancer cell survival [26,27]. Our finding is the first report indicating an association between phosphorylation of Lyric and heart failure. The NIF heart samples in this study displayed increased phosphorylation at lyric amino acid 298, whereas IF samples displayed a decrease in lyric phosphorylation at the same site (Table 4). Although no studies have established the role of phosphorylation at site 298 in the regulation of Lyric activity, other regions on the Lyric protein are involved in protein/protein interactions and appear to be regulated by phosphorylation events.

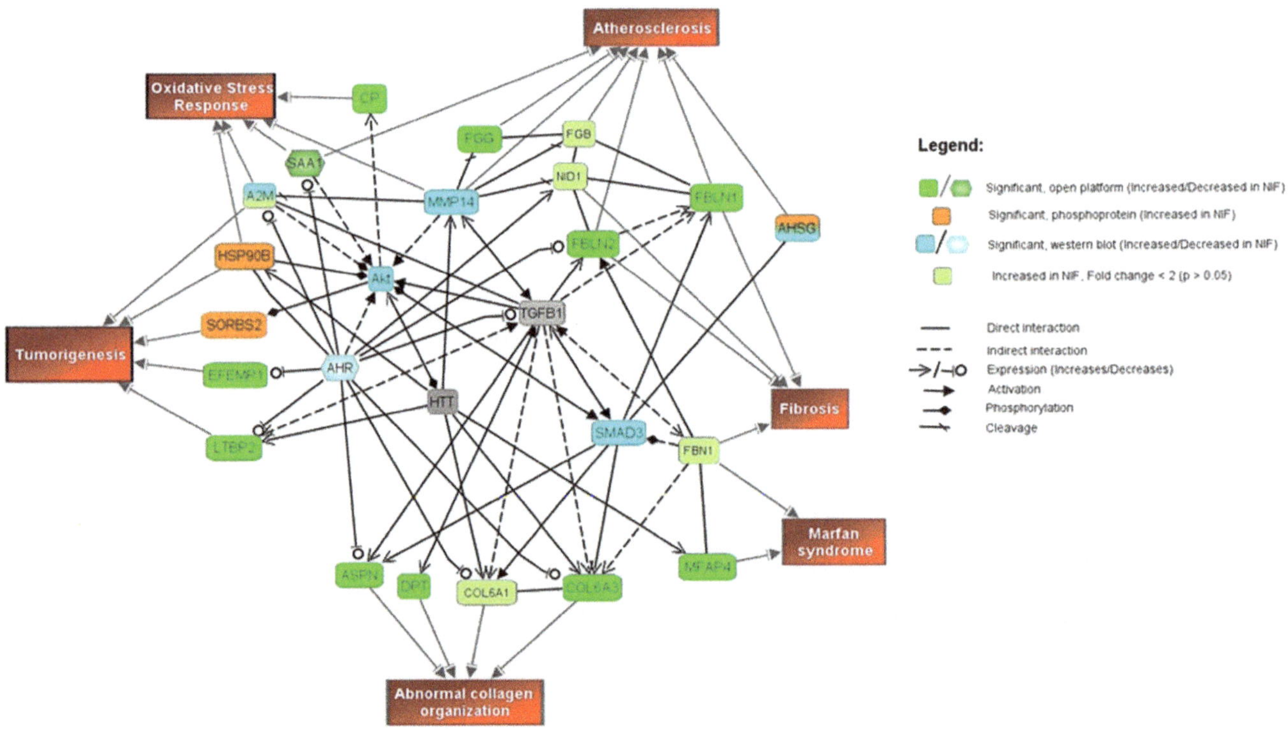

Figure 6. Interaction network of non-ischemic failing hearts. Relevant interactions of the differentially expressed proteins and their relationships with selected pathologies are depicted.

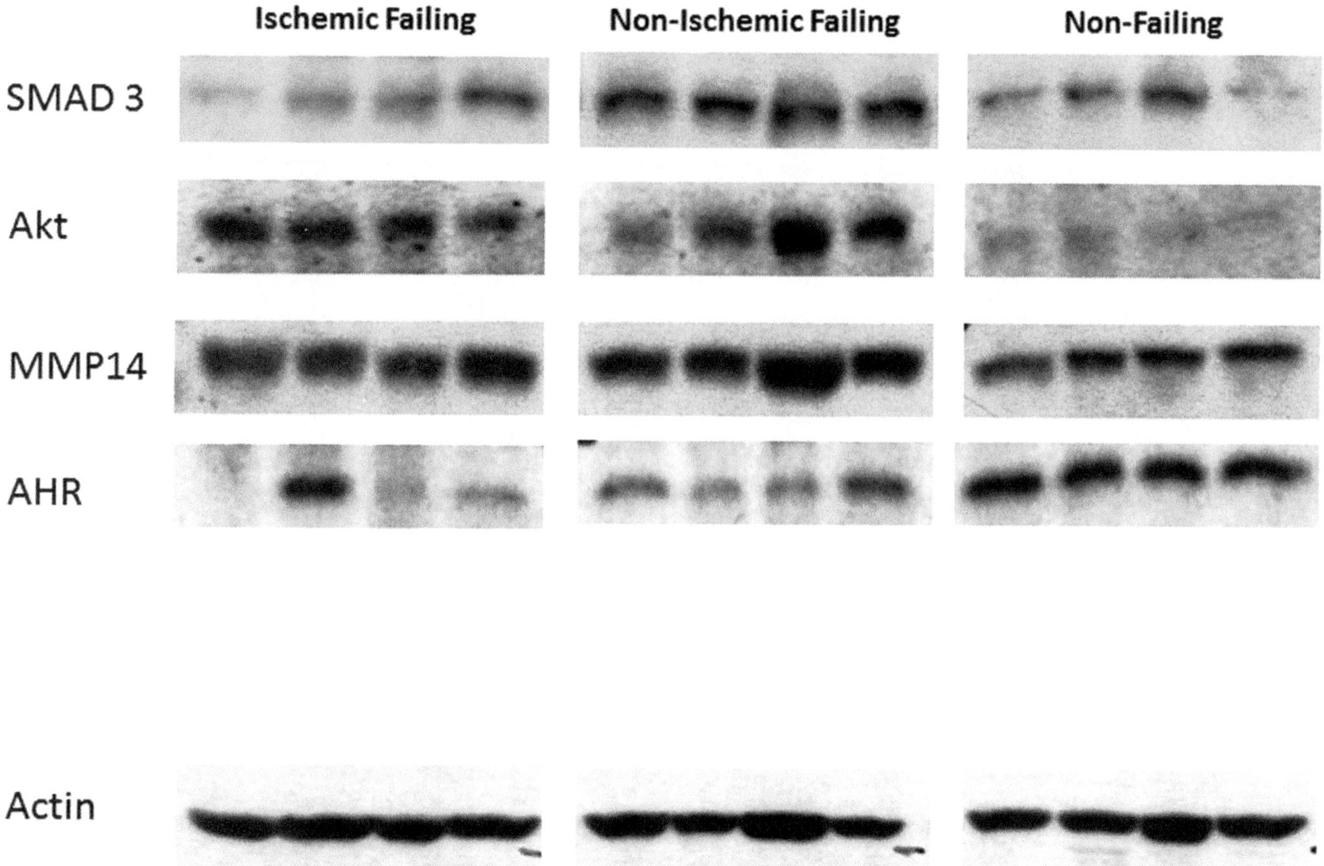

Figure 7. Western blot analysis of central proteins identified from pathway analysis. Protein extracts from IF, NIF, or NF samples (40 μg) were subjected to polyacrylamide gel electrophoresis. Replica nitrocellulose blots were incubated with anti- SMAD3, -AKT, -MMP14, -AHR or -sarcomeric actin.

Assuming that this phosphorylation/dephosphorylation of Lyric at 298 also functions as a toggle switch for protein binding, the increased phosphorylation in IF could be an attempt to recruit a partner transcription factor to activate cell growth in the viable myocardium to compensate for the injury already suffered. Conversely, dephosphorylation of the pro-growth Lyric protein could be contributing to progression of NIF heart failure by activating pro-cell death pathways or suppressing pro-cell growth pathways.

Leiomodin-1 is primarily expressed in smooth muscle, with some expression in the heart, and is speculated to play a role in cardiac hypertrophy and muscle contraction [28]. Phosphorylation of leiomodin-1 was suggested to be a mediator of the actin cytoskeleton formation in human trabecular meshwork cells [29]. Multiple amino acid sites on leiomodin-1 exhibited greater phosphorylation in the NIF samples than the IF samples, with differences ranging from 4 to 9 fold greater, depending on the site (Table 4). The presence of leiomodin-1 in the smooth muscle and the cytoskeleton links well to a pathological role in heart failure. Generation of mutants in leiomodin-1 unable to be phosphorylated at the amino acids revealed herein will be critical in determining the involvement of this relatively uncharacterized protein in the development of these two distinct types of heart failure.

Significantly different phosphorylation only seen in one HF etiology. Phosphorylation of basigin at serine 368 near the C-terminus was increased in IF (compared to NIF and NF). Basigin is a transmembrane glycoprotein that induces MMP activity and subsequent ECM breakdown that is associated with adverse tissue remodeling seen in many pathological conditions such as HF[30]. Basigin is also connected to energy metabolism by directly mediating monocarboxylate transporter (MCT) localization and activity in the sarcolemma. Dissociation of basigin from MCT1, the primary isoform in heart, reduces cellular lactate influx limiting lactate oxidation inside the cardiomyocyte [31]. Considering basigin-MCT1 interactions, the phosphorylation state of basigin could affect lactate influx into the cardiomyocyte and thus influence cardiac metabolism. In fact, the C-terminus of basigin is necessary for dimerization and association with MCT1 [32], and a serine-to-alanine mutation at serine 193 disrupted basigin dimerization and MMP2 induction [33]. This data suggests that phosphorylation of basigin may alter its activity and function, and could contribute to the increase in lactate pools seen in the IF. The role of differential phosphorylation states of basigin in heart failure deserves further attention.

POPD1, a member of the Popeye domain containing family, is a membrane protein abundantly expressed in the heart. POPD1 has been shown to play an important role in cardiac pacemaker cells, cellular adhesion, and cellular signaling, especially in times of

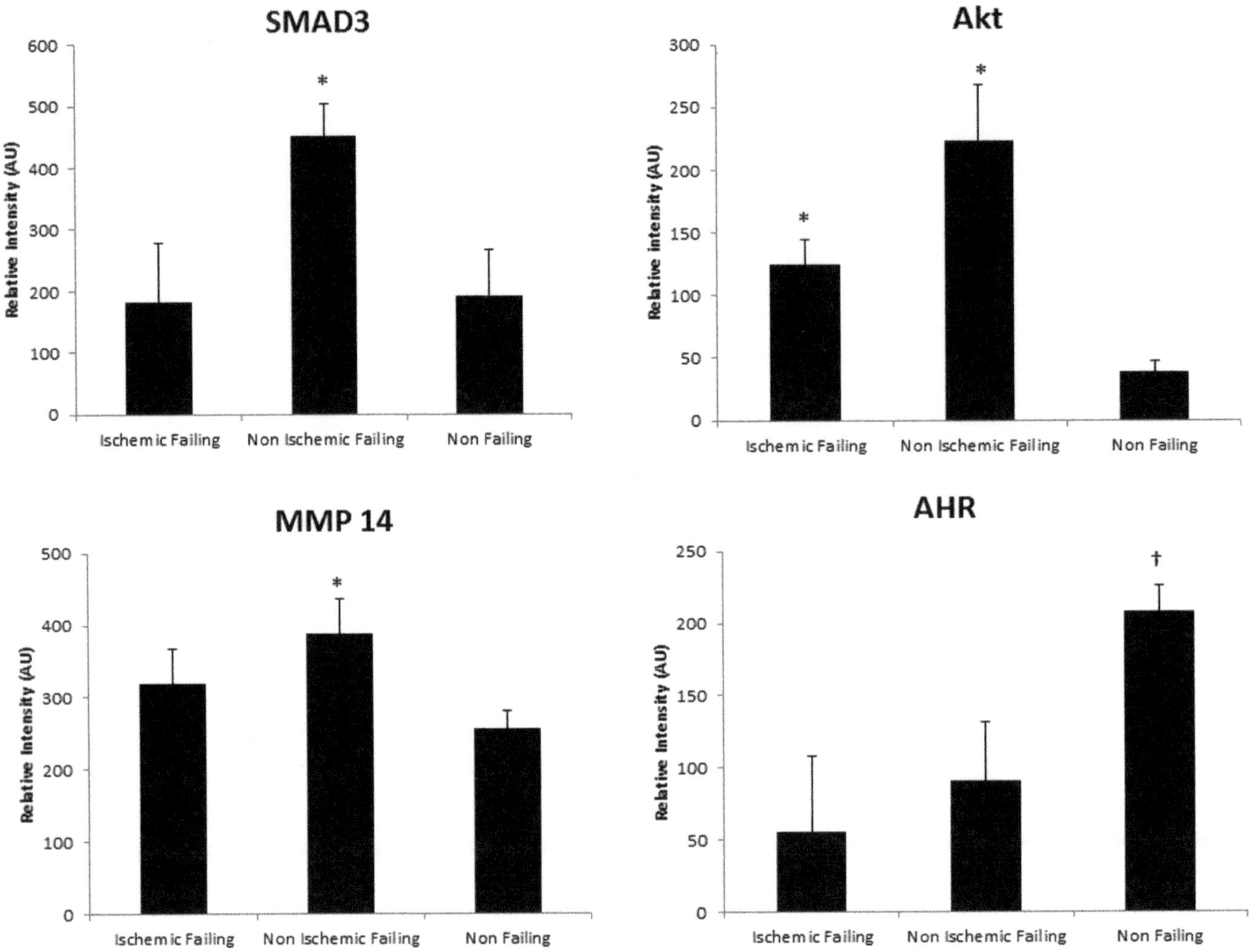

Figure 8. Quantitation of SMAD3, AKT, MMP14, and AHR as determined by densitometry analysis and expressed as relative intensity (arbitrary units (AU)) normalized to actin levels. *: significantly elevated relative to non-failing, †: significantly elevated relative to both NIF and IF.

stress [34,35]. Some literature suggest that POPD1 content is decreased in human heart failure [36]. While the overall abundance of POPD1 was not changed between the three groups in our data, POPD1 phosphorylation at 2 sites was diminished in NIF heart relative to NF heart, while phosphorylation at these sites was minimally changed in IF (Table 4). POPD1 phosphorylation has not been examined, but this protein is important in the RhoA signaling pathway, a key regulator of myosin light chain phosphorylation [37]. Myosin light chain phosphorylation is decreased when POPD1 is overexpressed, and a recent study demonstrated that the transition from compensated to decompensated heart failure is centrally mediated by a reduction in myosin light chain phosphorylation [38]. Interestingly, in our study, slow cardiac myosin regulatory light chain 2 (MLRV) was significantly less phosphorylated at serine 15 in NIF compared to IF heart (Table 4). Together, these findings suggest etiology-specific phosphorylation events in the RhoA/POPD1/MLRV pathway may play a role in the development of non-ischemic heart failure.

Multiple sites on SORBS2 exhibited increased phosphorylation in NIF samples compared to the other two groups (Table 4). SORBS2 is an adaptor protein that mediates interactions between structural proteins, membrane proteins, other signaling molecules, and actin filaments in cardiomyocytes [39]. From a mass spectrometry based proteomics approach, SORBS2 has been recently identified as a protein released from cardiac tissue immediately following acute myocardial infarction [40]. SORBS2 also promotes the ubiquitination and degradation of c-Abl, an important regulator of the actin cytoskeleton and apoptosis, [41] and alterations in SORBS2 activity by differential phosphorylation could activate the apoptotic cascade contributing to the development of non-ischemic heart failure. SORBS2 is expressed exclusively within the myofibril Z-bands, which link the sarcomeric contractile units together, and regulates the signaling cascade needed for proper force production and transmission in these contractile units [39,42]. Another sarcomeric protein that plays a key role in force transmission at the Z-line, titin, was differentially phosphorylated in NIF (Table 4). The phosphorylation of these two structural proteins may contribute to the disruption of the tightly regulated contractile apparatus leading to the cardiac contractile deficiencies in NIF.

Phosphorylation/dephosphorylation of PDH/ODPA is complex. The activity of PDH is regulated via phosphorylation of three

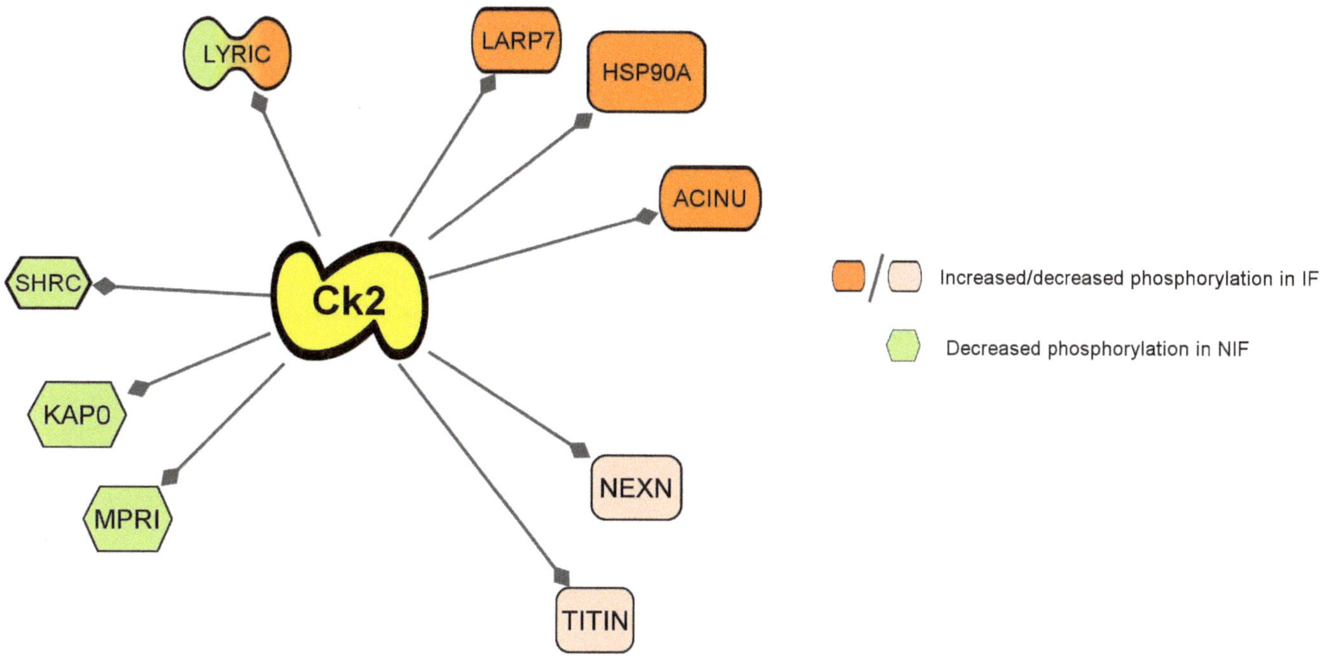

Figure 9. Casein kinase phosphorylation targets. Nine of the differentially phosphorylated proteins shown in Table 4 are possible targets of casein kinase.

serine resides (232, 293, and 300) [43]. *In vitro*, phosphorylation at a single site is sufficient to inactivate PDH, [43] and dephosphorylation by pyruvate dehydrogenase phosphatases activate PDH [44]. A decrease in phosphorylation of PDH at Ser 300 is observed in IF, while phosphorylation at Ser 293 is unchanged or only modestly changed. In non-failing, well-perfused heart, fatty acids provide 60–90% of the energy for ATP production, with the remaining 10–40% derived from carbohydrate (glucose and lactate) oxidation [45]. In the failing heart, the preferential fuel source switches to glucose from fatty acids. The marked decrease in PDH phosphorylation in IF supports the current dogma regarding the switch towards glucose, at least in IF, and suggests a mechanism by which this is occurring, namely reduction of PDH inhibition. Interestingly, PDH phosphorylation was not significantly changed in NIF hearts, suggesting that this shift in energy substrate is etiology specific. The trend in lower pyruvate levels in the IF tissue fits with our hypothesis that PDH activity is increased in IF. Despite the differences in pyruvate and PDH Ser 300 levels between HF etiologies, PDH enzyme activity was not statistically different between groups (data not shown, $p = 0.866$). In all, the data suggest that PDH activity may differentiate between NIF and IF, but additional studies will be required. Whether the increase in glucose oxidation within the ischemic heart represents a protective response to chronic ischemia or a maladaptive response that further stresses the ischemic heart remains unclear.

Role of Casein Kinase 2 in the development of heart failure: Etiology specific?

Of the 26 differently phosphorylated proteins, nine had sites that were predicted targets of casein kinase 2 (Ck2, Figure 9). Ck2 is a ubiquitous serine/threonine protein kinases thought to have over 300 protein substrates that modulate a variety of cellular processes, including cell cycle control, cellular differentiation, and proliferation [46]. Classified as a "messenger-independent kinase," Ck2 is a constitutively active kinase that is regulated through protein-protein interactions, localization, and extent of phosphorylation and oligomerization [46,47]. Ck2 activity has been shown to both induce hypertrophy and inhibit apoptosis within cardiomyocytes, primarily through its interaction with apoptosis repressor with caspase recruitment domain (ARC), histone deacetylases, and the tumor suppressor gene p27 [48–52]. Many studies have demonstrated that Ck2 activity is critical for ischemic and stress-induced cardiac hypertrophic growth [48–54].

The majority of significant Ck2-specific sites in the IF hearts were increasingly phosphorylated, while all of the significant phosphoproteins with Ck2-specific sites in the NIF group were all relatively dephosphorylated. Furthermore, Lyric, a protein showing etiology-specific differences in phosphorylation, is predicted to be a target of Ck2 [13].

The observation that many of these phosphorylation sites may be targets of Ck2 suggest that variation in Ck2 activity may point to a branching point between these two disease states. In ischemic heart failure, the initial injury and cardiomyocyte loss triggers pro-hypertrophic and anti-apoptotic pathways, of which Ck2 is a central player. This sustained cardiac hypertrophy, due in part to increased Ck2 activity, leads to maladaptive cardiac remodeling and eventually heart failure. Conversely, in non-ischemic heart disease, Ck2 activity is decreased, leading to increased apoptotic activity and suppression of pro-growth pathways. As such, modulation of Ck2 activity could be an etiology-specific treatment, although further analysis into the role of Ck2 in the development of ischemic and non-ischemic heart failure is needed.

Conclusions

This is the first study using a multi-'omics-driven systems biology approach to obtain a more integrated and comprehensive molecular assessment of the different etiologies of heart failure. Using an unbiased assessment of the unenriched and phosphoenriched proteomes of two HF etiologies, combined with selected metabolomics and Western blot analysis, the previously undocumented molecular fingerprints of the different heart failure etiologies were explored. These molecular differences between heart failure etiologies have enabled us to complement pathways believed to be involved in the development of HF in general. As our human heart repository becomes more robust in terms of increased specimen number and cohort size, the evaluation of additional post translational modifications (PTMs) and the use of multiple reaction monitoring [55] for more sensitive and precise quantitative analyses of these PTMs becomes achievable. Comprehensive understanding of the proteome of this common disease through study of human cardiac tissue from a robust biorepository will lead to better, more focused treatments, and ultimately improved patient outcomes.

Supporting Information

Excel File S1 The following information is contained within Excel File S1. Key sheet-Contains an index of the remainder of the excel file sheets, sample identifiers, patient ID, disease etiology, peptide modifications, and Modloc scoring criteria. ST1-peptide expression data from unbiased proteomics. ST2-protein expression data from unbiased proteomics. ST3-Phosphopeptide expression data from phospho-enriched proteomics. ST4-Differential Unbiased Protein Expression (Fold Changes, ANOVA) for unbiased proteomics. ST5-Differential Phosphopeptide Expression (Fold Changes, ANOVA).

Methods S1 Supplemental Materials and Methods.

Table S1 Unenriched protein expression profiles.

Table S2 Phosphoenriched peptide expression profiles.

Table S3 Expression profile of 68 unenriched overlapping proteins.

Table S4 Differential phosphorylation of proteins in NIF and IF heart.

Acknowledgments

We acknowledge Carolina Donor Services for facilitating the acquisition of unused donor hearts. We kindly acknowledge Dr. Robert Lefkowitz for the use of the LTQ-Orbitrap in phosphoproteomics experiments.

Author Contributions

Conceived and designed the experiments: JWT EJS VAB MDH MAM VP DEB. Performed the experiments: MAS MKHH LWN JWT EJS BJF CDT KAH ORI WLN GPL KMS MWF. Analyzed the data: MAS MKKH LWN JWT EJS BJF KMS LS MDH MWF VP DEB. Contributed reagents/materials/analysis tools: CAM VP. Contributed to the writing of the manuscript: MAS MKKH LWN JWT EJS BJF LS CAM DEB.

References

1. Roger VL, Go AS, Lloyd-Jones DM, Benjamin EJ, Berry JD, et al. (2012) Heart disease and stroke statistics–2012 update: a report from the American Heart Association. Circulation 125: e2–e220.
2. Lloyd-Jones DM, Larson MG, Leip EP, Beiser A, D'Agostino RB, et al. (2002) Lifetime risk for developing congestive heart failure: the Framingham Heart Study. Circulation 106: 3068–3072.
3. Levy D, Kenchaiah S, Larson MG, Benjamin EJ, Kupka MJ, et al. (2002) Long-term trends in the incidence of and survival with heart failure. N Engl J Med 347: 1397–1402.
4. Roger VL, Go AS, Lloyd-Jones DM, Benjamin EJ, Berry JD, et al. (2012) Executive summary: heart disease and stroke statistics–2012 update: a report from the American Heart Association. Circulation 125: 188–197.
5. Margulies KB, Bednarik DP, Dries DL (2009) Genomics, transcriptional profiling, and heart failure. J Am Coll Cardiol 53: 1752–1759.
6. Sharma P, Cosme J, Gramolini AO (2012) Recent advances in cardiovascular proteomics. J Proteomics.
7. Gonzalez A, Lopez B, Beaumont J, Ravassa S, Arias T, et al. (2009) Cardiovascular translational medicine (III). Genomics and proteomics in heart failure research. Rev Esp Cardiol 62: 305–313.
8. Klawitter J, Klawitter J, Agardi E, Corby K, Leibfritz D, et al. (2013) Association of DJ-1/PTEN/AKT- and ASK1/p38-mediated cell signalling with ischaemic cardiomyopathy. Cardiovasc Res 97: 66–76.
9. Soderblom EJ, Philipp M, Thompson JW, Caron MG, Moseley MA (2011) Quantitative label-free phosphoproteomics strategy for multifaceted experimental designs. Anal Chem 83: 3758–3764.
10. Weng L, Dai H, Zhan Y, He Y, Stepaniants SB, et al. (2006) Rosetta error model for gene expression analysis. Bioinformatics 22: 1111–1121.
11. Piacentino V, 3rd, Milano CA, Bolanos M, Schroder J, Messina E, et al. (2012) X-linked inhibitor of apoptosis protein-mediated attenuation of apoptosis, using a novel cardiac-enhanced adeno-associated viral vector. Hum Gene Ther 23: 635–646.
12. Jensen MV, Joseph JW, Ilkayeva O, Burgess S, Lu D, et al. (2006) Compensatory responses to pyruvate carboxylase suppression in islet beta-cells. Preservation of glucose-stimulated insulin secretion. J Biol Chem 281: 22342–22351.
13. Wong YH, Lee TY, Liang HK, Huang CM, Wang TY, et al. (2007) KinasePhos 2.0: a web server for identifying protein kinase-specific phosphorylation sites based on sequences and coupling patterns. Nucleic Acids Res 35: W588–594.
14. Jourdan-Lesaux C, Zhang J, Lindsey ML (2010) Extracellular matrix roles during cardiac repair. Life Sci 87: 391–400.
15. Vilahur G, Cubedo J, Casani L, Padro T, Sabate-Tenas M, et al. (2012) Reperfusion-triggered stress protein response in the myocardium is blocked by post-conditioning. Systems biology pathway analysis highlights the key role of the canonical aryl-hydrocarbon receptor pathway. Eur Heart J.
16. Bujak M, Ren G, Kweon HJ, Dobaczewski M, Reddy A, et al. (2007) Essential role of Smad3 in infarct healing and in the pathogenesis of cardiac remodeling. Circulation 116: 2127–2138.
17. Chaanine AH, Hajjar RJ (2011) AKT signalling in the failing heart. Eur J Heart Fail 13: 825–829.
18. Rosello-Lleti E, Alonso J, Cortes R, Almenar L, Martinez-Dolz L, et al. (2012) Cardiac protein changes in ischaemic and dilated cardiomyopathy: a proteomic study of human left ventricular tissue. J Cell Mol Med 16: 2471–2486.
19. Barallobre-Barreiro J, Didangelos A, Schoendube FA, Drozdov I, Yin X, et al. (2012) Proteomics analysis of cardiac extracellular matrix remodeling in a porcine model of ischemia/reperfusion injury. Circulation 125: 789–802.
20. de Vega S, Iwamoto T, Yamada Y (2009) Fibulins: multiple roles in matrix structures and tissue functions. Cell Mol Life Sci 66: 1890–1902.
21. Argraves WS, Greene LM, Cooley MA, Gallagher WM (2003) Fibulins: physiological and disease perspectives. EMBO Rep 4: 1127–1131.
22. Argraves WS, Tanaka A, Smith EP, Twal WO, Argraves KM, et al. (2009) Fibulin-1 and fibrinogen in human atherosclerotic lesions. Histochem Cell Biol 132: 559–565.
23. Hu B, Thirtamara-Rajamani KK, Sim H, Viapiano MS (2009) Fibulin-3 is uniquely upregulated in malignant gliomas and promotes tumor cell motility and invasion. Mol Cancer Res 7: 1756–1770.
24. Sottrup-Jensen L (1989) Alpha-macroglobulins: structure, shape, and mechanism of proteinase complex formation. J Biol Chem 264: 11539–11542.
25. French K, Yerbury JJ, Wilson MR (2008) Protease activation of alpha2-macroglobulin modulates a chaperone-like action with broad specificity. Biochemistry 47: 1176–1185.
26. Zhang N, Wang X, Huo Q, Li X, Wang H, et al. (2013) The oncogene metadherin modulates the apoptotic pathway based on the tumor necrosis factor superfamily member TRAIL (Tumor Necrosis Factor-related Apoptosis-inducing Ligand) in breast cancer. J Biol Chem 288: 9396–9407.
27. Kim JY, Welsh EA, Oguz U, Fang B, Bai Y, et al. (2013) Dissection of TBK1 signaling via phosphoproteomics in lung cancer cells. Proc Natl Acad Sci U S A 110: 12414–12419.
28. Kostyukova AS (2007) Leiomodin/tropomyosin interactions are isoform specific. Arch Biochem Biophys 465: 227–230.
29. Clark R, Nosie A, Walker T, Faralli JA, Filla MS, et al. (2013) Comparative genomic and proteomic analysis of cytoskeletal changes in dexamethasone-treated trabecular meshwork cells. Mol Cell Proteomics 12: 194–206.
30. Huet E, Gabison EE, Mourah S, Menashi S (2008) Role of emmprin/CD147 in tissue remodeling. Connect Tissue Res 49: 175–179.

31. Wilson MC, Meredith D, Fox JE, Manoharan C, Davies AJ, et al. (2005) Basigin (CD147) is the target for organomercurial inhibition of monocarboxylate transporter isoforms 1 and 4: the ancillary protein for the insensitive MCT2 is EMBIGIN (gp70). J Biol Chem 280: 27213–27221.
32. Wilson MC, Meredith D, Halestrap AP (2002) Fluorescence resonance energy transfer studies on the interaction between the lactate transporter MCT1 and CD147 provide information on the topology and stoichiometry of the complex in situ. J Biol Chem 277: 3666–3672.
33. Cui HY, Guo T, Wang SJ, Zhao P, Dong ZS, et al. (2012) Dimerization is essential for HAb18G/CD147 promoting tumor invasion via MAPK pathway. Biochem Biophys Res Commun 419: 517–522.
34. Hager HA, Bader DM (2009) Bves: ten years after. Histol Histopathol 24: 777–787.
35. Froese A, Breher SS, Waldeyer C, Schindler RF, Nikolaev VO, et al. (2012) Popeye domain containing proteins are essential for stress-mediated modulation of cardiac pacemaking in mice. J Clin Invest 122: 1119–1130.
36. Gingold-Belfer R, Bergman M, Alcalay Y, Schlesinger H, Aravot D, et al. (2011) Popeye domain-containing 1 is down-regulated in failing human hearts. Int J Mol Med 27: 25–31.
37. Russ PK, Kupperman AI, Presley SH, Haselton FR, Chang MS (2010) Inhibition of RhoA signaling with increased Bves in trabecular meshwork cells. Invest Ophthalmol Vis Sci 51: 223–230.
38. Warren SA, Briggs LE, Zeng H, Chuang J, Chang EI, et al. (2012) Myosin light chain phosphorylation is critical for adaptation to cardiac stress. Circulation 126: 2575–2588.
39. Sanger JM, Wang J, Gleason LM, Chowrashi P, Dube DK, et al. (2010) Arg/Abl-binding protein, a Z-body and Z-band protein, binds sarcomeric, costameric, and signaling molecules. Cytoskeleton (Hoboken) 67: 808–823.
40. Kakimoto Y, Ito S, Abiru H, Kotani H, Ozeki M, et al. (2013) Sorbin and SH3 domain-containing protein 2 is released from infarcted heart in the very early phase: proteomic analysis of cardiac tissues from patients. J Am Heart Assoc 2: e000565.
41. Soubeyran P, Barac A, Szymkiewicz I, Dikic I (2003) Cbl-ArgBP2 complex mediates ubiquitination and degradation of c-Abl. Biochem J 370: 29–34.
42. Frank D, Kuhn C, Katus HA, Frey N (2006) The sarcomeric Z-disc: a nodal point in signalling and disease. J Mol Med (Berl) 84: 446–468.
43. Korotchkina LG, Patel MS (1995) Mutagenesis studies of the phosphorylation sites of recombinant human pyruvate dehydrogenase. Site-specific regulation. J Biol Chem 270: 14297–14304.
44. Karpova T, Danchuk S, Kolobova E, Popov KM (2003) Characterization of the isozymes of pyruvate dehydrogenase phosphatase: implications for the regulation of pyruvate dehydrogenase activity. Biochim Biophys Acta 1652: 126–135.
45. Lopaschuk GD, Ussher JR, Folmes CD, Jaswal JS, Stanley WC (2010) Myocardial fatty acid metabolism in health and disease. Physiol Rev 90: 207–258.
46. Bolanos-Garcia VM, Fernandez-Recio J, Allende JE, Blundell TL (2006) Identifying interaction motifs in CK2beta–a ubiquitous kinase regulatory subunit. Trends Biochem Sci 31: 654–661.
47. Veis A, Sfeir C, Wu CB (1997) Phosphorylation of the proteins of the extracellular matrix of mineralized tissues by casein kinase-like activity. Crit Rev Oral Biol Med 8: 360–379.
48. Tan WQ, Wang JX, Lin ZQ, Li YR, Lin Y, et al. (2008) Novel cardiac apoptotic pathway: the dephosphorylation of apoptosis repressor with caspase recruitment domain by calcineurin. Circulation 118: 2268–2276.
49. Li PF, Li J, Muller EC, Otto A, Dietz R, et al. (2002) Phosphorylation by protein kinase CK2: a signaling switch for the caspase-inhibiting protein ARC. Mol Cell 10: 247–258.
50. Eom GH, Cho YK, Ko JH, Shin S, Choe N, et al. (2011) Casein kinase-2alpha1 induces hypertrophic response by phosphorylation of histone deacetylase 2 S394 and its activation in the heart. Circulation 123: 2392–2403.
51. Murtaza I, Wang HX, Feng X, Alenina N, Bader M, et al. (2008) Down-regulation of catalase and oxidative modification of protein kinase CK2 lead to the failure of apoptosis repressor with caspase recruitment domain to inhibit cardiomyocyte hypertrophy. J Biol Chem 283: 5996–6004.
52. Hauck L, Harms C, An J, Rohne J, Gertz K, et al. (2008) Protein kinase CK2 links extracellular growth factor signaling with the control of p27(Kip1) stability in the heart. Nat Med 14: 315–324.
53. Kim SO, Baines CP, Critz SD, Pelech SL, Katz S, et al. (1999) Ischemia induced activation of heat shock protein 27 kinases and casein kinase 2 in the preconditioned rabbit heart. Biochem Cell Biol 77: 559–567.
54. Konecny F, Zou J, Husain M, von Harsdorf R (2012) Post-myocardial infarct p27 fusion protein intravenous delivery averts adverse remodelling and improves heart function and survival in rodents. Cardiovasc Res 94: 492–500.
55. Liebler DC, Zimmerman LJ (2013) Targeted quantitation of proteins by mass spectrometry. Biochemistry 52: 3797–3806.

3

Temporal Profile and Mechanisms of the Prompt Sympathoexcitation following Coronary Ligation in Wistar Rats

Luciana Mesquita Passamani[1,2], Ana Paula Abdala[1], Davi José de Almeida Moraes[3], Karla Nívea Sampaio[4], José Geraldo Mill[2], Julian Francis Richmond Paton[1]*

1 School of Physiology & Pharmacology, Bristol Heart Institute, Medical Sciences Building, University of Bristol, Bristol, United Kingdom, **2** Department of Physiological Sciences, Health Sciences Center, Federal University of Espírito Santo, Vitória, Espírito Santo, Brazil, **3** Department of Physiology, School of Medicine of Ribeirão Preto, University of São Paulo, Ribeirão Preto, São Paulo, Brazil, **4** Department of Pharmaceutical Sciences, Health Sciences Center, Federal University of Espírito Santo, Vitória, Espírito Santo, Brazil

Abstract

Our aim was to assess the timing and mechanisms of the sympathoexcitation that occurs immediately after coronary ligation. We recorded thoracic sympathetic (tSNA) and phrenic activities, heart rate (HR) and perfusion pressure in Wistar rats subjected to either ligation of the left anterior descending coronary artery (LAD) or Sham operated in the working heart-brainstem preparation. Thirty minutes after LAD ligation, tSNA had increased (basal: 2.5±0.2 µV, 30 min: 3.5±0.3 µV), being even higher at 60 min (5.2±0.5 µV, $P<0.01$); while no change was observed in Sham animals. HR increased significantly 45 min after LAD ($P<0.01$). Sixty minutes after LAD ligation, there was: (i) an augmented peripheral chemoreflex - greater sympathoexcitatory response (50, 45 and 27% of increase to 25, 50 and 75 µL injections of NaCN 0.03%, respectively, when compared to Sham, $P<0.01$); (ii) an elevated pressor response (32±1 versus 23±1 mmHg in Sham, $P<0.01$) and a reduced baroreflex sympathetic gain (1.3±0.1 versus Sham 2.0±0.1%.mmHg^{-1}, $P<0.01$) to phenylephrine injection; (iii) an elevated cardiac sympathetic tone (ΔHR after atenolol: −108±8 versus −82±7 bpm in Sham, $P<0.05$). In contrast, no changes were observed in cardiac vagal tone and bradycardic response to both baroreflex and chemoreflex between LAD and Sham groups. The immediate sympathoexcitatory response in LAD rats was dependent on an excitatory spinal sympathetic cardiocardiac reflex, whereas at 3 h an angiotensin II type 1 receptor mechanism was essential since Losartan curbed the response by 34% relative to LAD rats administered saline ($P<0.05$). A spinal reflex appears key to the immediate sympathoexcitatory response after coronary ligation. Therefore, the sympathoexcitatory response seems to be maintained by an angiotensinergic mechanism and concomitant augmentation of sympathoexcitatory reflexes.

Editor: Dinender K. Singla, University of Central Florida, United States of America

Funding: This work was supported by The British Heart Foundation and "Coordenação de Aperfeiçoamento de Pessoal de Nível Superior - CAPES". The funders had no role in study design, data collection and analysis, decision to publish, or preparation of the manuscript.

Competing Interests: The authors have declared that no competing interests exist.

* Email: Julian.F.R.Paton@Bristol.ac.uk

Introduction

Coronary artery ligation is accepted to mimic myocardial infarction (MI) causing sympathetic nervous system over activity [1], [2]. Although the enhanced sympathetic activity provides initially inotropic support to the heart, maintaining cardiac output and arterial pressure following MI, it is also associated with the pathogenesis of ventricular arrhythmias [3]–[5] and sudden cardiac death [6]. Further, the sustained sympathoexcitation may contribute to the cardiac pathology leading to progressive cardiac remodelling and development of heart failure [7]–[9]. Thus, a thorough understanding of timing of the sympathoactivation and any change in the mechanisms for it may be important for improving future treatment strategies, e.g. the appropriate timing of medication to antagonise sympathetic effects on the vasculature versus the heart may be essential for maintaining arterial pressure but preventing cardiac arrhythmias/sudden cardiac death.

Most of our knowledge on changes in cardiovascular autonomic balance has been obtained days after MI or later in the course of chronic heart failure, using indirect methodological approaches such as measuring plasma catecholamine levels [10], heart rate variability (HRV) and cardiovagal baroreflex sensitivity [11]. Little information about the time course and contributing mechanisms of sympathetic changes immediately following a MI exists (i.e. acute phase). Sequential and direct measurements of sympathetic drive are essential to elucidate these issues. In this regard, a number of chronic studies have shown a multifactorial process for sympathetic modulation after MI, which may include: cardiac vagal and cardiac sympathetic afferents [12], [13], changes in peripheral neural reflexes (peripheral chemoreceptor reflex) [14], sympathetic neural remodelling [15] and activation of brain angiotensinergic mechanisms [16]. However, the importance and sequence of activation of these mechanisms immediately following MI have not been characterized. Our hypothesis was that there would be a sustained and immediate (within 30 min) increase in sympathetic activity and reduction in cardiac vagal tone post coronary ligation and that multiple time-dependent mechanisms underpin the sympathoexcitation. Thus, the purpose of this study was to determine when the autonomic imbalance occurred after ligation of the left anterior descending coronary artery (LAD) to mimic MI, and the underlying mechanisms.

Methods

Animals

Experiments were performed on male Wistar rats (60–100 g) using an anaesthetic-free preparation with a preserved functional brainstem – the working heart-brainstem preparation (WHBP) [17], [18]. All surgical and experimental procedures were carried out in compliance with the United Kingdom Animals (Scientific Procedures) Act 1986 and were approved by the University of Bristol Animal Ethics Committee (Permit number: PPL 30/3121).

WHBP and nerve recordings

Animals were pre-treated with heparin sodium (1000 units, i.p.) and deeply anaesthetized with isoflurane (5%, vaporized in 95% $O_2-5\%$ CO_2), until loss of the paw withdrawal reflex. Following sub-diaphragmatic transection, rats were exsanguinated and anaesthesia terminated. Preparations were submerged in ice-chilled Ringer solution (composition in mM: 1.25 $MgSO_4.7H_2O$, 1.25 KH_2PO_4, 3.0 KCl, 25.0 $NaHCO_3$, 125.0 NaCl, 2.5 $CaCl_2.2H_2O$ and 10 D-glucose), decerebrated pre-collicularly and a 6.0 suture passed around LAD. The preparation was placed into a recording chamber and a double-lumen catheter inserted into the descending aorta for retrograde perfusion. The second lumen of the catheter was used to monitor perfusion pressure (PP). The perfusate was carbogen gassed (to pH 7.4), warmed {31°C; which was optimal for viability as originally described by Paton [18]} Ringer solution containing Ficoll 70 (1.25%), which was recirculated using a peristaltic roller pump. Neuromuscular blockade was established using vecuronium bromide (2 mg/mL; Organon). Mean PP was >60 mmHg achieved by adjusting flow rate (20–22 mL/min) and addition of arginine vasopressin (20–60 µL of 5 µM; Sigma). Heart rate (HR) was derived from the ECG. The left phrenic and thoracic sympathetic nerves (T8–T10) were recorded simultaneously with bipolar suction electrodes. Minutes after the onset of perfusion an augmenting (i.e. eupnoeic) pattern of phrenic nerve activity was achieved. All signals were amplified, band-pass filtered (0.5–5 kHz) and acquired using a CED 1401 A/D Converter and analyzed using Spike2 software (Cambridge Electronic Design).

Coronary ligation in situ and measurement of area at risk

After baseline recordings of phrenic (PNA) and thoracic sympathetic nerve activities (tSNA), HR, ECG and PP, either LAD ligation was carefully performed without affecting nerve recordings; or the suture remained untied in Sham operated preparations. At the end of each experiment, the heart was rapidly excised and via the ascending aorta perfused with 1% Evans blue dye (Sigma) to indicate the myocardial area at risk as reported previously [19], [20]. Once perfusion was completed, the atria were removed. After overnight fixation in 10% formalin, the ventricles were cut in five transverse slices and digitally photographed and analyzed using ImageJ software. The area at risk was determined as the percentage of Evans blue non-stained area relative to the entire left ventricle area. In all Sham operated rats, no cardiac area at risk was observed.

Experimental protocols

Our aim was to examine changes in respiratory and cardiovascular autonomic tone and its reflex control immediately after coronary ligation (total: n = 76; see Figure 1). Six experimental protocols were performed 60 minutes post LAD ligation and in Sham animals: (I) Peripheral chemoreceptors were stimulated using three doses of sodium cyanide (0.03% solution; 25, 50 and 75 µL bolus) injected into the aorta; being each injection separated by 10 min. The chemoreflex was quantified by measuring the increase in central respiratory rate, the maximum bradycardia and the percentage increase in tSNA during a 5s period at the peak of the chemoreflex sympathetic response compared to an equivalent control period. (II) The baroreceptor reflex was stimulated using phenylephrine (30 µg bolus, i.a., Sigma). The sympathetic (non-cardiac) baroreflex gain was quantified as percentage inhibition of sympathetic activity/ Δpressure ($\%.mmHg^{-1}$). The percentage of sympathoinhibition was obtained from the ratio of mean tSNA during the peak of the PP increase against the mean activity from a preceding equivalent time period, at an equivalent stage of the respiratory cycle. The bradycardic baroreflex gain was quantified as ΔHR/Δpressure ($bpm.mmHg^{-1}$). (III) Cardiac sympathetic tone was assessed by adding atenolol to the perfusate (20 µg/mL, Sigma) to block cardiac β1-adrenoceptors and inferred from the HR change. (IV) Bilateral cervical vagotomy was performed to measure the cardiac vagal tone as expressed by the HR change. (V) Angiotensin II type 1 receptor (AT1R) antagonist, Losartan potassium (Sigma), was used to evaluate the role of an AT1R in the initiation and maintenance of sympathetic activity post LAD ligation. Either Losartan (40 µM, n = 10) or saline (control, n = 9) was added to the perfusate 1 h and re-applied 2 h post LAD ligation and tSNA recorded up to 3 h after LAD ligation. Half the dose of Losartan used in this study is able to block angiotensin II effects in the mediation of the baroreceptor reflex in the nucleus of the solitary tract [21]. (VI) The spinal cord was fully transected at the first cervical level and the tSNA response measured before (15–20 min) and after (60 min) LAD ligation (n = 5) and in Sham animals (n = 5) to assess contribution of spinal reflexes in generation of sympathetic activity. In a seventh group (Protocol VII), the left ventricular pressure (LVP) was continuously recorded using a PE-10 cannula inserted into the left ventricle via its apex before and post LAD ligation. In the first four protocols (LAD n = 21 and Sham n = 19), basal cardiorespiratory parameters and tSNA were evaluated. The tSNA signal was rectified and integrated (50 ms time constant) and noise levels subtracted before analysis. The mean tSNA (µV) was taken from one minute of recording before (Basal) and at 15, 30, 45 and 60 min post LAD ligation or Sham operated animals. Respiratory-sympathetic activity modulation was evaluated at baseline, 30 and 60 min post LAD ligation and in Sham groups. Phrenic-triggered mean integrated tSNA was carried out and analyzed during: late expiration (Late E), inspiration (I), post-inspiration (PI) and mid-expiration (Mid E). The time duration of Late E, I, PI and Mid E was based on the duration of the inspiratory phrenic burst [22].

Statistical analysis

All data are expressed as means ± S.E.M. Data were analyzed using one-way ANOVA for repeated measures, followed by Tukey's post hoc test and Student's paired and unpaired t-Test with the level of significance set at $P<0.05$.

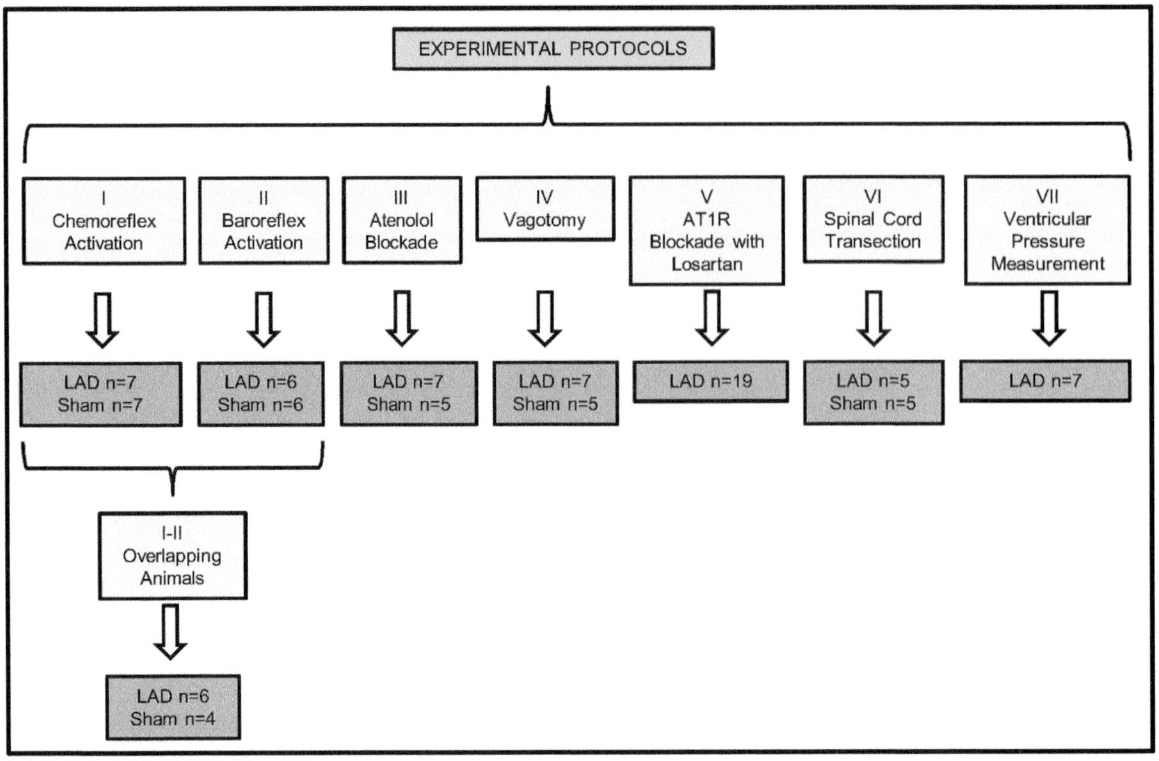

Figure 1. Schematic representation of experimental protocolos performed after LAD ligation or sham surgery. The number of tested animals per group is shown. LAD, left anterior descending coronary artery.

Results

Area at risk, ECG and hemodynamic changes following coronary ligation in situ

The LAD ligation induced transient ECG changes (Figures 2A and 2B) in many preparations (13 of 21 animals) consistent with MI; 11 animals exhibited arrhythmias post ligation and 2 animals showed atrioventricular block. These disturbances lasted up to 34.0±4.6 min when sinus rhythm returned. The myocardial area at risk was 36.3±1.1% of the left ventricle (n = 21, Figure 2C). The LAD ligation led to hemodynamic changes of the left ventricle (n = 7, see Figure 2D and Table 1).

Baseline changes in cardiorespiratory parameters and tSNA post coronary ligation

Within 30 min post LAD ligation, mean tSNA increased (45.4±6.7%, reaching 117.2±17.5% by 60 min, $P<0.01$) while HR increased by 45 min (2.8±0.7%, and 3.3±0.7% at 60 min, $P<0.01$) [Figures 3 (Ai) and 3 (Aiii); n = 21, $P<0.01$] compared to Sham rats [Figures 3 (Bi) and 3 (Biii); n = 19, $P>0.05$]. No changes in PP were found over 60 min post LAD ligation and in Sham rats [Figures 3 (Aii) and 3 (Bii)]; PNA frequency increased in both rat groups to a similar level [Figures 3 (Aiv) and 3 (Biv), $P<0.01$].

Peripheral chemoreceptor reflex

The sympathoexcitatory component of the response to peripheral chemoreceptor activation was greater 60 min post LAD ligation compared to Sham (Figure 4; n = 7 per group, $P<0.01$, unpaired t-Test) at all doses of cyanide tested (25, 50 and 75 μL: 49.7, 45.3 and 26.8% of increase, respectively). Despite exacerbation of the sympathetic response, there were no differences in peripheral chemoreflex evoked changes in PP, RR or HR.

Baroreceptor reflex

Both the pressor effect and the sympathetic (non-cardiac) baroreflex gain evoked by phenylephrine were significantly

Table 1. Hemodynamic parameters before and minutes after LAD ligation in situ (n = 7).

	Before	1 min	30 min	60 min
LVSP (mmHg)	71.1±5.9	70.6±3.4	69.0±3.5	66.9±3.7
LVEDP (mmHg)	7.5±1.4	13.2±2.0**	14.7±2.6**	14.9±2.4**
LV +dP/dT (mmHg.s^{-1})	1794±173	1559±107*	1530±111*	1460±107**
LV −dP/dT (mmHg.s^{-1})	−1462±187	−1275±133	−1298±141	−1254±140

*$P<0.05$ and **$P<0.01$ compared to Before. LVSP, left ventricular systolic pressure; LVEDP, left ventricular end-diastolic pressure; LV dP/dT, maximum rate of LVP rise and fall.

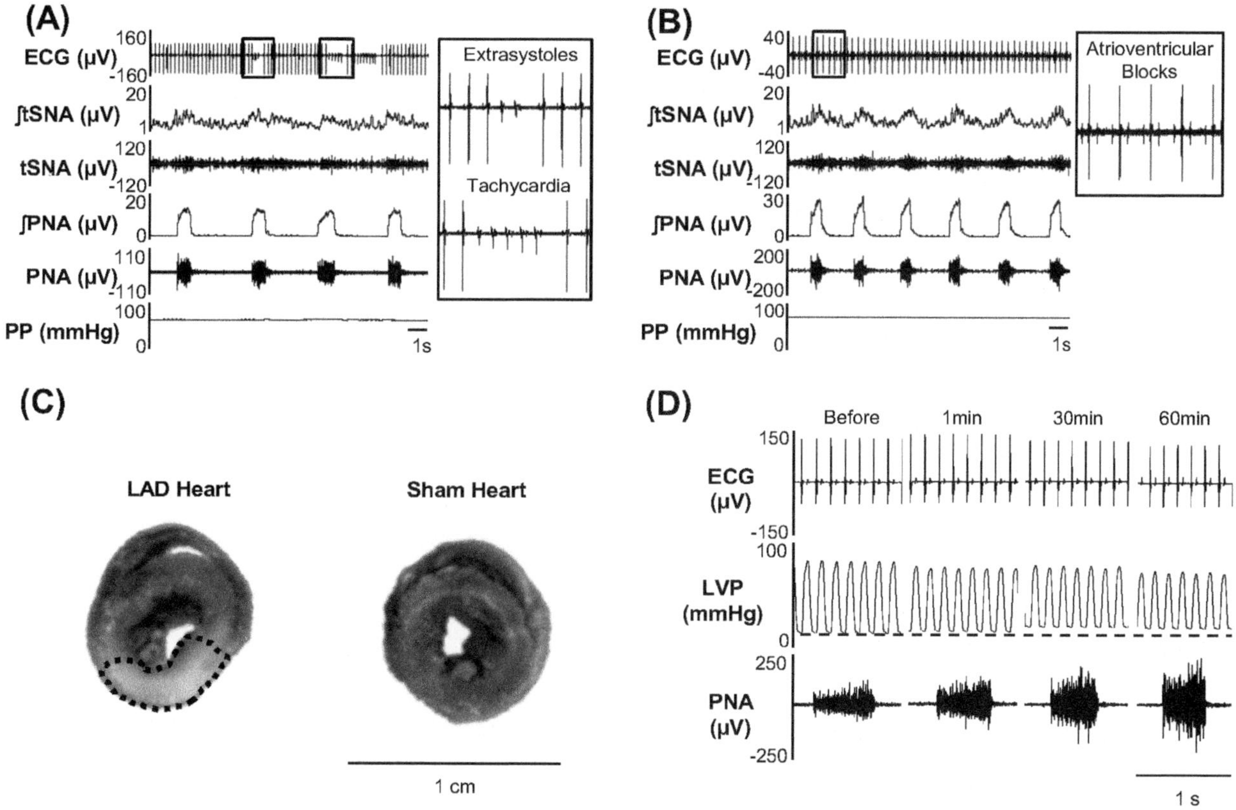

Figure 2. Representative traces from rats showing LVP and transient ECG changes post LAD ligation. (A) Extra-systoles and tachycardia occurred post LAD ligation in some rats. (B) Atrioventricular block starting shortly post LAD ligation. These changes in the ECG lasted 34.0±4.6 min. (C) Median cross-sections of Evans blue dye-stained hearts. The LAD heart cross-section (left) had a safe blue-marked area versus a myocardial area at risk that did not absorb the dye (outlined pale area), contrasting with the Sham heart completely stained blue. (D) Recording showing LVP before and 1, 30, and 60 min post LAD ligation.

different 60 min after LAD ligation versus Sham rats (Figures 5A and 5B; n = 6 each group, P<0.01, unpaired t-Test). The pressor response to phenylephrine was increased (LAD 31.5±1.3 versus Sham 23.1±1.2 mmHg, P<0.01) while the baroreflex gain was depressed (LAD 1.3±0.1 versus Sham 2.0±0.1%.mmHg^{-1}; n = 6 per group, P<0.01). The baroreflex bradycardia was unaffected after LAD ligation (Figure 5C).

Cardiac sympathetic and vagal tones

The cardiac sympathetic tone was elevated post LAD ligation. There was a greater fall in HR in LAD rats compared to Sham group (−107.8±8.0, n = 7, versus −81.6±7.4 bpm, n = 5; P<0.05, unpaired t-Test) after atenolol. Cardiac vagal tone (assessed by bilateral vagotomy) was unaffected by LAD ligation (11.6±1.8, n = 7, versus Sham 13.9±2.4 bpm, n = 5; P>0.05, unpaired t-Test). The level of mean tSNA was also not attenuated by bilateral vagotomy (before LAD ligation: 2.9±0.2; 60 min after LAD ligation/before vagotomy: 4.3±0.3; and 15 min after vagotomy: 7.2±0.6 μV), ruling out a vagal mechanism for sympathoexcitation post LAD ligation.

Mechanisms for sympathoexcitation post coronary ligation Angiotensin II. We assessed whether AT1R were important for the sympathoexcitation post LAD ligation. The mean level of tSNA became different from 3 h onwards (33.8% of difference) between Losartan (n = 10) and Control (n = 9) LAD groups (Figure 6A; *P<0.05, unpaired t-Test) suggesting that an AT1R mediated mechanism was functioning from this time point. The mean level of PP was maintained stable for both groups ruling out any confounding baroreceptor influence.

Spinal cord transection. Given that the angiotensinergic mechanism occurred ~3 h post LAD ligation, we sought other mechanisms that could contribute to the initiation of sympathoexcitation. We assessed whether a spinal mechanism underpinned sympathoexcitation post LAD ligation. In spinal transected rats, tSNA was higher within 30 min post LAD ligation (2.7±0.2 versus basal 1.6±0.2 μV, P<0.01, n = 5; Figure 6C) compared to Sham operated (1.4±0.4 versus basal 1.2±0.3 μV, P>0.05, n = 5; Figure 6B). As seen in the spinal cord intact rats, the increase in mean tSNA continued to climb post LAD ligation with time (i.e. 3.9±0.5 μV by 60 min; P<0.01). In terms of HR, there was a significant drop after spinal transection. Although there was no change in HR at 60 min post LAD ligation in the spinal transected group, it decreased at 60 min in the Sham transected group (P<0.01, see Figure S1 in Supplemental data), suggesting sympathoactivation in the LAD group. The increase in sympathetic activity evoked by LAD ligation at 30, 45, and 60 min of spinal transected rats (LAD: 73.7±11.7, 112.0±15.5, and 147.6±23.9%, respectively; n = 5) was the same as that seen in spinal intact rats (45.4±6.7, 78.7±11.7, and 117.3±17.5%, respectively; n = 21, P>0.05, unpaired t-Test) (Figure 6D).

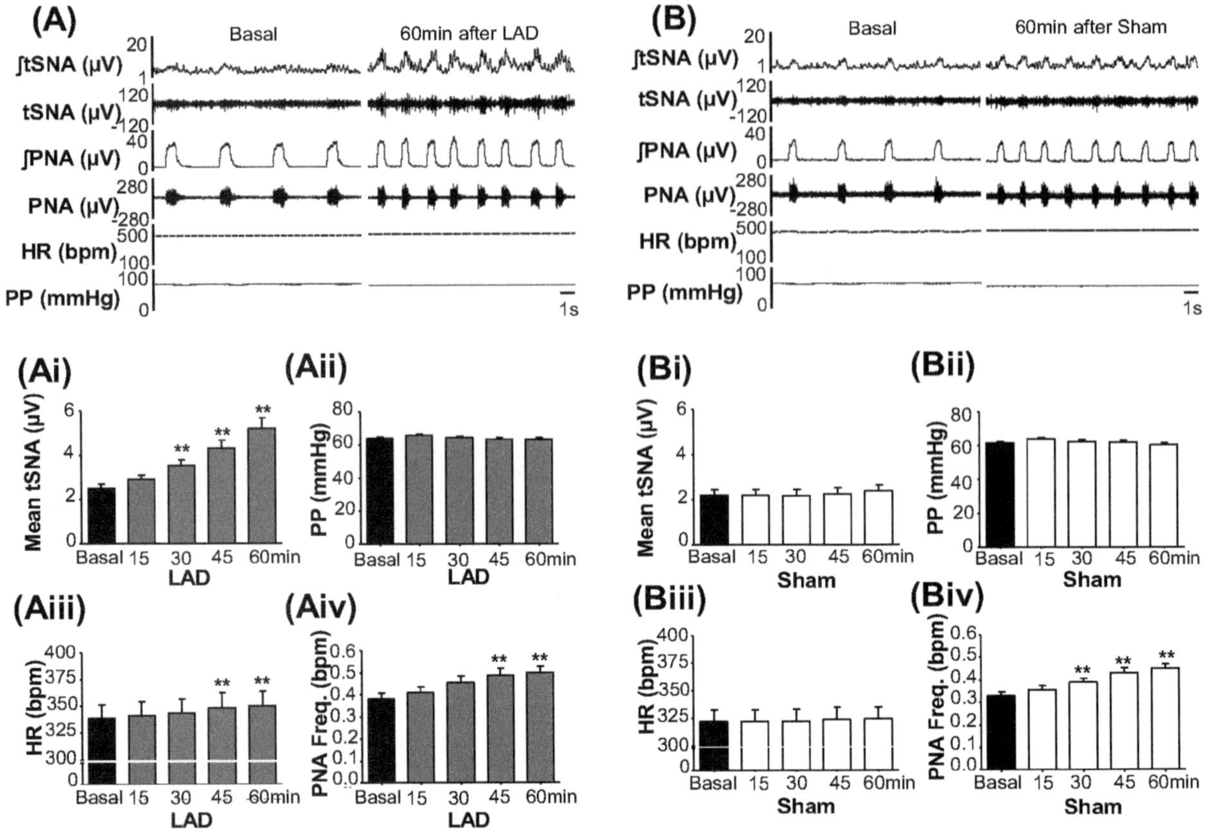

Figure 3. Baseline changes post LAD ligation. Typical traces of raw and integrated tSNA and PNA, ECG and PP before (Basal) and up to 60 min post LAD ligation (A) and in Sham operated (B). Means of tSNA, PP, HR and PNA frequency before (Basal) and at 15, 30, 45 and 60 min post LAD ligation (Ai, Aii, Aiii and Aiv, respectively, n = 21) and Sham operated (Bi, Bii, Biii and Biv, respectively, n = 19). **P<0.01 compared to Basal.

Respiratory-sympathetic activity modulation post coronary ligation

Measuring the mean tSNA from four phases of respiratory cycle – late expiration (Late E), inspiration (I), post-inspiration (PI) and mid-expiration (Mid E) 30 and 60 min after LAD ligation (n = 21) and in Sham (n = 19), we observed that tSNA was higher in all expiratory (Late E, Mid E and PI) and inspiratory (I) phases in the LAD group [P<0.01 compared to basal; see Figure S2(A) in Supplemental data], with no changes in Sham group [P>0.05 compared to basal; Figure S2(B)]. The magnitude of these increases was similar between the respiratory phases in LAD group [P>0.05; Figure S2(A)]. These data indicate that the increased strength of respiratory coupling to sympathetic outflow after LAD ligation is non-selective.

Discussion

The chronic over active sympathetic nervous system post coronary artery ligation has been intensively researched. In contrast, the acute responses of the autonomic nervous system, their onset and mechanisms following MI remain to be well clarified. In the last decades, studies have reported sudden (in the first minute) cardiac afferent and efferent sympathetic responses to transient ischaemia via short-term coronary occlusion in anaesthetized cats [23]–[27] and dogs [28]. However, these studies failed to show sustained activation of afferent discharge and the multiple time-dependent reflex responses and underlying mechanisms mediating these responses in the following minutes post-occlusion. Thus, the present study addresses these deficits of knowledge and provides the first evidence in the rat showing a sustained sympathetic hyperactivity very early following permanent LAD ligation. The thoracic sympathetic activity was increased significantly at 30 min post-occlusion and continued rising over 60 min in our preparation. Although we did not measure the cardiac sympathetic outflow directly, both the increase in basal HR and enhanced bradycardia post atenolol following LAD ligation supports an elevated cardiac sympathetic discharge.

Timing of autonomic imbalance post coronary ligation

Most experimental studies in humans and animals models have used indirect methods/indices to provide information about changes in the balance of autonomic activity after MI; this reflects the technical difficulty of obtaining direct measurements of autonomic nervous activity. Some studies have investigated plasma catecholamine levels [10], [29] [32] and norepinephrine spillover [33] in patients with recent MI, HRV in patients weeks/months after MI [1], [34], [35] or baroreflex sensitivity in patients with recent MI (<28 days) [11]. Although these methodologies estimate autonomic activity indirectly, direct measurements of sympathetic nervous activity in animal models are critical to clarify both the precise time course and degree of sympathetic activation post MI as well as investigate the underlying mechanisms.

Graham et al. [2] have obtained directly muscle sympathetic nerve activity (MSNA) measurements at 2 to 4 days, which were repeated at 3 months and 6 months after uncomplicated acute MI

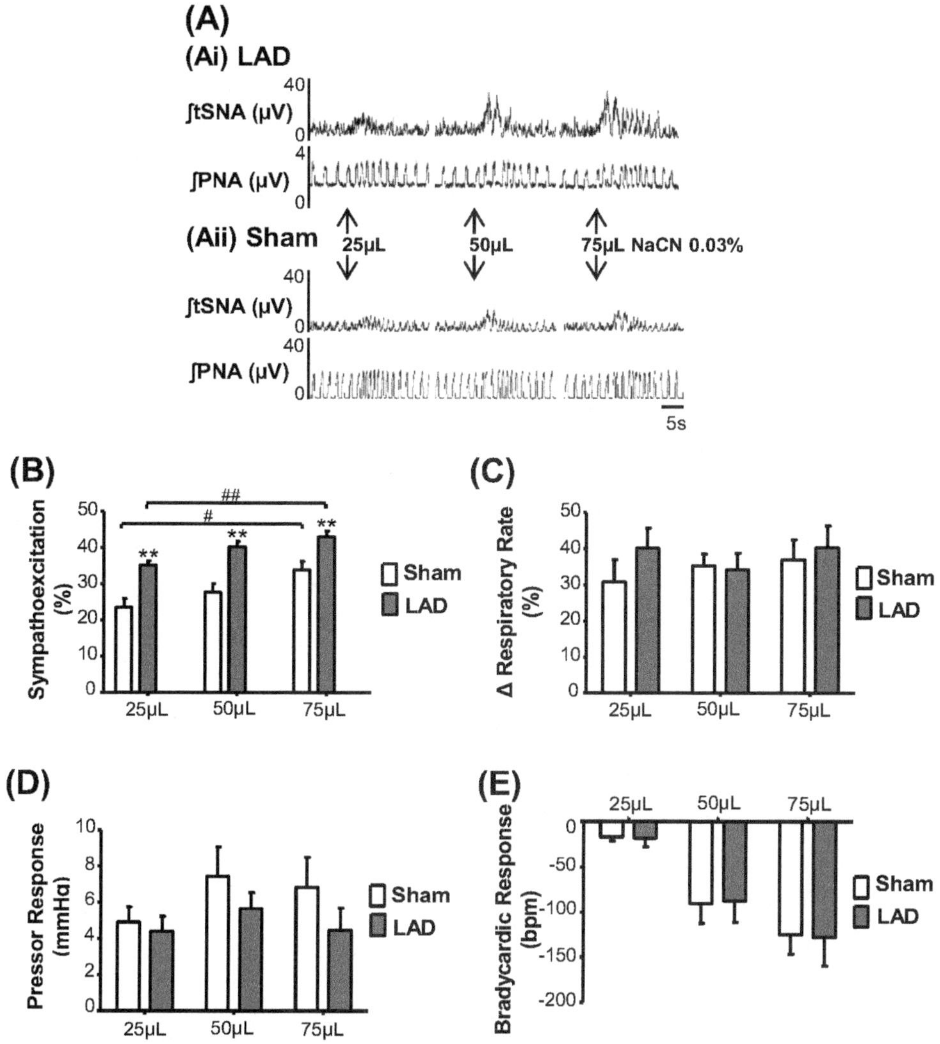

Figure 4. Peripheral chemoreflex responses post LAD ligation. Three doses of sodium cyanide (0.03% solution; 25, 50 and 75 μL, i.a.) were given 60 min post LAD ligation and in Sham operated (n = 7 each group). (A) Recordings of a LAD rat (Ai) and a Sham rat (Aii) showing sympathoexcitation at all doses. (B) Change in sympathoexcitatory response (**$P<0.01$ compared to Sham). Difference in the magnitude of sympathoexcitation between doses used in the study ($^{\#}P<0.05$ and $^{\#\#}P<0.01$). No changes in chemoreflex evoked responses in respiratory rate (C), pressor (D), and bradycardia (E).

in patients. The mean frequency of MSNA was increased 2 to 4 days (first measurement point of the study) post MI and this change lasted for at least 6 months, demonstrating a protracted sympathetic hyperactivity. However, the exact onset of sympathetic over activity was not shown. In contrast, Jardine et al. [36] demonstrated sequential measurement of sympathetic activity before and after (hourly for 3 h and then daily to 7 days) MI in a conscious ovine model. Cardiac sympathetic nerve activity was increased significantly at 60 min following coronary ligation, peaked at 120 min and sustained for 7 days post MI. These data are similar to the time course we observed in the rat. Despite using different experimental approaches, both the latter and the present study were performed in mammals free of the depressant effects of anaesthetics.

Baro- and chemo- reflex sympathetic responses

In accordance with the increase observed in basal sympathetic activity, the sympathetic components of two major homeostatic reflexes were also altered within 60 min post LAD ligation. We observed a greater chemoreflex evoked sympathoexcitation and depressed sympathetic (non-cardiac) baroreflex gain (i.e. impaired sympathoinhibition), suggesting up-modulation of pro-sympathetic reflex pathways, which is consistent with studies where renal sympathetic nerve activity was measured in pacing-induced chronic heart failure rabbits [37] and heart failure (6–8 weeks after MI) rats [38]; these studies suggest that peripheral chemoreflex sensitivity may be a contributory mechanism to the tonic elevation in sympathetic activity as found in conditions of hypertension [39], [40].

Cardiac vagal tone and its reflex activation

In contrast to widespread sympathoactivation following LAD ligation, we found that both baseline cardiac vagal tone and reflex bradycardia evoked from both the peripheral chemo- and baroreceptors were unaffected. Variable information is available regarding both tonic and reflex cardiac parasympathetic modulation immediately post infarction. Some studies in humans and cats suggest cardiac vagal over activity in the first minutes/hours

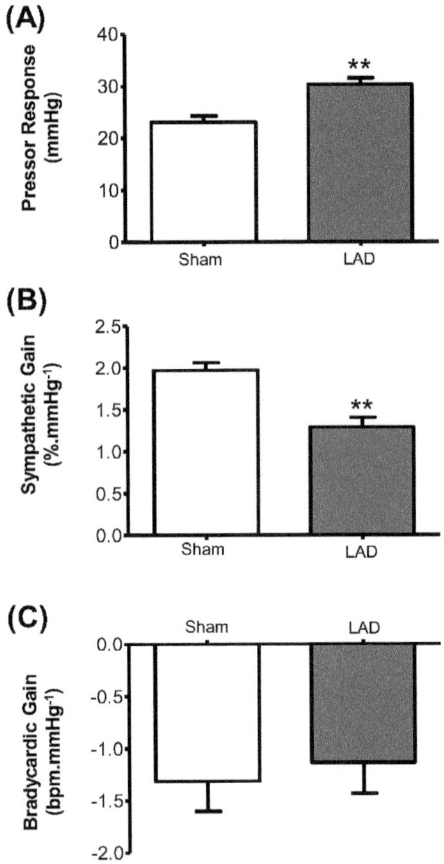

Figure 5. Baroreceptor reflex responses post LAD ligation. Phenylephrine (30 µg, i.a.) was given 60 min post LAD ligation and in Sham rats (n = 6 each group). (A) and (B) Changes in phenylephrine evoked pressor response and sympathetic gain (**P<0.01 compared to Sham). (C) No change in bradycardic gain.

following MI [41], [42]. In these studies, vagal over activity was more frequent during inferior infarction whereas sympathetic overactivity occurred in anterior infarction (comparable to coronary ligation of the present study). This may be explained by a preferential distribution of vagal afferents in the inferoposterior wall of the left ventricle that could reflexly drive up cardiac vagal activity. In addition, Lombardi et al. [1] showed sympathetic excitation and a reduced vagal modulation in HR variability (a vagal tone "marker") at approximately 3 h after MI in humans. We did not confirm any change in vagal tone at 1 h post coronary ligation in the in situ rat. The absence of impaired tonic cardiac vagal activity may be due to our early time evaluation or a species difference. In contrast to our finding, a marked impairment of cardiac baroreflex sensitivity has been well established in patients with chronic heart failure (CHF) [43], [44] but the exact timing of these measurements post MI is not reported. In sum, taking our evidence and that reported previously it appears that immediately after MI cardiac vagal tone is preserved and may increase dependent upon exactly where the infarct has occurred {posterior versus anterior circulation [45]}. This activity may be important in tempering any adverse effects of excessive cardiac sympathetic activity.

Mechanisms initiating sympathetic activation post coronary ligation

The role of the brain renin-angiotensin II system (RAS) in modulating sympathetic outflow and baroreflex sensitivity [46] in heart disease [47] is well established. Evidence supports that central RAS acting via AT1R modulates sympathetic activity in CHF: (i) Wang & Ma [48] have shown an elevated concentration of angiotensin II in cerebrospinal fluid in dogs with pacing-induced CHF. (ii) AT1R expression is up-regulated in the nucleus of the solitary tract, subfornical organ and paraventricular nucleus after CHF in rats [49] and the rostral ventro-lateral medulla (RVLM) of rabbits after pacing-induced CHF [50]. (iii) Losartan attenuated the AT1R up-regulation in CHF rabbits [50]. (iv) Central blockade of AT1R reduced sympathetic activity and increased baroreflex sensitivity in CHF rabbits [51], [52]. (v) In Wistar rats, both intracerebroventricular infusion and systemic administration of Losartan reduced sympathetic hyperactivity and left ventricular end-diastolic pressure in heart failure induced by coronary artery ligation [16].

Our data revealed that an angiotensinergic mechanism mediated via AT1R underpins the elevation in sympathetic outflow which is functionally detected from 3 h post LAD ligation. Evidence reveals AT1R located in circumventricular organs (eg, subfornical organ), hypothalamic paraventricular nucleus and the supraoptic nucleus are activated following MI and cause sympathoexcitation [53]. Our study was performed in a precollicularly decerebrated preparation devoid of the hypothalamic regions, with no functioning blood-brain barrier. Nevertheless, AT1R expression is up-regulated in CHF in the nucleus of the solitary tract [49] and the RVLM [50], [54], [55]; such brainstem areas were preserved and functional in our preparation. Evidence has shown that AT1R up-regulation involves reactive oxygen species in CHF [56]. Furthermore, the existence of brain tissue angiotensin II is also demonstrated by endogenous angiotensinogen synthesis in astrocytes within the medulla oblongata [57]. Thus, we suggest that angiotensinergic activation of brainstem nuclei may be sufficient to sustain sympathetic hyperactivity 3 h after coronary ligation. Certainly, this time course would be consistent with the time for protein synthesis [58] and we assume this to be the case for the AT1R. An increased angiotensinergic mechanism within the NTS could well account for both the elevated peripheral chemoreflex and depressed baroreflex response as we have described before [59]–[61], whereas those in the RVLM could account for the heightened sympathetic discharge.

The initiating mechanism triggering sympathetic over activity after cardiac ischaemia in rats may include a spinal sympathetic cardiocardiac reflex. This reflex was firstly reported by Malliani et al. [25] after coronary ligation in cats. Brown [23] demonstrated that cardiac sympathetic afferent nerve fibres are activated during myocardial ischaemia. Preganglionic sympathetic neurons were shown to become excited post MI, which was sustained after both vagotomy and spinal transection proving a spinal reflex [25]. In our experiments with spinal transection, increased sympathetic activity post LAD ligation was also observed as in intact animals, and HR was maintained and did not fall as seen in the control group, suggesting increased cardiac sympathetic tone. Thus, given the negative data with Losartan at 1 h post LAD ligation, we can propose a non-angiotensinergic spinal mechanism for initiating the increase in sympathetic outflow post coronary ligation.

Besides the cardiac sympathetic afferents, arterial baroreceptor reflex may be altered simultaneously during myocardial ischaemia, because of their unloading triggering reflex increases in efferent sympathetic nerve activity [62]. However, the perfusion pressure

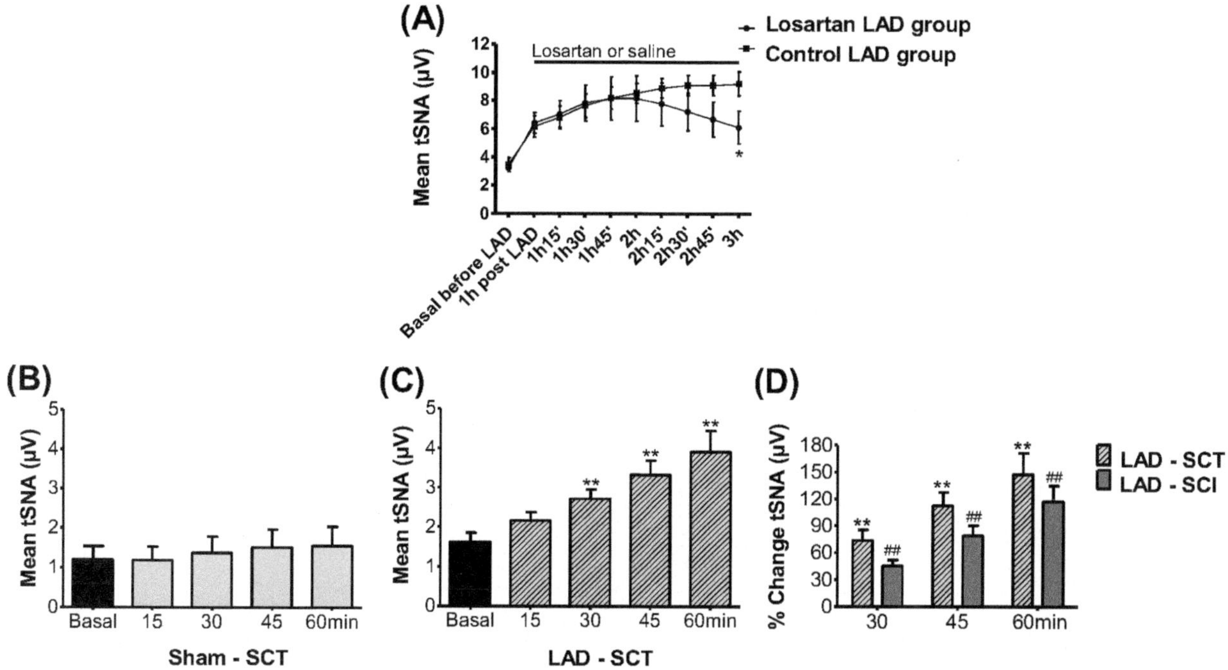

Figure 6. Mechanisms of sympathoexcitation post LAD ligation. (A) The Losartan effect (40 µM added to the perfusate) on the level of tSNA from 1 h to 3 h post LAD ligation (Losartan LAD group: n = 10; Control LAD group: n = 9). The level of mean tSNA was lower at 3 h post LAD ligation in Losartan LAD group (*P<0.05 compared to Control LAD group). (B), (C) and (D) Evaluation of sympathetic activity after spinal cord transection (SCT): Means of tSNA before (Basal) and at 15, 30, 45, and 60 min after LAD ligation (C; n = 5) and in Sham rats (B; n = 5). (D) Percentage of change in mean tSNA at 30, 45 and 60 min after LAD ligation in spinal transected rats (LAD – SCT; n = 5, **P<0.01 compared to respective basal value) and spinal cord intact rats (LAD – SCI; n = 21, ##P<0.01 compared to respective baseline). There was no change between the percent increases of both groups (P>0.05).

was maintained constant during LAD ligation, excluding the role of these receptors in our preparation.

Functional relevance of prompt sympathetic activation post-MI

The present findings indicate selective up-regulation of sympathetic activity with no change in cardiac vagal tone or reflex modulation. It is reasonable to assume that this initial modulation leads to a protective effect to the heart supporting cardiac function [5]. Although long term sympathetic nervous system activation is detrimental to cardiac function in heart failure [5], [63], in the first moments post MI it compensates for cardiac contractility dysfunction. In addition, increased [64], [65] or preserved vagal control (as found in the present study) in the early phase of acute myocardial ischaemia would exert an antiarrhythmic effect, reducing overall mortality.

In summary, our work shows both increased basal sympathetic drive and chemoreflex sympathoactivation but no changes in vagal regulation in the first hour following coronary artery ligation. Both spinal cord mechanisms and later elevated angiotensinergic activity contribute to increased sympathetic activity generation, some of which is directed to the heart. A detailed knowledge of any mechanisms that are responsible for the autonomic responses following cardiac ischaemia may assist in the temporal design of future effective pharmacological interventions.

Supporting Information

Figure S1 HR changes post LAD ligation in spinal animals. Means of HR before (Basal before SCT) and after (Basal after SCT) spinal cord transection, and in the following 15, 30, 45 and 60 min post LAD ligation (B; LAD – SCT group, n = 5) and in Sham operated (A; Sham – SCT group, n = 5). **P< 0.01, *P<0.05 and ##P<0.01.

Figure S2 Respiratory-sympathetic activity coupling. Phrenic-triggered mean integrated tSNA from four respiratory phases – late expiration (Late E), inspiration (I), post-inspiration (PI) and mid-expiration (Mid E) – before (Basal) and at 30 and 60 min post LAD ligation (A; n = 21) and in Sham (B; n = 19). **, ##, &&, ††P<0.01 compared to respective baseline; the magnitude of increase at 30 and 60 min in relation to baseline is given in percentage.

Acknowledgments

We thank Professor Benedito Honório Machado for expert advice (University of São Paulo, Ribeirão Preto/SP/Brazil) and Wioletta Pijacka for technical assistance (University of Bristol, Bristol/UK).

Author Contributions

Conceived and designed the experiments: JFRP. Performed the experiments: LMP. Analyzed the data: LMP KNS JGM DJAM APA JFRP. Contributed reagents/materials/analysis tools: APA JFRP. Contributed to the writing of the manuscript: LMP JGM KNS JFRP.

References

1. Lombardi F, Sandrone G, Spinnler MT, Torzillo D, Lavezzaro GC, et al. (1996) Heart rate variability in the early hours of an acute myocardial infarction. Am J Cardiol 77: 1037–1044.
2. Graham LN, Smith PA, Stoker JB, Mackintosh AF, Mary DA (2002) Time course of sympathetic neural hyperactivity after uncomplicated acute myocardial infarction. Circulation 106: 793–797.
3. Pantridge JF, Webb SW, Adgey AA (1981) Arrhythmias in the first hours of acute myocardial infarction. Prog Cardiovasc Dis 23: 265–278.
4. Jardine DL, Charles CJ, Frampton CM, Richards AM (2007) Cardiac sympathetic nerve activity and ventricular fibrillation during acute myocardial infarction in a conscious sheep model. Am J Physiol Heart Circ Physiol 293: H433–439.
5. Floras JS (2009) Sympathetic nervous system activation in human heart failure: clinical implications of an updated model. J Am Coll Cardiol 54: 375–385.
6. Brunner-La Rocca HP, Esler MD, Jennings GL, Kaye DM (2001) Effect of cardiac sympathetic nervous activity on mode of death in congestive heart failure. Eur Heart J 22: 1136–1143.
7. Cohn JN, Levine TB, Olivari MT, Garberg V, Lura D, et al. (1984) Plasma norepinephrine as a guide to prognosis in patients with chronic congestive heart failure. N Engl J Med 311: 819–823.
8. Kaye DM, Lefkovits J, Jennings GL, Bergin P, Broughton A, et al. (1995) Adverse consequences of high sympathetic nervous activity in the failing human heart. J Am Coll Cardiol 26: 1257–1263.
9. Bristow M (2003) Antiadrenergic therapy of chronic heart failure: surprises and new opportunities. Circulation 107: 1100–1102.
10. McAlpine HM, Cobbe SM (1988) Neuroendocrine changes in acute myocardial infarction. Am J Med 84: 61–66.
11. La Rovere MT, Bigger JT Jr, Marcus FI, Mortara A, Schwartz PJ (1998) Baroreflex sensitivity and heart-rate variability in prediction of total cardiac mortality after myocardial infarction. ATRAMI (Autonomic Tone and Reflexes After Myocardial Infarction) Investigators. Lancet 351: 478–484.
12. Malliani A, Montano N (2002) Emerging excitatory role of cardiovascular sympathetic afferents in pathophysiological conditions. Hypertension 39: 63–68.
13. Fu LW, Longhurst JC (2009) Regulation of cardiac afferent excitability in ischemia. Handb Exp Pharmacol: 185–225.
14. Schultz HD, Li YL (2007) Carotid body function in heart failure. Respir Physiol Neurobiol 157: 171–185.
15. Cao JM, Chen LS, KenKnight BH, Ohara T, Lee MH, et al. (2000) Nerve sprouting and sudden cardiac death. Circ Res 86: 816–821.
16. Huang BS, Ahmad M, Tan J, Leenen FH (2009) Chronic central versus systemic blockade of AT (1) receptors and cardiac dysfunction in rats post-myocardial infarction. Am J Physiol Heart Circ Physiol 297: H968–975.
17. St-John WM, Paton JF (2000) Characterizations of eupnea, apneusis and gasping in a perfused rat preparation. Respir Physiol 123: 201–213.
18. Paton JF (1996) A working heart-brainstem preparation of the mouse. J Neurosci Methods 65: 63–68.
19. Huang CH, Kim SJ, Ghaleh B, Kudej RK, Shen YT, et al. (1999) An adenosine agonist and preconditioning shift the distribution of myocardial blood flow in conscious pigs. Am J Physiol 276: H368–375.
20. Huang CH, Tsai SK, Chiang SC, Wang YY, Chih CL, et al. (2011) Brief pressure overload preconditions rabbit myocardium independent of adenosine receptor activation. Ann Thorac Surg 92: 1727–1732.
21. Boscan P, Allen AM, Paton JF (2001) Baroreflex inhibition of cardiac sympathetic outflow is attenuated by angiotensin II in the nucleus of the solitary tract. Neuroscience 103: 153–160.
22. Zoccal DB, Simms AE, Bonagamba LG, Braga VA, Pickering AE, et al. (2008) Increased sympathetic outflow in juvenile rats submitted to chronic intermittent hypoxia correlates with enhanced expiratory activity. J Physiol 586: 3253–3265.
23. Brown AM (1967) Excitation of afferent cardiac sympathetic nerve fibres during myocardial ischaemia. J Physiol 190: 35–53.
24. Brown AM, Malliani A (1971) Spinal sympathetic reflexes initiated by coronary receptors. J Physiol 212: 685–705.
25. Malliani A, Schwartz PJ, Zanchetti A (1969) A sympathetic reflex elicited by experimental coronary occlusion. Am J Physiol 217: 703–709.
26. Lombardi F, Casalone C, Della Bella P, Malfatto G, Pagani M, et al. (1984) Global versus regional myocardial ischaemia: differences in cardiovascular and sympathetic responses in cats. Cardiovasc Res 18: 14–23.
27. Ninomiya I, Matsukawa K, Honda T, Nishiura N, Shirai M (1986) Cardiac sympathetic nerve activity and heart rate during coronary occlusion in awake cats. Am J Physiol 251: H528–537.
28. Felder RB, Thames MD (1981) The cardiocardiac sympathetic reflex during coronary occlusion in anesthetized dogs. Circ Res 48: 685–692.
29. Griffiths J, Leung F (1971) The sequential estimation of plasma catecholamines and whole blood histamine in myocardial infarction. Am Heart J 82: 171–179.
30. Siggers DC, Salter C, Fluck DC (1971) Serial plasma adrenaline and noradrenaline levels in myocardial infarction using a new double isotope technique. Br Heart J 33: 878–883.
31. Videbaek J, Christensen NJ, Sterndorff B (1972) Serial determination of plasma catecholamines in myocardial infarction. Circulation 46: 846–855.
32. Karlsberg RP, Cryer PE, Roberts R (1981) Serial plasma catecholamine response early in the course of clinical acute myocardial infarction: relationship to infarct extent and mortality. Am Heart J 102: 24–29.
33. McCance AJ, Forfar JC (1989) Cardiac and whole body [3H] noradrenaline kinetics in ischaemic heart disease: contrast between unstable anginal syndromes and pacing induced ischaemia. Br Heart J 61: 238–247.
34. Lombardi F, Sandrone G, Pernpruner S, Sala R, Garimoldi M, et al. (1987) Heart rate variability as an index of sympathovagal interaction after acute myocardial infarction. Am J Cardiol 60: 1239–1245.
35. Bigger JT Jr, Fleiss JL, Rolnitzky LM, Steinman RC, Schneider WJ (1991) Time course of recovery of heart period variability after myocardial infarction. J Am Coll Cardiol 18: 1643–1649.
36. Jardine DL, Charles CJ, Ashton RK, Bennett SI, Whitehead M, et al. (2005) Increased cardiac sympathetic nerve activity following acute myocardial infarction in a sheep model. J Physiol 565: 325–333.
37. Sun SY, Wang W, Zucker IH, Schultz HD (1999) Enhanced peripheral chemoreflex function in conscious rabbits with pacing-induced heart failure. J Appl Physiol (1985) 86: 1264–1272.
38. Wang WZ, Gao L, Wang HJ, Zucker IH, Wang W (2008) Interaction between cardiac sympathetic afferent reflex and chemoreflex is mediated by the NTS AT1 receptors in heart failure. Am J Physiol Heart Circ Physiol 295: H1216–H1226.
39. McBryde FD, Abdala AP, Hendy EB, Pijacka W, Marvar P, et al. (2013) The carotid body as a putative therapeutic target for the treatment of neurogenic hypertension. Nat Commun 4: 2395.
40. Paton JF, Sobotka PA, Fudim M, Engelman ZJ, Hart EC, et al. (2013) The carotid body as a therapeutic target for the treatment of sympathetically mediated diseases. Hypertension 61: 5–13.
41. Webb SW, Adgey AA, Pantridge JF (1972) Autonomic disturbance at onset of acute myocardial infarction. Br Med J 3: 89–92.
42. Cerati D, Schwartz PJ (1991) Single cardiac vagal fiber activity, acute myocardial ischemia, and risk for sudden death. Circ Res 69: 1389–1401.
43. Goldstein RE, Beiser GD, Stampfer M, Epstein SE (1975) Impairment of autonomically mediated heart rate control in patients with cardiac dysfunction. Circ Res 36: 571–578.
44. Thames MD, Kinugawa T, Smith ML, Dibner-Dunlap ME (1993) Abnormalities of baroreflex control in heart failure. J Am Coll Cardiol 22: 56A–60A.
45. Meller ST, Gebhart GF (1992) A critical review of the afferent pathways and the potential chemical mediators involved in cardiac pain. Neuroscience 48: 501–524.
46. Reid IA (1992) Interactions between ANG II, sympathetic nervous system, and baroreceptor reflexes in regulation of blood pressure. Am J Physiol 262: E763–778.
47. DiBona GF, Jones SY, Brooks VL (1995) ANG II receptor blockade and arterial baroreflex regulation of renal nerve activity in cardiac failure. Am J Physiol 269: R1189–1196.
48. Wang W, Ma R (2000) Cardiac sympathetic afferent reflexes in heart failure. Heart Fail Rev 5: 57–71.
49. Yoshimura R, Sato T, Kawada T, Shishido T, Inagaki M, et al. (2000) Increased brain angiotensin receptor in rats with chronic high-output heart failure. J Card Fail 6: 66–72.
50. Liu D, Gao L, Roy SK, Cornish KG, Zucker IH (2006) Neuronal angiotensin II type 1 receptor upregulation in heart failure: activation of activator protein 1 and Jun N-terminal kinase. Circ Res 99: 1004–1011.
51. Murakami H, Liu JL, Zucker IH (1997) Angiotensin II blockade [corrected] enhances baroreflex control of sympathetic outflow in heart failure. Hypertension 29: 564–569.
52. Liu JL, Zucker IH (1999) Regulation of sympathetic nerve activity in heart failure: a role for nitric oxide and angiotensin II. Circ Res 84: 417–423.
53. Huang BS, Leenen FH (2009) The brain renin-angiotensin-aldosterone system: a major mechanism for sympathetic hyperactivity and left ventricular remodeling and dysfunction after myocardial infarction. Curr Heart Fail Rep 6: 81–88.
54. Gao L, Wang WZ, Wang W, Zucker IH (2008) Imbalance of angiotensin type 1 receptor and angiotensin II type 2 receptor in the rostral ventrolateral medulla: potential mechanism for sympathetic overactivity in heart failure. Hypertension 52: 708–714.
55. Zucker IH, Schultz HD, Patel KP, Wang W, Gao L (2009) Regulation of central angiotensin type 1 receptors and sympathetic outflow in heart failure. Am J Physiol Heart Circ Physiol 297: H1557–1566.
56. Liu D, Gao L, Roy SK, Cornish KG, Zucker IH (2008) Role of oxidant stress on AT1 receptor expression in neurons of rabbits with heart failure and in cultured neurons. Circ Res 103: 186–193.
57. Bunnemann B, Fuxe K, Metzger R, Bjelke B, Ganten D (1992) The semi-quantitative distribution and cellular localization of angiotensinogen mRNA in the rat brain. J Chem Neuroanat 5: 245–262.
58. MacDougall JD, Gibala MJ, Tarnopolsky MA, MacDonald JR, Interisano SA, et al. (1995) The time course for elevated muscle protein synthesis following heavy resistance exercise. Can J Appl Physiol 20: 480–486.
59. Paton JF, Kasparov S (1999) Differential effects of angiotensin II on cardiorespiratory reflexes mediated by nucleus tractus solitarii - a microinjection study in the rat. J Physiol 521 Pt 1: 213–225.

60. Kasparov S, Paton JF (1999) Differential effects of angiotensin II in the nucleus tractus solitarii of the rat–plausible neuronal mechanism. J Physiol 521 Pt 1: 227–238.
61. Polson JW, Dampney RA, Boscan P, Pickering AE, Paton JF (2007) Differential baroreflex control of sympathetic drive by angiotensin II in the nucleus tractus solitarii. Am J Physiol Regul Integr Comp Physiol 293: R1954–1960.
62. Felder RB, Thames MD (1979) Interaction between cardiac receptors and sinoaortic baroreceptors in the control of efferent cardiac sympathetic nerve activity during myocardial ischemia in dogs. Circ Res 45: 728–736.
63. Petersson M, Friberg P, Eisenhofer G, Lambert G, Rundqvist B (2005) Long-term outcome in relation to renal sympathetic activity in patients with chronic heart failure. Eur Heart J 26: 906–913.
64. Vanoli E, De Ferrari GM, Stramba-Badiale M, Hull SS Jr, Foreman RD, et al. (1991) Vagal stimulation and prevention of sudden death in conscious dogs with a healed myocardial infarction. Circ Res 68: 1471–1481.
65. Rosenshtraukh L, Danilo P Jr, Anyukhovsky EP, Steinberg SF, Rybin V, et al. (1994) Mechanisms for vagal modulation of ventricular repolarization and of coronary occlusion-induced lethal arrhythmias in cats. Circ Res 75: 722–732.

4

PARP-Inhibitor Treatment Prevents Hypertension Induced Cardiac Remodeling by Favorable Modulation of Heat Shock Proteins, Akt-1/GSK-3β and Several PKC Isoforms

Laszlo Deres[1,2], Eva Bartha[1], Anita Palfi[1], Krisztian Eros[1,2], Adam Riba[1,2], Janos Lantos[3], Tamas Kalai[4], Kalman Hideg[4], Balazs Sumegi[2,5,6], Ferenc Gallyas[5,6], Kalman Toth[1], Robert Halmosi[1,2]*

1 First Department of Medicine, Division of Cardiology, University of Pécs, Pécs, Hungary, **2** Szentagothai Janos Research Center, University of Pécs, Medical School, Pécs, Hungary, **3** Department of Surgical Research and Techniques, University of Pécs, Pécs, Hungary, **4** Department of Organic and Medicinal Chemistry, University of Pécs, Pécs, Hungary, **5** Department of Biochemistry and Medical Chemistry, Medical School, University of Pécs, Pécs, Hungary, **6** MTA-PTE Nuclear-Mitochondrial Interactions Research Group, Pécs, Hungary

Abstract

Spontaneously hypertensive rat (SHR) is a suitable model for studies of the complications of hypertension. It is known that activation of poly(ADP-ribose) polymerase enzyme (PARP) plays an important role in the development of postinfarction as well as long-term hypertension induced heart failure. In this study, we examined whether PARP-inhibitor (L-2286) treatment could prevent the development of hypertensive cardiopathy in SHRs. 6-week-old SHR animals were treated with L-2286 (SHR-L group) or placebo (SHR-C group) for 24 weeks. Wistar-Kyoto rats were used as aged-matched, normotensive controls (WKY group). Echocardiography was performed, brain-derived natriuretic peptide (BNP) activity and blood pressure were determined at the end of the study. We detected the extent of fibrotic areas. The amount of heat-shock proteins (Hsps) and the phosphorylation state of Akt-1^{Ser473}, glycogen synthase kinase (GSK)-$3\beta^{Ser9}$, forkhead transcription factor $(FKHR)^{Ser256}$, mitogen activated protein kinases (MAPKs), and protein kinase C (PKC) isoenzymes were monitored. The elevated blood pressure in SHRs was not influenced by PARP-inhibitor treatment. Systolic left ventricular function and BNP activity did not differ among the three groups. L-2286 treatment decreased the marked left ventricular (LV) hypertrophy which was developed in SHRs. Interstitial collagen deposition was also decreased by L-2286 treatment. The phosphorylation of extracellular signal-regulated kinase (ERK)$1/2^{Thr183\text{-}Tyr185}$, Akt-$1^{Ser473}$, GSK-$3\beta^{Ser9}$, $FKHR^{Ser256}$, and PKC ε^{Ser729} and the level of Hsp90 were increased, while the activity of PKC $\alpha/\beta II^{Thr638/641}$, $\zeta/\lambda^{410/403}$ were mitigated by L-2286 administration. We could detect signs of LV hypertrophy without congestive heart failure in SHR groups. This alteration was prevented by PARP inhibition. Our results suggest that PARP-inhibitor treatment has protective effect already in the early stage of hypertensive myocardial remodeling.

Editor: Rajesh Gopalrao Katare, University of Otago, New Zealand

Funding: The work was supported by Hungarian National Research Foundations (OTKA F-46594, OTKA K-73738, OTKA K-81123, OTKA NN-109841). This research was realized in the frames of SROP 4.2.1.B-10/2/KONV-2010-0002, 4.2.4. A/2-11-1-2012-0001. The funders had no role in study design, data collection and analysis, decision to publish, or preparation of the manuscript.

* Email: dr.halmosi.robert@gmail.com

Introduction

Left ventricular hypertrophy (LVH) represents the heart's response to increased biomechanical stress such as arterial hypertension or valvular heart disease. Cardiac hypertrophy has traditionally been considered a compensatory mechanism required to normalize wall tension and to maintain cardiac output. However, recent clinical studies as well as several animal models have shown that cardiac hypertrophy is rather a maladaptive process, ultimately leading to heart failure (HF) and sudden cardiac death independent of the underlying cause of hypertrophy [1].

Both physiologic and pathologic stimulation-induced cellular adaptations of the heart are typically initiated by stress-responsive signaling pathways, which serve as central transducers of cardiac hypertrophic growth and/or ventricular dilation. These signaling pathways include extracellular signal-regulated protein kinases (ERK), p38 mitogen-activated protein kinases (p38-MAPK), c-Jun NH_2-terminal kinases (JNK) and several protein kinase C (PKC) isoforms [2]. These pathways and the Akt-1/glycogen synthase kinase-3β (GSK-3β) signaling cascade have all been demonstrated to alter their activation state in response to hypertrophic stimuli, and may therefore contribute to myocardial remodeling [3].

The poly(ADP-ribose) polymerase (PARP) enzyme becomes activated in response to DNA single-strand breaks that can be excessive as a response to free radicals and oxidative cell damage. PARP is an energy-consuming enzyme that transfers ADP-ribose to nuclear proteins. As a result of this process, the intracellular

NAD^+ and ATP levels decrease remarkably resulting in cell dysfunction and cell death via the necrotic route. Therefore, PARP-activation contributes to the pathogenesis of various cardiovascular diseases including endothelial dysfunction, ischemia-reperfusion injury and myocardial infarction, as well as HF. Several studies reported that endothelial dysfunction associated with hypertension also depends on PARP activity and can be prevented by its pharmacological inhibition [4,5].

It has been shown previously that our experimental agent, an isoquinoline derivative PARP-inhibitor, L-2286 (Fig. 1) had a beneficial effect against oxidative cell damage, against ischemia-reperfusion injury and the development of postinfarction or long-term high blood pressure-induced heart failure. Although the molecule have a slight scavenger characteristic, its forementioned effects were mediated mainly by influencing the Akt-1/GSK-3β, MAPK and PKC signal transduction factors [3,6,7].

Hypertension in spontaneously hypertensive rat (SHR) is similar to that of human in numerous ways such as the occurence of long-term, stable LVH followed by a transition to HF [8,9,10]. It makes SHR a useful tool for studying the development of LVH [9] and HF, well separated from each other in time. Therefore, our present study aimed to clarify whether pharmacological PARP-inhibition has protective effect in an SHR model against the development of the early stage of hypertensive cardiac remodeling.

Materials and Methods

Ethics Statement

The investigation conforms to the Guide for the Care and Use of Laboratory Animals published by the U.S. National Insitutes of Health (NIH Publication No. 85-23, revised 1996), and was approved by the Animal Research Review Committee of the University of Pecs, Medical School.

Experimental protocol

Six weeks old male WKY-strain Wistar Kyoto and spontaneously hypertensive rats (Charles River Laboratories, Budapest, Hungary) were used. Animals were kept under standard conditions throughout the experiment; 12 h light-dark cycle, water and rat chow provided ad libitum. SHRs were randomly divided into two groups; SHR-L and SHR-C. SHR-L group was treated with L-2286 (2-[(2-piperidin-1-ylethyl)thio]quinazolin-4(3*H*)-one), a water-soluble PARP-inhibitor (5 mg/b.w. in kg/day, n = 12), while SHR-C group received only placebo (n = 11, SHR-C) p. os for 24 weeks [11,12]. WKY rats were used as age-matched controls (n = 10). Dosage of L-2286 administered in drinking water was based on preliminary data about the volume of daily consumption [3,6]. At the beginning and at the end of the 24-week-long period, echocardiographic measurements were performed. Invasive blood pressure measurements were carried out on 3 rats of each group at the end of the study. These rats were anesthetized with ketamine hydrochloride (Richter Gedeon Ltd., Budapest, Hungary) intraperitoneally and a polyethylene catheter (Portex, London, UK) was inserted into their left femoral artery. Systolic, diastolic and

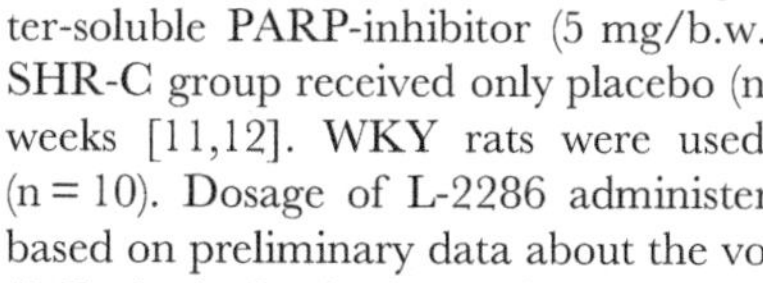

Figure 1. Chemical structure of L-2286 (2-[(2-Piperidine-1-ylethyl)thio]quinazolin-4(3H)-one).

mean arterial blood pressure was determined by CardioMed System CM-2005 (Medi-Stim AS, Oslo, Norway). Animals were euthanized with an overdose of ketamine hydrochloride intraperitoneally and heparinized with sodium heparin (100 IU/rat i.p., Biochemie GmbH, Kundl, Austria). After the sacrifice, blood was collected to determine the concentration of plasma brain-derived natriuretic peptide (BNP), and hearts were removed, the atria and great vessels were trimmed from the ventricles and weight of the ventricles was measured, which was then normalized to body mass (index of cardiac hypertrophy). The lung wet weight-to-dry weight ratio (an index of pulmonary congestion) was also measured in 7–9 experimental animals [3]. Hearts were freeze-clamped and were stored at −70°C or fixed in 10% formalin. In order to detect the extent of fibrotic areas, histologic samples were stained with Masson's trichrome. The phosphorylation state of Akt-1/GSK-3β, MAPK and PKC signaling molecules were monitored by Western blotting.

Determination of plasma B-type natriuretic peptide

Blood samples were collected into Lavender Vacutainer tubes containing EDTA and aprotinin (0.6 IU/ml of blood), and were centrifuged at 1600 g for 15 minutes at 4°C to separate the plasma. Supernatants were collected and kept at −70°C. BNP-45 were determined by enzyme immunoassay method as the manufacturer proposed (BNP-45, Rat EIA Kit, Phoenix Pharmaceuticals Inc., CA, USA).

Histology

Ventricles fixed in formalin were embedded in paraffin, and 5 μm thick sections were cut from base to apex. Sectiones were stained with Masson's trichrome staining to detect the interstitial fibrosis, and quantified by the NIH ImageJ image processing program as described previously [3].

Western blot analysis

Fifty milligrams of heart samples were homogenized in ice-cold 50 mM Tris buffer, pH 8.0 containing protease inhibitor cocktail 1:100, and 50 mM sodium vanadate (Sigma-Aldrich Co., Budapest, Hungary), and were harvested in 2x concentrated sodium dodecyl sulphate (SDS)-polyacrylamide gel electrophoresis sample buffer. Proteins were separated on 10% or 12% SDS-polyacrylamide gel and transferred to nitrocellulose membranes. After blocking (2 h with 3% nonfat milk in Tris-buffered saline), membranes were probed overnight at 4°C with primary antibodies recognizing the following antigenes: phospho-specific Akt-1/protein kinase B-α Ser^{473} (1:1000), Actin (1:10000), phospho-specific glycogen synthase kinase (GSK)-3β Ser^{9} (1:1000), phospho-specific extracellular signal-regulated kinase (ERK 1/2) Thr^{202}-Tyr^{204} (1:1000), phospho-specific p38 mitogen-activated protein kinase (p38-MAPK) Thr^{180}-Gly-Tyr^{182} (1:1000), phospho-specific c-Jun N-terminal kinase (JNK) Thr^{183}-Tyr^{185} (1:1000), phospho-specific protein kinase C (PKC) (pan) βII Ser^{660} (1:1000), phospho-specific protein kinase C α/βII (PKC α/βII) $Thr^{638/641}$ (1:1000), phospho-specific protein kinase C δ (PKC δ) Thr^{505} (1:1000), phospho-specific protein kinase C ζ/λ (PKC ζ/λ) $Thr^{410/403}$ (1:1000), phospho-specific protein kinase C ε (PKC ε) Ser^{729} (1:1000), anti-poly(ADP-ribose) (anti-PAR, 1:5000), phospho-Foxo1A (forkhead transcription factor, FKHR Ser^{256}, 1:1000), Heat shock protein 72 (Hsp72, 1:20000), Heat shock protein 90 (Hsp90, 1:1000). Antibodies were purchased from Cell Signaling Technology (Beverly, MA, USA) except from actin, which was bought from Sigma-Aldrich Co, (Budapest, Hungary), phospho-specific PKC ε, which was purchased from Upstate (London, UK), anti-PAR, which was purchased from Alexis

Table 1. Effect of L-2286 treatment on gravimetric parameters and on plasma BNP in SHR.

	WKY	SHR-C	SHR-L
SAP^{30w}, (mmHg)	129±7	192±9[b]	186±5[b]
DAP^{30w}, (mmHg)	89±5	127±8[b]	125±4[b]
MAP^{30w}, (mmHg)	103±7	149±5[b]	146±7[b]
BW^{6w} (g)	71.01±1.89	72.02±2.36	69.9±3.21
BW (g)	393±14.01	323.8±11.27[a]	321.86±6.8[a,c]
WV (g)	1.16±0.17	1.45±0.18[b]	1.24±0.24[b,c]
WV/BW (mg/g)	2.95±0.17	4.48±0.12[b]	3.85±0.15[b,c]
Lung wet weight/dry weight	4.84±0.92	4.79±0.84	4.77±0.99
p-BNP (ng/ml)	2.19±0.011	2.33±0.034	2.31±0.031

WKY: normotensive age-matched control rats, n = 7, SHR-C: SHR age-matched control rats, n = 8, SHR-L: SHR treated with L-2286 for 24 weeks, n = 9. SAP, DAP, MAP^{30w}: systolic, diastolic and mean arterial blood pressure at 30-week-old age (n = 3 from each group). BW^{6w}: body weight of 6-week-old rats, BW: body weight, WV: weights of ventricles, BNP: plasma b-type natriuretic peptide. Values are means±S.E.M.
[a]<0.01 (vs. WKY group),
[b]<0.05 (vs. WKY group),
[c]<0.05 (vs. SHR-C).

Biotechnology (London, UK), Hsp90, which was bought from Santa Cruz Biotechnology (Wembley, UK), Hsp72, which was purchased from StressGene Biomol GmbH (Hamburg, Germany). Membranes were washed six times for 5 min in Tris-buffered saline, pH 7.5 containing 0.2% Tween before addition of goat anti-rabbit horseradish peroxidase-conjugated secondary antibody (1:3000 dilution, Bio-Rad, Budapest, Hungary). The antibody-antigen complexes were visualized by means of enhanced

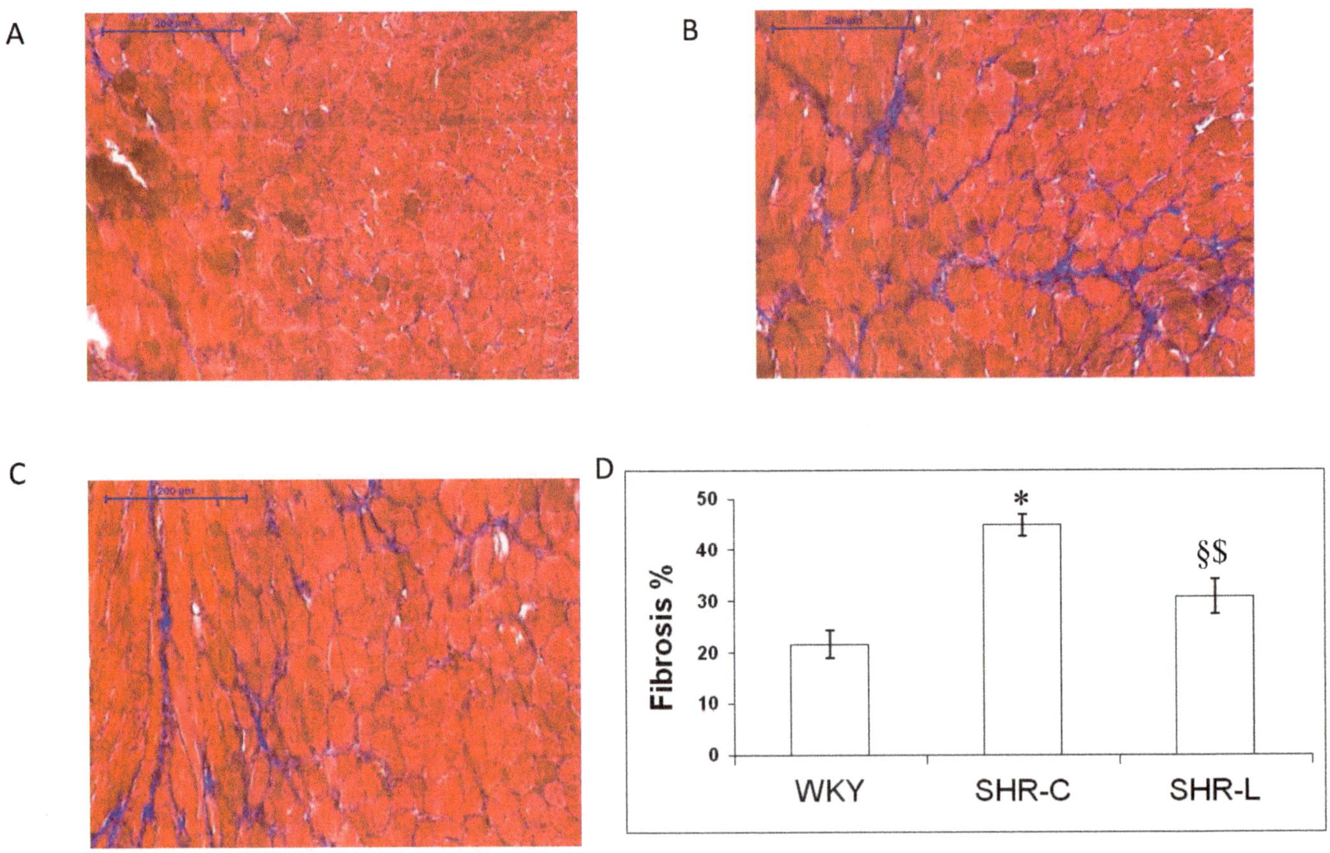

Figure 2. L-2286 treatment decreased the deposition of interstitial collagen. Sections stained with Masson's trichrome (n = 5). Scale bars mean 200 μm. Magnifications 10-fold. WKY (A): normotensive age-matched control rats. SHR-C (B): 30 week-old spontaneously hypertensive rats, SHR-L (C): 30 week-old spontaneously hypertensive rats treated with L-2286 for 24 week. D: Denzitometric evaluation of the sections is shown. *p<0.01 vs. WKY, §p<0.05 vs. WKY, $p<0.05 vs. SHR-C.

Table 2. L-2286 treatment moderately influenced the echocardiographic parameters in 6 weeks old SHRs.

	WKY	SHR-C	SHR-L
EF (%)^{6w}	67.26±0.525	68.4±1.77	68.23±1.81
FS^{6w}	38.63±4.47	38.03±5.52	39.35±4.15
LVEDV^{6w} (ml)	147.27±13.88	149.56±16.78	149.11±14.43
LVESV^{6w} (ml)	46.63±4.47	48.03±5.52	47.35±5.45
Septum^{6w} (mm)	1.2±0.07	1.18±0.05	1.17±0.12
PW^{6w} (mm)	1.19±0.07	1.16±0.067	1.14±0.04
LV mass^{6w} (uncorrected)	344.14±35.49	351.66±36.23	354.77±33.23

WKY: normotensive age-matched control rats, n = 7, SHR-C: SHR age-matched control rats, n = 8, SHR-L: n = 9, SHR treated with L-2286 for 24 weeks.EF^{6w}: ejection fraction, FS^{6w}: fractional shortening, LVEDV^{6w}: left ventricular (LV) end-diastolic volume, LVESV^{6w}: LV end-systolic volume, Septum^{6w}: thickness of septum, PW^{6w}: thickness of posterior wall, LV mass^{6w}: weights of LVs.

chemiluminescence. After scanning, results were quantified by NIH ImageJ program. Pixel densities of bands were normalized to that of the loading controls.

Noninvasive evaluation of cardiac functions and dimensions

At the start of the experiment, all animals were examined by echocardiography to exclude rats with any heart abnormalities. Transthoracic two-dimensional echocardiography was performed under inhalation anesthesia at the beginning of the experiment and on the day of sacrifice. Rats were lightly anesthetized with a mixture of 1.5% isoflurane (Forane, Abbott Laboratories, Hungary) and 98.5% oxygen. The chest of animals was shaved, acoustic coupling gel was applied and warming pad was used to maintain normothermia. Rats were imaged in the left lateral decubitus position. Cardiac dimensions and functions were measured from short- and long-axis views at the mid-papillary level by a VEVO 770 high-resolution ultrasound imaging system (VisualSonics, Toronto, Canada) equipped with a 25 MHz transducer. LV fractional shortening (FS), ejection fraction (EF), LV end-diastolic volume (LVEDV), LV end-systolic volume (LVESV), and the thickness of septum and posterior wall were determined. FS (%) was calculated by $100x((LVID_d-LVID_s)/LVID_d)$ (LVID: LV inside dimension; d: diastolic; s: systolic), EF (%) was calculated by 100x((LVEDV-LVESV)/LVEDV), relative wall thickness (RWT) was calculated by (PW thickness + interventricular septal thickness)/$LVID_d$.

Statistical analysis

All data are expressed as mean±SEM. First of all the homogeneity of the groups was tested by F-test (Levene's test). There were no significant differences among the groups. Comparisons among groups were made using one-way ANOVA (SPSS for Windows 11.0). For post hoc comparison Bonferroni test was chosen. Values of $p<0.05$ were considered statistically significant.

Results

Effect of L-2286 on normotensive WKY rats was also examined, but the investigated parameters did not differ significantly from the non-treated WKY animals. Therefore, data of L-2286 treated WKY rats were not shown to avoid unnecessary redundancies.

Effect of PARP inhibition on gravimetric parameters of spontaneously hypertensive rats

Body weights did not differ significantly among the three groups (WKY: 71.01±0.11 g, SHR-C: 72.03±2.36 g, SHR-L:

Table 3. L-2286 treatment moderately influenced the echocardiographic parameters in 30 weeks old SHRs.

	WKY	SHR-C	SHR-L
EF (%)^{30w}	69.1±2.4	68.72±2.1	69.01±3.2
FS^{30w}	39.8±1.9	39.04±1.85	40.57±2.66
LVEDV^{30w} (ml)	279.18±18.18	335.87±10.36^{a}	326.94±9.18^{a}
LVESV^{30w} (ml)	85.77±8.56	96.85±10.36^{a}	99.81±11.85^{a}
Septum^{30w} (mm)	1.43±0.04	1.93±0.04^{a}	1.79±0.05^{a,b}
PW^{30w} (mm)	1.54±0.08	2.15±0.12^{a}	1.87±0.03^{a,b}
RWT^{30w}	0.38±0.05	0.504±0.02^{a}	0.445±0.012^{a,b}
LV mass^{30w} (uncorrected)	1002.81±59.5	1370.35±79.87^{a}	1121.13±53.23^{a,b}
LV mass^{30}/BW^{30} (mg/g)	2.73±0.7	4.23±0.8^{a}	3.70±0.3^{a,b}

WKY: normotensive age-matched control rats, n = 7, SHR-C: SHR age-matched control rats, n = 8, SHR-L: n = 9, SHR treated with L-2286 for 24 weeks.EF^{30w}: ejection fraction, F^{30w}: fractional shortening, LVEDV^{30w}: left ventricular (LV) end-diastolic volume, LVESV^{30w}: LV end-systolic volume, Septum^{30w}: thickness of septum, PW^{30w}: thickness of posterior wall, RWT^{30w}: relative wall thickness, LV mass^{30w}: weights of LVs. Values are mean±S.E.M.

^{a}p<0.05 (vs. WKY group),

^{b}p<0.05 (vs. SHR-C group).

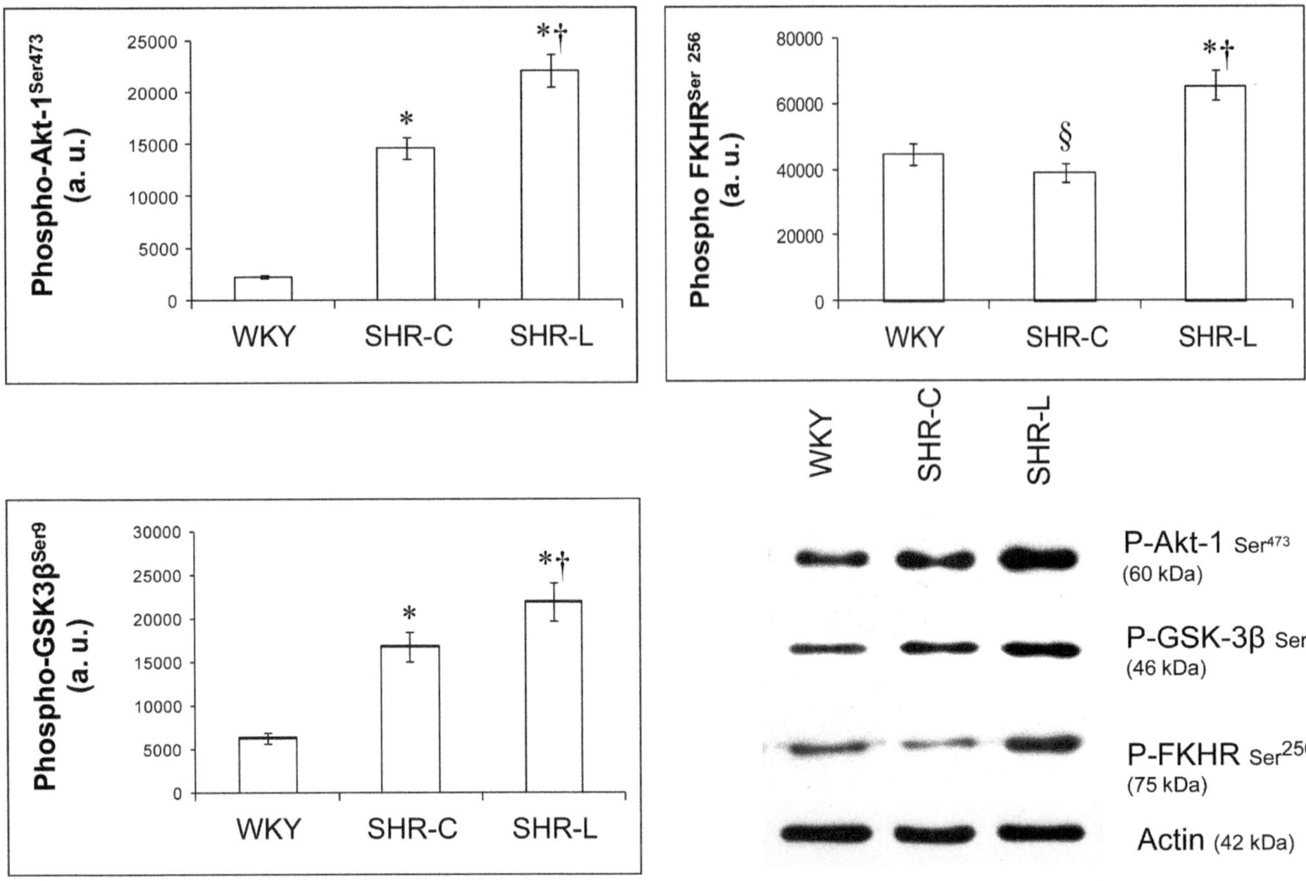

Figure 3. Effect of L-2286 treatment on Akt-1^{Ser473}/GSK-3β^{Ser9}, FKHR^{Ser256} pathway. Representative Western blot analysis of Akt-1^{Ser473}, GSK-3β^{Ser9}, FKHR^{Ser256} phosphorylation and densitometric evaluation is shown (n = 4). Actin was used as loading control. Values are means±S.E.M. WKY: normotensive age-matched control rats. SHR-C: 30 week-old spontaneously hypertensive rats, SHR-L: 30 week-old spontaneously hypertensive rats treated with L-2286 for 24 weeks. $^{*}p<0.01$ vs. WKY, $^{\dagger}p<0.01$ vs. SHR-C, $^{\S}p<0.05$ vs. WKY.

69.92±3.21 g, 6-week-old rats) at the beginning of our study. However, at the end of the 24-week-long treatment period, body weights of WKY group were significantly higher than those of SHR-C and SHR-L groups (WKY: 392.7±14.01 g, SHR-C: 323.8±11.27 g, SHR-L: 321.9±6.84 g, $p<0.01$ WKY vs. SHR groups, 30-week-old rats). The degree of myocardial hypertrophy was determined by ventricular weight to body weight ratio (WV/BW, mg/g). This parameter was significantly increased in SHR groups compared to the WKY group (WV/BW: WKY: 2.95±0.17, SHR-C: 4.48±0.12, SHR-L: 3.85±0.15, $p<0.05$ WKY vs. SHR groups). Similar results were obtained in case of weights of ventricles (WV, WKY: 1.16±0.17 g, SHR-C: 1.45±0.18 g, SHR-L: 1.24±0.24 g, $p<0.05$ WKY vs. SHR groups). The WV and WV/BW ratios were significantly decreased by L-2286 treatment ($p<0.05$ SHR-L vs. SHR-C). The lung wet weight-to-dry weight ratio was not elevated significantly in SHR-C and SHR-L compared to WKY groups (Table 1). All these results indicate the presence of cardiac hypertrophy without congestive heart failure in the SHR-C group that was ameliorated in the SHR-L group.

L-2286 treatment did not influence the levels of plasma BNP and blood pressure

Slightly elevated plasma BNP levels were found both in SHR-C and SHR-L groups (not significant vs. WKY group). Although plasma BNP level was a little higher in SHR-C group than in SHR-L group, this difference was also not statistically significant (Table 1). In both SHR groups, blood pressure was significantly elevated compared to the WKY group ($p<0.05$). L-2286 treatment did not decrease significantly the elevated blood pressure (Table 1).

L-2286 decreased the interstitial collagen deposition in the myocardium

Histological analysis revealed slight interstitial collagen deposition in the WKY group. Chronic high blood pressure caused significantly higher collagen deposition in SHR-C rats that was significantly diminished ($p<0.05$) in the SHR-L group (Fig. 2).

PARP inhibition decreased the left ventricular hypertrophy in spontaneously hypertensive rats

At the beginning of the study the echocardiographic parameters of the three groups did not differ significantly from each other (Table 2). At the age of 30 weeks there was no significant difference in LV systolic functions (EF and FS) between the WKY and SHR groups. Heart rate did not differ significantly during the anesthesia among the groups. LVESV and LVEDV were increased significantly in SHRs ($p<0.05$ WKY vs. SHR-C and SHR-L), and these unfavorable alterations were not reduced by L-2286 treatment. The thickness of the septum, and the posterior

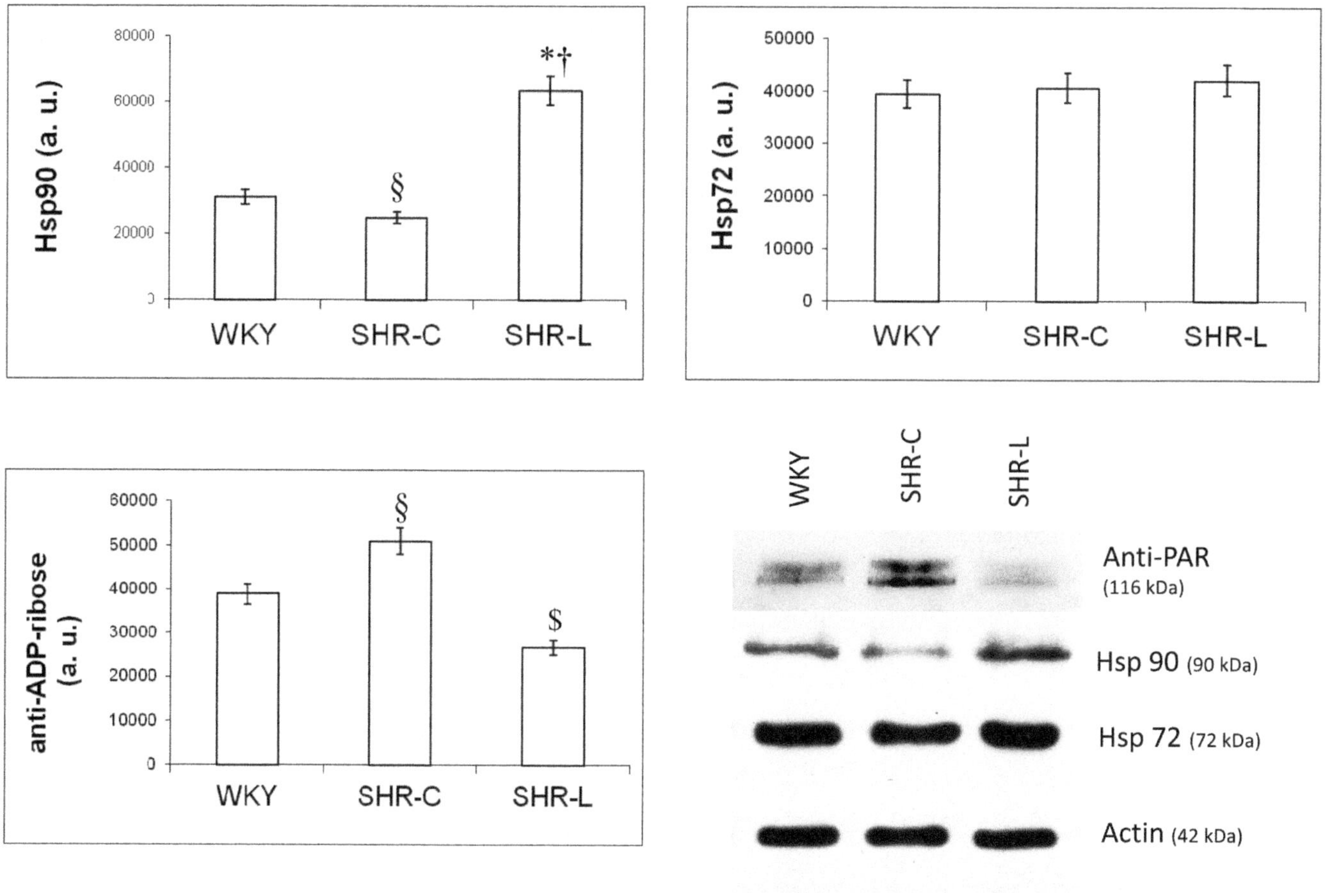

Figure 4. Effect of L-2286 treatment on the level of Hsp72, 90 and poly(ADP-ribos)ylation. Representative Western-blot analysis of Hsp72, 90, anti-PAR and densitometric evaluations are shown (n = 4). Actin was used as loading control. Values are means±S.E.M. WKY: normotensive age-matched control rats. SHR-C: 30 week-old spontaneously hypertensive rats, SHR-L: 30 week-old spontaneously hypertensive rats treated with L-2286 for 24 weeks. $^{*}p<0.01$ vs. WKY, $^{\dagger}p<0.01$ v.s SHR-C, $^{\S}p<0.05$ vs. WKY, $^{\$}p<0.05$ vs. SHR-C.

wall and the relative wall thickness were also increased in SHR groups (indicating the presence of ventricular hypertrophy) comparing to the WKY group ($p<0.05$), and these parameters could be significantly reduced by the administration of L-2286 ($p<0.05$ SHR-C vs. SHR-L group) (Table 3).

Effect of L-2286 treatment on poly-ADP-ribosylation as well as on the phosphorylation state of Akt-1^{Ser473}/GSK-3β^{Ser9} and FKHR^{Ser256}

Akt-1^{Ser473} was moderately phosphorylated in WKY group. In SHR-C group, the phosphorylation of Akt-1^{Ser473} was more pronounced ($p<0.01$ vs. WKY). Moreover, in SHR-L rats the L-2286 treatment caused further elevation in Akt-1^{Ser473} phosphorylation ($p<0.01$ vs. WKY and SHR-C groups) (Fig. 3). The same result was obtained in the case of GSK-3β^{Ser9} phosphorylation (Fig. 3).

Another target protein of Akt-1^{Ser473} (besides GSK3β^{Ser9}) is FKHR^{Ser256}. Consistently with the result of Akt-1^{Ser473} phosphorylation, the strongest phosphorylation (therefore inhibition) could be observed in SHR-L group ($p<0.01$ vs. SHR-C and WKY). The lowest phosphorylation and therefore the highest activity of FKHR was seen in SHR-C group ($p<0.05$ vs. WKY, Fig. 3). To detect the effectivity of L-2286, the ADP-ribosylation of the samples were analysed by Western-blot. The lowest degree of ADP-ribosylation was present in SHR-L group, and the most pronounced ADP-ribosylation was seen in SHR-C group ($p<0.05$ vs. WKY) (Fig. 4).

Effect of L-2286 on the amount of Hsp72 and 90

There was no significant difference among the three groups in the level of Hsp72. On the other hand, the level of Hsp90 was elevated in SHR-L group compared to WKY and SHR-C groups ($p<0.01$ SHR-L vs. WKY or SHR-C groups), and the lowest amount of this protein was present in WKY samples (Fig. 4).

Effect of L-2286 administration on MAPKs

Phosphorylation of p38-MAPK$^{Thr180\text{-}Gly\text{-}Tyr182}$, ERK 1/2$^{Thr183\text{-}Tyr185}$ and JNK was the lowest in the WKY group compared to SHR-C and SHR-L groups (p38-MAPK$^{Thr180\text{-}Gly\text{-}Tyr182}$: $p<0.01$ vs. SHR groups, ERK 1/2: $p<0.05$ vs. SHR groups, JNK: $p<0.05$ vs. SHR groups). In the case of p38-MAPK$^{Thr180\text{-}Gly\text{-}Tyr182}$, ERK 1/2$^{Thr183\text{-}Tyr185}$ and JNK, their phosphorylation was elevated in both SHR-C and SHR-L groups, but there were no significant differences between the two SHR groups (Fig. 5, JNK: data not shown).

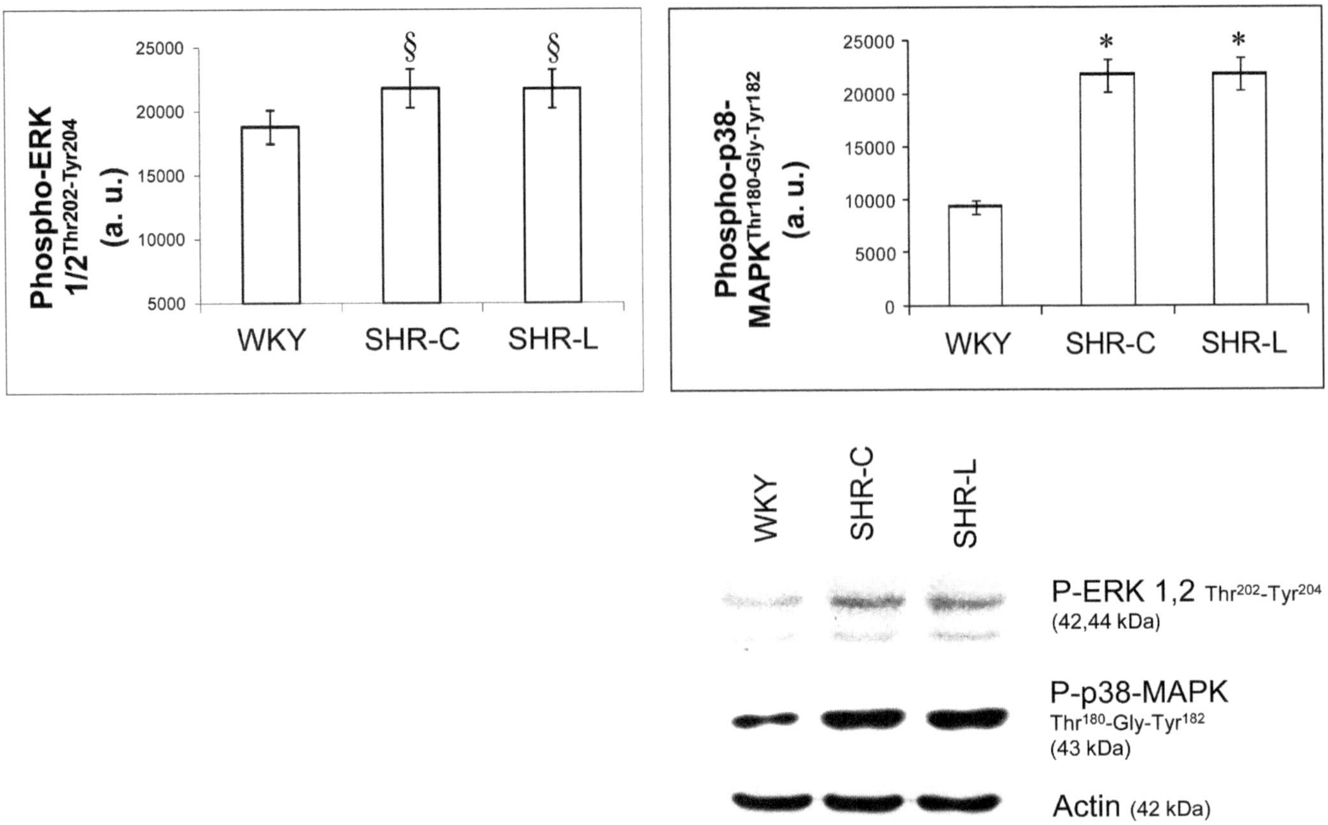

Figure 5. Effect of L-2286 on the phosphorylation state of MAPK pathway. Representative Western blot analysis of ERK 1/2$^{Thr183\text{-}Tyr185}$, and p38-MAPK$^{Thr180\text{-}Gly\text{-}Tyr182}$ phosphorylation and densitometric evaluation is shown (n = 4). Actin was used as loading control. Values are means±S.E.M. WKY: normotensive age-matched control rats. SHR-C: 30 week-old spontaneously hypertensive rats, SHR-L: 30 week-old spontaneously hypertensive rats treated with L-2286 for 24 weeks. $^{\S}p<0.05$ vs. WKY $^{*}p<0.01$ vs. WKY.

Influence of L-2286 treatment on the phosphorylation state of several PKC isoforms

The overall (pan) phosphorylation of PKC (pan βII^{Ser660}) was low in the WKY group and became significantly higher in SHR-C and SHR-L groups ($p<0.01$ WKY vs. SHR groups). Administration of L-2286 could not affect the phosphorylation state of PKC pan βII Ser^{660} in SHR-L group compared to the SHR-C group (Fig. 6).

The lowest phosphorylation could be observed in the WKY group in case of PKC $\alpha/\beta II^{Thr638/641}$, δ^{Thr505}, $\zeta/\lambda^{Thr410/403}$ and ε^{Ser729} ($p<0.01$ vs. SHR groups). As PKC ζ antibody, we used a combined antibody (i.e. PKC ζ/λ Thr$^{410/403}$), which did not discriminate between PKC ζ and λ; PKC λ being structurally highly homologous to PKC ζ in the COOH-terminal end of the molecule [12]. L-2286 treatment decreased significantly the phosphorylation of PKC $\alpha/\beta II^{Thr638/641}$ and ζ, while it could increase the phosphorylation of ε^{Ser729} (PKC $\alpha/\beta II^{Thr638/641}$, ζ, ε^{Ser729}: $p<0.01$, SHR-L vs. SHR-C) (Fig. 6,7). In the case of PKC δ^{Thr505} there was no significant difference between the SHR groups (Fig. 7).

Discussion

The major findings of this study are that chronic inhibition of nuclear PARP enzyme reduces excessive ADP-ribosylation of nuclear proteins, beneficially influences the intracellular signaling pathways and thus prevents the development of cardiac hypertrophy, which is an early consequence of hypertension. We used the SHR model that is a relevant animal model of essential hypertension in humans [13]. Our study began at a very early age (6-week-old) of SHRs, because at this age the blood pressure of animals is still normal and the hearts show no signs of remodeling. However, by the end of the study (30 weeks), marked signs of hypertensive cardiopathy develop in SHRs.

Previously, we have proved that PARP-inhibition could inhibit the transition of hypertensive cardiopathy to end-stage heart failure [6], but there is no data about the role of PAPR-inhibitors against the development of early consequences of hypertension.

Hypertension is a major risk factor for cardiovascular mortality and morbidity, and it is associated with left ventricular hypertrophy and diastolic dysfunction and later with systolic dysfunction and it can lead to heart failure. There is a strong correlation between left ventricular mass and the development of cardiovascular pathogies [14]. The development of long-term hypertension-induced myocardial remodeling can be explained by different mechanism in the literature, but generally, oxidative stress and abnormal signaling are considered as molecular basis of the disease. Peroxynitrite and other reactive species induce oxidative DNA damage and consequent activation of the nuclear enzyme PARP. In related animal models of the disease, pharmacological inhibition of PARP provides significant therapeutic benefits [15].

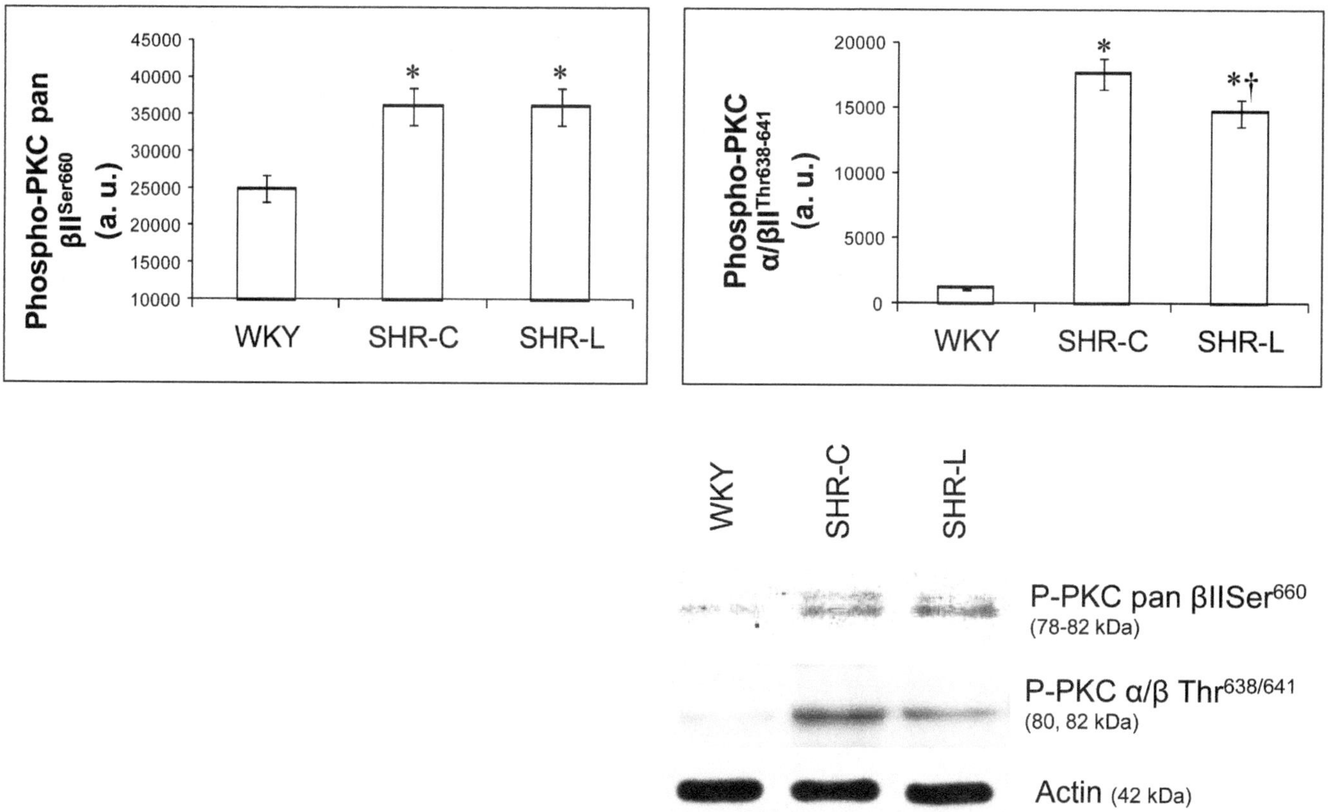

Figure 6. Effect of L-2286 administration on the activity of PKC isoenzymes. Representative Western blot analysis of PKC pan βII^{Ser660} and PKC $\alpha/\beta II^{Thr638/641}$ phosphorylation and densitometric evaluations are shown (n=4). Values are means±S.E.M. WKY: normotensive age-matched control rats. SHR-C: 30 week-old spontaneously hypertensive rats, SHR-L: 30 week-old spontaneously hypertensive rats treated with L-2286 for 24 weeks. *p<0.01 vs. WKY, †p<0.01 vs. SHR-C.

PARP inhibition and gravimetric parameters in SHR

Significant LV hypertrophy develops by the age of 3 months in SHR animals but it is more often studied closer to 6 months of age [16]. In our SHR rats myocardial hypertrophy developed, as increased WV/BW ratio could be observed. We could not observe any obvious signs of HF, because BNP activity and the index of pulmonary congestion was not elevated compared to the WKY group.

PARP inhibition and interstitial collagen deposition in SHR

Chronic hypertension leads to excessive collagen deposition (fibrosis) as part of the process of cardiovascular remodeling. In our previous studies, when SHR or postinfarcted animals exhibited overt heart failure, L-2286 also prevented interstitial fibrosis and adverse structural remodeling [3,6]. In the present study, our results suggest that PARP inhibitor treatment can exert marked antifibrotic effect already in this early stage of hypertensive heart disease.

PARP inhibition and echocardiographic parameters

In our experiment the systolic LV function was not decreased in SHR rats during the 24-week-long treatment. It is in accordance with several other studies [8,9,10] involving different experimental models of pressure overload-induced hypertrophy. During the development of hypertension, alterations in LV geometry may also occur as an adaptation to increased pressure overload. In hypertensive patients, LV geometry can be classified into four patterns on the basis of LV mass index and RWT and these patterns have been shown to be closely related to LV function and to patients' prognosis [17,18,19]. In this study, increased RWT and increased WV/BW were found, which indicates concentric LV hypertrophy [9]. L-2286 treatment decreased significantly the signs of left ventricular hypertrophy (wall thickness and RWT) even though the elevated blood pressure of SHR rats was not influenced by PARP inhibition.

L-2286 treatment and the activity of Akt-1^{Ser473}/ GSK3β^{Ser9} and FKHR^{Ser256} pathway

Previous works demonstrated that PARP inhibitors can induce the phosphorylation and activation of Akt-1 in reperfused myocardium, thus raising the possibility that the protective effect of PARP inhibition can be mediated through the activation of the prosurvival phosphatidylinositol-3-kinase (PI3-kinase)/Akt-1 pathway [20]. Akt-1 is a key molecule in the signaling cascade of physiological hypertrophy [21]. Recent results demonstrate an important role of Akt/m-TOR signaling in cardiac angiogenesis, whose disruption contributes to the transition from hypertrophy to HF [1]. In our experiment, the phosphorylation of Akt-1^{Ser473} was far the lowest in WKY group and the highest in SHR-L group. Phosphorylation and therefore the inhibition of GSK-3β^{Ser9} and Foxo1 (FKHR) (downstream targets of Akt-1) [22,23] were also determined. This showed the same pattern as the phosphorylation of Akt-1. The similar results were obtained in our studies using

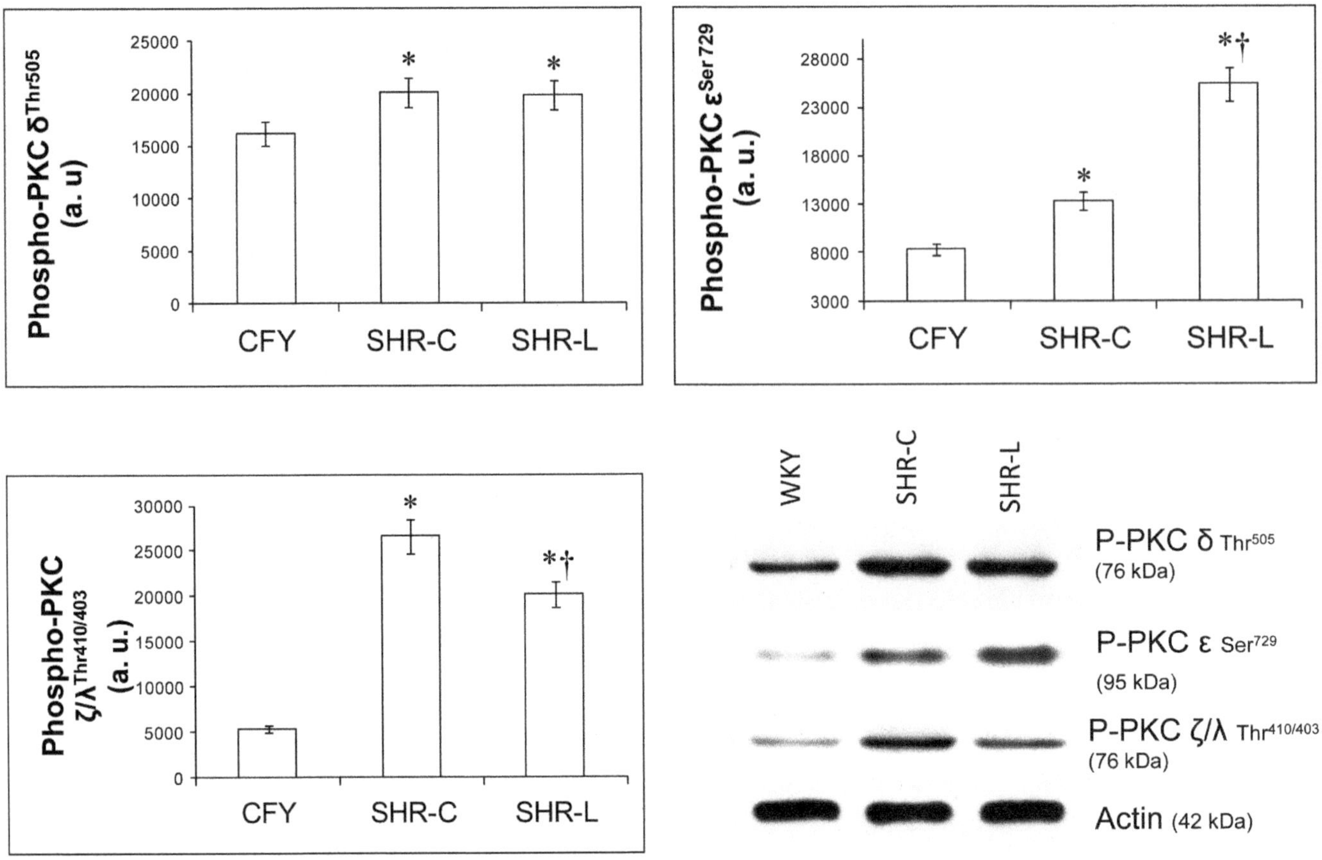

Figure 7. Effect of L-2286 administration of PKC isoenzymes. Representative Western blot analysis of PKC δ^{Thr505}, ε^{Ser729} and $\zeta/\lambda^{Thr410/403}$ phosphorylation and densitometric evaluation is shown (n = 4). Actin was used as loading control. Values are means±S.E.M. WKY: normotensive age-matched control rats. SHR-C: 30 week-old spontaneously hypertensive rats, SHR-L: 30 week-old spontaneously hypertensive rats treated with L-2286 for 24 weeks. $^{*}p<0.01$ vs. WKY, $^{\dagger}p<0.01$ vs. SHR-C.

PARP inhibitors [20,24] or by suppressing PARP-1 activation by siRNA technique [25]. These results may indicate that SHR-C animals tried to compensate for the adverse effects of chronic hypertension, but failed to do so. On the other hand, L-2286 treatment further elevated Akt activation that could, at least partially, account for the beneficial changes in the cardial remodeling of the SHR-L animals.

L-2286 administration and levels of Hsp 72 and 90

Cellular stress leads to the expression of Hsp's [26]. They are known to protect the myocardium from the damaging effects of ischemia and reperfusion [27]. According to the results of Jiang et al [27] and Shinohara et al [28] the Hsp's can preserve the mitochondrial respiratory function and structure which are damaged in case of cell death. The flux of pro-apoptotic proteins can be induced by various stimuli, one of them is the decreased level of ATP. This can be induced by overactivation of PARP-1, which consumes too much ATP in certain pathologic conditions [29]. In case of Hsp90 in our study, the level of it was increased by long-term L-2286 treatment. Besides the activation of Akt-1^{Ser473}, this can contribute to the cell survival in L-2286 treated rats. The level of Hsp72 was not influenced significantly by L-2286 administration in our investigation.

L-2286 administration and MAPKs in young SHR

Previous works demonstrated that PARP inhibitors have a moderate effect on MAPKs in acute phase of myocardial infarction and in postinfarction heart failure [3,20]. MAPKs are ubiquitously expressed and their activation is observed in different heart diseases, including hypertrophic cardiomyopathy, dilated cardiomyopathy, and ischemic/reperfusion injury in human and animal models [30]. In our study, the phosphorylation of p38-$MAPK^{Thr180\text{-}Gly\text{-}Tyr182}$, JNK and ERK $1/2^{Thr183\text{-}Tyr185}$ was elevated both in SHR-C and SHR-L groups. Our results are consistent with the results of Kacimi et Gerdes [31] using spontaneously hypertensive heart failure (SHHF) rats. L-2286 treatment did not influence the phosphorylation of p38-MAPK and JNK. The role of JNK and p38-MAPK-signaling in cardiac hypertrophy is not fully clarified [1]. However, both p38-MAPK and JNK transduction cascades have been implicated in the regulation of hypertrophic response as well as cardiomyopathy and HF [32]. JNK activity was not altered by L-2286 treatment in SHR animals, similarly to Hsp72 level. This result is in accordance with previous data [28] demonstrating that Hsp72 downregulates JNK by accelerating its dephosphorylation.

The elevated blood pressure may induced ERK activation [33]. Accordingly, activation of ERK1/2 was the lowest in WKY group, and was higher in SHR-C. Phosphorylation of ERK1/2 was not

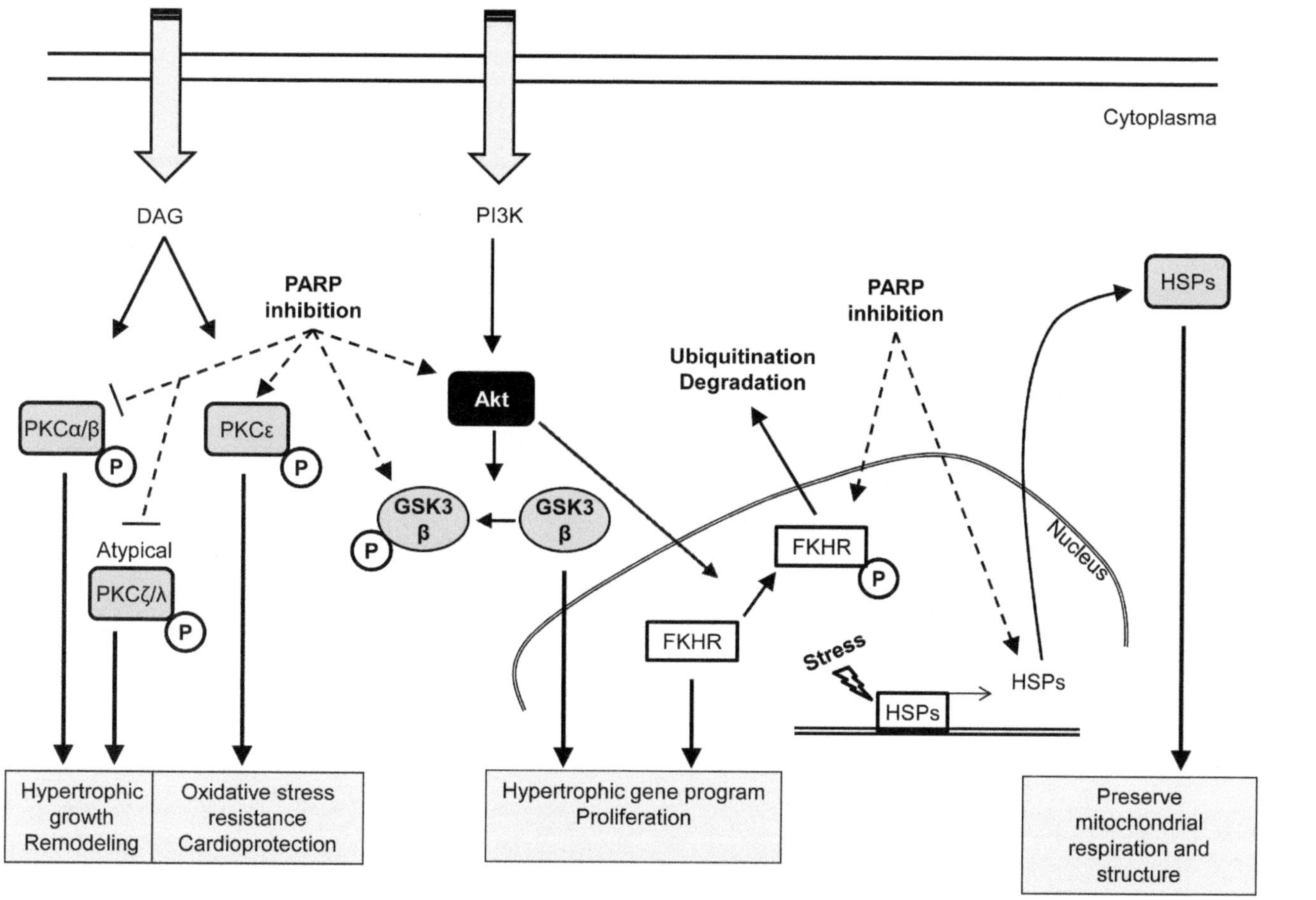

Figure 8. Summary of pathway alterations due to L-2286 treatment.

elevated by L-2286 administration in this study. The in vivo role of ERK in cardiac hypertrophy has been demonstrated in several genetically engineered animal models. Cardiac-specific expression of constitutively activated MEK1 promotes cardiac hypertrophy without compromised function or long-term animal survival, suggesting that activation of ERK activity promotes a compensated form of hypertrophy [30]. All these results suggest that MAPK activation did not participate significantly in mediating the adverse cardiac effects of chronic hypertension in our model.

PARP inhibition and PKC pathways in young SHR

PARP inhibitors were found to affect PKC isoenzymes [3,17]. The levels of all PKC isoforms increased in SHR groups compared to the WKY group in our study. Our results are in agreement with Koide et al. [34] using Dahl Salt-Sensitive rats in cardiac hypertrophy stage. Recent studies suggested that PKC is critically involved in the development of cardiac remodeling and HF. The data also suggest that individual PKC isoforms have different effects on cell signaling pathways, variously leading to changes in cardiac contractility, hypertrophic response and tolerance to myocardial ischaemia in the heart [34].

Activation of PKC pan βII^{Ser660} and δ^{Thr505} were not altered by L-2286 treatment, while activation of $\alpha/\beta II^{Thr638/641}$ and $\zeta/\lambda^{Thr410/403}$ were attenuated and activation of ε^{Ser729} was augmented by L-2286. These alterations can mediate – at least partly – the favourable cardiovascular effects of L-2286, similarly as it was found in previous works [3,20].

PKC α is the most extensively expressed among the myocardial PKC isoforms, and it is a key regulator of cardiomyocyte hypertrophic growth [35,36]. PKC α was sufficient to stimulate cell hypertrophy [37]. Transgenic mice overexpressing PKC β2 exhibited cardiac hypertrophy and decreased LV performance; this depressed cardiac function improved after the administration of a PKC β-selective inhibitor [38]. Previous reports suggest that PKC α and β and PKC ζ/λ are involved in the development of cardiac hypertrophy and HF. Additionally, PKC ε plays a role in physiological hypertrophic responses [34,39], has cardioprotective effect [40] and by interacting with Akt-1 and affecting Bcl-2 promote vascular cytoprotection [41]. Accordingly, in our study, both the activity of Akt-1^{Ser473} and PKCε^{Ser729} were elevated by L-2286 administration.

Conclusions

In our study, we examined the effect of a PARP inhibitor (L-2286) in SHR at the stage of LV hypertrophy. L-2286 exerted a beneficial effect on the progression of myocardial hypertrophy (thickness of PW and septum, RWT) and myocardial fibrosis. In the background of these changes, we did not observe any blood pressure lowering effect of PARP-inhibition. According to our results, PARP-inhibition can exert this antihypertrophic effect due to the activation of several prosurvival (especially Akt-1/GSK-3β, FKHR, PKCε and Hsp90) and the inhibition of prohypertrophic (PKC- α/βII, - ζ/λ) protein kinases (Fig.8).

Acknowledgments

We are grateful for Bertalan Horvath and Laszlo Giran for their excellent technical support.

Author Contributions

Conceived and designed the experiments: LD EB AP TK KH BS FG KT RH. Performed the experiments: LD EB KE AR. Analyzed the data: LD KE GF SB KT RH. Contributed reagents/materials/analysis tools: JL TK KH. Wrote the paper: LD EB RH.

References

1. Luedde M, Katus HA, Frey N (2006) Novel molecular targets in the treatment of cardiac hypertrophy. Recent Pat Cardiovasc Drug Discov 1: 1–20.
2. Baines CP, Molkentin JD (2005) STRESS signaling pathways that modulate cardiac myocyte apoptosis. J Mol Cell Cardiol 38: 47–62.
3. Palfi A, Toth A, Hanto K, Deres P, Szabados E, et al. (2006) PARP inhibition prevents postinfarction myocardial remodeling and heart failure via the protein kinase C/glycogen synthase kinase-3β pathway. J Mol Cell Cardiol 41: 149–159.
4. Szabó Cs, Pacher P, Zsengellér Zs, Vaslin A, Komjáti K, et al. (2004) Angiotensi II-mediated endothelial dysfunction: role of poly(ADP-ribose) polymerase activation. Mol Med 10: 28–35.
5. Pacher P, Mabley JG, Soriano FG, Liaudet L, Szabó C (2002) Activation of poly(ADP-ribose) polymerase contributes to the endothelial dysfunction associated with hypertension and aging. Int J Mol Med 9: 659–664.
6. Bartha E, Solti I, Kereskai L, Lantos J, Plozer E, et al. (2009) PARP inhibition delays transition of hypertensive cardiopathy to heart failure in spontaneously hypertensive rats. Cardiovasc Res 83: 501–510.
7. Racz B, Hanto K, Tapodi A, Solti I, Kalman N, et al. (2010) Regulation of MKP-1 expression and MAPK activation by PARP-1 in oxidative stress: a new mechanism for the cytoplasmic effect of PARP-1 activation. Free Radic Biol Med 49: 1978–1988.
8. Ito N, Ohishi M, Yamamoto K, Tatara Y, Shiota A, et al. (2007) Renin-Angiotensin inhibition reverses advanced cardiac remodeling in aging spontaneously hypertensive rats. Am J Hypertens 20: 792–799.
9. Kokubo M, Uemura A, Matsubara T, Murohara T (2005) Noninvasive evaluation of the time course of change in cardiac function in spontaneously hypertensive rats by echocardiography. Hypertens Res 28: 601–609.
10. Meurrens K, Ruf S, Ross G, Schleef R, van Holt K, et al. (2007) Smoking accelerates the progression of hypertension-induced myocardial hypertrophy to heart failure in spontaneously hypertensive rats. Cardiovasc Res 76: 311–322.
11. Kulcsar Gy, Kalai T, Osz E, Sar CP, Jeko J, et al. (2006) Synthesis and study of new 4-quinazolinone inhibitors of the DNA repair enzyme poly(ADP-ribose) polymerase (PARP). Arkivoc IV:121–131.
12. Hideg K, Kálai T, Sümegi B (2003) Quinazoline derivates and their use for preparation of pharmaceutical compositions having PARP-Enzyme inhibitory effect. WO2004/096779, Hung Pat PO301173.
13. Pfeffer JM, Pfeffer MA, Mirsky I, Braunwald E (1982) Regression of left ventricular hypertrophy and prevention of left ventricular dysfunction by captopril in the spontaneously hypertensive rat. Proc Natl Acad Sci U S A. 79(10):3310–4.
14. Lip GY, Felmeden DC, Li-Saw-Hee FL, Beevers DG (2000) Hypertensive heart disease. A complex syndrome or a hypertensive 'cardiomyopathy'? Eur Heart J; 21: 1653–1665.
15. Pacher P, Szabo C (2008) Role of the peroxynitrite-poly(ADP-ribose) polymerase pathway in human disease. Am J Pathol 173: 2–13.
16. McCrossan ZA, Billeter R, White E (2004) Transmural changes in size, contractile and electrical properties of SHR left ventricular myocytes during compensated hypertrophy. Cardiovasc Res 63: 283–292.
17. Cooper RS, Simmons BE, Castaner A, Santhanam V, Ghali J, et al. (1990) Left ventricular hypertrophy is associated with worse survival independent of ventricular function and number of coronary arteries severely narrowed. Am J Cardiol. 65(7):441–445.
18. Levy D, Garrison RJ, Savage DD, Kannel WB, Castelli WP (1990) Prognostic implications of echocardiographically determined left ventricular mass in the Framingham Heart Study. N Engl J Med. 322: 1561–1566.
19. Koren MJ, Devereux RB, Casale PN, Savage DD, Laregh JH (1991) Relation of left ventricular mass and geometry to morbidity and mortality in uncomplicated essential hypertension. Ann Intern Med. 114: 345–352.
20. Pálfi A, Tóth A, Kulcsár G, Hantó K, Deres P, et al. (2005) The role of Akt and MAP kinase systems in the protective effect of PARP inhibition in Langendorff perfused and in isoproterenol-damaged rat hearts. J Pharmacol Exp Ther 315: 273–282.
21. Taniike M, Yamaguchi O, Tsujimoto I, Hikoso S, Takeda T, et al. (2008) Apoptosis signal-regulating kinase 1/p38 signaling pathway negatively regulates physiological hypertrophy. Circulation 117: 545–552.
22. Li HH, Willis MS, Lockyer P, Miller N, MCDonough H, et al. (2007) Atrogin-1 inhibits Akt-dependent cardiac hypertrophy in mice via ubiquitin-dependent coactivation of Forkhead proteins. J Clin Invest 117: 3211–3223.
23. Ni YG, Berenji K, Wang N, Oh M, Sachan N, et al. (2006) Foxo transcription factors blunt cardiac hypertrophy by inhibiting calcineurin signaling. Circulation 114: 1159–1168.
24. Kovacs K, Toth A, Deres P, Kalai T, Hideg K, et al. (2006) Critical role of PI3-kinase/Akt activation in the PARP inhibitor induced heart function recovery during ischemia-reperfusion. Biochem Pharmacol 71: 441–452.
25. Tapodi A, Debreceni B, Hanto K, Bognar Z, Wittmann I, et al. (2005) Pivotal role of Akt activation in mitochondrial protection and cell survival by poly(ADP-ribose)polymerase-1 inhibition in oxidative stress. J Biol Chem 280: 35767–3575.
26. Sőti Cs, Nagy E, Giricz Z, Vígh L, Csermely P, et al. (2005) Heat shock proteins as emerging therapeutic targets. Br J Pharmacol 146: 769–780.
27. Jiang B, Xiao W, Shi Y, Liu M, Xiao X (2005) Heat shock pretreatment inhibited the release of Smac/DIABLO from mitochondria and apoptosis induced by hydrogen peroxide in cardiomyocytes and C_2C_{12} myogenic cells. Cell Stress Chaperons 10: 252–262.
28. Shinohara T, Takahashi N, Kohno H, Yamanaka K, Ooie T, et al. (2007) Mitochondria are targets for geranylgeranylacetone-induced cardioprotection against ischemia-reperfusion in rat heart. Am J Physiol Heart Circ Physiol 293:H1892–H1899.
29. Pacher P, Szabó C (2007) Role of poly(ADP-ribose) polymerase 1 (PARP-1) in cardiovascular diseases: The therapeutic potential of PARP inhibitors. Cardiovasc Drug Rev 25: 235–260.
30. Wang Y (2007) Mitogen-Activated Protein Kinases in heart development and diseases. Circulation 116: 1413–1423.
31. Kacimi R, Gerdes AM (2003) Alterations in G protein and MAP Kinase signaling pathways during cardiac remodeling in hypertension and heart failure. Hypertension 41: 968–977.
32. Liang Q, Molkentin JD (2003) Redefining the roles of p38 and JNK signaling in cardiac hypertrophy: dichotomy between cultured myocytes and animal models. J Mol Cell Cardiol 35: 1385–1394.
33. Bogoyevitch MA (2000) Signalling via stress-activated mitogen-activated protein kinases in the cadriovascular system. Cardiovas Res 45: 826–842.
34. Koide Y, Tamura K, Suzuki A, Kitamura K, Yokoyama K, et al. (2003) Differential induction of protein kinase C isoforms at the cardiac hypertrophy stage and congestive heart failure stage in Dahl salt-sensitive rats. Hypertens Res 26: 421–426.
35. Dorn GW II, Force T (2005) Protein kinase cascades in the regulation of cardiac hypertrophy. J Clin Invest 115: 527–537.
36. García-Hoz C, Sánchez-Fernández G, García-Escudero R, Fernández-Velasco M, Palacios-García J, et al. (2012) Protein Kinase C (PKC)ζ-mediated $G\alpha_q$ Stimulation of ERK5 Protein Pathway in Cardiomyocytes and Cardiac Fibroblasts JBiolChem. 287: 7792–7802.
37. Braz JC, Bueno OF, De Windt LJ, Molkentin JD (2002) PKC alpha regulates the hypertrophic growth of cardiomyocytes through extracellular signal-regulated kinase1/2 (ERK1/2) J. Cell Biol. 156: 905–919.
38. Takeishi Y, Chu G, Kirkpatrick DM, Li Z, Wakasaki H, et al. (1998) In vivo phosphorylation of cardiac troponin I by protein kinase Cbeta2 decreases cardiomyocyte calcium responsiveness and contractility in transgenic mouse hearts. J Clin Invest. 102: 72–78.
39. Inagaki K, Iwanaga Y, Sarai N, Onozawa Y, Takenaka H, et al. (2002) Tissue angiotensin II during progression or ventricular hypertrophy to heart failure in hypertensive rats; differential effects on PKC epsilon and PKC beta. J Mol Cell Cardiol. 34: 1377–1385.
40. Dorn GW II, Souroujon MC, Liron T, Chen CH, Gray MO, et al. (1999) Sustained in vivo cardiac protection by a rationally designed peptide that causes epsilon protein kinase C translocation. Proc Natl Acad Sci USA 96: 12798–12803.
41. Steinberg R, Harari OA, Lidington EA, Boyle JJ, Nohadani M, et al. (2007) A protein kinase Cepsilon-anti-apoptotic kinase signalling complex protects human vascular endothelial cells against apoptosis through induction of Bcl-2. J Biol Chem 282: 32288–32297.

5

Impact of Combined Clenbuterol and Metoprolol Therapy on Reverse Remodelling during Mechanical Unloading

Manoraj Navaratnarajah*, Urszula Siedlecka, Michael Ibrahim, Carin van Doorn, Gopal Soppa, Ajay Gandhi, Adarsh Shah, Punam Kukadia, Magdi H. Yacoub, Cesare M. Terracciano

Harefield Heart Science Centre, Imperial College London, National Heart and Lung Institute, Laboratory of Cellular Electrophysiology, Harefield Hospital, Harefield, Middlesex, United Kingdom

Abstract

Background: Clenbuterol (Cl), a β_2 agonist, is associated with enhanced myocardial recovery during left ventricular assist device (LVAD) support, and exerts beneficial remodelling effects during mechanical unloading (MU) in rodent heart failure (HF). However, the specific effects of combined Cl+β_1 blockade during MU are unknown.

Methods and Results: We studied the chronic effects (4 weeks) of β_2-adrenoceptor (AR) stimulation via Cl (2 mg/kg/day) alone, and in combination with β_1-AR blockade using metoprolol ((Met), 250 mg/kg/day), on whole heart/cell structure, function and excitation-contraction (EC) coupling in failing (induced by left coronary artery (LCA) ligation), and unloaded (induced by heterotopic abdominal heart transplantation (HATx)) failing rat hearts. Combined Cl+Met therapy displayed favourable effects in HF: Met enhanced Cl's improvement in ejection fraction (EF) whilst preventing Cl-induced hypertrophy and tachycardia. During MU combined therapy was less beneficial than either mono-therapy. Met, not Cl, prevented MU-induced myocardial atrophy, with increased atrophy occurring during combined therapy. MU-induced recovery of Ca^{2+} transient amplitude, speed of Ca^{2+} release and sarcoplasmic reticulum Ca^{2+} content was enhanced equally by Cl or Met mono-therapy, but these benefits, together with Cl's enhancement of sarcomeric contraction speed, and MU-induced recovery of Ca^{2+} spark frequency, disappeared during combined therapy.

Conclusions: Combined Cl+Met therapy shows superior functional effects to mono-therapy in rodent HF, but appears inferior to either mono-therapy in enhancing MU-induced recovery of EC coupling. These results suggest that combined β_2-AR simulation +β_1-AR blockade therapy is likely to be a safe and beneficial therapeutic HF strategy, but is not as effective as mono-therapy in enhancing myocardial recovery during LVAD support.

Editor: Yiru Guo, University of Louisville, United States of America

Funding: The authors are grateful to the Magdi Yacoub Institute (HSC 87/04) for financial support. The funders had no role in study design, data collection and analysis, decision to publish, or preparation of the manuscript.

Competing Interests: The authors have declared that no competing interests exist.

* Email: manonava@hotmail.com

Introduction

The use of LVADs in end stage HF continues to expand [1]. LVADs are used primarily as "bridge to transplantation". In a minority of patients they have been used as a "bridge to recovery" (BTR), where sufficient functional recovery of the failing heart is achieved, allowing device removal. However, explantation rates remain universally low (≤10%) [2,3].

HF-associated remodelling is a complex series of whole heart, cellular, molecular, structural and functional changes affecting various pathways, including EC coupling, the extracellular matrix (ECM), apoptosis and adrenergic receptor signalling [4]. Previously thought to be uni-directional, such adverse remodelling is now considered reversible, a process termed reverse remodelling. Pharmacological intervention induces mild reversal of HF remodelling, demonstrating functional and prognostic benefit [5–7], however, a more substantial degree of reverse remodelling is achieved via LVAD [8]. Despite profound LVAD-induced reverse remodelling, functional myocardial recovery is rare. This disparity is proposed to arise due to negative MU-induced changes occurring during prolonged unloading [9,10]. Indeed, in animals and humans, initial contractile recovery of failing hearts is seen to subsequently worsen during prolonged MU [3,11]. Time dependent worsening of EC coupling [12], Ca^{2+} handling [11] and myocardial atrophy [13] are proposed negative drivers of contractile performance.

"Combination therapy" describes a strategy in which pharmacotherapy is combined with LVAD support, to enhance LVAD–induced positive remodelling and/or combat LVAD-induced "negative" remodelling [10]. In our institute this strategy - the "Harefield Protocol" - successfully enhanced rates of functional recovery (>63%) in patients with dilated cardiomyopathy [14,15]. In this unique protocol, the β_2-adrenoceptor (AR) agonist Cl was employed alongside conventional HF pharmacotherapy, primarily as an agent to prevent myocardial atrophy. Cl's ability to induce physiological cardiac hypertrophy [16] mandated its inclusion in this protocol, but whether anti-atrophic properties contributed to enhancing functional recovery is unclear [17]. Hence, Cl's precise role in enhancing functional recovery remains poorly defined and controversial. Beyond hypertrophic effects, Cl demonstrates other wide-ranging favourable whole heart/cellular functional, structural, metabolic, cell-survival, EC coupling and gene expression effects in non-failing [16,18], failing [19,20] and unloaded [19,21] hearts.

BTR remains controversial, but the clinical success of combination therapy (14, 15) justifies continued scrutiny of this strategy. Therefore, the search for other novel pharmacological strategies aimed at enhancing LVAD-induced functional recovery continues, and we have recently shown the pacemaker current inhibitor ivabradine and Met to show positive effects on myocardial size, EC coupling and the ECM during mechanical unloading in rodent HF [22].

The efficacy of β-AR blockade in HF therapy is established [4,6,23] and is predominantly secondary to blockade of detrimental β_1-AR signalling [4]. Greater understanding of the roles played by β_1-/β_2-AR signalling indicates distinct and often opposing physiological and pathological actions on cardiac structure and function [24], with chronic β_1-AR signalling associated with pro-apoptotic and maladaptive remodelling [25] and chronic β_2-AR signalling with cardio-protective actions, improved function and myocyte viability [26,27]. Supporting this, combined β_1-AR blockade (Met) and β_2-AR stimulation (fenoterol) has shown synergistic beneficial remodelling effects in rodent HF [24], although lack of synergy (Cl+Met) has also been demonstrated [20]. These studies instituted pharmacotherapy early after LCA ligation (<3 weeks) and combined drug effects in an established rodent HF model remain unknown. β_2-AR stimulation (Cl) demonstrates positive effects during MU in rodent studies [19,28], however, the specific effects of combined β_2-AR stimulation and β_1-AR blockade remain unstudied within this setting.

In this study, we report for the first time the chronic effects of combined β_2-AR stimulation (Cl) and β_1-AR blockade (Met) on reverse remodelling during MU in a rodent HF model. In particular, we have examined the drug effects on whole heart/cell size, function, EC coupling and T-tubule structure in a rat model of established HF, 12 weeks post LCA ligation, and during MU using HATx.

Methods

Ethics Statement

The investigation conformed to the Guide for the care and Use of Laboratory Animals published by the US National Institutes of Health (NIH publication No 85–23, revised 1996). Experiments were approved by the Harefield Heart Science Centre ethics review panel.

(For extended methods please refer to Methods S1).

Animal models

Induction of heart failure. HF was induced via permanent LCA ligation as previously described [11,19–22,24]. Animals were anaesthetised with isoflurane (5% induction, 1.5% maintenance) mixed with O_2 (2–3 L/min), intubated and mechanically ventilated via rodent ventilator, and a left thoracotomy performed. The pericardium was opened and heart visualised, the proximal LCA was identified and a suture (6–0 prolene) placed underneath the artery and lightly tied. Heamostasis was achieved and the chest closed. Sham operated animals underwent the identical protocol but the suture was not tied. Acute 24 hour mortality was 25% in the LCA ligation group and 0% in the sham group. Male syngeneic Lewis rats (10 weeks old ~200 g, Harlan, UK) were used for all experiments to avoid the need for immunosuppression following subsequent heterotopic abdominal transplant (HATx) in the mechanical unloading (MU) groups. 1 week after surgery LV dimensions and function (ejection fraction (EF)) were assessed by transthoracic echocardiography (TTE) (Acuson Sequoia^{TM} 256; Acuson, USA), as previously described [18–21,24]. LAD ligation animals with an EF less than 40% were included in the study, as in our experience animals with baseline function greater than this were unlikely to develop severe dysfunction 12 weeks following surgery. 12 weeks following LCA ligation the presence of severe cardiac dysfunction was confirmed via repeat TTE, and animals were randomised to groups (n = 8). All groups had similar average EF and variability. 3 month mortality was 1% following LCA ligation and 0% in sham group. TTE was performed under general anaesthesia with isoflurane 1%, mixed with O_2 (2–3 L/min) to provide adequate sedation but minimal cardiac depression. Experiments were not performed in non-failing hearts as these show an exaggerated atrophic response during unloading compared with failing hearts [29].

In order to test the effects of pharmacotherapy (Cl and/or Met) in combination with MU, failing hearts (12 weeks after LCA ligation) were transplanted into the abdomen of syngeneic male Lewis rats (weight ~250 g) as previously described [11–13,19], for a period of 4 weeks. In brief, both animals (recipient and donor) were anaesthetised with isoflurane (5% induction, 1% maintenance) mixed with O_2 (2–3 L/min), and self-ventilated throughout the procedure. The failing heart was removed from the donor animal under cardioplegic arrest, and the donor aorta anastomosed to the recipient abdominal aorta and the donor pulmonary artery to the recipient inferior vena cava. Total ischaemic time was <40 minutes and operative mortality <4%, with no deaths occurring in any of the treatment groups during the 4 week treatment period.

Recipients were then assigned to 4 treatment groups: (1) Cl (Sigma, England) 2 mg/kg/day via subcutaneous infusion using osmotic minipump (Model 2002, Alzet), (2) Met (Sigma, England) 250 mg/kg/day in drinking water, (3) Met 250 mg/kg/day +Cl 2 mg/kg/day via drinking water and osmotic minipump respectively, (4) no drug treatment (MUHF+Cl, MUHF+Met, MUHF+MetCl and MUHF, respectively). Animals in Met-treated and MUHF group also received an osmotic minipump containing normal saline. All groups contained 8 animals and treatment duration was 4 weeks. At end of treatment Cl levels in blood were measured as previously described [18], with no difference between the different groups treated (in μM: HF+Cl = 0.17+/−0.01, n = 8; MUHF+Cl = 0.17+/−0.01, n = 8; HF+MetCl = 0.16+/−0.01; n = 8; MUHF+MetCl = 0.16+/−0.02, n = 8; p = 0.93).

In order to test the effects of Cl and Met in non-transplanted failing hearts, HF animals were randomly allocated to 4 treatment groups: (1) Cl 2 mg/kg/day, (2) Met 250 mg/kg/day, (3) combined Met+Cl treatment, (4) no drug treatment (HF+Cl, HF+Met, HF+MetCl and HF, respectively). Drug administration was via drinking water and osmotic minipump, exactly as described above. At the end of the treatment period *in vivo* heart function was measured via repeat TTE.

We have compared the effects of Met during mechanical unloading with those of ivabradine in a previously published study [22]. Therefore, we have included this data here for comparison with the effects of Cl and combined MetCl therapy. The data acquired from the Met group are contemporary and obtained in otherwise identical conditions to the data for the Cl and MetCl groups.

In-vivo assessment of heart rate. 4 animals per treatment group received implantable ECG telemetry transmitters (CA-F40 Data Sciences International, Minneapolis, MN) on day 0 of the 4 week treatment period, for *in vivo* HR and arrhythmia studies. Animals underwent continuous 24 hour ECG recording at weekly intervals during the treatment period. *In vivo* ECG recordings were acquired using Dataquest ART 3.1 software (Data Sciences International, Minneapolis, MN), and offline HR/arrhythmia analysis performed using ECG-Auto 2.4 software (EMKA, France).

Animal anaesthesia, analgesia and euthanasia. Adequacy of anaesthesia during all procedures was monitored by loss of reflexes, degree of muscle relaxation and respiration rate. Respiration rate and body temperature were monitored throughout all procedures and body temperature maintained at 37°C, via heating mat. Analgesia was provided by subcutaneous (SC) injection of vetergesic (buprenorphine), just prior to skin incision. For LCA ligation and implantation of telemetry device a single dose of 0.03 mg/kg was utilised, and for heterotopic abdominal heart transplant both the donor and recipient received a single dose of 0.05 mg/kg. Post-operative condition of the rats was monitored, and repeat SC injection administered as required (0.01–0.05 mg/kg) every 12 hours during the first week post-operative week. At the end of the 4 week treatment period animals were sacrificed via schedule 1 cervical dislocation. In each group, 4 hearts were utilised for acute cellular experiments, and 4 for histological analysis.

Cardiomyocyte studies

LV cardiomyocytes were isolated by standard enzymatic digestion for 8–10 minutes using collagenase (1 mg/ml, Worthington, USA) and hyaluronidase (0.6 mg/ml, Sigma, England) [19] and used within 6 h.

Assessment of sarcomere shortening and calcium handling. Simultaneous assessment of sarcomere shortening and Ca^{2+} handling in field stimulated cardiomyocytes was performed using an inverted microscope (TE 200), Ionoptix system (Ionoptix Corporation, USA) and the Ca^{2+} sensitive, single-excitation dual emission fluorescent dye Indo-1 AM (Molecular Probes, USA). In addition, sarcoplasmic reticulum (SR) Ca^{2+} uptake (SERCA) and sodium-calcium exchanger (NCX) contribution to Ca^{2+} extrusion were assessed using rapid caffeine application as previously described [19].

Assessment of electrophysiological parameters. Cells were studied using a MultiClamp 700A (Axon Instruments) in whole cell patch configuration. Current-voltage relationships for L-type Ca^{2+} current were studied and normalized to cell capacitance, as previously described [19].

Assessment of cell volume, t tubules and calcium sparks with confocal microscopy. Cell volume and t-tubule organisation were studied using the membrane binding dye di-8-Anepps (Molecular Probes, Eugene, OR, USA) and the Zeiss Axiovert microscope (Carl Zeiss, Oberkochen, Germany) with an LSM 510 confocal attachment. In addition, local changes in Ca^{2+} levels were assessed using the fluorescent dye Fluo-4 AM (Molecular Probes, USA) and the same confocal microscope as previously described [29].

Statistical analysis

Statistical comparison of data was performed using one-way analysis of variance followed by Bonferroni post-hoc test for individual significant differences, or Student's t-test where appropriate. All statistical analyses were performed using Prism 4 software (Graph-Pad Software, Inc.) and $P<0.05$ was considered significant. Data are expressed as mean ±SEM [n], where n is the number of cells unless otherwise specified. All of the experiments were performed using a minimum of four animals, unless otherwise stated.

Results

Heart rate

There was no difference in average HR between sham-operated and HF group at any time point (mean HR (bpm) at 4 weeks: sham 332±4.8 vs. HF 329±5.5; $P>0.05$). HR of transplanted failing hearts (MUHF) was significantly lower (~20%) than that of non-transplanted failing hearts at all time-points (**Figure 1A**). Cl caused a consistent increase in HR (~12%) at all time-points during MU, with Met either alone, or in combination with Cl reducing HR by approximately 15% (**Figure 1A**). Assessment of HR of non-transplanted failing hearts revealed similar drug effects: Cl caused a significant increase in HR (~10%) compared to HF group during first 3 weeks of therapy, but this effect was not present at week 4. Met caused significant and equivalent HR reduction (~20%) either alone, or in combination with Cl, compared to HF group at all-time points (**Figure 1B**).

LV function

LCA ligation induced LV dysfunction after 12 weeks (time of randomisation), characterised by reduced LVEF (%): sham 83.3±0.8 vs. HF 37.6±0.7; reduced LVFS (%): sham 48.3±0.7 vs. HF 16.6±0.5; and LV chamber dilatation (diastolic diameter (cm)): sham 0.60±0.03 vs. HF 0.98±0.04, $P<0.001$ for all parameters.

No difference in these parameters was detected between treatment groups prior to commencing therapy (**Figure 2A and B**). *In-vivo* function of transplanted failing hearts was not assessed, but that of non-transplanted hearts was assessed via repeat TTE at the end of the 4 week treatment period. Cl improved contractile function of non-transplanted failing hearts, and improvement in LVEF was enhanced further by combination with Met (**Figure 2A and B**). Met-induced increase in EF and FS was not statistically significant.

Cardiac and cardiomyocyte size

LCA ligation induced cardiac and cellular hypertrophy, shown by increased total HW, HW:BW ratio and cardiomyocyte volumes, compared to sham-operated group (**Table 1**). MU of failing hearts induced myocardial atrophy at whole heart and cardiomyocyte level, with both HW and cardiomyocyte volumes falling below those of sham values (**Figure 3A and B**). HW of MUHF group was ~40% smaller than that of HF group and ~17% smaller than sham, with cell volume being ~55% lower than in HF group and ~26% smaller than sham volumes. Cl had no effect on myocardial atrophy. Met prevented both whole heart and cellular atrophy, restoring mean HW and cardiomyocyte volumes to sham values, whilst combined MetCl therapy worsened MU-induced atrophy (**Figure 3A and B**).

In non-transplanted failing hearts Cl augmented cardiac hypertrophy, an effect that disappeared during combined MetCl therapy (**Figure 3C**). At a cellular level Met induced partial regression of cellular hypertrophy, but this effect was also lost during combined MetCl therapy (**Figure 3D**).

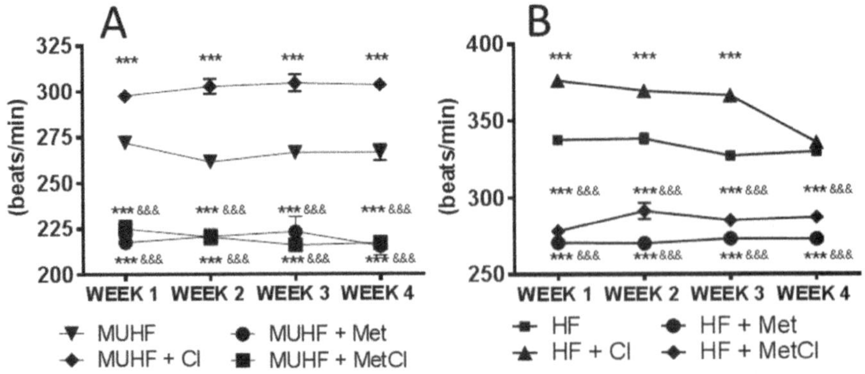

Figure 1. Average HR of mechanically unloaded failing hearts (MUHF) (A) and non-transplanted failing hearts (B) measured using telemetry devices (n = 4 per group). Cl increased HR significantly at all time-points during MU, whereas Met caused equal HR reduction either alone, or in combination with Cl at all time-points during MU. ***P<0.001 vs. MUHF and &&&P<0.001 vs. MUHF+Cl. Cl increased HR in-non-transplanted failing hearts significantly but this effect was lost at week 4. Met caused equal HR reduction in-non-transplanted failing hearts either alone, or in combination with Cl, at all time-points. ***P<0.001 vs. HF and &&&P<0.001 vs. HF+Cl.

Cardiomyocyte EC coupling

MU-induced recovery of deranged EC coupling. LCA ligation caused impaired cardiomyocyte contractility and deranged Ca^{2+} cycling: speed of sarcomeric contraction, relaxation and Ca^{2+} release, along with Ca^{2+} transient amplitude were all decreased, sarcomeric contraction amplitude remaining unchanged (**Figure 4 A–E**). MU normalised speed of sarcomeric contraction and this effect was further enhanced by Cl, with Met and MetCl therapy having no added effect (**Figure 4B**). MU partially improved speed of relaxation, and this effect was antagonised by Met, with no additional observed changes following Cl and MetCl treatment (**Figure 4C**). In addition, MU recovered Ca^{2+} transient amplitude, speed of Ca^{2+} release and SR Ca^{2+} content, and this recovery was further enhanced by both Cl and Met mono-therapy equally, but not by combined MetCl treatment (**Figure 4 D–F**).

An increased SR Ca^{2+} leak, secondary to altered RyR function, is one mechanism contributing to reduced SR Ca^{2+} load in HF [30]. Ca^{2+} sparks are complex entities regulated by multiple factors, and represent a measure of diastolic SR Ca^{2+} release [29]. Ca^{2+} spark frequency was increased in HF group compared to sham group suggesting increased SR Ca^{2+} leak ((sparks/100 μm/sec): sham 0.80±0.17 [37] vs. HF 3.00±0.34 [40]; P<0.001). MU normalised HF-induced increase in Ca^{2+} spark frequency (sparks/100 μm/sec): MUHF 0.82±0.13 [36] vs. HF 3.00±0.48 [40]; P< 0.001. This recovery was unaffected by either Cl or Met mono-

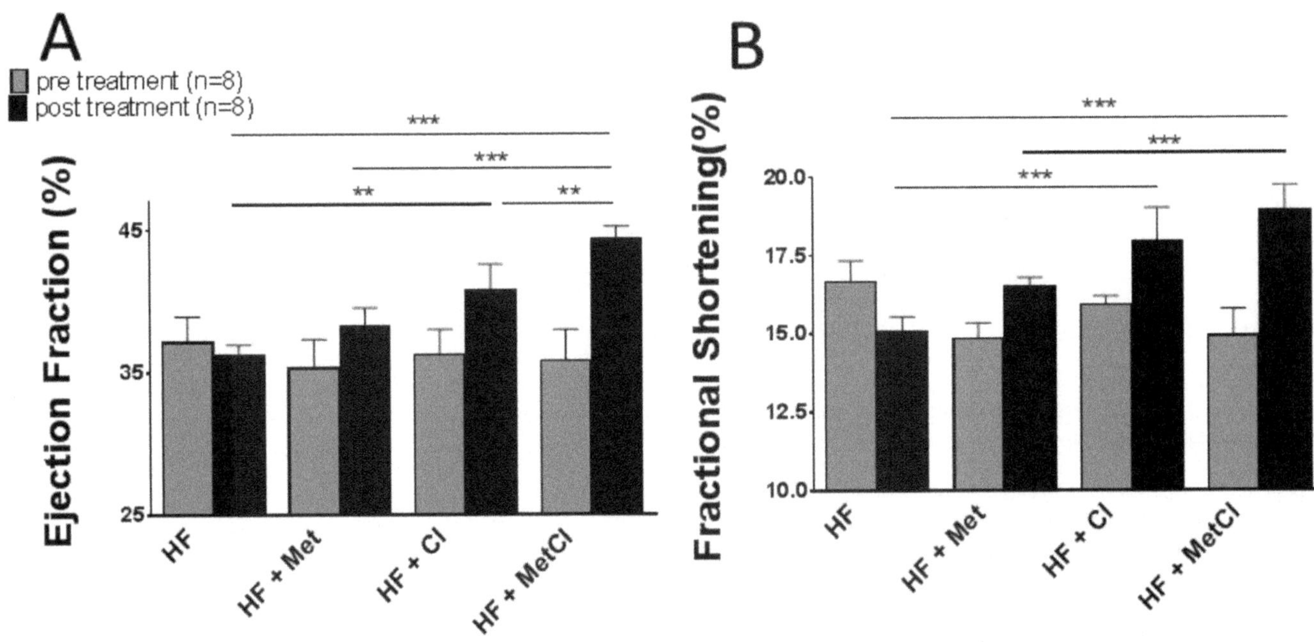

Figure 2. Effect of Cl, Met and combined MetCl therapy on contractile function in non-transplanted failing hearts, EF (A) and FS (B): No difference in baseline values in treatment groups was seen (light grey bars). Average values at end of treatment period are shown (black bars): Cl-treated group showed improved EF and FS compared to untreated HF group, and improvement in EF was further enhanced in MetCl group. Met-induced improvement in EF and FS was not statistically significant. ***P<0.001 (n = 8 per group).

Table 1. Anatomical and cell volume data (16 weeks after LCA ligation).

	Sham	HF
N	8	8
Body weight (g)	386±5.6	415±6.2**
Heart weight (g)	1.2±0.05	1.6±0.05***
Heart weight/Body weight ×1000	3.0±0.1	3.6±0.1***
Cell volume (μm^3)	36248±12012	59705±13508***

**P<0.01,
***P<0.001 vs. sham.

therapy, but abolished by combined MetCl therapy (sparks/100 μm/sec): MUHF+Cl 1.67±0.27 [35] vs. MUHF+Met [30] 1.70±0.26; P>0.05, both P>0.05 vs. MUHF, and P<0.001 vs. MUHF+MetCl [30] 3.51±0.36; P<0.001 vs. MUHF and P>0.05 vs. HF. MU also caused recovery of HF-induced depression of L-type Ca^{2+} current and t-tubule density (**Figure 5**). However, this recovery was largely antagonised by all three drug treatments; with only maintenance of L-type Ca^{2+} current recovery occurring in the combined MetCl-treated group (**Figure 5A and B**).

Effects of Cl and Met on deranged EC coupling in non-transplanted failing hearts. Met therapy, either alone or in combination with Cl normalised speed of sarcomeric contraction, relaxation and Ca^{2+} release, along with Ca^{2+} transient amplitude, while Cl mono-therapy displayed no effect (**Figure 6B–E**). Met, Cl and combined MetCl therapy all recovered SR Ca^{2+} content,

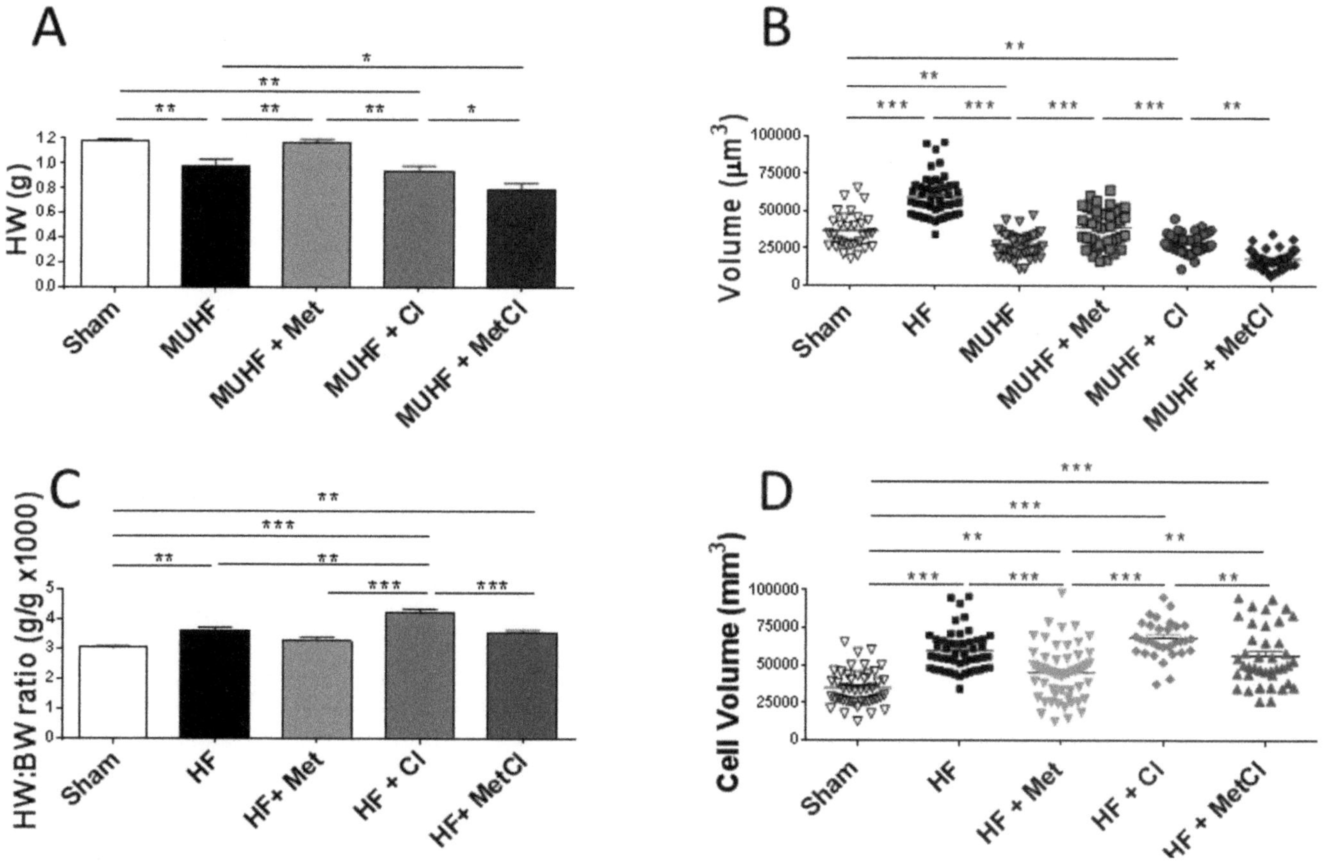

Figure 3. Effect of Cl, Met and combined MetCl treatment on heart weight (HW) (A) and cardiomyocyte volume measured using confocal microscopy (B) during unloading (MUHF). Prevention of MU-induced cardiac and cardiomyocyte atrophy is achieved by Met and not Cl, with combined MetCl therapy increasing atrophy. *P<0.05, **P<0.01 and ***P<0.001, (HW and cardiomyocyte volume data acquired from 8 and 4 hearts per group, respectively). Effect of Cl, Met and combined MetCl therapy on heart weight:body weight ratio (HW:BW) (C) and cardiomyocyte volume (D). HF-induced cardiac hypertrophy was enhanced by Cl therapy but this effect disappeared during combined MetCl therapy. HF-induced myocyte hypertrophy was partially attenuated by Met, but this effect was lost during combination MetCl therapy (HW and cardiomyocyte volume data acquired from 8 and 4 hearts per group, respectively).

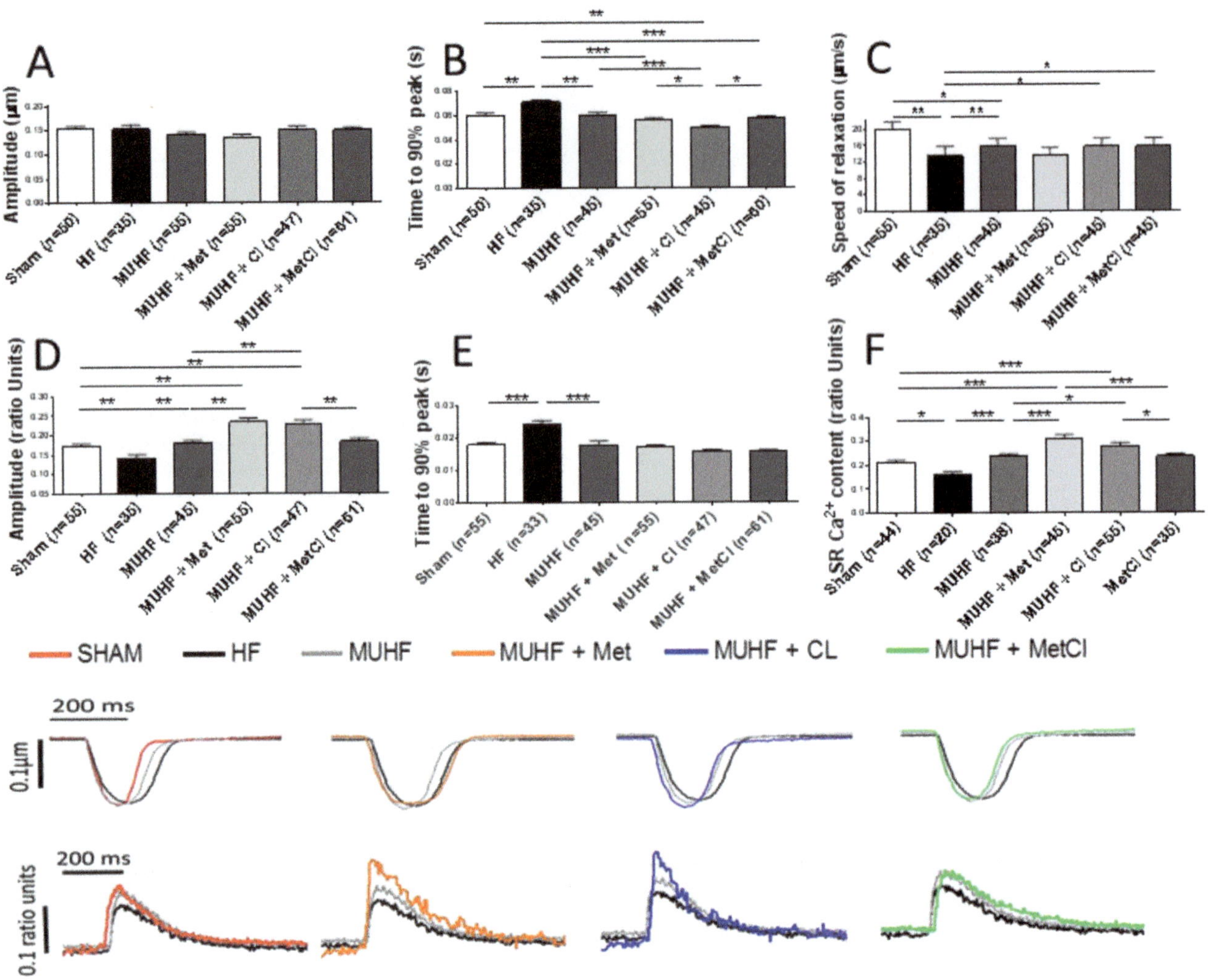

Figure 4. Effects of Cl, Met and MetCl therapy on cardiomyocyte contractility (A–C) and Ca^{2+} handling (D–F) during mechanical unloading (MUHF), measured using Indo-1 and Ionoptix system. Cl's enhancement of MU-induced recovery of speed of sarcomeric contraction (B) and Met's antagonism of MU-induced improvement in speed of relaxation (C) are shown. Cl and Met's enhancement of MU-induced recovery of Ca^{2+} transient amplitude (D), speed of Ca^{2+} release (E) and SR Ca^{2+} content (F), and lack of enhancement during combined MetCl therapy is shown. *$P<0.05$, **$P<0.01$ and ***$P<0.001$. Representative traces of sarcomeric contractions (G) and Ca^{2+} transients (H) are shown.

with the greatest improvement seen following Met therapy (**Figure 6F**). Cl alone caused significant reduction in spark frequency (HF+Cl 1.10±0.17 [30]; $P<0.01$ vs. HF), whereas spark frequency was no different to HF in the Met or MetCl-treated groups (HF+Met 2.10±0.22 [30] and HF+MetCl 2.00±0.32 [32], both groups $P>0.05$ vs. HF). Drug therapies had differing effects on L-type Ca^{2+} current and t-tubule density. HF-induced depression of both these parameters was normalised by Cl; Met therapy alone, or in combination with Cl showed no effect (**Figure 7**).

Discussion

In the first part of this study we showed that Met but *not* Cl prevented MU-induced myocardial atrophy, with combined MetCl therapy worsening atrophic remodelling. MU induced recovery of deranged EC coupling, with either Cl *or* Met mono-therapy, but *not* combined MetCl therapy, broadly enhancing this recovery. MU-induced recovery of Ca^{2+} transient amplitude, speed of Ca^{2+} release and SR Ca^{2+} content was enhanced by Cl *or* Met mono-therapy equally. However, these positive effects, together with Cl's enhancement of speed of sarcomeric contraction, were lost during combined MetCl therapy, along with MU-induced recovery of Ca^{2+} spark frequency.

The second part of this study showed combined β_2-AR stimulation (Cl) and β_1-AR blockade (Met) to improve depressed whole heart function in HF, to a greater degree than either mono-therapy. Cl's improvement in LVEF was enhanced by Met, but the mechanisms underlying this superiority appeared independent of cellular EC coupling. Met and Cl mono-therapy displayed distinct EC coupling effects. Met's effects were more favourable than those of Cl, with lack of evidence supporting additive or synergistic benefit, and more suggestive of selected antagonism during combined therapy. Met alone, and in combination with Cl normalised speed of sarcomeric contraction, relaxation, Ca^{2+} release and Ca^{2+} transient amplitude, and enhanced SR Ca^{2+} content; whereas Cl mono-therapy improved SR Ca^{2+} content to a lesser degree than Met, and normalised deranged Ca^{2+} spark frequency, L-type Ca^{2+} current and t-tubule density, positive effects that were lost during combined MetCl therapy. Of note,

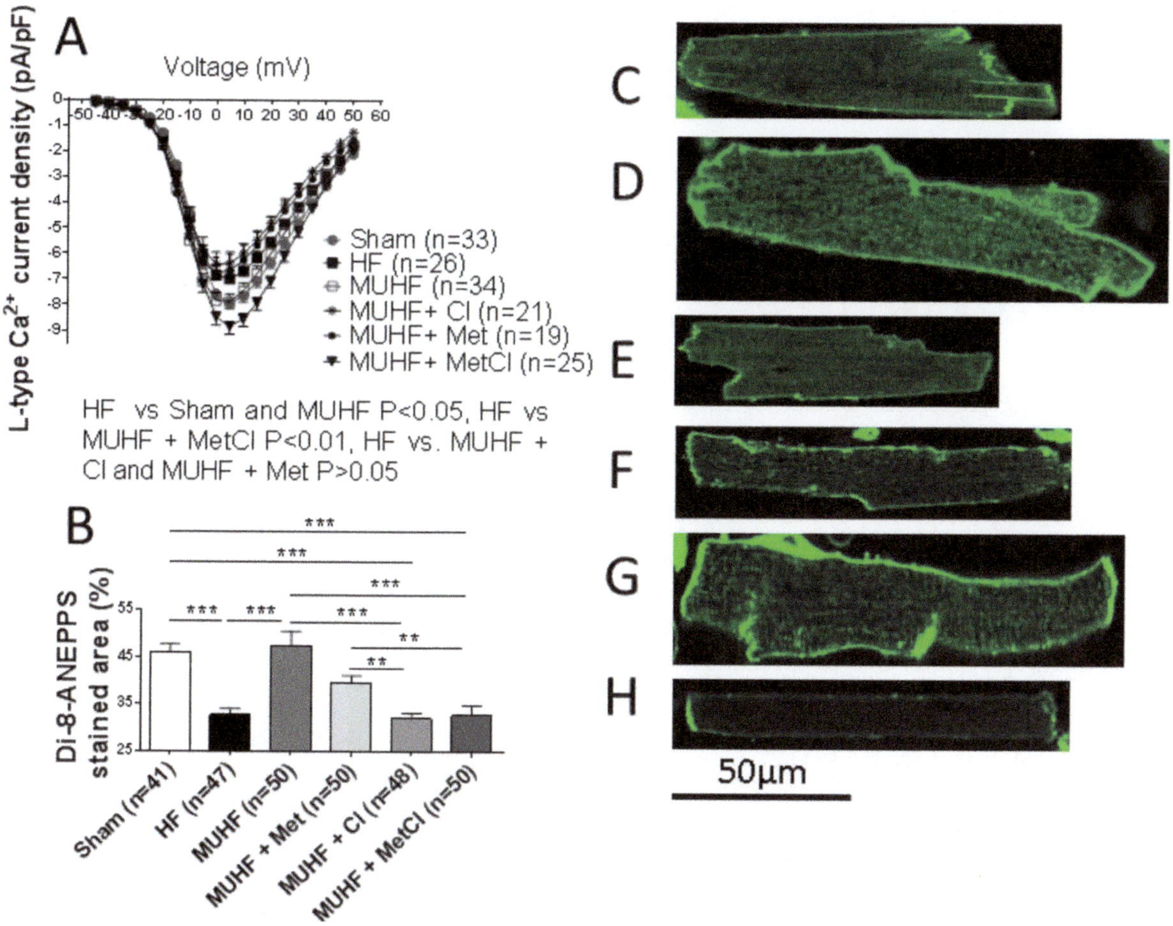

Figure 5. MU-induced recovery of depressed L-type Ca^{2+} current (A) and t-tubule density (B). Maintenance of L-type Ca^{2+} current recovery by combined MetCl therapy, and antagonism of such recovery by Cl or Met mono-therapy (A) is shown, along with antagonism of t-tubule density recovery by all treatments (B). *P<0.05, **P<0.01 and ***P<0.001. Representative di-8-Anepps stained cells from sham (C), HF (D), MUHF (E), MUHF+Cl (F), MUHF+Met (G) and MUHF+MetCl (H) groups are shown. Data for the Met group has been previously published [22] and added here for comparison.

undesirable Cl-induced hypertrophic/chronotropic effects were prevented during combined therapy.

These results suggest that A) Cl's success in enhancing functional recovery in LVAD-supported patients is unrelated to myocardial size, and reliant on positive EC coupling effects, B) combined β_2-AR stimulation +β_1-AR blockade is likely to be a safe and beneficial HF therapeutic pharmacological strategy and C) either the strategy of β_2-AR stimulation *or* β_1-AR blockade is likely to be superior to that of combined β_2-AR stimulation +β_1-AR blockade in enhancing functional recovery during LVAD support. This is, however, in contrast with the current clinical experience with β_1-AR blockade in patients with LVADs and could be explained by the type and degree of adverse remodelling obtained in our models. It cannot be excluded that subpopulations of LVAD patients with specific, lower degrees of dysfunction may benefit from this pharmacological treatment and more clinical studies are warranted.

Combined β_2-AR stimulation and β_1-AR blockade during mechanical unloading

Myocardial atrophy. LVAD-mediated unloading of failing ventricles regresses cardiac and cellular hypertrophy [8]. Whether such regression progresses during prolonged clinical LVAD support towards myocardial "atrophy" i.e. decreased cardiac and cell size to sub-normal values, remains controversial [31]. In contrast, convincing experimental data derived mainly from rodent studies employing HATx clearly demonstrate atrophy of normal [13,28] and failing [11] hearts. It must be emphasised that in this context atrophy relates to decreased size and not function.

A key question surrounding Cl is whether anti-atrophic properties contributed to enhanced recovery rates produced by the Harefield Protocol [18]. Findings of similar myocyte size in both explanted and non-recovered patients treated by this protocol, suggest Cl's pro-recovery effects were unrelated to myocardial size [17]. This present study reinforces this prospect. We show Cl to be ineffective in preventing myocardial atrophy associated with prolonged unloading (4 weeks), and this agrees with previous work [28] in non-failing rat hearts undergoing 2 weeks unloading. In contrast, we previously showed Cl to limit regression of rodent HF myocyte hypertrophy during short-term unloading (1 week) [19]. However, such a brief period of MU, during which atrophic remodelling is regarded as being sub-maximal [11,13] was considered inadequate, and a poor representation of prolonged clinical LVAD support.

As we have previously shown [22], Met prevented myocardial atrophy, but this effect was lost during combined MetCl therapy

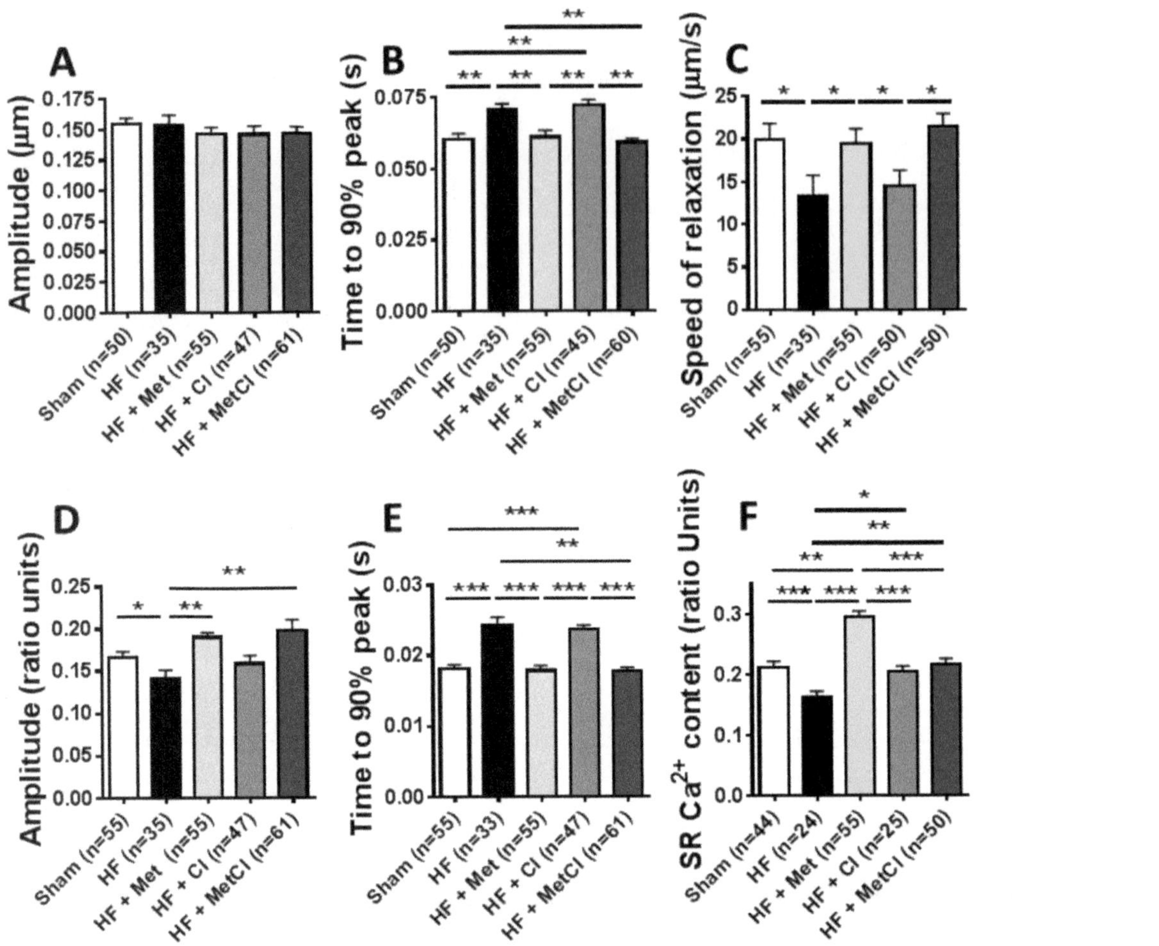

Figure 6. Effects of Cl, Met and MetCl therapy on cardiomyocyte contractility (A–C) and Ca^{2+} handling (D–F) from non-transplanted failing hearts, measured using Indo-1 and Ionoptix system are shown. Full recovery of speed of sarcomeric contraction (B), relaxation (C), Ca^{2+} transient amplitude (D) and speed of Ca^{2+} release (E) caused by Met therapy, either alone or in combination with Cl, and lack of improvement following Cl mono-therapy is shown. Superiority of Met mono-therapy in recovering depressed SR Ca^{2+} content is also shown (F). *$P<0.05$, **$P<0.01$ and ***$P<0.001$.

with actual worsening of atrophy. The latter observation is unexpected, if compared with the effects of the combined therapy in normally-loaded hearts; this can be due to additional detrimental consequences of mechanical unloading and require to be further studied. Atrophic remodelling is complex and the multiple pathways involved poorly defined [32]. The ubiquitin proteosome, calpain, lysosomal proteolysis and authophagy systems, and mTOR IGF-1/PI3K/AKT and ERK-1 pathways are all altered during MU [32]. These growth regulatory pathways, along with the TGF-β, CAMKII and calcineurin/NFAT hypertrophic signalling pathways, known components under β-AR influence [33], may represent Met's route of action, and augmentation of myocyte number (not assessed in this study) via regenerative mechanisms is another possibility. This finding is particularly important as, to date, no pharmacotherapy has proven effective in attenuating myocardial atrophy, with success via haemodynamic loading strategies alone [34], re-emphasising the critical importance of load in regulation of cardiac mass [13]. Such loading, potentially brought about by HR reduction and subsequent augmentation of LV filling, may have driven Met's anti-atrophic actions; but the lack of effect during combined MetCl therapy, despite an equivalent reduction in HR, makes this mechanism unlikely.

EC coupling during mechanical unloading. LVAD support induces reversal/alteration in expression and function of numerous Ca^{2+} handling elements adversely remodelled during HF. Recovery of SR Ca^{2+} content, L-type Ca^{2+} current fast inactivation and Ca^{2+} transient amplitude is seen [35], and these parameters show positive correlation with functional recovery in patients treated with the Harefield Protocol [17]. LVAD-induced enhanced SERCA 2A expression [36] and stabilisation of RyR function [37] are potentially involved mechanisms.

In the present study, MU recovered HF-induced deranged EC coupling with normalisation of Ca^{2+} transient amplitude, speed of Ca^{2+} release and sarcomeric contraction, SR Ca^{2+} content, Ca^{2+} spark frequency, L-type Ca^{2+} current amplitude and t-tubule density. Drug effects on this recovery were not clear-cut but overall, the positive effects of either mono-therapy disappeared during combined therapy. MU-induced recovery of Ca^{2+} transient amplitude, speed of Ca^{2+} release and SR Ca^{2+} content, proven markers of recovery during LVAD support [17], were equally enhanced by Cl and Met mono-therapy, with Cl also enhancing speed of sarcomeric contraction. These effects were lost during

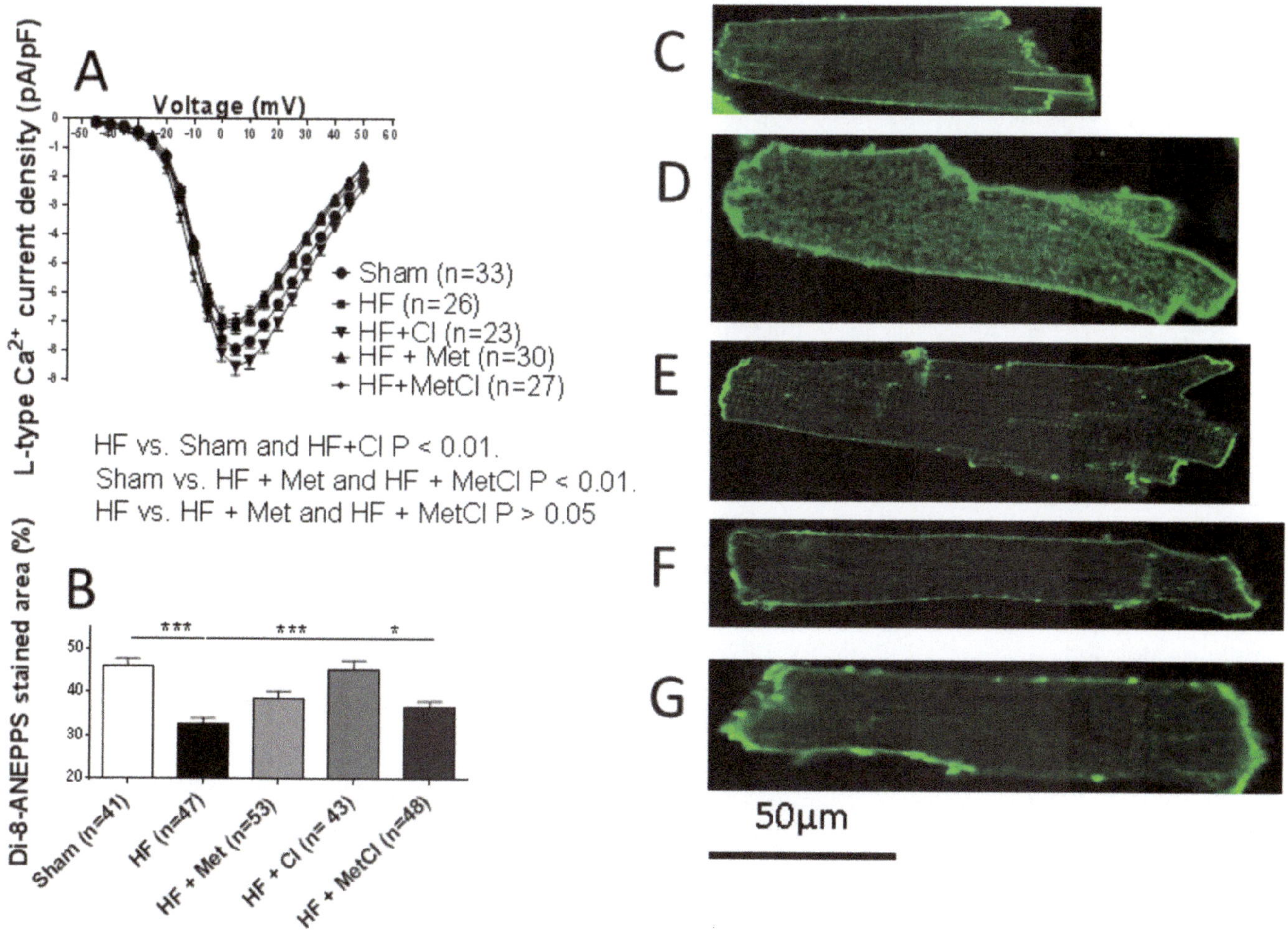

Figure 7. Full recovery of HF-induced depression of L-type Ca^{2+} current (A) and t-tubule density (B) caused by Cl, and lack of improvement in these parameters following Met and MetCl therapy are shown. ***$P<0.001$. Representative di-8-Anepps stained cells from sham (C), HF (D), HF+Cl (E), HF+Met (F) and HF+MetCl (G) groups. Data for the Met group has been previously published [22] and added here for comparison.

combined therapy along with MU-induced recovery of RyR function (normalised Ca^{2+} spark frequency).

Cl's effects may originate from improved myofilament sensitivity [19] and SERCA2a expression [28] previously shown during MU. MU is associated with increased β_2-AR mRNA expression [21] and adenoviral mediated β_2-AR overexpression with improved function following MU [38]. These findings, coupled with results from our study, re-enforce the rationale for the use of Cl/ β_2-AR agonists during LVAD support. Specific study of β_1-AR blockade during MU is lacking. Hence, mechanisms driving Met's effects are speculative. Enhancement of MU-induced recovery of β-AR responsiveness [35] and/or RyR and SERCA/phospholamban function/phosphorylation/expression [36,37], proven actions of β-blockers in non-unloaded failing myocardium [4] may be involved. Despite mainly beneficial effects during MU, the antagonism of L-type Ca^{2+} current and t-tubule density recovery highlight potentially unwanted effects of Cl and Met, the significance of which requires further investigation.

Combined β_1-AR blockade and β_2-AR stimulation in heart failure

β-adrenergic signalling. Deranged β-adrenergic signalling is instrumental in HF pathogenesis [4]. Selective down-regulation/ de-sensitisation of β_1-ARs promotes relative augmentation of β_2: β_1-ARs ratio and signalling [4,39]. Down-regulation of β_1-AR signalling is thought protective against heightened sympathetic stimulation, and the clinical efficacy of β_1-AR blockade is proven [4,6,23].

Augmented β_2-AR signalling is also considered cardio-protective [24], and the idea that β_2-AR agonism may be beneficial in clinical HF is long-standing [40], but remains controversial and poorly studied in humans. Undesirable β_2-AR agonist effects such as elevation of HR and arrhythmia risk shown by certain studies [41,42], along with fears over increasing LV mass, both independent prognostic risk factors in cardiac disease [43,44] tempered enthusiasm for using β_2-AR agonists in HF therapy. These factors, coupled with expanding evidence supporting β-blocker efficacy [4,6,23], and the phenomenon of β_2-AR agonist tachyphylaxis, rendered the notion of therapeutic β_2-AR agonism illogical and unsound. Hence, little clinical data exists regarding

β_2-AR agonist administration within this context, with data derived from a few small, non-randomised studies in HF patients [45–46] and chronic lung disease patients with HF, receiving β_2-AR agonist therapy [42,47]. Results are unclear, showing both sustained [42,45] and transient [46] improvements in cardiac function, as well as negative functional effects [47].

This study re-enforces the concept that β_2-AR agonism represents a beneficial HF therapeutic strategy, albeit alongside that of clinically proven β_1-AR blockade [24]. Cl's undesirable effects of cardiac hypertrophy and tachycardia were inhibited by Met with no evidence of pro-arrhythmic behaviour (**Figure S1 in Methods S1**). Combined MetCl therapy displayed superior improvement in whole heart systolic function to either mono-therapy, although a cellular mechanism explaining this superiority was not apparent. Met and Cl showed different positive EC coupling effects with evidence of selected antagonism rather than synergy. Met's improvement of cellular contraction, relaxation, Ca^{2+} release, Ca^{2+} transient amplitude, and SR Ca^{2+} was not enhanced by Cl. T-tubule disruption uncouples the normally tight relationship between L-type Ca^{2+} channels and RyRs, reducing EC coupling efficiency [48]. Cl improved this coupling shown by recovery of L-type Ca^{2+} current and t-tubule density, along with RyR function (normalised Ca^{2+} spark frequency). Such improvements appeared not to alter cellular contractility, but were abolished by Met.

Additive anti-apoptotic effects of either Cl [20] or fenoterol [24] in combination with Met, demonstrated by previous rodent HF studies [20,24] may be responsible for the whole heart functional effects. Such a mechanism is plausible, as opposing actions of the two β-adrenergic signalling pathways on cell survival is recognised; β_1-AR signalling broadly promoting apoptosis [25] and β_2-AR signalling driving improved myocyte viability [26,27]. Restoration of Ca^{2+} handling protein expression e.g SERCA2a or RyR [18,20], myo-filament sensitivity [19] and myocardial stiffness/diastolic function [49] represent other properties of Cl and Met, that may underpin the augmented function seen during combined therapy; and afterload (blood pressure (BP)) reduction is another. However, at similar doses to those used in this study, chronic Met [20,50], Cl [20] or combined therapy [20] has not been seen to significantly alter BP. β_2-AR agonist tachyphylaxis is recognised following chronic administration [24,45]. Temporal functional effects were not assessed in this study, and whether tachyphylaxis occurred is unknown. The loss of Cl's chronotropic effect at week 4 suggests it may have done. In a longer rodent HF study (1 year), Met was shown to prevent β_2-AR agonist (fenoterol) tachyphylaxis (caused by decreased β_2-AR density), producing extension of fenoterol's positive functional effects. Such a process may also explain the findings from our, albeit shorter study.

Conclusions

In conclusion, our study shows that Met but not Cl prevented MU-induced myocardial atrophy, with atrophic worsening during combined therapy. Cl and Met broadly enhanced MU-induced recovery of deranged EC coupling, but this enhancement was lost during combined therapy. These results suggest that A) Cl's success in enhancing functional recovery in LVAD-supported patients is unrelated to myocardial size and reliant on positive EC coupling effects and B) either the strategy of β_2-AR stimulation *or* β_1-AR blockade is likely to be superior to that of combined β_2-AR stimulation $+\beta_1$-AR blockade in enhancing functional recovery during LVAD support. Such findings warrant further investigation.

In the second part of this study, we show for the first time in a model of established rodent HF that combined β_2-AR simulation (Cl) $+\beta_1$-AR blockade (Met) displays superior functional effects to either mono-therapy, and undesirable Cl-induced hypertrophic/chronotropic effects are prevented by Met. Mechanisms underlying this superiority appeared independent of cellular EC coupling and require further investigation. These results suggest that this pharmacological strategy is likely to be safe and beneficial in HF therapy.

Limitations

Met was used in this study to facilitate comparison with previous studies using this rodent HF model. Bisoprolol and not Met is used in the Harefield Protocol. As such, findings from this study may not be directly applicable to this specific clinical scenario.

Supporting Information

Methods S1 A detailed description of Material and Methods is provided. The file also contains Figure S1 showing the ventricular ectopic (VE) rate in sham, failing and treated failing hearts.

Author Contributions

Conceived and designed the experiments: MN US MI AS AG CVD PK CT GS MY. Performed the experiments: MN US MI AS AG CVD PK CT GS MY. Analyzed the data: MN US MI AS AG CVD PK CT GS MY. Contributed reagents/materials/analysis tools: MN US MI AS AG CVD PK CT GS MY. Wrote the paper: MN MI US.

References

1. Kirklin JK, Naftel DC, Kormos RL, Stevenson LW, Pagani FD, et al. (2011) Third INTERMACS Annual Report: the evolution of destination therapy in the United States. J Heart Lung Transplant 30:115–123. doi: 10.1016/j.healun.2010.12.001.
2. Mancini DM, Beniaminovitz A, Levin H, Catanese K, Flannery M, et al. (1998) Low incidence of myocardial recovery after left ventricular assist device implantation in patients with chronic heart failure. Circulation 98:2383–2389. doi: 10.1161/01.CIR.98.22.2383.
3. Maybaum S, Mancini D, Xydas S, Starling RC, Aaronson K, et al. (2007) Cardiac improvement during mechanical circulatory support: a prospective multicenter study of the LVAD Working Group. Circulation 115:2497–2505. doi: 10.1161/CIRCULATIONAHA.106.633180.
4. Bristow MR (2011) Treatment of chronic heart failure with beta-adrenergic receptor antagonists: a convergence of receptor pharmacology and clinical cardiology. Circ Res 109:1176–1194. doi: 10.1161/CIRCRESAHA.111.245092.
5. Colucci WS, Packer M, Bristow MR, Gilbert EM, Cohn JN, et al. (1996) Carvedilol inhibits clinical progression in patients with mild symptoms of heart failure, US Carvedilol Heart Failure Study Group. Circulation 94:2800–2806. doi: 10.1161/01.CIR.94.11.2800.
6. Lechat P, Escolano S, Golmard JL, Lardoux H, Witchitz S, et al. (1997) Prognostic value of bisoprolol-induced hemodynamic effects in heart failure during the Cardiac Insufficiency BIsoprolol Study (CIBIS). Circulation. 96:2197–2205. doi: 10.1161/01.CIR.96.7.2197.
7. St John SM, Pfeffer MA, Plappert T, Rouleau JL, Moye LA, et al. (1994) Quantitative two-dimensional echocardiographic measurements are major predictors of adverse cardiovascular events after acute myocardial infarction. The protective effects of captopril. Circulation 89:68–75. doi: 10.1161/01.CIR.89.1.68.
8. Margulies KB (2002) Reversal mechanisms of left ventricular remodeling: lessons from left ventricular assist device experiments. J Card Fail 8:S500–S505. doi:10.1054/jcaf.2002.129264.
9. Klotz S, Jan Danser AH, Burkhoff D (2008) Impact of left ventricular assist device (LVAD) support on the cardiac reverse remodeling process. Prog Biophys Mol Biol 97:479–496. doi: 10.1016/j.pbiomolbio.2008.02.002.

10. Yacoub MH, Tansley P, Birks EJ, Banner NR, Khaghani A, et al. (2001) A novel combination therapy to reverse end-stage heart failure. Transplant Proc 33:2762–2764. doi: 2132/jtrans.proc.2001.1321.
11. Oriyanhan W, Tsuneyoshi H, Nishina T, Matsuoka S, Ikeda T, et al. (2007) Determination of optimal duration of mechanical unloading for failing hearts to achieve bridge to recovery in a rat heterotopic heart transplantation model. J Heart Lung Transplant 26:16–23. doi:10.1016/j.healun.2006.10.016.
12. Ito K, Nakayama M, Hasan F, Yan X, Schneider MD, et al. (2003) Contractile reserve and calcium regulation are depressed in myocytes from chronically unloaded hearts. Circulation 107:1176–1182. doi: 10.1161/01.CIR.000005 1463.72137.96.
13. Korecky B, Masika M (1991) Use of heterotopically isotransplanted rat heart to study the effect of load on cardiac mass. J Cardiovasc Pharmacol 17 Suppl 2:S105. doi: 17.1314/JCardPh.12123.
14. Birks EJ, Tansley PD, Hardy J, George RS, Bowles CT, et al. (2006) Left ventricular assist device and drug therapy for the reversal of heart failure. N Engl J Med 355:1873–1884. doi: 10.1056/NEJMoa053063.
15. Birks EJ, George RS, Hedger M, Bahrami T, Wilton P, et al. (2011) Reversal of severe heart failure with a continuous-flow left ventricular assist device and pharmacological therapy: a prospective study. Circulation 123:381–390. doi: 10.1161/CIRCULATIONAHA.109.933960.
16. Wong K, Boheler KR, Bishop J, Petrou M, Yacoub MH (1998) Clenbuterol induces cardiac hypertrophy with normal functional, morphological and molecular features. Cardiovasc Res 37:115–122. doi: 10.1016/S0008-6363(97)00190-9.
17. Terracciano CM, Hardy J, Birks EJ, Khaghani A, Banner NR, et al. (2004) Clinical recovery from end-stage heart failure using left-ventricular assist device and pharmacological therapy correlates with increased sarcoplasmic reticulum calcium content but not with regression of cellular hypertrophy. Circulation 109:2263–2265. doi: 10.1161/01.CIR.0000129233.51320.92.
18. Soppa GK, Smolenski RT, Latif N, Yuen AH, Malik A, et al. (2005) Effects of chronic administration of clenbuterol on function and metabolism of adult rat cardiac muscle. Am J Physiol Heart Circ Physiol 288:H1468–H1476. doi: 10.1152/ajpheart.00624.2004.
19. Soppa GK, Lee J, Stagg MA, Felkin LE, Barton PJ, et al. (2008) Role and possible mechanisms of clenbuterol in enhancing reverse remodelling during mechanical unloading in murine heart failure. Cardiovasc Res 77:695–706. doi: 10.1093/cvr/cvm106. Epub 2008 Jan 4.
20. Xydas S, Kherani AR, Chang JS, Klotz S, Hay I, et al. (2006) Beta(2)-Adrenergic stimulation attenuates left ventricular remodeling, decreases apoptosis, and improves calcium homeostasis in a rodent model of ischemic cardiomyopathy. J Pharmacol Exp Ther 317:553–561. doi: 10.1124/jpet.105.099432.
21. Tsuneyoshi H, Oriyanhan W, Kanemitsu H, Shiina R, Nishina T, et al. (2005) Heterotopic transplantation of the failing rat heart as a model of left ventricular mechanical unloading toward recovery. ASAIO J 51:116–120. doi: 10.1097/01.MAT.0000150325.05589.8B.
22. Navaratnarajah M, Ibrahim M, Siedlecka U, Van Doorn C, Shah A, et al. (2013) Influence of ivabradine on reverse remodelling during mechanical unloading. Cardiovasc Res 97:230–239. doi: 10.1093/cvr/cvs318.
23. Waagstein F, Bristow MR, Swedberg K, Camerini F, Fowler MB, et al. (1993) Beneficial effects of metoprolol in idiopathic dilated cardiomyopathy. Metoprolol in Dilated Cardiomyopathy (MDC) Trial Study Group. Lancet 342:1441–1446. doi: 11.321.lanc/1993.21.
24. Ahmet I, Krawczyk M, Zhu W, Woo AY, Morrell C, et al. (2008) Cardioprotective and survival benefits of long-term combined therapy with beta2 adrenoreceptor (AR) agonist and beta1 AR blocker in dilated cardiomyopathy postmyocardial infarction. J Pharmacol Exp Ther 325:491–499. doi: 10.1124/jpet.107.135335.
25. Zheng M, Zhu W, Han Q, Xiao RP (2005) Emerging concepts and therapeutic implications of beta-adrenergic receptor subtype signaling. Pharmacol Ther 108:257–268. doi:10.1016/j.pharmthera.2005.04.006.
26. Zhu WZ, Zheng M, Koch WJ, Lefkowitz RJ, Kobilka BK, et al. (2001) Dual modulation of cell survival and cell death by beta(2)-adrenergic signaling in adult mouse cardiac myocytes. *Proc* Natl Acad Sci U S A 98:1607–1612. doi: 10.1073/pnas.98.4.1607.
27. Zhu WZ, Wang SQ, Chakir K, Yang D, Zhang T, et al. (2003) Linkage of beta1-adrenergic stimulation to apoptotic heart cell death through protein kinase A-independent activation of Ca2+/calmodulin kinase II. J Clin Invest 111:617–625. doi:10.1172/JCI16326.
28. Tsuneyoshi H, Oriyanhan W, Kanemitsu H, Shiina R, Nishina T, et al. (2005) Does the beta2-agonist clenbuterol help to maintain myocardial potential to recover during mechanical unloading? Circulation 112:I51–I56. doi: 10.1161/CIRCULATIONAHA.104.525097.
29. Ibrahim M, Al Masri A, Navaratnarajah M, Siedlecka U, Soppa GK, et al. (2010) Prolonged mechanical unloading affects cardiomyocyte excitation-contraction coupling, transverse-tubule structure, and the cell surface. FASEB J 24:3321–3329. doi: 10.1096/fj.10-156638.
30. Bers DM (2006) Altered cardiac myocyte Ca regulation in heart failure. Physiology. (*Bethesda*) 21:380–387. doi: 10.1152/physiol.00019.2006.
31. Drakos SG, Kfoury AG, Hammond EH, Reid BB, Revelo MP, et al. (2010) Impact of mechanical unloading on microvasculature and associated central remodeling features of the failing human heart. J Am Coll Cardiol 56:382–391. doi: 10.1016/j.jacc.2010.04.019.
32. Baskin KK, Taegtmeyer H (2011) Taking pressure off the heart: the ins and outs of atrophic remodelling. Cardiovasc Res 90:243–250. doi: 10.1093/cvr/cvr06.
33. Zhao M, Fajardo G, Urashima T, Spin JM, Poorfarahani S, et al. (2011) Cardiac pressure overload hypertrophy is differentially regulated by {beta}-adrenergic receptor subtypes. Am J Physiol Heart Circ Physiol 301:H1461–H1470. doi: 10.1152/ajpheart.00453.2010.
34. Wang J, Marui A, Ikeda T, Komeda M (2008) Partial left ventricular unloading reverses contractile dysfunction and helps recover gene expressions in failing rat hearts. Interact Cardiovasc Thorac Surg 7(1):27–31. doi: 10.1510/icvts.2007.165563.
35. Dipla K, Mattiello JA, Jeevanandam V, Houser SR, Margulies KB (1998) Myocyte recovery after mechanical circulatory support in humans with end-stage heart failure. Circulation 97:2316–2322. doi: 10.1161/01.CIR.97.23.2316.
36. Heerdt PM, Holmes JW, Cai B, Barbone A, Madigan JD, et al. (2000) Chronic unloading by left ventricular assist device reverses contractile dysfunction and alters gene expression in end-stage heart failure. Circulation. 2000 102:2713–2719. doi: 10.1161/01.CIR.102.22.2713.
37. Marx SO, Reiken S, Hisamatsu Y, Gaburjakova M, Gaburjakova J, et al. (2001) Phosphorylation-dependent regulation of ryanodine receptors: a novel role for leucine/isoleucine zippers. J Cell Biol 153:699–708. doi: 10.1083/jcb.153.4.699.
38. Tevaearai HT, Eckhart AD, Walton GB, Keys JR, Wilson K, et al. (2002) Myocardial gene transfer and overexpression of beta2-adrenergic receptors potentiates the functional recovery of unloaded failing hearts. Circulation 106:124–129. doi: 10.1161/01.CIR.0000020220.79105.FD.
39. Brodde OE (1991) Beta 1- and beta 2-adrenoceptors in the human heart: properties, function, and alterations in chronic heart failure. Pharmacol Rev 43:203–242. doi: 6.43.PhRev/5321.
40. Irmer M, Wollschlager H, Just H (1981) Treatment of severe congestive heart failure with the beta-agonist fenoterol (author's transl). Klinn Wochenschr 59:639–645. doi: 54.32111.KLW.1.
41. Dawson JR, Bayliss J, Norell MS, Canepa-Anson R, Kuan P, et al. (1982) Clinical studies with beta 2 adrenoceptor agonists in heart failure. Eur Heart J 3:135–141. doi: 32.3121/eurheartj/ehn421.
42. Matera MG, Martuscelli E, Cazzola M (2010) Pharmacological modulation of beta-adrenoceptor function in patients with coexisting chronic obstructive pulmonary disease and chronic heart failure. Pulm Pharmacol Ther 23:1–8. doi: 10.1016/j.pupt.2009.10.001.
43. Kolloch R, Legler UF, Champion A, Cooper-Dehoff RM, Handberg E, et al. (2008) Impact of resting heart rate on outcomes in hypertensive patients with coronary artery disease: findings from the INternational VErapamil-SR/trandolapril STudy (INVEST). Eur Heart J 29:1327–1334. doi: 10.1093/eurheartj/ehn123.
44. Levy D, Garrison RJ, Savage DD, Kannel WB, Castelli WP (1990) Prognostic implications of echocardiographically determined left ventricular mass in the Framingham Heart Study. N Engl J Med 322:1561–1566. doi: 10.1056/NEJM199005313222203.
45. Awan NA, Needham K, Evenson MK, Hermanovich J, Joye JA, et al. (1981) Therapeutic efficacy or oral pirbuterol in severe chronic congestive heart failure: acute hemodynamic and long-term ambulatory evaluation. Am Heart J 102:555–563. PMID: 7270402.
46. Colucci WS, Alexander RW, Mudge GH, Rude RE, Holman BL, et al. (1981) Acute and chronic effects of pirbuterol on left ventricular ejection fraction and clinical status in severe congestive heart failure. Am Heart J 102: 564–568. PMID: 6115573.
47. Au DH, Udris EM, Fan VS, Curtis JR, McDonell MB, et al. (2003) Risk of mortality and heart failure exacerbations associated with inhaled beta-adrenoceptor agonists among patients with known left ventricular systolic dysfunction. Chest 123:1964–1969. doi:10.1378/chest.123.6.1964.
48. Song LS, Sobie EA, McCulle S, Lederer WJ, Balke CW, et al. (2006) Orphaned ryanodine receptors in the failing heart. Proc Natl Acad Sci U S A 103:4305–4310. doi: 10.1073/pnas.0509324103.
49. Hon JK, Steendijk P, Petrou M, Wong K, Yacoub MH (2001) Influence of clenbuterol treatment during six weeks of chronic right ventricular pressure overload as studied with pressure-volume analysis. J Thorac Cardiovasc Surg 22:767–774. doi:10.1067/mtc.2001.114354.
50. Wei S, Chow LT, Sanderson JE (2000) Effect of carvedilol in comparison with metoprolol on myocardial collagen postinfarction. J Am Coll Cardiol 36:276–281. doi.org/10.1016/S0735-1097(00)00671-9.

6

Circulating Levels of Tumor Necrosis Factor-Alpha Receptor 2 Are Increased in Heart Failure with Preserved Ejection Fraction Relative to Heart Failure with Reduced Ejection Fraction: Evidence for a Divergence in Pathophysiology

Brendan N. Putko[1,2], Zuocheng Wang[1,2], Jennifer Lo[1,2], Todd Anderson[3], Harald Becher[1,2], Jason R. B. Dyck[2,4], Zamaneh Kassiri[2,5], Gavin Y. Oudit[1,2]*, on behalf of the Alberta HEART Investigators

1 Division of Cardiology, Department of Medicine, University of Alberta, Edmonton, Alberta, Canada, **2** Mazankowski Alberta Heart Institute, University of Alberta, Edmonton, Alberta, Canada, **3** Libin Cardiovascular Institute, University of Calgary, Calgary, Alberta, Canada, **4** Department of Pediatrics, University of Alberta, Edmonton, Alberta, Canada, **5** Department of Physiology, University of Alberta, Edmonton, Alberta, Canada

Abstract

Background: Various pathways have been implicated in the pathogenesis of heart failure (HF) with preserved ejection fraction (HFPEF). Inflammation in response to comorbid conditions, such as hypertension and diabetes, may play a proportionally larger role in HFPEF as compared to HF with reduced ejection fraction (HFREF).

Methods and Results: This study investigated inflammation mediated by the tumor necrosis factor-alpha (TNFα) axis in community-based cohorts of HFPEF patients (n = 100), HFREF patients (n = 100) and healthy controls (n = 50). Enzyme-linked immunosorbent assays were used to investigate levels of TNFα, its two receptors (TNFR1 and TNFR2), and a non-TNFα cytokine, interleukin-6 (IL-6), in plasma derived from peripheral blood samples. Plasma levels of TNFα and TNFR1 were significantly elevated in HFPEF relative to controls, while levels of TNFR2 were significantly higher in HFPEF than both controls and HFREF. TNFα, TNFR1 and TNFR2 were each significantly associated with at least two of the following: age, estimated glomerular filtration rate, hypertension, diabetes, smoking, peripheral vascular disease or history of atrial fibrillation. TNFR2 levels were also significantly associated with increasing grade of diastolic dysfunction and severity of symptoms in HFPEF.

Conclusions: Inflammation mediated through TNFα and its receptors, TNFR1 and TNFR2, may represent an important component of a comorbidity-induced inflammatory response that partially drives the pathophysiology of HFPEF.

Editor: John Calvert, Emory University, United States of America

Funding: This work was funded by the Canadian Institutes of Health Research, MOP-86602, http://www.cihr-irsc.gc.ca/e/193.html. The funders had no role in study design, data collection and analysis, decision to publish, or preparation of the manuscript.

Competing Interests: The authors have declared that no competing interests exist.

* E-mail: gavin.oudit@ualberta.ca

Introduction

Heart failure (HF) continues to have a significant clinical burden with a high mortality and morbidity, and has a worse one-year prognosis than cancer [1]. There are several classification schemes in HF; however, a common clinical approach involves classifying ambulatory patients with chronic HF into HF with preserved (≥ 50%) or reduced left-ventricular ejection fraction (<50%; HFPEF or HFREF, respectively) [1,2]. HFPEF presently accounts for approximately 40% of HF diagnoses, with a rising incidence, and mortality and morbidity comparable to HFREF [3–5]. Despite similarities in outcomes, it appears that HFPEF and HFREF represent distinct groups, with many pathophysiological differences, along the continuum of the HF [6]. Indeed, differential responses to therapeutic interventions between these two groups strongly support this concept. Clinical trials have validated angiotensin-converting enzyme inhibitors (ACEi), angiotensin II-receptor blockers (ARB), beta-adrenergic receptor antagonists (beta-blockers) and mineralocorticoid receptor antagonists (MRA) as therapeutics in HFREF [1]. Conversely, trials of ACEi, ARB, beta-blockers, MRA and phosphodiesterase-5 inhibitor failed to show any consistent and significant improvement in the clinical outcomes of patients with HFPEF.

Biomarker studies have differentially implicated various pathways in HF, including fibrosis and extracellular matrix remodeling, oxidative and cardiomyocyte stress, and inflammation [7–12]. A recent report showed that circulating tumor necrosis factor-alpha (TNFα) receptor 1 (TNFR1) levels are significant predictors of incident HF, in particular for HFPEF versus HFREF [13]. Circulating TNFα and its two receptors (TNFR1 and TNFR2) are elevated in patients with heart failure relative to controls [6,14]. The study presented herein expands on previous work by exploring associations between diastolic dysfunction or heart failure severity, and plasma levels of TNFα, TNFR1 and TNFR2, as well as a non-TNFα family cytokine, interleukin-6 (IL-6), in community-based cohorts of healthy controls, and ambulatory HFPEF and HFREF patients. Using well-defined HF cohorts, we set out to elucidate some elements of the mechanisms that drive HFPEF and HFREF. Our novel findings suggest that elevated plasma levels of TNFα receptors, in particular TNFR2, are more closely linked to the pathophysiology of HFPEF than HFREF.

Methods

Ethics statement

This study conforms with the conventions outlined in the Declaration of Helsinki, it received internal ethics board approval at the Universities of Alberta and Calgary for use of human subjects, and all subjects gave written informed consent [15].

Patient recruitment and baseline analysis

As part of a prospective clinical study, the Alberta HEART (Heart Failure Etiology and Analysis Research Team) project, community-based, ambulatory patients with clinical diagnoses of HF and healthy age- and gender-matched controls (n = 50) were consecutively recruited for comprehensive clinical, echocardiographic and biomarker analyses during a three-year period beginning in 2010 through the end of 2012. Blood pressure was recorded sitting or recumbent, and detailed clinical data were compiled at the time of enrollment. Transthoracic echocardiograms were performed using the Phillips IE33 ultrasound platform. Echocardiograms were interpreted by cardiologists with specialized echocardiography training who were blinded to both the clinical classification and biomarker analyses. LVEF was assessed using Simpson's biplane method of disks. HF patients were adjudicated as HFREF (n = 100) or HFPEF (n = 100) using an LVEF cutoff of 50%, according to clinical practice guidelines [1,2]. Adjudication of New York Heart Association (NYHA) functional class and primary etiology of HF were determined by cardiologists blinded to biomarker analyses. Grading of diastolic dysfunction was performed by blinded members of the authorship team based on previously published guidelines [16]. LA volume index, lateral e' and medial e' were used as a binary classifier for diastolic dysfunction, after which E/A ratio, or average E/e' ratio, for patients in AFib, was used to ascertain grade in those determined to have diastolic dysfunction. Diastolic dysfunction analyses could not be performed due to poor echocardiographic visualization in 9 HFPEF patients and 14 HFREF patients, and a further 1 HFPEF patient and 7 HFREF patients were excluded from diastolic function analyses due to the presence of severe mitral regurgitation (MR).

BNP levels were assessed as previously described using an Alere Triage reagent pack (Alere Inc., Ottawa, ON, CAN) read in an automated DxI 800 immunoanalyzer (Beckman-Coulter, Fullerton, CA, USA) at provincial heath laboratories in the province of Alberta [17]. Serum levels of creatinine and lipid profiles were available in study subjects' health records as part of their clinical evaluation. Inclusion criteria for healthy controls were as follows: no history of cardiovascular or renal disease, hypertension, diabetes, or atrial fibrillation; and no prescriptions for antiarrhythmics; ACEi; ARB; beta-blockers; digoxin; loop or thiazide diuretics; or MRA. Exclusion criteria for all study groups were any of the following: age less than 18 years; known malignancy, with expected survival time less than one year; pregnancy within the previous six months; recent cardiac event, including acute MI and decompensated HF; moderate or severe pulmonary hypertension; or severe mitral or aortic valvular stenosis.

Plasma biomarker analyses

Blood for plasma analysis was collected during a one-day baseline enrolment which included the acquisition of the echocardiograms and ECGs. Patients were rested and sitting while blood was collected into cooled lithium-heparin tubes, which were immediately placed on ice prior to plasma fractionation and deep freezing at ≤−75°C. Commercially-available enzyme-linked immunosorbent assay (ELISA) kits for TNF-α, TNFR1, TNFR2 and IL-6 (catalogue no. 's STA00C, SRT100, SRT200 and S6050, respectively, R&D Systems, MN, USA) were used as previously described [18,19]. Absorbance was measured at 450 nm with the wavelength correction set to 540 nm for all assays using a SpectraMax M5 Plate Reader (Molecular Devices, CA, USA). Detection rates for the ELISAs were 72.4%, 100%, 100% and 81.2%, respectively. The inter- and intra-assay coefficients of variation were 13.1% and 9.5% (n = 4); 7.0% and 5.2% (n = 4); 5.3% and 3.5% (n = 4); and 8.0% and 6.3% (n = 4), respectively.

Plasma ACE2 activity was measured using a previously established immunofluorescence protocol [20]. Lithium heparin anti-coagulated platelet-free plasma samples were diluted to a final ratio of 30:70 in plasma assay buffer: 1 M NaCl (Sigma Chem. Co., MO, USA), 75 mM Tris-HCl (Invitrogen, CA, USA) and 5 mM $ZnCl_2$ (Sigma Chem. Co., MO, USA) at pH 6.5. Assay buffer was made to contain various protease inhibitors: 10 μM captopril (ACE inhibitor; Sigma Chem. Co., MO, USA); 5 μM amastatin (aminopeptidase inhibitor; Sigma Chem. Co., MO, USA); and Protease Inhibitor Cocktail (Sigma Chem. Co., MO, USA) dissolved to achieve a concentration of 10 μM bestatin (aminopeptidase inhibitor), 1 μM E-64 [N-(trans-Epoxysuccinyl)-L-leucine-4-guanidinobutylamide; cysteine protease inhibitor], 770 nM pepstatin A (aspartyl protease inhibitor), 154 μM AEBSF [4-(20aminoethyl)benzenesulfonyl fluoride hydrochloride; serine protease inhibitor], 75 nM phosphoramidon (neprilysin inhibitor), 15 nM aprotinin (serine protease inhibitor) and 75 nM leupeptin (cysteine, serine and threonine proteases inhibitor). The use of protease inhibitors in the buffer solution was meant to ensure that the fluorogenic substrate and specific ACE2 inhibitor (both described below), which are integral to the assay, were not cleaved by other proteases naturally present in human plasma. Samples were incubated with Dnp-quenched Mca-containing fluorogenic substrate (catalogue no. ES007, R&D Systems, MN, USA) at a final concentration of 10 μM at 37°C. To find the fluorescence increase due to ACE2 activity, plasma samples were assayed both in the presence and absence of the specific linear ACE2 inhibitor, DX600 (catalogue no. 002-26, Phoenix Pharmaceuticals, CA, USA). Fluorescence was measured with excitation and emission settings at 320 nm and 405 nm, respectively, using SpectraMax M5 plate reader (Molecular Devices, CA, USA). The maximal fluorescence increase due to ACE2 activity was determined from the maximum fluorescence difference between inhibited and uninhibited aliquots; this was normalized to a standard curve for Mca-containing fluorescent peptide (catalogue no. M-1975, Bachem, CA, USA) and scaled for time of measurement and plasma volume over 24 hours, with 1 hour as the baseline. All ACE2 enzymatic activity values herein are expressed in pmol/hr/mL, which describes the amount of substrate turned over per unit time per unit volume of plasma. Inter- and intra-assay coefficients of variation were 10.2% and 7.5% (n = 10), respectively.

Data analysis

Continuous data in tables are expressed as median with interquartile range (IQR) in parentheses. Continuous data in figures are expressed as box and whisker plots on a logarithmic scale to account for non-normal distributions, where boxes represent IQR with median as a bisecting line, while whiskers represent the minimum and maximum values. Categorical data are expressed as percentages. All categorical data were compared using Pearson Chi-square tests, while continuous variables analyzed by category were compared using Mann-Whitney U Test or Kruskal-Wallis Test with Mann-Whitney U Test for pairwise comparisons, where appropriate. Associations between categorical factors or continuous covariates and circulating inflammatory markers were tested using binary logistic or linear regression analyses, respectively, with log-transformed inflammatory marker levels to account for non-normal distributions. Associations between increasing grade of diastolic dysfunction or NYHA functional class and plasma biomarkers were tested using ordinal logistic regression analyses with log-transformed inflammatory marker levels. Forest plots are used to graphically display results from logistic regression analyses. A p-value$<$0.05 was considered significant for all statistical analyses. Statistical analyses were conducted using SPSS Statistics Version 20 (IBM, NY, USA). Obesity was defined as BMI$\geq$30 kg/m^2 per WHO criteria [21]. Estimated glomerular filtration rate (eGFR) was calculated by the revised four-variable Modification of Diet in Renal Disease equation [22]. Left-ventricular hypertrophy (LVH) was defined as left-ventricular mass index (LVMI) $\geq$115 g/m^2 for males and $\geq$ 95 g/m^2 for females per previously published criteria [23].

Results

Baseline clinical profile and assessments of heart function

Demographic and clinical information for the control, HFPEF and HFREF groups is displayed in Table 1. In this study, the HF patient populations recapitulated observations in previous reports [3–5,24]. The study subjects were predominantly of white race in all study groups (Table 1). HFPEF patients were older (p = 0.003), and significantly more were obese (p = 0.016) and hypertensive than HFREF patients, while neither HF group had different gender ratios (p = 0.210), histories of diabetes, peripheral vascular disease (p = 0.234) or atrial fibrillation (AFib; Table 1). Interestingly, total cholesterol (p = 0.774), triglycerides (p = 0.656) and total cholesterol:high-density lipoprotein (HDL) ratio (p = 0.187) were not significantly different between HF phenotypes, despite differences in obesity prevalence (Table 1). Ischemic etiology was more prevalent in HFREF than HFPEF, but both groups were on evidence-based therapeutic regimens (Table 1). Importantly, drugs that can affect inflammation were comparably used by the two HF groups: NSAID use was equivalent and statin use was not significantly different (p = 0.438; Table 1). NYHA functional class distribution was also not significantly different between the HFPEF and HFREF groups (Table 1).

Heart rates did not differ significantly between controls or the two HF groups; however, a significantly greater number of HFPEF patients were in AFib on the day of study than HFREF patients (p = 0.018; Table 2). The HFREF group had significantly lower LVEF compared to control and HFPEF groups, while both HFPEF and HFREF had greater LV posterior wall thickness (LVPW; p$<$0.001 for both) and mass index (LVMI; p$<$0.001 for both); left atrial volume index (LA volume index; p$<$0.001 for both); and average E/e' ratio (p$<$0.001 for both) compared to control (Table 2). LVPW (p$<$0.05), and left ventricular end diastolic and systolic dimensions (LVEDD and LVESD, respectively; p$<$0.001 for both) were significantly different between the two HF groups (Table 2). The distributions of grades of diastolic dysfunction were also significantly different (p = 0.043), which might be due to the high prevalence of AFib acting as a confounder in this analysis (Table 2). Significantly more HFREF subjects had left-ventricular hypertrophy (LVH) than HFPEF subjects (p$<$0.001; Table 2).

Circulating inflammatory markers in healthy control, HFPEF and HFREF

Compared to control, plasma levels of TNFα were only significantly elevated in HPFEF, while levels of TNFR1 and TNFR2 were significantly elevated in both HFPEF and HFREF (Figure 1A–C). Meanwhile, IL-6 was not significantly different between control and the HF groups (Figure 1D). Interestingly, TNFR2 was significantly elevated in HFPEF relative to HFREF, while TNFα and TNFR1 were non-significantly elevated in HFPEF (Figure 1A–C). We explored the relationship between age, eGFR, sex, obesity, LVH, hypertension, diabetes, smoking status, peripheral vascular disease or history of atrial fibrillation with TNFα, TNFR1, TNFR2 and IL-6 in the combined HF group (Table 3). Advanced age was significantly associated with elevated TNFR1 and TNFR2, and low eGFR was significantly associated with elevated TNFα in addition to its two receptors (Table 3). TNFα, TNFR1 and TNFR2 increased differentially in response to smoking status or comorbid conditions, such as hypertension and diabetes, but were always associated with at least two covariates, while IL-6 was not associated with any covariate (Table 3). Sex, obesity and LVH were not significantly associated with any of the inflammatory markers (Table 3).

Modulators of inflammatory markers in HFPEF and HFREF

We investigated how the inflammatory markers in this study related to two clinically-relevant and commonly-used ordinal quantifications of disease status in HF: grade of diastolic dysfunction and NYHA functional class. We investigated these associations using ordinal logistic regression analyses. Elevated TNFR2 was significantly associated with increasing grade of diastolic dysfunction in HFPEF, but not in HFREF, while TNFR1 was not associated with diastolic dysfunction in either HF group (Figure 2A). Interestingly, elevated TNFR1 and TNFR2 levels were significantly associated with increasing NYHA functional class in both HPFEF and HFREF (Figure 2A). Neither TNFα, nor IL-6 were significantly associated with diastolic dysfunction or symptom severity in either HFPEF or HFREF (data not shown). LA volume index was not associated with plasma TNFR1 or TNFR2 levels in HFPEF (r = 0.110, p = 0.298; and r = 0.170, p = 0.105, respectively) or HFREF (r = 0.083, p = 0.443; and r = 0.056, p = 0.607, respectively). Plasma levels of TNFR1 and TNFR2 were weakly, but significantly, associated with average E/e' ratio in HFPEF (Figure 2B & C), but not HFREF (r = 0.215, p = 0.053; and r = 0.112, p = 0.318, respectively). Given that AFib can confound diastolic dysfunction analyses, we investigated associations between TNFR1 or TNFR2 and LA volume index or average E/e' ratio, as alternative measures of diastolic function that can be used for patients in AFib [25].

Increased activity of TNFα converting enzyme (TACE), a sheddase involved in proteolytic processing of TNFα, TNFRs, and angiotensin-converting enzyme 2 (ACE2) might represent a mechanism of increased circulating TNFα and TNFRs in HF [26,27]. ACE2 is a counter-regulatory homologue of angiotensin-

Table 1. Baseline clinical data.

Demographics	HC	HFPEF	HFREF	p-value
Number	50	100	100	---
Age, years	54 (52–62)	72 (63–79)	65 (59–73)	<0.001
Sex: male, %	48	62	71	0.029
Race: white, %	86	85	90	0.701
Physical Characteristics				
Obese, %	22	59	42	<0.001
Systolic BP	122 (115–136)	128 (118–141)	119 (104–132)	0.005
Diastolic BP	74 (67–78)	71 (63–79)	72 (64–80)	0.449
Medical History				
Smoker, %	18	61	52	<0.001
HTN, %	N/A	78	60	0.006
DM, %	N/A	46	36	0.134
PVD, %	0	10	5	0.071
AFib, %	N/A	52	40	0.089
NYHA Class, %				0.072
I	N/A	12	22	
II	N/A	56	47	
III	N/A	32	28	
IV	N/A	0	3	
Primary Etiology of HF, %				<0.001
Ischemic	N/A	14	37	
Non-ischemic	N/A	86	63	
Laboratory Values				
BNP, pg/mL	16 (11–28)	76 (44–236)	162 (79–398)	<0.001
SrCR, μM	72 (59–85)	99 (79–138)	96 (82–116)	<0.001
Total Cholesterol, mM	5.4 (4.8–5.8)	3.8 (3.2–4.4)	3.6 (3.0–4.4)	<0.001
Triglycerides, mM	1.3 (0.8–1.6)	1.2 (0.9–1.8)	1.3 (0.9–2.4)	0.662
Cholesterol: HDL Ratio	3.9 (3.1–4.5)	3.3 (2.8–4.3)	3.6 (2.9–4.5)	0.276
eGFR, mL/min/1.73 m^2	76 (62–85)	57 (41–78)	59 (48–72)	<0.001
Medication				
Antiarrhythmic, %	N/A	11	7	0.323
ACEi or ARB, %	N/A	86	89	0.521
Beta-blocker, %	N/A	30	36	0.367
Digoxin, %	N/A	11	16	0.301
Loop diuretic, %	N/A	78	68	0.111
MRA, %	N/A	19	38	0.003
NSAIDs, %	0	8	8	0.118
Thiazide diuretic, %	N/A	12	7	0.228
Statin, %	2	73	68	<0.001

Abbreviations: HC, healthy control; HFPEF, heart failure (HF) with preserved ejection fraction; HFREF, HF with reduced ejection fraction; BP, blood pressure; HTN, hypertension; DM, diabetes; PVD, peripheral vascular disease; AFib, history of atrial fibrillation; NYHA, New York Heart Association; BNP, B-type natriuretic peptide; SrCr, serum creatinine; HDL, high-density lipoprotein; eGFR, estimated glomerular filtration rate; ACEi, angiotensin converting enzyme inhibitor; ARB, angiotensin II receptor antagonist; MRA, mineralocorticoid receptor antagonist; and NSAIDs, non-steroidal anti-inflammatory drugs. See Methods section for details on how parameters were obtained. P-value represents Mann-Whitney U Test, Kruskal-Wallis Test or Chi-square Test where appropriate. Number was not tested, as the sample sizes were selected *a priori*.

converting enzyme (ACE) and a major regulator of endothelial function and myocardial fibrosis [28–30]. Since the membrane-bound localization of TACE poses a limitation in assessing its levels or activity in the plasma, we measured plasma ACE2 activity as a surrogate, as it increases with increased TACE activity [31]. Previous reports of plasma ACE2 activity showed an association with clinically diagnosed HFREF, symptom severity and worsening clinical outcomes [20,32]. In our HFPEF cohort, plasma ACE2 activity was significantly elevated relative to control

Table 2. Electrocardiogram and Echocardiography.

	HC	HFPEF	HFREF	p-value
HR, bpm	65 (60–76)	65 (60–78)	65 (60–76)	0.757
AFib, %	0	43	23	<0.001
LVEF, %	63 (60–67)	59 (54–63)	35 (27–41)	<0.001
LVEDD, cm	4.4 (4.1–4.6)	4.8 (4.3–5.2)	5.9 (5.4–6.4)	<0.001
LVESD, cm	2.8 (2.5–3.2)	3.1 (2.8–3.6)	4.7 (3.8–5.6)	<0.001
LVPW, cm	0.9 (0.8–1.0)	1.1 (1.0–1.2)	1.0 (0.9–1.1)	<0.001
LVMI, g/m^2				
Female	62 (54–69)	89 (78–111)	103 (80–119)	<0.001
Male	74 (56–87)	105 (83–119)	129 (104–152)	<0.001
LVH, %	6	34	60	<0.001
LA index, mL/m^2	23 (19–27)	34 (28–43)	37 (30–50)	<0.001
MR, %				<0.001
None	38	45	32	
Trace/mild	12	43	41	
Moderate	0	11	20	
Severe	0	1	7	
E-wave velocity, cm/s	74 (67–82)	87 (73–107)	76 (60–97)	<0.001
Medial E/e' ratio	9 (8–11)	14 (10–17)	15 (11–20)	<0.001
Lateral E/e' ratio	7 (6–8)	10 (8–13)	11 (8–16)	<0.001
Average E/e' ratio	8 (7–10)	12 (9–15)	13 (10–18)	<0.001
A-wave velocity, cm/s	68 (61–78)	79 (63–96)	74 (55–89)	0.052
E/A ratio	1.0 (0.8–1.2)	0.9 (0.8–1.3)	1.0 (0.6–1.6)	0.745
Grade: diastolic dysfunction*, %				<0.001
0 (Normal)	94	34	14	
1 (Impaired relaxation)	4	25	31	
2 (Pseudonormal filling)	2	24	34	
3 (Restrictive filling)	0	17	21	

Abbreviations: HC, healthy control; HFPEF, heart failure (HF) with preserved ejection fraction; HFREF, HF with reduced ejection fraction; HR, heart rate; AFib, atrial fibrillation based on ECG; LVEF, left-ventricular ejection fraction; LVEDD, left-ventricule (LV) end diastolic diameter; LVESD, LV end systolic diameter; LVPW, LV posterior wall thickness; LVMI, LV mass indexed to body surface area (BSA); LVH, left-ventricular hypertrophy; LA index, left-atrial volume indexed to BSA; MR, mitral regurgitation; E-wave, early diastolic wave velocity; e', mitral valve annular velocity as measured medially or laterally by way of tissue Doppler imaging; and A-wave, late diastolic velocity due to atrial systole. See Methods section for details on how parameters were obtained. P-value represents Kruskal-Wallis Test or Chi-square Test where appropriate.*Grade of diastolic dysfunction excluding those patients with severe MR or poor visualization on echocardiography.

(Figure 3A); however, it was not associated with increasing grade of diastolic dysfunction or NYHA class (Figure 3B).

Discussion

In this comparative analysis of healthy controls, and HF patients with preserved or reduced left-ventricular ejection fraction, we found that our cohorts recapitulated previous characterizations, whereby, HFPEF subjects were more likely to be older, hypertensive and obese [3–5,24]. Similarly, AFib was prevalent in both HF groups, which follows the trend observed in the MAGGIC meta-analysis [5]. Furthermore, the primary etiology of HF was much less likely to be ischemic in the HFPEF group. Despite differences in comorbidities, age and HF etiology the NYHA class distribution was similar between HFREF and HFPEF, which indicates that the two patient populations experienced significant burden of disease. Additionally, both groups had cardiac hypertrophy and exhibited marked diastolic dysfunction. In patients without marked systolic dysfunction, a greater prevalence of comorbidities might account for the similarity in symptoms between HFPEF and HFREF.

Improvement in exercise capacity in a cohort of HFPEF patients after an exercise training regimen was largely mediated by peripheral improvements, which suggests a systemic component to HFPEF, including skeletal muscle dysregulation [33]. Indeed, a recent model of HFPEF suggests that comorbidity-mediated systemic inflammation, results in coronary microvascular endothelial dysfunction, myocardial hypertrophy and fibrosis, and skeletal muscle dysregulation to produce the HFPEF phenotype [6]. We investigated TNFα and its receptors (TNFR1 and TNFR2) as one component of comorbidity-driven inflammation, and included IL-6 as non-TNF-family cytokine for comparison. We expand on previous work in HF: our data showed that levels of TNFα and TNFR1 were significantly increased in HFPEF relative control but not HFREF, while TNFR2 was significantly increased relative to both control and HFREF [14]. Plasma IL-6 levels were very comparable between HFPEF and HFREF, which suggests that TNFα-mediated inflammation might be a point of pathophysiological difference between HF phenotypes.

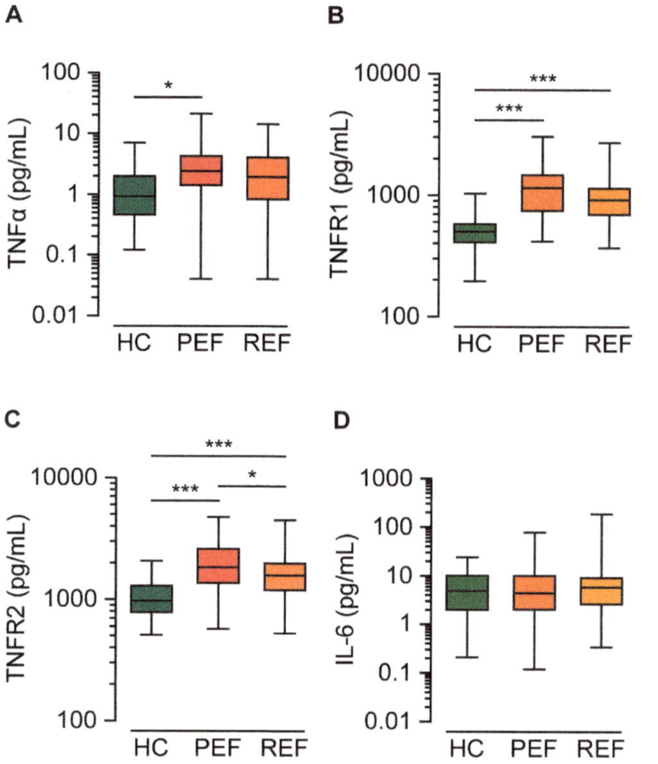

Figure 1. Circulating inflammatory markers in healthy control (HC), HFPEF (PEF) and HFREF (REF). Box and whisker plots show the relative distributions of TNF-α (A), TNFR1 (B), TNFR2 (C) and IL-6 (D) levels. * P<0.05, *** P<0.001 for Kruskal-Wallis Test with pairwise comparisons.

We found that low eGFR, hypertension, smoking status and history of atrial fibrillation were significantly associated with elevated TNFα levels, while elevated TNFR1 levels were associated with aging, low eGFR, hypertension, diabetes and PVD, and elevated TNFR2 levels were associated with aging, low eGFR, diabetes and atrial fibrillation. The advanced age and greater prevalence of comorbidities in the HFPEF population could drive the observed elevation in circulating inflammatory markers relative to HFREF. Indeed, non-cardiac comorbidities are more prevalent in HFPEF, with a larger fraction of adverse clinical outcomes attributable to non-cardiac events compared to HFREF [34]. Likewise, increased TNFα-axis inflammation has been linked to an increased risk of adverse cardiovascular and all-cause outcomes in HF [18,35,36]. Altogether, these data are congruent with the paradigm for HFPEF that includes comorbidities-driven dysregulation of TNFα-mediated signaling [6,34].

Our finding that circulating TNFR2 levels are significantly associated with increasing average E/e' ratio and grade of diastolic dysfunction in HFPEF, but not in HFREF, suggests a greater role for TNFα-mediated inflammation in this cohort. However, we found that TNFR1 and TNFR2 levels were significantly associated with increasing NYHA class in both HF phenotypes, which shows that part of the HFREF phenotype can also be attributed to inflammation. The association of diastolic dysfunction and symptoms with TNFR2 in HFPEF is consistent with findings in experimental models, as the TNFR1/TNFR2 axis is involved in mediating divergent effects: TNFR1 has been implicated in adverse cardiac remodeling and adipogenesis, while TNFR2

Table 3. Univariate correlations of biomarkers with continuous and binary covariates.

	Marker							
	TNFα		TNFR1		TNFR2		IL-6	
Continuous	R	p-value	R	p-value	R	p-value	R	p-value
Age	0.077	0.331	0.204	0.004	0.161	0.023	0.038	0.617
eGFR	0.187	0.020	0.534	<0.001	0.433	<0.001	0.082	0.280
Binary	**OR (95%CI)**	**p-value**	**OR (95%CI)**	**p-value**	**OR (95%CI)**	**p-value**	**OR (95%CI)**	**p-value**
Sex	1.68 (0.87–3.23)	0.121	0.60 (0.13–2.76)	0.513	0.50 (0.11–2.26)	0.368	1.42 (0.78–2.57)	0.251
Obese	1.40 (0.75–2.62)	0.294	2.27 (0.54–9.60)	0.266	1.84 (0.45–7.60)	0.397	1.17 (0.67–2.05)	0.578
LVH	1.68 (0.84–3.36)	0.142	0.69 (0.16–2.99)	0.622	0.46 (0.11–1.95)	0.290	1.13 (0.64–1.99)	0.677
HTN	2.04 (1.04–4.00)	0.038	11.59 (2.21–60.75)	0.004	3.24 (0.69–15.18)	0.136	0.64 (0.34–1.19)	0.162
DM	1.58 (0.82–3.04)	0.172	20.21 (4.05–100.96)	<0.001	11.29 (2.42–52.75)	0.002	0.97 (0.55–1.71)	0.918
Smoker	2.00 (1.04–3.82)	0.037	1.68 (0.39–7.13)	0.485	3.57 (0.84–15.24)	0.085	0.95 (0.54–1.67)	0.857
PVD	1.04 (0.35–3.12)	0.944	23.63 (1.30–430.17)	0.037	11.78 (0.68–204.67)	0.090	1.04 (0.37–2.92)	0.942
AFib	1.97 (1.01–3.81)	0.045	4.09 (0.94–17.77)	0.060	4.81 (1.12–20.74)	0.035	0.90 (0.52–1.58)	0.716

Abbreviations: eGFR, estimated glomerular filtration rate; LVH, left-ventricular hypertrophy; HTN, hypertension; DM, diabetes mellitus; PVD, peripheral vascular disease; and AFib, history of atrial fibrillation. See Methods section for details on how parameters were obtained.

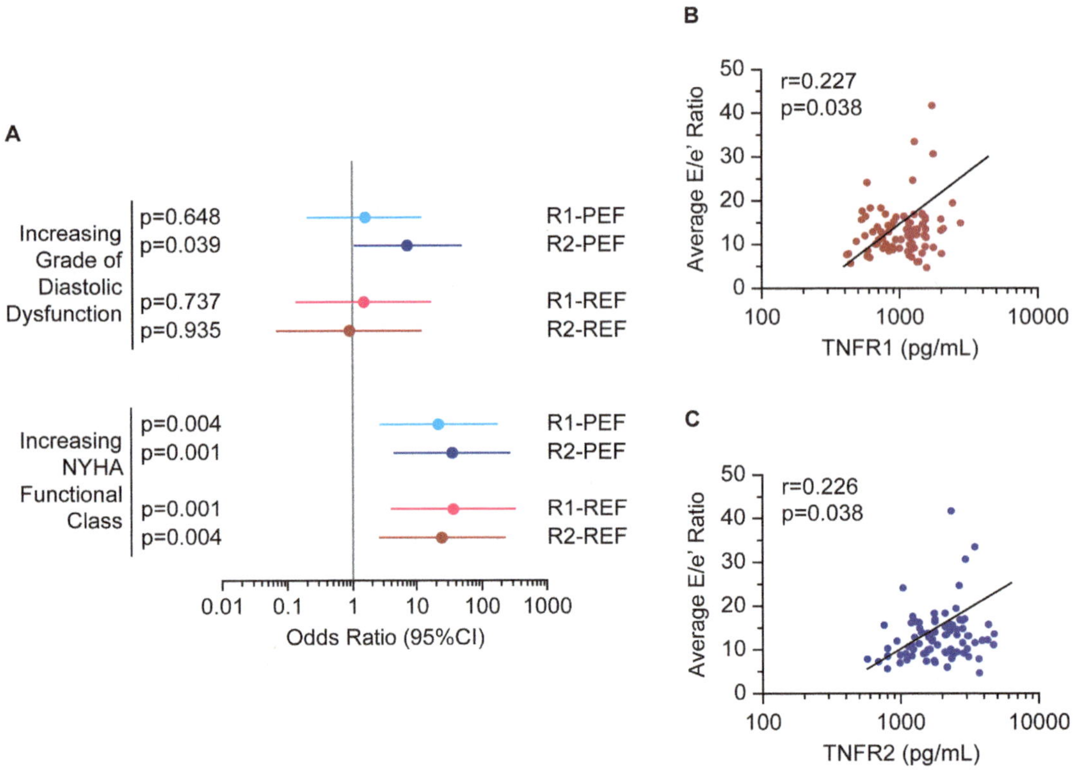

Figure 2. Associations of TNFR1 and TNFR2 with disease parameters. Forest plots show odds ratios and 95% confidence intervals (95%CI) for TNFR1 (R1) or TNFR2 (R2) as predictors of increasing grade of diastolic dysfunction or NYHA class in HFPEF (PEF) or HFREF (REF) (A). Scatterplots show average E/e' ratio as a function of TNFR1 (B) or TNFR2 (C) in HFPEF.

antagonizes the pathological effects of TNFR1, and also stimulates angiogenesis [37–40]. TNFR1 and TNFR2 also mediate opposite effects on phospholamban and SERCA2, key Ca^{2+} handling proteins involved in myocardial relaxation [37,41]. An increase in circulating TNFR2 levels might reflect a loss of protective signaling mechanisms due to tissue shedding of TNFR2, thereby leading to the correlation between circulating TNFR2 levels and diastolic dysfunction and symptoms in HFPEF.

The differential role of TNFRs might explain why TNFα is not associated with function or symptoms: the variable response to TNFα is mediated at the receptor level. Congruent with a recent report, we found TNFα was not strongly associated with either HF phenotype; however, Marti *et al.* implicate TNFR1, while our study implicates TNFR2 in HFPEF [13]. The key difference between the two studies is that Marti *et al.* explored risk of incident HF, while we examined existing HF populations. Indeed, we found TNFR1 to be associated with the greatest number of HF risk factors, which is congruent with a role for TNFR1 in precipitating incident HFPEF. Meanwhile, our data show that TNFR2 might then be a better biomarker for gauging severity of established HFPEF.

Circulating fragments of TNFα, TNFR1 and TNFR2 are generated from full, transmembrane proteins through the activity of TACE [26,27]. We hypothesized that increased circulating

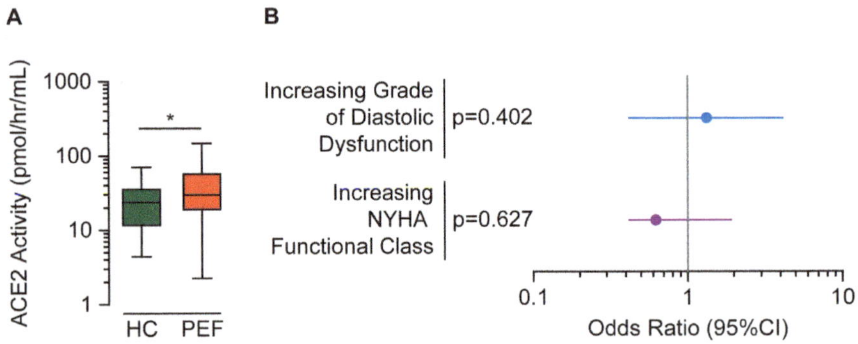

Figure 3. Angiotensin-converting enzyme 2 (ACE2) activity in HFPEF, and comparison with disease parameters. Box and whisker plots compare the distribution of plasma ACE2 activity in healthy control (HC) and HFPEF (PEF) (A). Forest plots show odds ratio and 95% confidence interval (95%CI) for ACE2 as predictor of increasing grade of diastolic dysfunction or NYHA class in HFPEF (B). * P<0.05 for Mann Whitney U test.

levels of TNFR1 and TNFR2 might reflect increased activity of TACE. ACE2 is also a substrate of TACE, and plasma ACE2 activity increases in conjunction with increased TACE activity [26,31]. Since TACE is membrane-bound, as a surrogate of TACE-activity we measured plasma ACE2 activity in HFPEF patients relative to healthy controls. Previous work showed a significant association between ACE2 and symptom severity and adverse clinical outcomes in patients with HFREF [20,32]. We found significantly elevated plasma ACE2 activity in HFPEF as compared to healthy controls, but no association to diastolic dysfunction or symptoms. This is congruent with the idea that elevated ACE2 activity is a consequence of the drivers of HFPEF, rather than an effector as may be the case in HFREF [20,32].

Conclusion

Taking our data together with previous reports indicates that the TACE/TNFα/TNFR1/TNFR2 inflammatory axis is a part of the pathogenesis of HFPEF [7–10,37–40]. In the context of the failure of TNFα antagonism as a therapeutic tool in HF, our data suggest that a downstream approach involving TNFR1 inhibition or TNFR2 potentiation may represent a more effective therapeutic approach for patients with HFPEF [42].

Limitations

Our study, while larger than most other studies that compared levels of TNFα and its receptors in HFPEF versus HFREF, is still relatively small in terms of clinical studies. Indeed, TNFα might also be informative with respect to differentiating HFPEF from HFREF, but our study cannot resolve whether this is the case. In addition, the results reported herein represent a single cross-section across healthy controls, and HFPEF and HFREF patients, so follow-up measurements are not included, nor are outcomes data. Further studies with a longitudinal component will be important for implicating various molecules or pathways in the pathophysiological development of HF, for which work by Marti *et al.* is a strong contribution [13]. Finally, our results only provide correlative evidence of whether these biochemical markers are primary mediators of the HF syndrome, or end-effectors of pathogenic processes. Indeed, while a conglomerate of evidence points towards an interplay between plasma and tissue levels for TNFR1 and TNFR2—shedding increases plasma levels at the expense of tissue levels—direct tissue and plasma comparisons from the same subjects will be necessary to determine the relative effects of proteolytic processing and changes in expression.

Acknowledgments

This work was completed on behalf of the Alberta HEART team of investigators: Todd Anderson*, Libin Cardiovascular Institute of Alberta, Department of Cardiac Sciences, University of Calgary, Calgary, AB; Harald Becher*, Mazankowski Alberta Heart Institute, Department of Medicine, University of Alberta, Edmonton, AB; Jason Dyck*, Department of Pediatrics, University of Alberta, Edmonton, AB; Zamaneh Kassiri*, Department of Physiology, University of Alberta, Edmonton, AB; Gavin Oudit*, Mazankowski Alberta Heart Institute, Department of Medicine, University of Alberta, Edmonton, AB; Justin Ezekowitz, Mazankowski Alberta Heart Institute, Department of Medicine, University of Alberta, Edmonton, AB; Mark Haykowsky, Faculty of Rehabilitation Medicine, University of Alberta, Edmonton, AB; Ian Paterson, Mazankowski Alberta Heart Institute, Department of Medicine, University of Alberta, Edmonton, AB; Finlay McAlister, Department of Medicine, University of Alberta, Edmonton, AB; Hank Duff, Libin Cardiovascular Institute of Alberta, Department of Cardiac Sciences, University of Calgary, Calgary, AB; Padma Kaul, Department of Medicine, University of Alberta, Edmonton, AB; Jonathan Howlett, Libin Cardiovascular Institute of Alberta, Department of Cardiac Sciences, University of Calgary, Calgary, AB; Israel Belenkie, Libin Cardiovascular Institute of Alberta, Department of Cardiac Sciences, University of Calgary, Calgary, AB; Alexander Clark, Faculty of Nursing, University of Alberta, Edmonton, AB; Matthias Friedrich, Montreal Heart Institute, Departments of Cardiology and Radiology, Université de Montréal, Montréal, QC; Sarah Weeks, Libin Cardiovascular Institute of Alberta, Department of Cardiac Sciences, University of Calgary, Calgary, AB; Daniel Kim, Mazankowski Alberta Heart Institute, Department of Medicine, University of Alberta, Edmonton, AB; Merril Knudtson, Libin Cardiovascular Institute of Alberta, Department of Cardiac Sciences, University of Calgary, Calgary, AB; Michelle Noga, Department of Radiology and Diagnostic Imaging, University of Alberta, Edmonton, AB; Richard Schulz, Departments of Pediatrics and Pharmacology, University of Alberta, Edmonton, AB; Hude Quan, Libin Cardiovascular Institute of Alberta, Department of Cardiac Sciences, University of Calgary, Calgary, AB; Richard Thompson, Department of Biomedical Engineering, University of Alberta, Edmonton, AB; Peter Light, Alberta Diabetes Institute, Department of Pharmacology, University of Alberta, Edmonton, AB; James White, Libin Cardiovascular Institute of Alberta, Department of Cardiac Sciences, University of Calgary, Calgary, AB; and Gary Lopaschuk, Department of Pediatrics, University of Alberta, Edmonton, AB. Gavin Oudit is the HEART team member to whom correspondence regarding this study should be addressed. *Contributing authors.

The authors wish to sincerely thank all of participants in this study. The authors also wish to thank Kelly Narine, Marleen Irwin, Darlene Ramadan and Leslie Jackson Carter, for data organization, and Mohua Podder for guidance with statistical analyses.

Author Contributions

Conceived and designed the experiments: BNP ZW JL GYO. Performed the experiments: BNP ZW JL. Analyzed the data: BNP ZW JL HB GYO. Contributed reagents/materials/analysis tools: JD ZK GYO. Wrote the paper: BNP ZW JL TA JD ZK GYO. Contributed critical review and insight into data analysis: TA HB JD ZK GYO. Facilitated patient data acquisition: TA JD.

References

1. Yancy CW, Jessup M, Bozkurt B, Butler J, Casey DE Jr, et al. (2013) 2013 ACCF/AHA Guideline for the Management of Heart Failure: A Report of the American College of Cardiology Foundation/American Heart Association Task Force on Practice Guidelines. Circulation 128: e240–327.
2. Paulus WJ, Tschope C, Sanderson JE, Rusconi C, Flachskampf FA, et al. (2007) How to diagnose diastolic heart failure: a consensus statement on the diagnosis of heart failure with normal left ventricular ejection fraction by the Heart Failure and Echocardiography Associations of the European Society of Cardiology. Eur Heart J 28: 2539–2550.
3. Owan TE, Hodge DO, Herges RM, Jacobsen SJ, Roger VL, et al. (2006) Trends in prevalence and outcome of heart failure with preserved ejection fraction. N Engl J Med 355: 251–259.
4. Bhatia RS, Tu JV, Lee DS, Austin PC, Fang J, et al. (2006) Outcome of heart failure with preserved ejection fraction in a population-based study. N Engl J Med 355: 260–269.
5. Meta-analysis Global Group in Chronic Heart Failure (MAGGIC) (2012) The survival of patients with heart failure with preserved or reduced left ventricular ejection fraction: an individual patient data meta-analysis. Eur Heart J 33: 1750–1757.
6. Paulus WJ, Tschope C (2013) A novel paradigm for heart failure with preserved ejection fraction: comorbidities drive myocardial dysfunction and remodeling through coronary microvascular endothelial inflammation. J Am Coll Cardiol 62: 263–271.
7. Cheng JM, Akkerhuis KM, Battes LC, van Vark LC, Hillege HL, et al. (2013) Biomarkers of heart failure with normal ejection fraction: a systematic review. Eur J Heart Fail 15: 1350–1362.
8. Ho JE, Liu C, Lyass A, Courchesne P, Pencina MJ, et al. (2012) Galectin-3, a marker of cardiac fibrosis, predicts incident heart failure in the community. J Am Coll Cardiol 60: 1249–1256.

9. Zile MR, Desantis SM, Baicu CF, Stroud RE, Thompson SB, et al. (2011) Plasma biomarkers that reflect determinants of matrix composition identify the presence of left ventricular hypertrophy and diastolic heart failure. Circ Heart Fail 4: 246–256.
10. Santhanakrishnan R, Chong JP, Ng TP, Ling LH, Sim D, et al. (2012) Growth differentiation factor 15, ST2, high-sensitivity troponin T, and N-terminal pro brain natriuretic peptide in heart failure with preserved vs. reduced ejection fraction. Eur J Heart Fail 14: 1338–1347.
11. van Veldhuisen DJ, Linssen GC, Jaarsma T, van Gilst WH, Hoes AW, et al. (2013) B-type natriuretic Peptide and prognosis in heart failure patients with preserved and reduced ejection fraction. J Am Coll Cardiol 61: 1498–1506.
12. Putko BN, Yogasundaram H, Oudit GY (2014) The harbinger of mortality in HFPEF: do GDF-15 levels reflect tandem, deterministic effects of fibrosis and inflammation? Can J Cardiol 30: 264–266.
13. Marti CN, Khan H, Mann DL, Georgiopoulou VV, Bibbins-Domingo K, et al. (2014) Soluble Tumor Necrosis Factor Receptors and Heart Failure Risk in Older Adults: The Health, Aging, and Body Composition Study. Circ Heart Fail 7: 5–11.
14. Niethammer M, Sieber M, von Haehling S, Anker SD, Munzel T, et al. (2008) Inflammatory pathways in patients with heart failure and preserved ejection fraction. Int J Cardiol 129: 111–117.
15. Rickham PP (1964) Human Experimentation. Code of Ethics of the World Medical Association. Declaration of Helsinki. Br Med J 2: 177.
16. Nagueh SF, Appleton CP, Gillebert TC, Marino PN, Oh JK, et al. (2009) Recommendations for the evaluation of left ventricular diastolic function by echocardiography. J Am Soc Echocardiogr 22: 107–133.
17. Bionda C, Bergerot C, Ardail D, Rodriguez-Lafrasse C, Rousson R (2006) Plasma BNP and NT-proBNP assays by automated immunoanalyzers: analytical and clinical study. Ann Clin Lab Sci 36: 299–306.
18. Dunlay SM, Weston SA, Redfield MM, Killian JM, Roger VL (2008) Tumor necrosis factor-alpha and mortality in heart failure: a community study. Circulation 118: 625–631.
19. Valgimigli M, Ceconi C, Malagutti P, Merli E, Soukhomovskaia O, et al. (2005) Tumor necrosis factor-alpha receptor 1 is a major predictor of mortality and new-onset heart failure in patients with acute myocardial infarction: the Cytokine-Activation and Long-Term Prognosis in Myocardial Infarction (C-ALPHA) study. Circulation 111: 863–870.
20. Epelman S, Tang WH, Chen SY, Van Lente F, Francis GS, et al. (2008) Detection of soluble angiotensin-converting enzyme 2 in heart failure: insights into the endogenous counter-regulatory pathway of the renin-angiotensin-aldosterone system. J Am Coll Cardiol 52: 750–754.
21. Haslam DW, James WP (2005) Obesity. Lancet 366: 1197–1209.
22. Levey AS, Coresh J, Greene T, Stevens LA, Zhang YL, et al. (2006) Using standardized serum creatinine values in the modification of diet in renal disease study equation for estimating glomerular filtration rate. Ann Intern Med 145: 247–254.
23. Zile MR, Gottdiener JS, Hetzel SJ, McMurray JJ, Komajda M, et al. (2011) Prevalence and significance of alterations in cardiac structure and function in patients with heart failure and a preserved ejection fraction. Circulation 124: 2491–2501.
24. Bursi F, Weston SA, Redfield MM, Jacobsen SJ, Pakhomov S, et al. (2006) Systolic and diastolic heart failure in the community. JAMA 296: 2209–2216.
25. Oh JK, Park SJ, Nagueh SF (2011) Established and novel clinical applications of diastolic function assessment by echocardiography. Circ Cardiovasc Imaging 4: 444–455.
26. Lambert DW, Yarski M, Warner FJ, Thornhill P, Parkin ET, et al. (2005) Tumor necrosis factor-alpha convertase (ADAM17) mediates regulated ectodomain shedding of the severe-acute respiratory syndrome-coronavirus (SARS-CoV) receptor, angiotensin-converting enzyme-2 (ACE2). J Biol Chem 280: 30113–30119.
27. Bell JH, Herrera AH, Li Y, Walcheck B (2007) Role of ADAM17 in the ectodomain shedding of TNF-alpha and its receptors by neutrophils and macrophages. J Leukoc Biol 82: 173–176.
28. D'Alessio A, Esposito B, Giampietri C, Ziparo E, Pober JS, et al. (2012) Plasma membrane microdomains regulate TACE-dependent TNFR1 shedding in human endothelial cells. J Cell Mol Med 16: 627–636.
29. Lovren F, Pan Y, Quan A, Teoh H, Wang G, et al. (2008) Angiotensin converting enzyme-2 confers endothelial protection and attenuates atherosclerosis. Am J Physiol Heart Circ Physiol 295: H1377–1384.
30. Zhong J, Basu R, Guo D, Chow FL, Byrns S, et al. (2010) Angiotensin-converting enzyme 2 suppresses pathological hypertrophy, myocardial fibrosis, and cardiac dysfunction. Circulation 122: 717–728.
31. Patel VB, Clarke N, Wang Z, Fan D, Parajuli N, et al. (2013) Angiotensin II induced proteolytic cleavage of myocardial ACE2 is mediated by TACE/ADAM-17: A positive feedback mechanism in the RAS. J Mol Cell Cardiol 66C: 167–176.
32. Epelman S, Shrestha K, Troughton RW, Francis GS, Sen S, et al. (2009) Soluble angiotensin-converting enzyme 2 in human heart failure: relation with myocardial function and clinical outcomes. J Card Fail 15: 565–571.
33. Haykowsky MJ, Brubaker PH, Stewart KP, Morgan TM, Eggebeen J, et al. (2012) Effect of endurance training on the determinants of peak exercise oxygen consumption in elderly patients with stable compensated heart failure and preserved ejection fraction. J Am Coll Cardiol 60: 120–128.
34. Ather S, Chan W, Bozkurt B, Aguilar D, Ramasubbu K, et al. (2012) Impact of noncardiac comorbidities on morbidity and mortality in a predominantly male population with heart failure and preserved versus reduced ejection fraction. J Am Coll Cardiol 59: 998–1005.
35. Cesari M, Penninx BW, Newman AB, Kritchevsky SB, Nicklas BJ, et al. (2003) Inflammatory markers and onset of cardiovascular events: results from the Health ABC study. Circulation 108: 2317–2322.
36. Feldman AM, Mann DL, She L, Bristow MR, Maisel AS, et al. (2013) Prognostic significance of biomarkers in predicting outcome in patients with coronary artery disease and left ventricular dysfunction: results of the biomarker substudy of the surgical treatment for ischemic heart failure trials. Circ Heart Fail 6: 461–472.
37. Defer N, Azroyan A, Pecker F, Pavoine C (2007) TNFR1 and TNFR2 signaling interplay in cardiac myocytes. J Biol Chem 282: 35564–35573.
38. Hamid T, Gu Y, Ortines RV, Bhattacharya C, Wang G, et al. (2009) Divergent tumor necrosis factor receptor-related remodeling responses in heart failure: role of nuclear factor-kappaB and inflammatory activation. Circulation 119: 1386–1397.
39. Romanatto T, Roman EA, Arruda AP, Denis RG, Solon C, et al. (2009) Deletion of tumor necrosis factor-alpha receptor 1 (TNFR1) protects against diet-induced obesity by means of increased thermogenesis. J Biol Chem 284: 36213–36222.
40. Luo Y, Xu Z, Wan T, He Y, Jones D, et al. (2010) Endothelial-specific transgenesis of TNFR2 promotes adaptive arteriogenesis and angiogenesis. Arterioscler Thromb Vasc Biol 30: 1307–1314.
41. Wu CK, Lee JK, Chiang FT, Yang CH, Huang SW, et al. (2011) Plasma levels of tumor necrosis factor-alpha and interleukin-6 are associated with diastolic heart failure through downregulation of sarcoplasmic reticulum Ca2+ ATPase. Crit Care Med 39: 984–992.
42. Chung ES, Packer M, Lo KH, Fasanmade AA, Willerson JT (2003) Randomized, double-blind, placebo-controlled, pilot trial of infliximab, a chimeric monoclonal antibody to tumor necrosis factor-alpha, in patients with moderate-to-severe heart failure: results of the anti-TNF Therapy Against Congestive Heart Failure (ATTACH) trial. Circulation 107: 3133–3140.

7

Qishenyiqi Protects Ligation-Induced Left Ventricular Remodeling by Attenuating Inflammation and Fibrosis *via* STAT3 and NF-κB Signaling Pathway

Chun Li[1]◈, Yong Wang[2]◈, Qi Qiu[3]◈, Tianjiao Shi[2], Yan Wu[2], Jing Han[2], Xingyun Chai[1], Wei Wang[2]*

1 Modern Research Center for Traditional Chinese Medicine, Beijing University of Chinese Medicine, Beijing, China, **2** Basic Medical College, Beijing University of Chinese Medicine, Beijing, China, **3** Anzhen Hospital of Capital Medical University, Beijing, China

Abstract

Aim: Qi-shen-yi-qi (QSYQ), a formula used for the routine treatment of heart failure (HF) in China, has been demonstrated to improve cardiac function through down-regulating the activation of the Renin-Angiotensin-Aldosterone System (RAAS). However, the mechanisms governing its therapeutic effects are largely unknown. The present study aims to demonstrate that QSYQ treatment can prevent left ventricular remodeling in heart failure by attenuating oxidative stress and inhabiting inflammation.

Methods: Sprague-Dawley (SD) rats were randomly divided into 6 groups: sham group, model group (LAD coronary artery ligation), QSYQ group with high dosage, middle dosage and low dosage (LAD ligation and treated with QSYQ), and captopril group (LAD ligation and treated with captopril as the positive drug). Indicators of fibrosis (Masson, MMPs, and collagens) and inflammation factors were detected 28 days after surgery.

Results: Results of hemodynamic alterations (dp/dt value) in the model group as well as other ventricular remodeling (VR) markers, such as MMP-2, MMP-9, collagen I and III elevated compared with sham group. VR was accompanied by activation of RAAS (angiotensin II and NADPHoxidase). Levels of pro-inflammatory cytokines (TNF-α, IL-6) in myocardial tissue were also up-regulated. Treatment of QSYQ improved cardiac remodeling through counter-acting the aforementioned events. The improvement of QSYQ was accompanied with a restoration of angiotensin II-NADPHoxidase-ROS-MMPs pathways. In addition, "therapeutic" QSYQ administration can reduce both TNF-α-NF-B and IL-6-STAT3 pathways, respectively, which further proves the beneficial effects of QSYQ.

Conclusions: Our study demonstrated that QSYQ protected LAD ligation-induced left VR via attenuating AngII -NADPH oxidase pathway and inhabiting inflammation. These findings provide evidence as to the cardiac protective efficacy of QSYQ to HF and explain the beneficial effects of QSYQ in the clinical application for HF.

Editor: Giovanni Li Volti, University of Catania, Italy

Funding: This study was financially supported, in part, by the Grants from the National Natural Science Foundation of China (No.81202788 and 81302908), the National Science & Technology Pillar Program (No. 2012BAI29B07), Beijing Natural Science Foundation (7142099), and Creation for Significant New Drugs Project of China (No. 2012ZX09103-201-011). The funders had no role in study design, data collection and analysis, decision to publish, or preparation of the manuscript.

Competing Interests: The authors have declared that no competing interests exist.

* Email: wangwei26960@126.com

◈ These authors contributed equally to this work.

Introduction

Heart failure (HF) is the ultimate consequence of a vast number of cardiovascular diseases. It is one of the leading causes of morbidity and mortality worldwide [1]. It is considered as an progressive yet irreversible process characterized by damaged pump performance and ventricular remodeling (VR) [2]. VR is also believed as the most essential mechanism for an HF occurrence [3]. Therefore, inhabiting VR early is increasingly becoming an effective way to postpone HF induced by myocardial infarction, hypertension and other cardiovascular diseases [4].

Recent clinical studies have indicated that the AngII-induced oxidative stress and inflammation are the critical mechanism of VR. As firstly, the Renin-Angiotensin-Aldosterone System (RAAS) can activate oxidative stress, thus contributing significantly to the deterioration of cardiovascular function, and eventually lead to myocardial remodeling [5]. In this pathway, NADPH oxidase is a crucial factor for bridging RAAS and oxidative stress progress by generating the reactive oxygen species (ROS) in virtual hypertrophy and remodeling of chronic HF. It is also a potential therapeutic target in HF cases [6,7]. Secondly, HF has been regarded, in the past decades, as a complex cascade of chronic inflammatory reactions that caused gradual cardiac depression [8]. Besides, recent extensive investigations revealed that cytokines, such as tumor necrosis factor-α (TNF-α) and interleukin-6 (IL-6) had important impacts on cardiac outcome as inflammatory markers [9]. Among them, TNF-α has been considered to have detrimental effects on myocardial function by NF-B and eventually

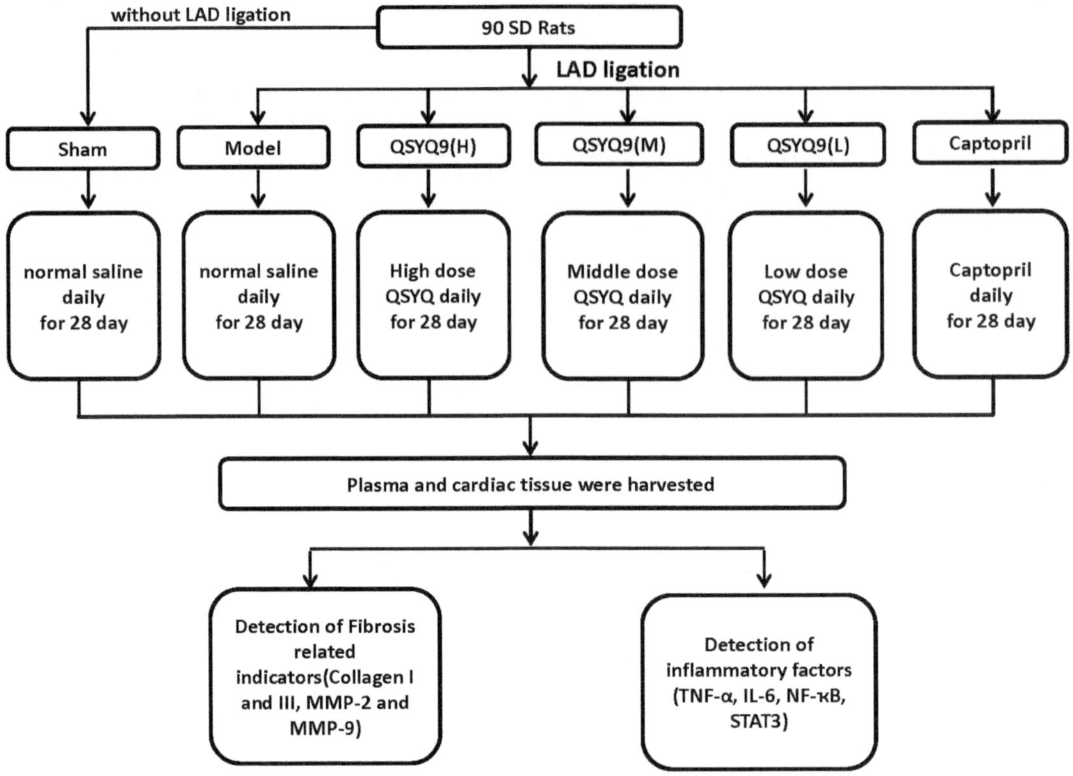

Figure 1. Study designs. Study designs. left anterior descending coronary artery (LAD) was ligated to induce the heart failure (HF) model. Sham groups were made following an identical procedure but without the actual tying of the polypropylene suture. The rats alive after sugery were divided into 5 groups randomly, 14 in model group, 14 in Captopril group and 14 in different dosages of QSYQ groups, respectively. The high dosage QSYQ [QSYQ (H)], middle [QSYQ (M)] and low [QSYQ (L)] groups were administered with QSYQ dissolving in water for 28 days by oral gavage at a total dosages of 9.33 g/kg (H), 4.67 g/kg (M) and 2.33 g/kg (L) of QSYQ on a daily bases. Captopril was given with a dosage of 5.83 mg/kg as a control drug.

result in VR [10]. Numerous studies have also shed light on the role of IL-6 in cardiovascular disease, as long-term IL-6 levels are highly associated with HF by prolongation of STAT signaling, especially STAT3, in cardiacmyocytes [11]. They are also applied as promising molecular targets to treat HF [12].

Traditional Chinese medicine (TCM) has been applied to treat HF for thousands of years, and some herbal formulas have been proven to be effective [13]. Qishenyiqi (QSYQ), one of the most well-known TCM formula, prepared from a composition of six herbs of TCM, including two star herbs, *Radix Astragali mongolici* ('huang-qi' in Chinese) and *Salvia miltiorrhizabunge* ('dan-shen' in Chinese), and four other adjunctive herbs: *Flos Lonicerae*, *Scrophularia*, *Radix Aconiti Lateralis Preparata*, and *Radix Glycyrrhizae*. This formula is widely manufactured in China in accordance with the China Pharmacopoeia standard of quality control [14], and is commonly applied in routine treatment of HF in China. Randomized, controlled clinical trials proved that it has a definite effect on improving heart function [15].

Our previous study demonstrated that QSYQ can ameliorate myocardial hypertrophy and remodeling by inhabiting the expression of angiotensin II (AngII) in LAD rats [16], improving hemorrheology in HF animals [17], and suppressing angiotensin II receptor levels [18]. However, whether it has protective effect on VR and its underlying mechanisms remained poorly defined. This paper demonstrates that QSYQ has the protective effects against VR in rats. Their targets are related to oxidative stress and inflammation by attenuating STAT3 and NF-κB signaling pathway.

Materials and Methods

1 Animals and grouping

Studies were performed in accordance with the Guide for the Care and Use of Laboratory Animals published by the National Institutes of Health (NIH Publications No. 85-23, revised 1996) and with approval of the Animal Care Committee of Beijing Medical Center. A total of 90 male SD rats in SPF grade were selected (purchased from Beijing Vital River Laboratory Animal Technology Co.Ltd.), weighted 240 g±10 g, and admitted into the study.

2 HF Model preparation and study designs

HF was induced by direct coronary ligation as described previously [16]. Before surgery, SD rats were anaesthetized with pentobarbital sodium at a dose of 50 mg/kg. After left thoracotomy and exposure of the heart, the left anterior descending coronary artery (LAD) was ligated with a 5.0 polypropylene suture (Surgipro, CT, USA) directly proximal to its main branching point. Sham groups were made following an identical procedure but without the actual tying of the polypropylene suture. After surgery, as soon as the restoration of spontaneous respiration, the rats were extubated and helped to recover under a heated lamp. They were fed with a standard diet and sufficient water and maintained on a 12 h light and dark cycle.

The overall mortality rate of model group rats during the entire experiment (28 days after ligation) was 20% to 30%. Among them, 9 rats died of the surgery,16 rats died the day after the surgery,

Table 1. Hemodynamic alterations in different groups ($\bar{x}\pm$ s).

Group	N	LVSP (mmHg)	LVEDP (mmHg)	HR (BPM)	MaxdP/dt (mmHg/s)	MindP/dt (mmHg/s)
Sham	10/10	211.90±20.032**	−28.36±12.129**	416.28±63.630	8389.01±1174.404**	−5362.59±978.656**
Model	14/14	162.87±8.997▲▲	−5.23±20.884▲▲	393.08±137.573	5527.27±703.294▲▲	−3511.02±403.734▲▲
QSYQ (H)	14/14	190.72±16.039*	−27.15±5.770**	404.41±62.745	7687.42±1162.700**	−4671.15±644.929*
QSYQ (M)	14/14	192.50±24.563*	−20.98±11.578*	416.78±69.329	7468.21±1297.474**	−4330.94±612.768
QSYQ (L)	14/14	190.03±22.892*	−23.95±11.442*	394.02±63.153	7450.21±1640.391**	−4493.49±1003.122*
Captopril	14/14	201.19±13.999**	−26.60±7.632**	418.13±39.357	7976.97±746.919**	−4563.19±1169.573*

▲▲$p<0.01$, vs sham group, vs sham group;
*$p<0.05$, vs model group,
**$p<0.01$, vs model group.

probably because of acute pump failure or lethal arrhythmias. The rats had serious clinical signs, such as short of breath, severe tachycardia. They were euthanized by the injection of 150 mg/kg sodium pentobarbital intraperitoneally. The rats alive were divided into 5 groups randomly, 14 in model group, 14 in Captopril group and 14 in different dosages of QSYQ groups, respectively. Meanwhile, 10 in sham group were investigated together. After the surgeries, all rats were weighed and administered with QSYQ, or normal saline or captopril by gastric perfusion every day for 28 days. The high dosage QSYQ [QSYQ (H)], middle [QSYQ (M)] and low [QSYQ (L)] groups were administered with QSYQ dissolving in water for 28 days by oral gavage at a total dosages of 9.33 g/kg (H), 4.67 g/kg (M) and 2.33 g/kg (L) of QSYQ (Beijing University of Chinese Medicine, Beijing, China) on a daily bases. The dosage choice was based on the recommended daily human dosage and the equivalent conversion between rats and human by body surface area as our previous study [19]. Captopril was given with a dosage of 5.83

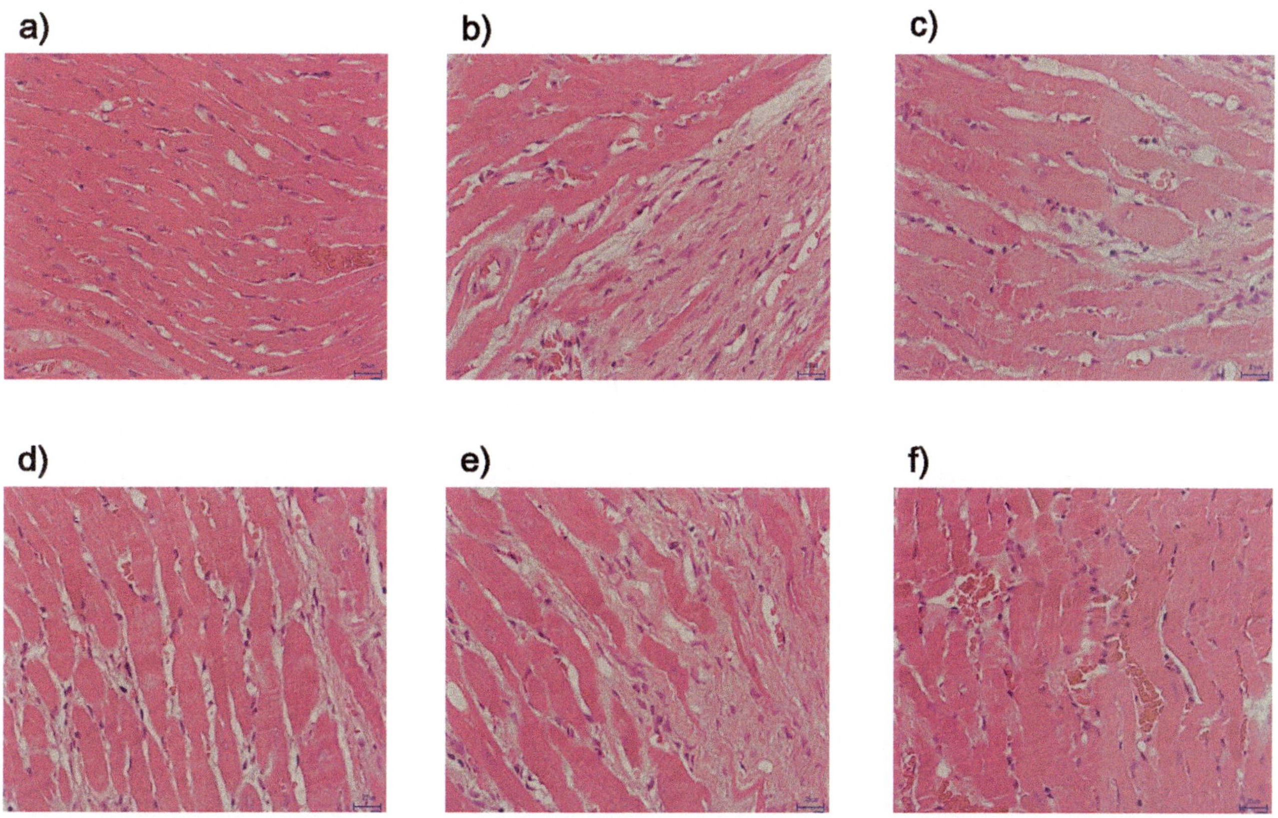

Figure 2. Effects of QSYQ on HE results after occlusion of the left anterior descending (LAD) artery in rats. Cardiomyocytes in the sham group were orderly arranged, and the nuclei were lightly stained and located in the center of muscle fibers. Thickening and lengthening of myocardial fibers could be observed in model group, wherein the nuclei were darkly stained. Cardiomyocyte hypertrophy, cellular degeneration and inflammatory cell infiltration were significantly improved in the different dosage of QSYQ group and Captopril group by contrast with those in the model group. a). cardiomyocytes in sham group; b). cardiomyocytes in model group; c) cardiomyocytes in QSYQ (H); d) cardiomyocytes in QSYQ (M); e) cardiomyocytes in QSYQ (L); f) cardiomyocytes in Captopril group.

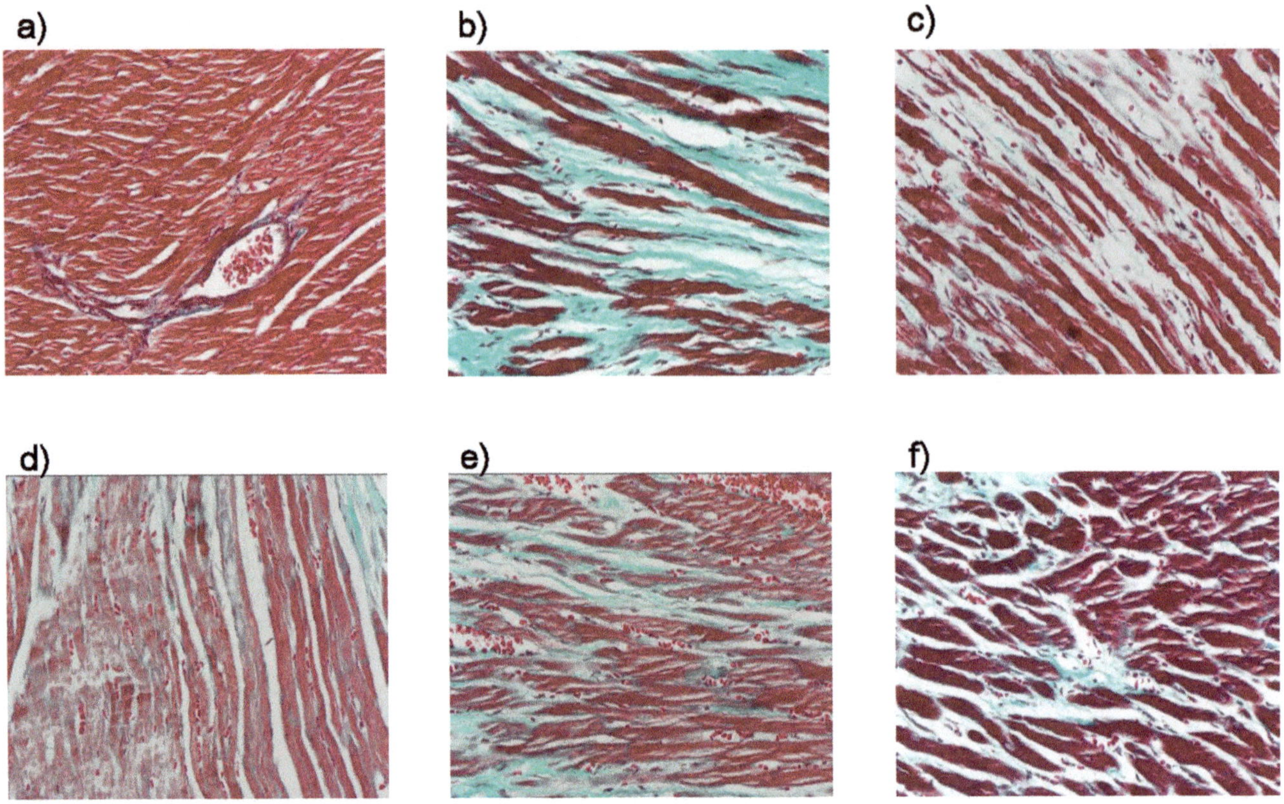

Figure 3. Effects of QSYQ on MASSON results after occlusion of the left anterior descending (LAD) artery in rats. Representative results of Masson trichrome staining of the left ventrentricle in sham group (a).; model group (b).; QSYQ (H) (c).; QSYQ (M) (d).; QSYQ (L) (e).; Captopril group (f). Blue staining indicates myocardial fibrosis. Masson trichrome staining revealed different degree fibrosis in different groups. In sham group, there were almost no fibrosis region. While in model group, there were significant fibrosis region. the increase was significantly attenuated in different dosage of QSYQ groups and Captopril group by contrast with those in the model group. n = 10~14 for each group.

mg/kg as a control drug. The sham group and the model groups received the same volume of water via oral gavage as the QSYQ vehicle. At the end of the study, all animals were anaesthetized using isoflurane (AbraxisBioScience, Richmond Hill, Ontario, Canada), followed by an overnight fast. The study designs were carried out as shown in **Figure 1.** Cardiac tissue samples were excised parallel to coronary sulcus, 3 mm apart from cardiac apex. All samples were frozen in liquid nitrogen immediately for further examinations.

3 Morphometric analysis

Myocardial tissues in the left ventricle (LV) of sacrificed rats (approximately 2 mm in thickness) were removed. Samples were fixed in 4% pre-cooled paraformaldehyde for 72 h and embedded in paraffin for histological studies. Paraffin-embedded tissues were sectioned into slices about 5 μm thicknesses. Masson's trichrome stain was performed to assess myocardial fibrosis. Images were visualized under an optical microscope at ×400 magnification.

4 Hemodynamic measurements in rats

LV performance was measured in rats anesthetized with 2% isoflurane as previously described [20,21]. A terminal hemodynamic study was performed 4 weeks (28±2 days) after sham operation or LAD ligation. In brief, under anesthesia, right carotid artery, left ventricular systolic and end-diastolic, diastolic and mean aortic pressures, MaxdP/dt, MindP/dt, and heart rate were recorded, using a system of PowerLab ML880 (AD Instrument, Australia).

5 Determination of superoxide dismutase (SOD) and malondialdehyde (MDA) by radioimmunoassay (RIA)

The plasma was homogenized in saline containing enzyme inhibitor (0.3 M EDTA-Na 10 uL, 0.34 M 8-hydroxyquinoline 10 uL, 0.32 M dimercaptopropanol 5 ul) (1 ml blood) on ice. The homogenate was centrifuged at 8000×g for 10 min. The supernatant was used for the determination of SOD and MDA using a RIA kit (Beijing Kangyuan Ruide Biotechnology Co. Ltd., Beijing, China) following the instructions of the company.

6 Measurement of plasma indicators by ELISA

Levels of TNF-α and IL-6 were quantified by commercial ELISA kits (Crystal Chem Inc., Downer's Grove, USA). Each assay was performed following related instructions. Standards at a series of concentrations were run in parallel with the samples. The concentrations in the samples were calculated in reference to the corresponding standard curves and were expressed as ng/mL.

7 Measurement of indicators by Western blot

The cardiac tissue was homogenized in RIPA buffer (50 mM TrisHCl Ph 7.4, 150 mM NaCl, 2 mM EDTA, 1% NP-40, 0.1% SDS) and total protein was extracted from this homogenate. The protein concentration in each sample extract was measured by a protein assay kit (Pierce Company, USA, lot number:

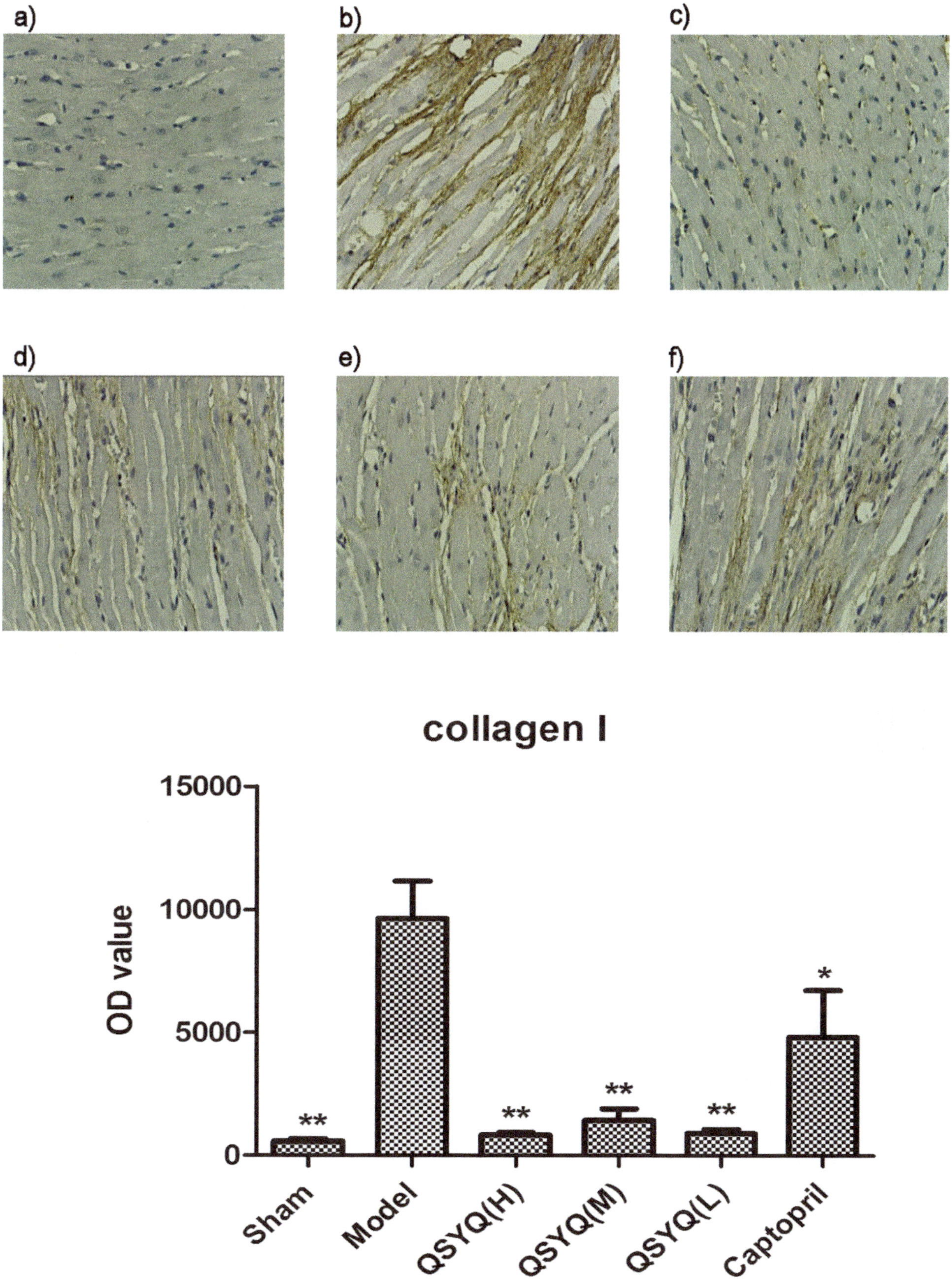

Figure 4. Results of Collagen I expression in different groups. The concentrations of collagens I in the model group (b) were obviously higher than those in sham group (a), indicating a cardiac remodeling in model rats. Whereas the levels of collagens I in high QSYQ (c), middle QSYQ (d) and low QSYQ groups (e) were remarkably lower than those in the model group. Captopril group (f) showed a same effect on suppressing the collagen

synthesis. n = 10~14 for each group. Quantitative analysis of collegen I was presented in (g). OD values represent the mean ± SD. *P<0.05 vs Model group, **P<0.01 vs Model group.

MB155207A) and then was adjusted to the same value in all samples with 2×4% SDS sample buffer. The samples were boiled for 5 mins followed by loading on a 12.5% SDS-PAGE gel (50 mg protein/10 uL per well) for electrophoresis using a Bio-Rad mini gel apparatus at 100 V for 2 h. The fractionated protein on the gel was transferred onto a NC membrane (Beijing PuLilai Gene Technology Co., Ltd, Beijing, China) and electrophoresed at 300 mA for 90 mins. The membrane was first probed with matrix metalloproteinase 2 (MMP2) or MMP9, NADPHoxidase, NF-κB or STAT3 primary antibody (Mouse monoclonal to MMP2, Abcam, USA. Ab3158; Rabbit monoclonal to MMP9, abcam, USA, Ab76003; Rabbit polyclonal to NADPH oxidase, Abcam, USA, Ab60940; Anti-NFκB, Abnova, PAB18492; Anti-NFκB p105/p50 antibody, pNFKB1, Abcam32360, Rabbit polyclonal to STAT3, Abcam, USA. Ab7966) and secondary antibody (donkey polyclonal secondary antibody to rabbit IgG-HRP, ab97064, Abcam, 1:5000), and then treated with ECL (ECL Plus western blotting detection reagent, GE Healthcare) for 1 min at room temperature. The bands in the membrane were visualized and analyzed by UVP BioImaging systems. After obtaining the MMP-2 (or MMP-9, NADPHoxidase, NF-κB, pNFKB1 or STAT3) blot density, the membrane was then treated by Restore Western Blot Stripping Buffer (Thermo Scientific) to remove the MMP-2 (or MMP-9, NADPHoxidase, NF-κB, pNFKB1 or STAT3) signals, followed by probing with glyceraldehyde-3-phosphate dehydrogenase (GAPDH) primary antibodies (GAPDH mouse monoclonal IgG, Ab8245, Abcam, 1:2000) using the same process as the MMP-2 antibody to get the MMP-9, NADPHoxidase, NF-κB, pNFKB1, STAT3 and GAPDH blot densities. The final reported data were normalized by GAPDH.

8 Measurement of indicators by Immunohistochemistry (IHC)

An avidin-biotin-peroxidase complex commercial method (cell & tissue staining kit, R&D Systems, Inc., USA) was used for IHC. Briefly, 4-mm-thick paraffin wax sections were mounted on slides, which were dried for 30 min in an oven (60–70 centigrade degree) and deparaffinized in xylene. The slides were then placed in changes of ethanol for 2 mins each. Washing in buffer solution was performed between steps. The slides were then placed in 3% hydrogenperoxide for 15 mins and were subsequently incubated in avidin block for 15 mins, biotin block for 15 mins, primary antibody (Anti-Collagen I antibody, Abcam, USA. ab34710; Anti-Collagen III antibody, Abcam, USA, ab7778) for 12 h at 4 centigrade degree, and biotinylated secondary antibody for 1 hour. The reagent incubation was performed with streptavidin peroxidase for 15 mins. A 1 min Mayer's hematoxylin counter stain was used. The slides were dehydrated, cleared with xylene, and mounted with permanent mounting medium. Finally pictures were analyzed by IPP 6.0 software.

9 Statistical analysis

All data were presented as mean ± standard deviation (SD). Statistical analysis was carried out on three or more groups by one-way analysis of variance (ANOVA) and Dunnetts' test. The values of $p<0.05$ were considered statistically significant.

Results

1 QSYQ treatment attenuated LAD-induced hemodynamic alterations

HF model group was associated with impaired diastolic and systolic LV functions, which were largely attenuated by the treatment with QSYQ for 28 d. As shown in **Table 1**, the indicators reflecting the LV systolic function including LV systolic pressure (LVSP) and Max dP/dt reduced by 23.14% and 34.11% respectively. When treated by different dosages of QSYQ, the values of two indicators were notably recovered ($p<0.05$–0.01). Compared to model group, the captopril group also exhibited a significant promoting effect on LVSP and Max dP/dt ($p<0.05$–0.01).

LV end-diastolic pressure (LVEDP) and Min dP/dt, which were associated with the LV diastolic function, showed a reverse changes. Compared with sham group, LVEDP in model group increased by 81.56%, Min dP/dt was also up-regulated by 34.53%, suggesting an injured diastolic function in model rats. QSYQ at dosage of 2.33 mg/kg, 4.67 mg/kg, and 9.33 mg/kg orally for 28 d could reduce LVEDP and Min dP/dt in different degree compared to model rats ($p<0.05$–0.01). The results showed protective effects of QSYQ on improving cardiac function. Captopril can also play the same action on these indicators ($p<$ 0.05–0.01). No difference was observed in heart rate (HR) among different groups.

2 Effects of QSYQ on MASSON

The HE-stained images of left ventricular tissue were shown in **Figures 2 and 3**, where cardiomyocytes in the sham group were orderly arranged, and the nuclei were lightly stained and located in the center of muscle fibers. Thickening and lengthening of myocardial fibers could be observed in model group, wherein the nuclei were darkly stained, and showing local tissue fibrosis. Cardiomyocyte hypertrophy, cellular degeneration and inflammatory cell infiltration were significantly improved in the different dosages of QSYQ groups and captopril group by contrast with those in the model group.

3 Effects of QSYQ on collagens I and II

The levels of collagens I and III were detected by IHC and the results were presented in **Figures 4–5**. The levels of collagens I and III in the model group were obviously higher than those in sham group, with an increasing of 1589.78% and 3359.57%, respectively, indicating a cardiac remodeling in model rats. Whereas the levels of these markers in different QSYQ groups were remarkably lower than those in the model group. Especially in collagen III, there is a dose-dependent manner in reduction rates. The captopril group showed the same effect on collagen synthesis ($p<0.01$).

To further confirm myocardial hypertrophy, two major indicators of LV remodeling, proteases MMP-2 and MMP-9, were detected by Western blot respectively. As revealed in **Figure 6.** Compared with sham (1.00±0.000), MMP-2 (1.46±0.080) and MMP-9 (1.64±0.226) were remarkably up-regulated in model group. Combined with IHC, the results indicated LV remodeling occurred in model rats. QSYQ (H) greatly suppressed myocardial hypertrophy and remodeling by MMP-2 (0.89±0.182) and MMP-9 (1.12±0.227). QSYQ (M) and QSYQ (L) also played the same effect on MMP-2 and MMP-9.

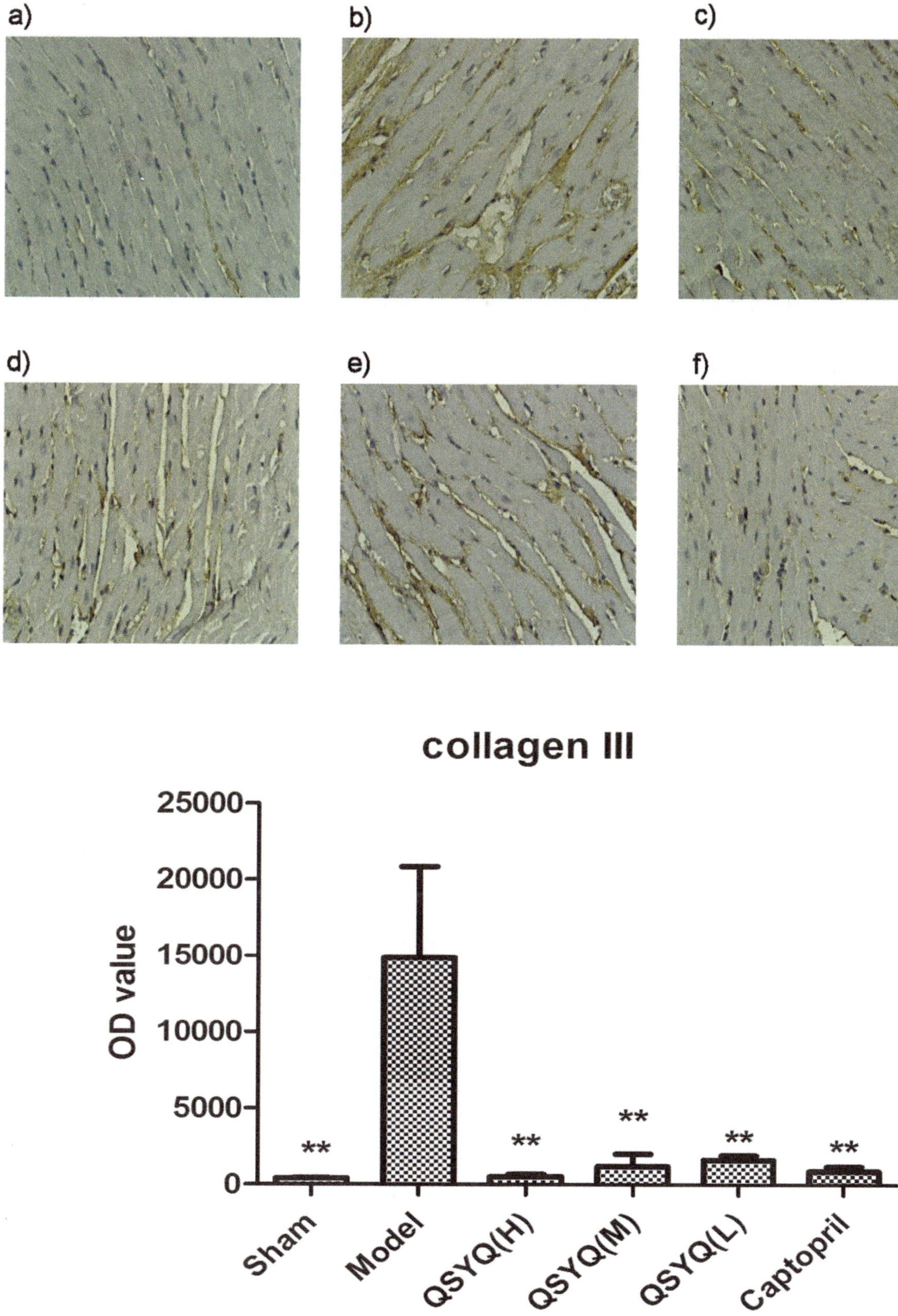

Figure 5. Results of Collagen III expression in different groups. The concentrations of collagens III in the model group (b) were obviously higher than those in sham group (a). Whereas the levels of collagens III in high QSYQ (c), middle QSYQ (d) and low QSYQ groups (e) were remarkably lower than that in the model group. There is a dosage-dependent manner. Captopril group (f) showed a same effect as QSYQ. Quantitative analysis of collegen III was presented in (g). n = 10~14 for each group. OD values represent the mean ± SD. *P<0.05 vsModel group, **P<0.01 vs Model group.

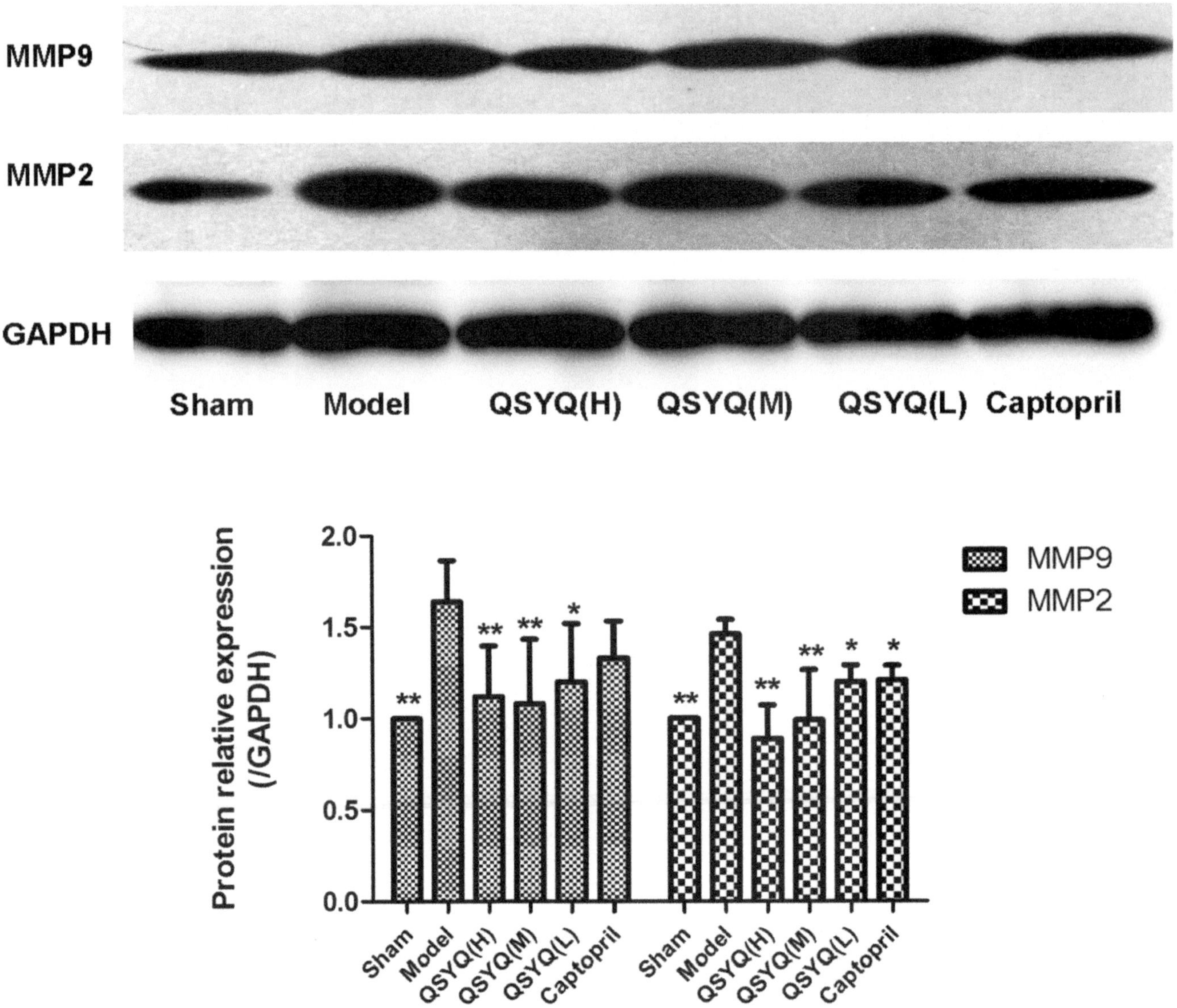

Figure 6. QSYQ treatment significantly decreased cardiac MMP-2 and MMP-9 in rats with HF. MMP-2 and MMP-9 were remarkably up-regulated in model group, indicating elevated degree of remodeling changes. QSYQ (H) greatly suppressed myocardial hypertrophy and remodeling by MMP-2 and MMP-9. QSYQ (M) and QSYQ (L) can also play the same effect. The captopril only suppressed expression of MMP-2, without significant effect on MMP-9. n = 10~14 for each group. Data were analyzed by one-way ANOVA, with p<0.05 indicating statistical significance. *p<0.05 and **p<0.01 vs. model group.

Table 2. Assessment of oxidative stress in different groups ($\bar{x}\pm$ s).

Group	N	SOD (U/mgprot)	MDA (nmol/mgprot)
Sham	10/10	145.87±14.807**	5.74±0.992*
Model	14/14	97.94±3.388▲▲	7.67±0.896▲
QSYQ (H)	14/14	148.70±32.041**	5.24±1.736*
QSYQ (M)	14/14	134.29±20.423**	5.13±1.044*
QSYQ (L)	14/14	117.62±22.356	5.32±1.274*
Captopril	14/14	111.17±19.954	5.50±0.943*

vs: compared with model, **p<0.05, **p<0.01; compared with sham, ▲p<0.05, ▲▲p<0.01.*

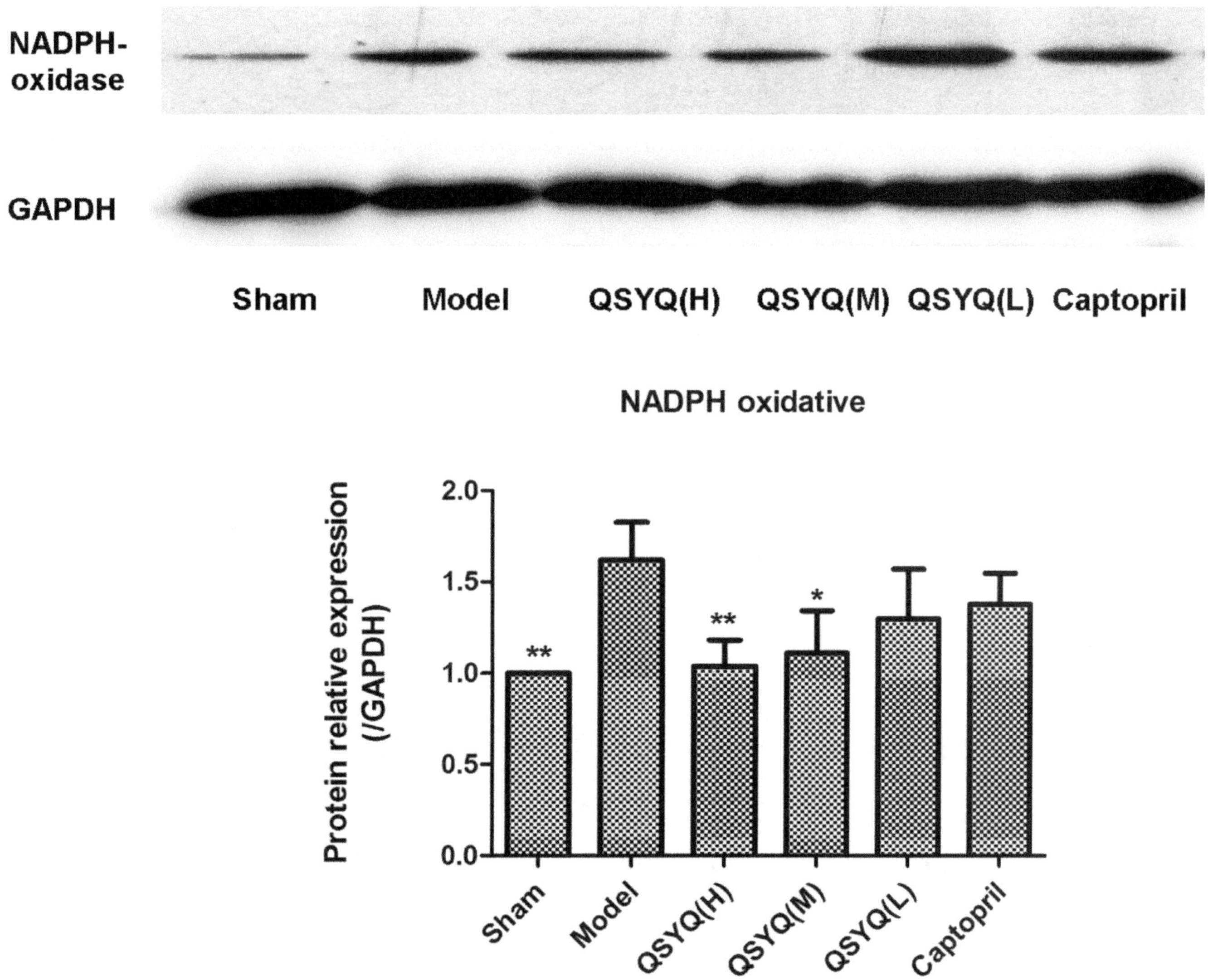

Figure 7. QSYQ treatment significantly decreased cardiac NADPHoxidase in rats with HF. The NADPHoxidase in model group was increased compared with sham group, while treated by QSYQ (H) and (M) doses, the levels showed 35.80% and 31.48% reduction, respectively. The treatment with QSYQ in low-dosage and captopril didn't improve the NADPHoxidase significantly. The effect of QSYQ on NADPHoxidase showed a dosage-dependent manner. n = 10~14 for each group. Data were analyzed by one-way ANOVA, with $p<0.05$ indicating statistical significance. *Differed significantly from the model group ($p<0.05$).

Table 3. Levels of inflammation indicators in different groups ($\bar{x}\pm$ s).

Group	N	IL-6 (pg/ml)	TNF-α (ng/ml)
Sham	10/10	218.08±65.418**	2.13±0.153**
Model	14/14	549.45±126.580▲▲	2.86±0.304▲▲
QSYQ (H)	14/14	250.70±65.140**	2.46±0.266*
QSYQ (M)	14/14	301.93±112.524**	2.25±0.419**
QSYQ (L)	14/14	346.67±32.633**	2.59±0.280
Captopril	14/14	318.32±70.427**	2.58±0.328

VS: compared with model, *$p<0.05$, **$p<0.01$; Compared with sham, ▲▲$p<0.01$.

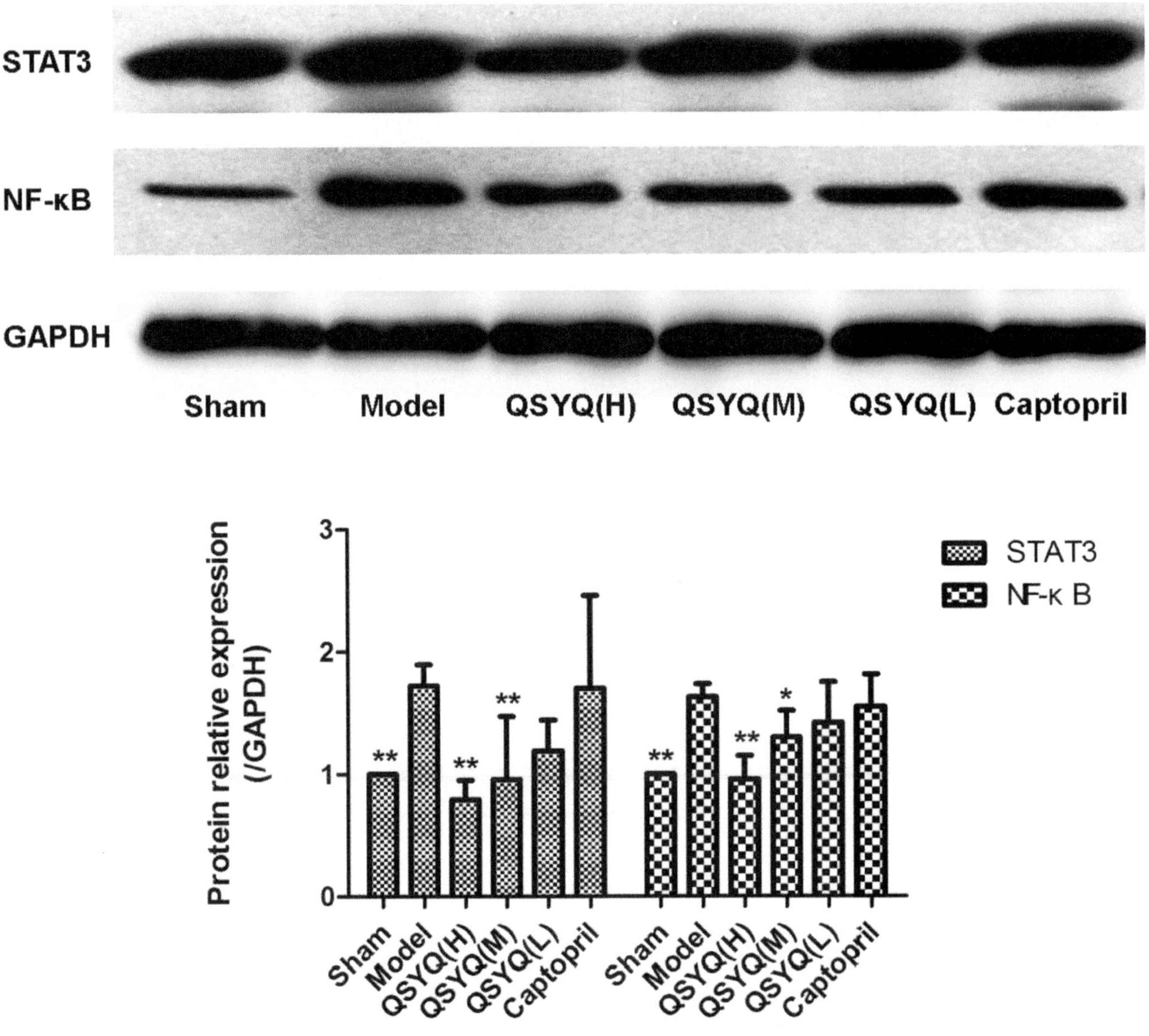

Figure 8. QSYQ significantly decreased cell signal transduction pathway factors of STAT3 and NF-κB in rats with HF. NF-κB in model group increased compared with sham, while treated by QSYQ (H) and (M) doses, the NF-κB level was significantly decreased. TheSTAT3 level in model group was up-regulated, while QSYQ at doses of 9.33 mg/kg (H) and 4.67 mg/kg (M) significantly decreased the STAT3 level respectively. After the administration of QSYQ (L) and captopril, the level of NF-κB and STAT3 had no statistical significance compared to model group. n = 10~14 for each group. Data were analyzed by one-way ANOVA, with $p<0.05$ indicating statistical significance. *Differed significantly from the model group ($p<0.05$).

Captopril only suppressed expression of MMP-2, but had no significant effect on MMP-9. Therefore, the results demonstrated that QSYQ could definitely inhibit myocardial remodeling in HF.

4 Effects of QSYQ on oxidative stress

Oxidative stress was evaluated by detection of MDA, SOD in plasma, and NADPHoxidase in the supernatant of cardiac tissue. As shown in **Table 2** and **Figure 7,** a significant increase on MDA level and decreasing on SOD activities in the model group were observed compared to the sham group. QSYQ (H) and (M) could significantly increase the levels of SOD (148.70±32.041, 134.29±20.423) ($p<0.01$), respectively, and decrease the levels of MDA (5.24±1.736 nd 5.13±1.044) respectively ($p<0.05$) (**Table 2**). QSYQ (L) and captopril had no significant effects on SOD, but both can significantly decreased the MDA level.

The Western blot results showed that the NADPHoxidase in model group (1.62±0.208) was increased by 62.40% ($p<0.05$) compared with sham group (1.00±0.000). While treated by QSYQ (H) and (M) doses, the NADPHoxidase level (1.04±0.142; 1.11±0.232) showed 35.80% and 31.48% reduction, respectively, compared to model group ($p<0.05$–0.01) (**Figure 7**). Low doses of QSYQ and captopril did not increase NADPH oxidase expression. Thus, the effect of QSYQ on NADPH oxidase expression was dose-dependent.

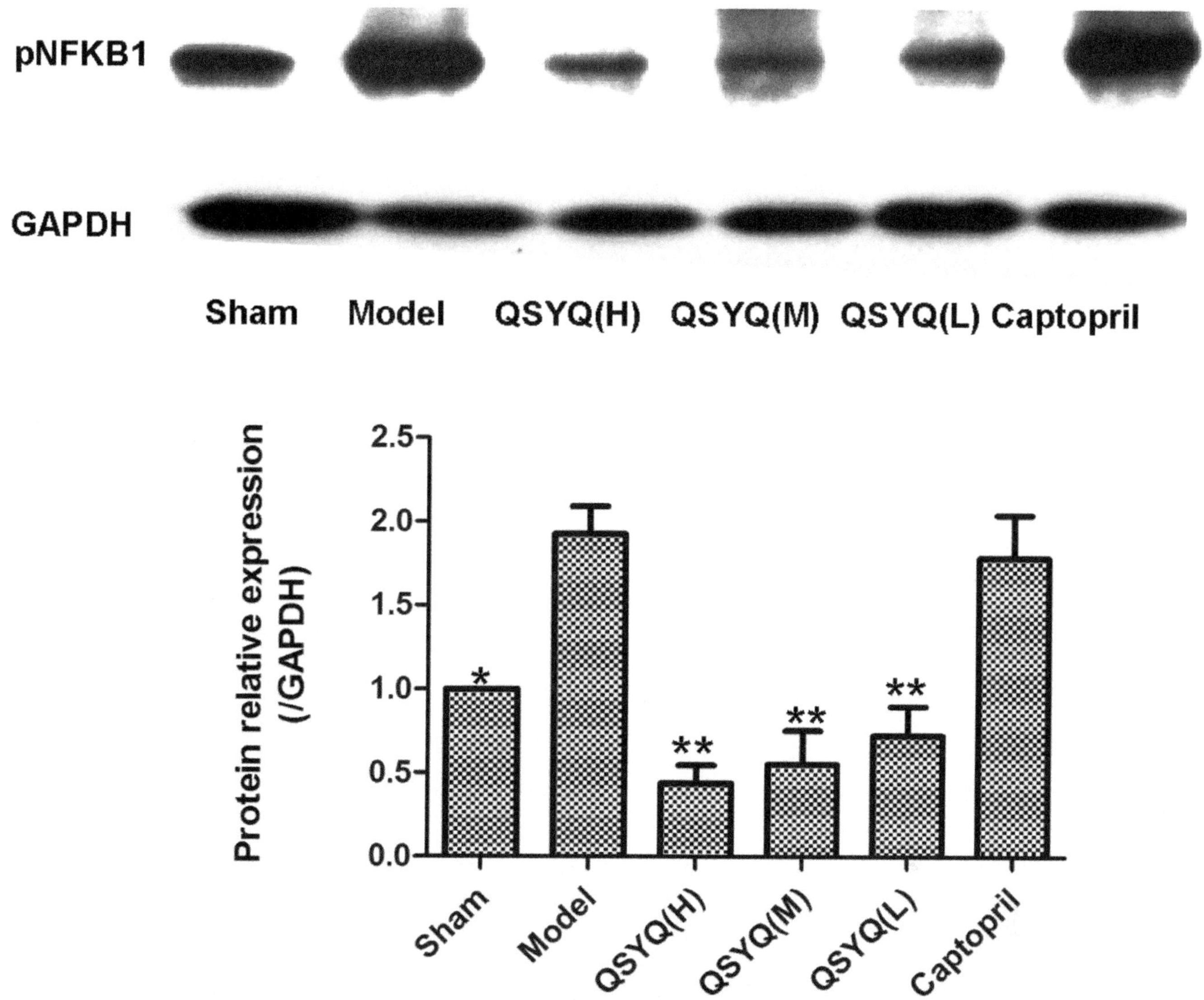

Figure 9. QSYQ significantly decreased cell signal transduction pathway factors of pNFKB1 in rats with HF. pNFKB1 in model group increased compared with sham, while treated by QSYQ (H), (M) and (L) doses, the pNFKB1 level was significantly decreased. In captopril group, the level of pNFKB1 had no statistical significance compared to model group. n = 10~14 for each group. Data were analyzed by one-way ANOVA, with $p<0.05$ indicating statistical significance. *Differed significantly from the model group ($p<0.05$), **Differed significantly from the model group ($p<0.01$).

5 QSYQ attenuated NF-κB activation and inflammation

The ELISA results showed that TNF-α and IL-6 were predominately up-regulated in model group by 38.78% and 60.30%, respectively. QSYQ (H) and (M) groups effectively down-regulated TNF-α by 13.98% and 21.32%, respectively. Meanwhile, they also could down-regulate IL-6 by 54.37% and 45.04% respectively. These results demonstrated a notable anti-inflammation efficacy of QSYQ. QSYQ (L) and captopril only reduced the expression of IL-6 ($p<0.05$), but had no significant effect on TNF-α (**Table 3**).

Moreover, the pathway protein NF-κB and pNFKB1 was also investigated. It's a critical signaling molecule which can mediate TNF-α producing apoptosis and oxidative stress. The NF-κB level in model group (1.63±0.107) increased by 63.41% ($p<0.05$) compared with sham group (1.00±0.000). QSYQ (H) and (M) dosages significantly decreased the NF-κB level to 0.96±0.190 and 1.30±0.217 ($p<0.05$–0.01), respectively. Surprisingly, the changes of pNFKB1 in different groups were more significant than NFκB. The results showed that in model group, the pNFKB1 were greatly activated (1.93±0.164) than in the sham group (1.00±0.000). QSYQ in different dosages can down-regulated the pNFKB1 in dose-dependent manner (0.438±0.109; 0.553±0.201; 0.724±0.176 respectively), which were consistent with the change of NF-κB. Captopril had no effect on the pNFKB1. (**Figure 8 and Figure 9**).

STAT3 mediated by IL-6 is another major cause to cardiac hypertrophy [22]. Interestingly, our present data displayed that theSTAT3 level in model group (1.72±0.177) was up-regulated by 71.71% ($p<0.05$) compared with sham (1.00±0.000). QSYQ (H) and (M) significantly decreased the STAT3 level to 0.79±0.161 and 0.96±0.512, respectively ($p<0.01$). (**Figure 8**).

After the administration of QSYQ (L) and captopril, the level of NF-κB and STAT3 had no statistical significance compared to model group ($P>0.05$). As the results shown, QSYQ not only

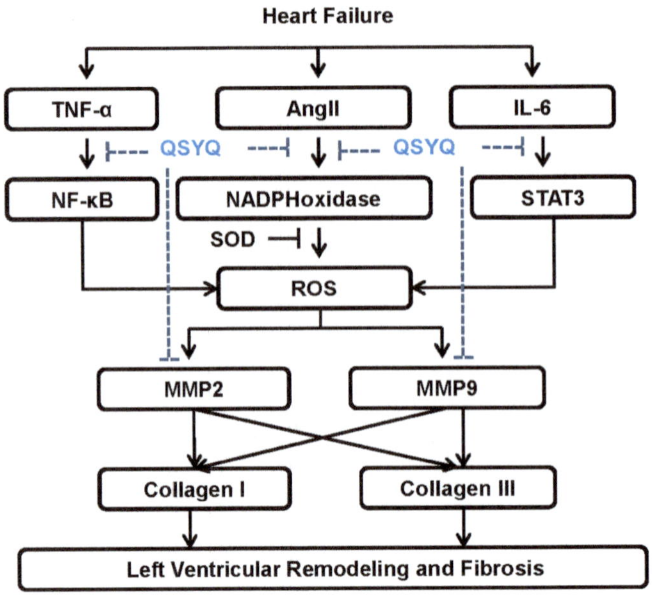

Figure 10. Protocol of the underlying mechanism of QSYQ in attenuating oxidative stress and inflammation signaling pathways in HF rats. QSYQ can reduce Left Ventricular Remodeling by Attenuating Inflammation and NADPH oxidase. It down-regulated the TNFα- NF-B and IL-6- STAT3 respectively to reduce the inflammation in heart failure. Futhermore, it also can supress the NADPH oxidase mediated oxidative stress injury to myocardial tissue. Finally, QSYQ can reduce the MMPs and collegen I and III in different degree and finally provide beneficial effects for clinical heart failure.

could improve the VR, but also evidently has a better efficacy on the anti-inflammation than captopril by depressing the TNF-α and IL-6.

Discussion

Accumulating evidence suggest that the increased oxidative stress coupled with activation of various downstream pro-inflammatory and cell death pathways play pivotal role on the development of complex alterations associated with HF [23]. However, despite of the accumulating knowledge in the past decades, the treatment of HF still remains poor and largely symptomatic [24].

Our research evaluated the effects of QSYQ treatment on myocardial dysfunction, inflammation, oxidative stress, and inter-related signaling pathways, using a rat model of LAD-induced HF. Since significant cardiac dysfunction as well as oxidative stress in this model occurs soon after the operation, with gradually increasing fibrosis and inflammation thereafter [25]. In the treatment protocol, we aimed to explore whether QSYQ can prevent the development of LAD ligation-induced left VR *via* attenuating oxidative stress and inhabiting inflammation.

Consistently with previous reports, the model group animals were characterized by declined diastolic and systolic myocardial performance such as hemodynamic alterations of LVSP, LVEDP, Max dP/dt, Min dP/dt, attenuated antioxidant defense (decreased SOD activity) coupled with increased myocardial ROS generation (up-regulation of MDA and NADPHoxidase). Our results were also in agreement with previous studies, demonstrating the enhanced activation of cardiac inflammatory markers, such as TNF-α and IL-6 and collagen contents associated with HF [10]. The LAD induced-ROS generation also activates pro-inflammatory pathways molecules such as NF-κB [26] and STAT3 [27,28], which reinforce, in turn, the expression of remodeling markers MMP-2 and MMP-9. QSYQ treatment was able to attenuate the oxidative stress and alterations of the above mentioned cardiac remodeling indicators (collagens I and III) as well as MMP-2 and MMP-9. Interestingly, it also depresses the activations of both TNFα-NF-κB and IL-6-STAT3 pathways. The beneficial effects of QSYQ could be explained, in part, by its potential anti-inflammatory properties. Our recent results suggested that QSYQ may exert potent effects on key pro-inflammatory cytokines, including IL-1 and C-reactive protein (CRP) *in vivo*. These results are also in support of the emerging role of the inflammation in the development and progression of HF [29,30].

The present study demonstrates that QSYQ, an ancient formula composed of six TCM, including two major herbs: Radix Astragali mongolici and Salvia miltiorrhiza Bunge, and four other adjunctive herbs, in a certain ratio, attenuate the cardiac remodeling by checking the MASSON and collagens I and III in HF rats. As shown in **Figure 10**, its cardioprotective efficacy is a comprehensive results by different pathway in a synergistic manner, including restoration of Ang II-NADPHoxidase-ROS-MMPs pathways and reduction of both TNF-α-NF-κB and IL-6-STAT3 pathways, thus to restore the hemodynamic parameters, normalize the cardiac function, and provide the comprehensive cardiac protective efficacy to HF.

Author Contributions

Conceived and designed the experiments: WW. Performed the experiments: CL Y. Wang QQ TS. Analyzed the data: CL Y. Wang. Contributed reagents/materials/analysis tools: Y. Wu JH. Wrote the paper: CL Y. Wang XC.

References

1. Armstrong PC, Kirkby NS, Zain ZN, Emerson M, Mitchell JA, et al. (2011) Thrombosis is reduced by inhibition of COX-1, but unaffected by inhibition of COX-2, in an acute model of platelet activation in the mouse. PLoS One 6: e20062.
2. Fertin M, Dubois E, Belliard A, Amouyel P, Pinet F, et al. (2012) Usefulness of circulating biomarkers for the prediction of left ventricular remodeling after myocardial infarction. The American journal of cardiology 110: 277–283.
3. Ahmad T, Fiuzat M, Felker GM, O'Connor C (2012) Novel biomarkers in chronic heart failure. Nature Reviews Cardiology 9: 347–359.
4. Kirkpatrick JN, Sutton MSJ (2012) Assessment of ventricular remodeling in heart failure clinical trials. Current heart failure reports 9: 328–336.
5. Khatib R, Joseph P, Briel M, Yusuf S, Healey J (2012) Blockade of the renin–angiotensin–aldosterone system (RAAS) for primary prevention of non-valvular atrial fibrillation: A systematic review and meta analysis of randomized controlled trials. International journal of cardiology.
6. Zhang M, Perino A, Ghigo A, Hirsch E, Shah AM (2013) NADPH oxidases in heart failure: poachers or gamekeepers? Antioxidants & Redox Signaling 18: 1024–1041.
7. Schröder K, Zhang M, Benkhoff S, Mieth A, Pliquett R, et al. (2012) Nox4 is a protective reactive oxygen species generating vascular NADPH oxidase. Circulation research 110: 1217–1225.
8. Gullestad L, Ueland T, Vinge LE, Finsen A, Yndestad A, et al. (2012) Inflammatory cytokines in heart failure: mediators and markers. Cardiology 122: 23–35.
9. Hohensinner PJ, Niessner A, Huber K, Weyand CM, Wojta J (2011) Inflammation and cardiac outcome. Current opinion in infectious diseases 24: 259–264.
10. Lecour S, James RW (2011) When are pro-inflammatory cytokines SAFE in heart failure? European heart journal 32: 680–685.
11. Li Y, Takemura G, Okada H, Miyata S, Maruyama R, et al. (2006) Reduction of inflammatory cytokine expression and oxidative damage by erythropoietin in chronic heart failure. Cardiovascular research 71: 684–694.
12. Rohini A, Agrawal N, Koyani CN, Singh R (2010) Molecular targets and regulators of cardiac hypertrophy. Pharmacological Research 61: 269–280.
13. Ferreira AS, Lopes AJ (2011) Chinese medicine pattern differentiation and its implications for clinical practice. Chinese Journal of Integrative Medicine 17: 818–823.
14. ChengTao H, Yi W, JianZhou L, Qian L, HaiBin Q, et al. (2009) Analysis of myocardial proteomic alteration after Qishenyiqi formula treatment in acute infarcted rat hearts. China Journal of Chinese Materia Medica 34: 1018–1021.
15. Dai G, Zhang B, Guo Z (2007) Application of central randomized system in project of clinical trial for secondary prevention of myocardial infarction by Qishen Yiqi Drop Pill]. Zhongguo Zhong xi yi jie he za zhi Zhongguo Zhongxiyi jiehe zazhi = Chinese journal of integrated traditional and Western medicine/ Zhongguo Zhong xi yi jie he xue hui, Zhongguo Zhong yi yan jiu yuan zhu ban 27: 653.
16. Wang Y, Li C, Ouyang Y, Yu J, Guo S, et al. (2012) Cardioprotective effects of Qishenyiqi mediated by angiotensin II type 1 receptor blockade and enhancing angiotensin-converting enzyme 2. Evidence-Based Complementary and Alternative Medicine 2012.
17. Lin Y, Qiu Q, Yang KX, Suo W, Chuo WJ, et al (2012) Effects of Yixin Jiedu Decoction on hemodynamic in Ameroid narrow ring caused heart failure small pigs. China Journal of Traditional Chinese Medicine and Pharmacy 5, 1280–1283.
18. Wang Y, Liu Z, Li C, Li D, Ouyang Y, et al. (2012) Drug target prediction based on the herbs components: the study on the multitargets pharmacological mechanism of qishenkeli acting on the coronary heart disease. Evidence-Based Complementary and Alternative Medicine 2012.
19. Wang Y, Li C, Ouyang Y, Shi T, Yang X, et al. (2013) QSYQ Attenuates Oxidative Stress and Apoptosis Induced Heart Remodeling Rats through Different Subtypes of NADPH-Oxidase. Evidence-Based Complementary and Alternative Medicine 2013.
20. Mukhopadhyay P, Bátkai S, Rajesh M, Czifra N, Harvey-White J, et al. (2007) Pharmacological inhibition of CB1 cannabinoid receptor protects against doxorubicin-induced cardiotoxicity. Journal of the American College of Cardiology 50: 528–536.
21. Pacher P, Nagayama T, Mukhopadhyay P, Bátkai S, Kass DA (2008) Measurement of cardiac function using pressure–volume conductance catheter technique in mice and rats. Nature protocols 3: 1422–1434.
22. Mir SA, Chatterjee A, Mitra A, Pathak K, Mahata SK, et al. (2012) Inhibition of signal transducer and activator of transcription 3 (STAT3) attenuates interleukin-6 (IL-6)-induced collagen synthesis and resultant hypertrophy in rat heart. Journal of Biological Chemistry 287: 2666–2677.
23. Rajesh M, Mukhopadhyay P, Bátkai S, Patel V, Saito K, et al. (2010) Cannabidiol attenuates cardiac dysfunction, oxidative stress, fibrosis, and inflammatory and cell death signaling pathways in diabetic cardiomyopathy. Journal of the American College of Cardiology 56: 2115–2125.
24. Kairouz V, Lipskaia L, Hajjar RJ, Chemaly ER (2012) Molecular targets in heart failure gene therapy: current controversies and translational perspectives. Annals of the New York Academy of Sciences 1254: 42–50.
25. Houser SR, Margulies KB, Murphy AM, Spinale FG, Francis GS, et al. (2012) Animal Models of Heart Failure A Scientific Statement From the American Heart Association. Circulation research 111: 131–150.
26. Wysong A, Couch M, Shadfar S, Li L, Rodriguez JE, et al. (2011) NF-κB Inhibition Protects against Tumor-Induced Cardiac Atrophy in Vivo. The American journal of pathology 178: 1059–1068.
27. Wang M, Zhang W, Crisostomo P, Markel T, Meldrum KK, et al. (2007) Endothelial STAT3 plays a critical role in generalized myocardial proinflammatory and proapoptotic signaling. American Journal of Physiology-Heart and Circulatory Physiology 293: H2101–H2108.
28. Kurdi M, Booz GW (2010) Deciphering STAT3 signaling in the heart: plasticity and vascular inflammation. Congestive Heart Failure 16: 234–238.
29. Hamid T, Gu Y, Ortines RV, Bhattacharya C, Wang G, et al. (2009) Divergent Tumor Necrosis Factor Receptor–Related Remodeling Responses in Heart Failure Role of Nuclear Factor-κB and Inflammatory Activation. Circulation 119: 1386–1397.
30. Bartunek J, Vanderheyden M (2012) Inflammation and related biomarkers in cardiovascular disease. Biomarkers 6: 1–3.

8

Speckle-Tracking Echocardiography Elucidates the Effect of Pacing Site on Left Ventricular Synchronization in the Normal and Infarcted Rat Myocardium

Michal Mor[1☯], Wesam Mulla[1☯], Sigal Elyagon[1], Hovav Gabay[1,2], Shani Dror[1], Yoram Etzion[1,3¶*], Noah Liel-Cohen[4¶]

1 Cardiac Arrhythmia Research Laboratory, Department of Physiology and Cell Biology, Faculty of Health Sciences, Ben-Gurion University of the Negev, Beer-Sheva, Israel, **2** Department of Emergency Medicine, Recanati School for Community Health Professions, Faculty of Health Sciences and PREPARED Center for Emergency Response Research, Ben-Gurion University of the Negev, Beer-Sheva, Israel, **3** Division of Internal Medicine, Soroka University Medical Center, Beer-Sheva, Israel, **4** Cardiology Department, Soroka University Medical Center, Beer-Sheva, Israel

Abstract

Background: Right ventricular (RV) pacing generates regional disparities in electrical activation and mechanical function (ventricular dyssynchrony). In contrast, left ventricular (LV) or biventricular (BIV) pacing can improve cardiac efficiency in the setting of ventricular dyssynchrony, constituting the rationale for cardiac resynchronization therapy (CRT). Animal models of ventricular dyssynchrony and CRT currently relay on large mammals which are expensive and not readily available to most researchers. We developed a methodology for double-site epicardial pacing in conscious rats. Here, following post-operative recovery, we compared the effects of various pacing modes on LV dyssynchrony in normal rats and in rats with ischemic cardiomyopathy.

Methods: Two bipolar electrodes were implanted in rats as follows: Group A (n = 6) right atrial (RA) and RV sites; Group B (n = 7) RV and LV sites; Group C (n = 8) as in group B in combination with left coronary artery ligation. Electrodes were exteriorized through the back. Following post-operative recovery, two-dimensional transthoracic echocardiography was performed during pacing through the different electrodes. Segmental systolic circumferential strain (Ecc) was used to evaluate LV dyssynchrony.

Results: In normal rats, RV pacing induced marked LV dyssynchrony compared to RA pacing or sinus rhythm, as measured by the standard deviation (SD) of segmental time to peak Ecc, SD of peak Ecc, and the average delay between opposing ventricular segments. LV pacing and, to a greater extend BIV pacing diminished the LV dyssynchrony compared to RV pacing. In rats with extensive MI, the effects of LV and BIV pacing were markedly attenuated, and the response of individual animals was variable.

Conclusions: Rodent cardiac pacing mimics important features seen in humans. This model may be developed as a simple new tool to study the pathophysiology of ventricular dyssynchrony and CRT.

Editor: Alena Talkachova, University of Minnesota, United States of America

Funding: This work was supported by a research grant from the Clalit Research Institute, Clalit health services, Israel (Yoram Etzion and Noah Liel-Cohen). The funders had no role in study design, data collection and analysis, decision to publish, or preparation of the manuscript.

Competing Interests: The authors have declared that no competing interests exist.

* E-mail: tzion@bgu.ac.il

☯ These authors contributed equally to this work.

¶ These authors also contributed equally to this work.

Introduction

Dyssynchronous contraction of the left ventricle (LV) can markedly worsen the outcome of heart failure (HF) independently of traditional risk factors [1,2]. This pathophysiology is often derived from or exacerbated by native conduction delay, such as left bundle branch block (LBBB) or artificial pacing of the right ventricle (RV) [3–5]. Based on QRS widening, it is estimated that at least 25–30% of patients with HF exhibit dyssynchronous LV contraction [6,7]. Clinical studies employing biventricular (BIV) pacing (cardiac resynchronization therapy; CRT) to treat HF patients with dyssynchronous contraction have revealed significant benefits in terms of contractile performance, improved quality of life, and long-term survival [8].

Although dyssynchronous heart failure (DHF) has been extensively studied in mechanical terms and although the clinical effectiveness of CRT is remarkable, there are multiple issues that remain ill-defined at present. It is, for example, estimated that around 30% of patients do not benefit from CRT, and the clinical criteria to identify CRT non-responders remain obscure and controversial. In addition, there is variability in individual patient vulnerability to DHF progression in response to conventional RV pacing, which is difficult to predict at present [4,9]. Only recently has the impact of dyssynchrony and BIV pacing on molecular signaling and the ionic properties of the myocardium been realized [9,10]. Animal studies have shown that DHF is associated with regional molecular changes (collectively termed 'molecular polarization'), including downregulation of Ca^{2+} handling proteins and connexin 43, activation of stress response kinases and increased expression of tumor necrosis factor in the lateral LV wall. Most of these changes can be reversed by CRT [11]. Additional studies identifying regional changes in ionic channels and multiple gene transcripts [12,13] have revealed a highly complicated picture in which multiple players are involved. Therefore, comprehensive understanding of the effects of various pacing modes at the molecular level will require extensive additional scientific efforts.

One of the problems hampering progress in this field of research is the lack of suitable animal models that can be utilized for routine experimentation. Current studies almost exclusively utilize large animals (mainly dogs) and are based on the implantation of human devices. Such an experimental setting is highly demanding. In addition, the large animal models can not be manipulated genetically, an issue that is becoming increasingly critical when it is necessary to reveal molecular mechanisms. While rat and mouse models are extensively used in research on HF [14], these animal models are largely missing in research on DHF and CRT, mainly due to technical difficulties in electrode implantation. Two independent studies using M-mode echocardiography have managed to demonstrate dyssynchrony between the septum and the LV lateral wall in the murine heart [13,15]. In addition, in the pioneering study of Bilchick et al. 2006 mice were implanted with a single pacing electrode on the RV free wall and were paced for seven days using an implanted miniature pacemaker. Using microarray analysis, this study demonstrated indications for molecular polarization as a result of prolonged RV pacing [13,15]. Thus, it appears that rodents may mimic important features that are seen in large mammals in regard to the mechanical effect of ventricular pacing. However, to the best of our knowledge, the mechanical effect of RV pacing as compared with LV and BIV pacing has not yet been defined in rodents.

In the present study, using an implanted device that was developed for pacing and recordings in conscious rodents [16], we acutely evaluated the effect of pacing site on LV synchronization in normal and infarcted rats following post operative recovery. We hypothesized that the mechanical effects of LV pacing and BIV pacing should be favorable compared to RV pacing. Elucidation of this issue seems critical in order to clarify whether rodent models may be further developed as simple experimental tools to study the molecular biology of DHF and CRT. Utilizing speckle-tracking 2-dimensional echocardiography, a method that has been repeatedly validated in rats for segmental strain analysis over the past decade [17–20], we confirmed the existence of mechanical dyssynchrony when RV pacing was applied. In addition, we elucidated the electrical and mechanical effects of LV pacing and BIV pacing. Overall, our results support the notion that the effects of pacing in rodents can recapitulate important features observed in large animal models and humans.

Methods

Ethics statement

All animal studies reported in this article were approved by the institutional ethics committee, Faculty of Health Sciences, Ben-Gurion University of the Negev, Israel. At the end of all experiments animals were killed using IV KCl injection under deep isoflurane anesthesia.

Implantable rat pacing device

The implantable device that was used to pace the heart at different locations was originally designed for long-term atrial pacing and recording in freely moving rats [16]. In this device, the electrical connections to the epicardial surface are achieved using miniature-bipolar hook electrodes, which have been described in detail previously [16]. The specific design of the miniature-bipolar hook electrode allows it to be positioned on a desired location on the epicardial surface of the atria or ventricles through a small lateral thoracotomy without the need of additional suturing [16]. The implantable device consists of an 8-pin 'female' connector that is attached by flexible insulated electrical wires to a set of two miniature bipolar hook electrodes (Figure 1a). Peripheral electrodes that are implanted on the back for pseudo ECG measurements also exist (Figure 1a,c). Before implantation, the 8-pin 'female' connector was covered with a latex sheath to prevent direct contact with the subcutaneous tissue during the operation. Electron beam radiation was applied for sterilization of the device before use.

Surgical procedures

Adult male Sprague-Dawley rats (250–300 g) were anesthetized (ketamine/xylazine 75/5 mg/kg, IP) and mechanically ventilated. The animals were placed supine on a warmed heating and under sterile conditions a skin incision in the left thorax was performed and a subcutaneous tunnel was extended posteriorly to the upper back of the animal. The 8-pin 'female' connector (covered with a latex sheath) was inserted through the subcutaneous tunnel. Thereafter, lateral thoracotomy was performed and the two miniature -bipolar hook electrodes were positioned as follows: Group A; on the right atrium (RA) and RV apex (RV). Group B; on the RV and on the posterobasal aspect of the left ventricle (LV). Group C; similar electrode implantation as in group B, as well as proximal left anterior descending coronary artery ligation to induce myocardial infarction (MI). In order to insert electrodes on the right side (for positioning on the RA and RV) a small subcutaneous tunnel was done in the chest wall through which the electrodes were moved to the right side of the thorax. The coronary artery was ligated by 6/0 surgical suture and MI was confirmed by the presence of regional cyanosis in the myocardial surface. Following chest closure, each animal was placed in a prone position and the back connector was exteriorized through the skin of the back (Figure 1B). Postoperative recovery and analgesia were done as described previously [16].

Cardiac pacing and echocardiograpy

Normal rats were evaluated 6–8 days following the surgical procedure. MI rats were evaluated 14 days following the surgical procedure. For the echocardiograpic analysis, each animal was sedated (isoflurane 1%) and placed on a heating pad. ECG recordings (Nihon Kodhen, RMC1100) were monitored online throughout the experiment and were also digitized and stored for offline analysis in each pacing mode (PCI-6024E, National Instruments, Austin, TX, USA). Electrical stimulation (2 ms square pulses) was applied through isolation units (Iso-Flex, AMPI, Israel) at a double diastolic threshold. The cycle length that was used to induce override pacing in the normal rats was set to 150 ms (400 bpm) which invariably induced override pacing in these animals. In the MI rats, baseline heart rate was sometimes slightly higher than 400 bpm. Therefore, the override pacing cycle length was set to 140 ms (428 bpm), which managed to override

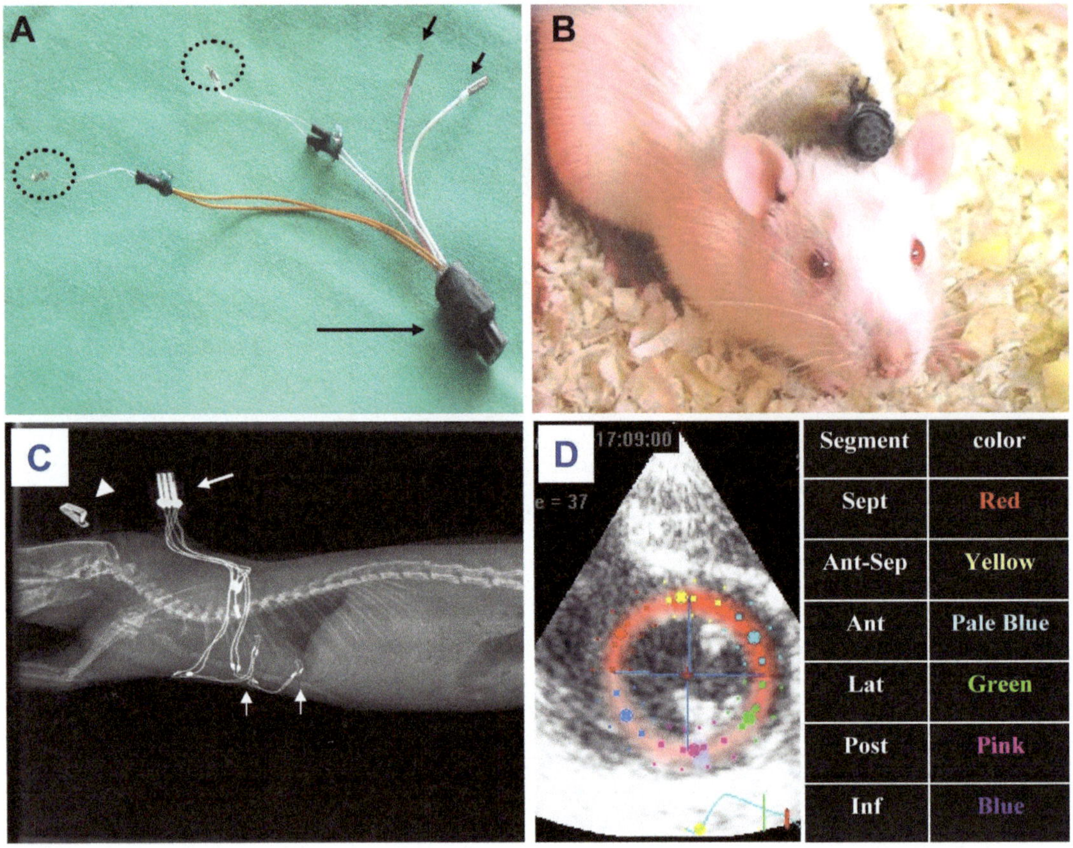

Figure 1. Experimental setup for LV strain analysis in paced rats. A: An implanted pacing device consisting of two miniature-bipolar hook electrodes (dotted circles). Long arrow; 8-pin back connector. Short arrows; peripheral electrodes for optional pseudo ECG measurements in conscious animals [16]. **B**: A rat with an exteriorized back connector following the implantation procedure. **C**: X-ray lateral view of an implanted rat. The two miniature-bipolar hook electrodes (vertical arrows at the bottom) were inserted on the RV and the LV as described in the text. The X-ray view is shown for illustration and was not utilized to access the position of the electrodes on the heart. D: Short axis mid-level echocardiographic view of an implanted rat and standard separation map of the LV into six segments for circumferential strain (Ecc) analysis.

the spontaneous heart rate of these animals. During BIV pacing, two independent isolation units were used for simultaneous but independent RV apical and LV pacing. A program developed by YE [16] was used to control data acquisition, electrical stimulation and off-line analysis. QT interval measurements were manually done off-line on the digital signals under high time and voltage magnification scales. These measurements were performed using dedicated cursors which marked the isoelectric line and stressed out the time of return of the ECG signal to this line. The measured QT intervals of five independent complexes were averaged in each condition to reduce sampling error. Two-dimensional transthoracic echocardiography was performed with a Vivid 7 echocardiography system (GE Healthcare, Milwaukee WI, USA) by short-axis mid-ventricular scans at the level of the papillary muscle tips. Images were obtained with a 10 S transducer (5.4~11.8 MHz) using an image depth of 2.5 cm and a frame rate of 225 frames/s as was repeatedly validated in the literature in rat studies [17-20]. The acquisition protocol was as follows: Following optimal positioning of the transducer on the chest wall, it was fixed in place by the operator, while 2D clips (20 s each) were sequentially recorded in sinus rhythm followed by override pacing at the different pacing sites. Of note, we took special care that the transducer will stay in the exact same position throughout the experiment to allow for accurate comparison between the different pacing modes in each animal. The procedure was always done by two experimentalist, one acquiring there echocardiography clips and the other controlling the pacing and confirming continuous electrical capture in each pacing mode. At the end of each experiment, the animal was sacrificed and correct positioning of the epicardial electrodes was confirmed by post mortem operation. Offline analysis of LV fractional area shortening (LV-FAS) was done by calculating the LV areas during maximal systole (LVAs) and during maximal diastole (LVAd) and then expressing LV-FAS as: (LVAd-LVAs)/LVAd×100.

Circumferential 2-dimensional strain analysis

Based on the existing literature in rodents, we restricted our current analysis to circumferential strain (Ecc) which is more reliable than radial strain in the small heart of rats [18,19]. Ecc was evaluated as described in the literature [17–19]. Briefly, analysis of mid-level short-axis images was done with dedicated software ("2D-strain", EchoPAC, GE healthcare, Vingmed, Norway). Endocardial border at end-systole and the region of interest from the endocardium to the epicardial edge were determined by the user (Figure 1d). Thereafter, an automatic speckle tracking analysis was performed for the short-axis images to track the motion of speckles contained within the region of interest on a frame-to-frame basis [21]. Ecc curves, expressed in percentage values as a function of time were exported to a customized program (MATLAB software, MathWorks) to calculate the time from onset of QRS to peak Ecc (time to peak Ecc) and the value of maximal Ecc (across the six mid-level segments (Figure 1d, Figure 2a). The values of maximal Ecc are shown as % of segmental length at onset QRS complex. At least five consecutive beats were analyzed under each pacing condition in each animal. Initial determination of the region of interest from the endocardium to the epicardial edge was performed under no pacing conditions and was kept as constant as possible during the different pacing conditions. Analysis of all rats in each group was done by a single observer (MM - normal rats, WM - MI rats). An independent observer who is highly experienced in echocardiographic methodologies including 2D strain analysis (NLC) confirmed the consistency of the analysis performed by the two observers.

Statistical analysis

Values are expressed as means ±SE. Due to the relatively small sample size in each group, analysis of the difference between pacing conditions was done using Kruskal-Wallis one way analysis of variance on ranks with Student-Neuman-Keuls post hoc test. All statistical tests were done using SigmaStat 3.1 (Systat Software, Inc, Point Richmond, CA). The criterion for significance was set at $P<0.05$.

Results

RV pacing versus RA pacing or sinus rhythm in normal rats

As a first step we aimed to compare the effect of RV pacing to both no pacing and RA pacing modes. This analysis was done in order to confirm that the override pacing itself does not induce rate-dependent LV dyssynchrony compared to the no pacing mode (sinus rhythm). For that purpose, group A (n = 6) was instrumented with a bipolar RA pacing electrode and a bipolar RV pacing electrode, and override pacing in these two locations (150 ms CL) was compared to the no pacing state. The obtained Ecc traces of the different LV segments typically demonstrated no major differences between RA pacing and sinus rhythm. In contrast, RV pacing invariably induced marked changes in the segmental strain pattern. The RV pacing typically produced an early systolic contraction in the inferior or posterior segments, which was associated, in some cases, with a clear stretching effect in opposing segments (Figure 2A). Summary of the segmental time to peak Ecc and the segmental peak Ecc patterns under the different pacing modes is presented figure 2B. Analysis of important global parameters derived from the segmental Ecc analysis under the different pacing modes is shown in Figure 3. The global time to peak Ecc was found to be slightly shorter during RA pacing compared to no pacing (85.6±4.1%, $p<0.05$) an was also shorter compared to RV pacing (Figure 3A). Global peak Ecc (Figure 3B) was not different between RA pacing and no pacing but was markedly attenuated during RV pacing (61.0±3.7% compared to no pacing, $p<0.01$ compared to both RA pacing and no pacing). While the Ecc analysis identified a marked effect of RV pacing on strain parameters, concurrent analysis of LV-FAS did not identify a significant effect of the different pacing modes on this parameter (Figure 3C, see discussion). Specific analysis of LV dyssynchrony variables indicated marked deleterious effects of RV pacing on all the calculated parameters, including standard deviation of time to peak Ecc (Figure 3D), standard deviation of peak Ecc (Figure 3E) and the average time difference between the peak Ecc of opposing segments (Delta TP opposing segments, Figure 3F). There was no statistical difference in these parameters between RA pacing and sinus rhythm.

Effects of different ventricular pacing modes in normal rats

In the next stage, we evaluated group B (n = 7) rats, which had bipolar pacing leads in the RV and LV. The effect of override pacing in these two locations alone or simultaneously (BIV pacing) was compared to the no pacing mode. In terms of electrical activity, the ECG recording indicated QRS prolongation during RV pacing as compared to LV and BIV pacing (Figure 4A). However, the unclear separation between the QRS and the T-wave in the rodent heart [22,23], did not allow quantitative analysis of QRS width during the various pacing modes. Nevertheless, an analysis of QT duration indicated marked QT prolongation during RV pacing (138.3±5.3%, $p<0.01$) as compared to the no pacing mode. This marked QT prolongation was reduced by LV pacing (124.9±2.9%) and even further reduced by BIV pacing (109.1±3.6%), as shown with detailed statistical analysis in Figure 4B. In addition, recordings of epicardial electrograms from the RV electrode when pacing the LV and vice versa, was performed in two animals from group B. These recordings supported a longer sequence of activation during RV pacing compared to LV pacing (Figure 4C).

We next evaluated the mechanical dyssynchrony during the various pacing modes. Summary of the segmental time to peak Ecc and the segmental peak Ecc under the different pacing modes in group B are presented figure 5. Analysis of important global parameters derived from the segmental Ecc analysis under the different pacing modes is shown in Figure 6. RV pacing significantly reduced both the global time to peak Ecc and the global peak Ecc as compared to no pacing. These parameters recovered significantly during LV and BIV pacing (Figure 6A, B). In addition, while a prominent increase in all the parameters of LV dyssynchrony was noted during RV pacing, LV pacing and particularly BIV pacing markedly improved all three parameters of LV dyssynchrony (Figure 6 D–E). Of note, the segmental pattern of the time to peak Ecc during RV pacing (Figure 5) was somewhat different from that observed in group A (Figure 2), possibly due to variability in the positioning of the RV electrode on the epicardial surface of the RV (see limitations section in our discussion). As in group A (Figure 3), we could not detect significant changes in LV-FAS during the different pacing modes (Figure 6C).

Effects of different ventricular pacing modes in rats with ischemic-induced heart failure

To elucidate the influence of ischemic HF on the electromechanical results of our model, group C (n = 8) was subjected to a combined procedure of electrode implantation and left coronary artery ligation. We analyzed the effect of pacing two weeks following surgery, at a time when prominent scar tissue and myocardial remodeling were present (Figure 7A, B). Out of the eight animals with confirmed MI, one had electrical capture only in the LV and was excluded from analysis. Two additional animals had electrical capture only in the RV and were therefore analyzed only in the no pacing and RV pacing modes. Final statistical analysis was done only on the five MI rats that exhibited electrical capture in both RV and LV sites. In electrophysiological terms, the MI rats demonstrated baseline prolongation of the QT interval compared to the normal rats (94.0±4.4 ms vs. 70.5±4.4 ms, $p<0.001$). However, the effect of pacing on the QT interval followed a similar trend to that in the normal rats. Indeed, RV pacing

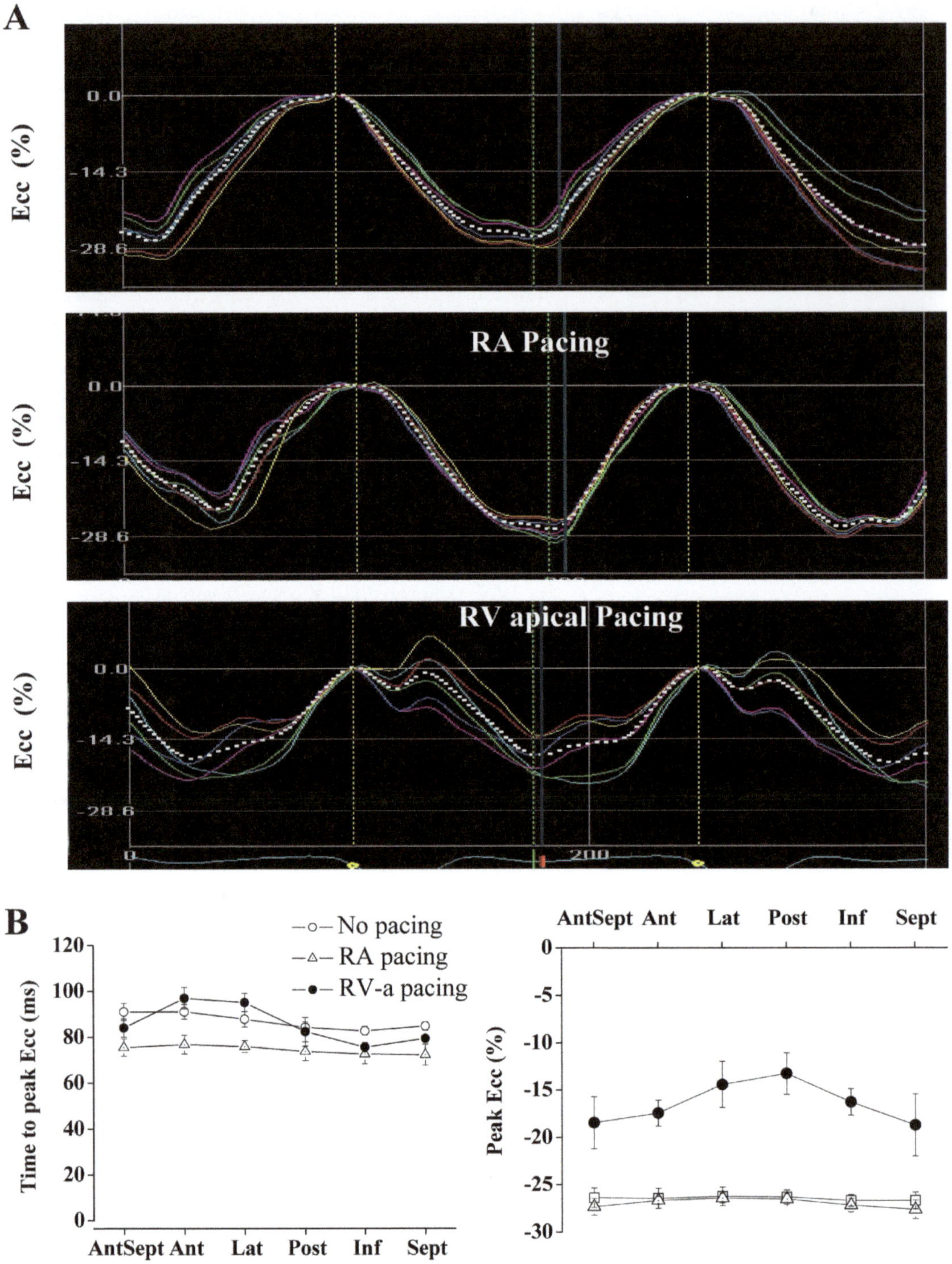

Figure 2. Segmental Ecc analysis during RA and RV pacing. A: Representative strain waveforms in an instrumented rat subjected to no pacing (upper), RA pacing (middle) and RV (lower). The colors of the different waveforms match those in the segmental map in Figure 1D. White dotted lines represent the global (average) strain of all six segments. **B**: Average segmental time to peak Ecc (left) and peak Ecc (right) in seven animals subjected no pacing, RA pacing, and RV pacing.

statistically increased the QT interval as compared with no pacing mode (118.6±3.7%, $p<0.05$), while the QT during LV and BIV pacing did not differ from sinus rhythm (113.9±4.7% and 106.2±3.9%, respectively, see details in Figure 7C).

Evaluation of segmental Ecc in group C revealed typical akinesia or dyskinesia in the anteroseptal, anterior and lateral segments at baseline (Figure 7D). No apparent effect of pacing on the magnitude and temporal pattern of the peak Ecc was observed in these rats (Figure 7E, Figure 8 A,B). In addition, while dyssynchrony parameters were much higher in the MI animals at baseline, there were no apparent effects of the different pacing modes on these parameters, excluding a non-significant tendency

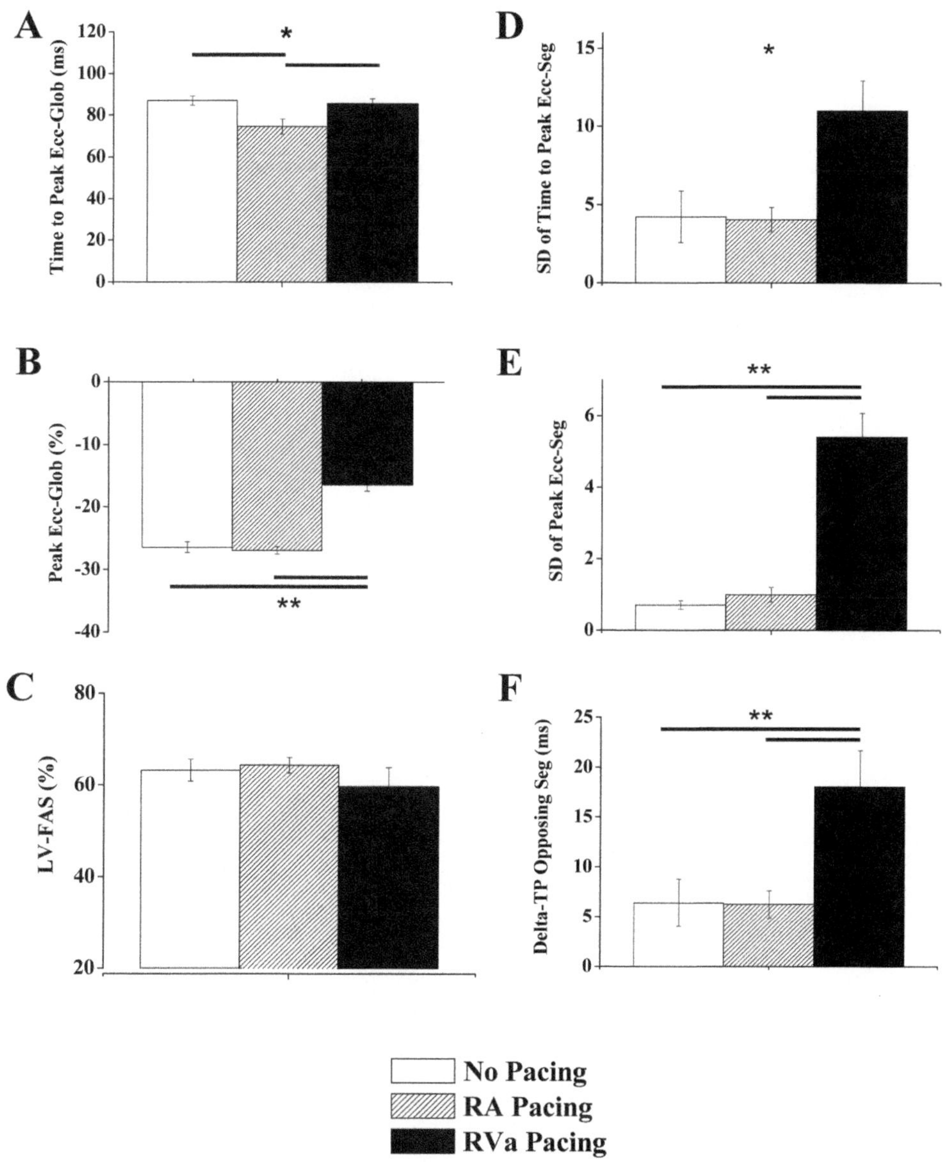

Figure 3. RV pacing induces marked LV dyssynchrony compared to RA pacing. Summary of echocardiographic parameters in group A subjected to no pacing, RA pacing, and RV pacing. **A**: Average time to peak Ecc of all six segments (global). **B**: Average peak Ecc of all six segments (global). **C**: LV fractional area shortening. **D**: Standard deviation of the time to peak Ecc of different segments. **E**: Standard deviation of the peak Ecc of different segments. **F**: Analysis of 'delta TP opposing segments', i.e., the average time difference between the peak Ecc of opposing segments. * $P < 0.05$, ** $P < 0.01$. Horizontal lines above\below the bar graphs indicate significant differences between pacing modes in the post-hoc analysis. Note that in **D** the Kruskal-Wallis test was significant. However, the post-hoc analysis could not reveal the source of difference between the groups.

to increase in the 'delta TP opposing segments' parameter during RV pacing (Figure 8 D–F). Looking more closely at the effect of pacing on the 'delta TP of opposing segments' in individual rats (Figure 9 A), we observed a consistent tendency for this parameter to increase during RV pacing in 6 out of the 7 evaluated animals. Compared with RV pacing the effects of LV pacing and BIV pacing on the delta TP of opposing segments were variable. While these pacing modes seemed to have a beneficial effect in some cases (e.g., animals 2 and 3), there was a worsening of this parameter in animal 5 when LV and BIV pacing were applied (Figure 9 A). An additional analysis specifically focusing on the two opposing segments that had maximal temporal dyssynchrony during RV pacing detected a rather similar pattern (Figure 9 B, C).

Discussion

The present study introduces a new model of ventricular pacing in an instrumented rat, which allowed us for the first time to systematically evaluate the effects of pacing site on LV synchronization in the rodent heart. We used speckle-tracking echocardiography analysis of Ecc, which has been reported to reliably and sensitively detect changes in LV dyssynchrony under various clinically relevant conditions in the rat heart [17–20]. The speckle-tracking echocardiographic methodology has previously been applied extensively in large animal models and in people and has been shown to be much more sensitive to changes in LV dyssynchrony than global echocardiographic measures, such as fractional shortening [24]. Therefore, in the present study, it is not

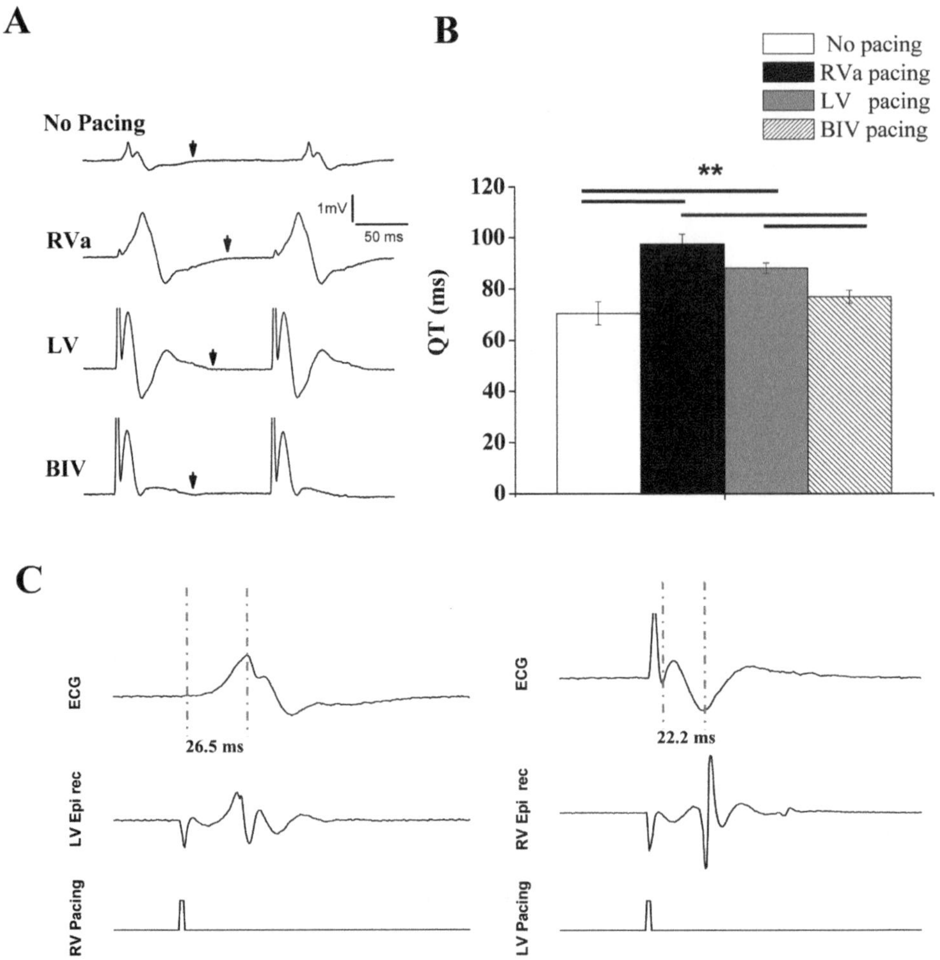

Figure 4. RV pacing induces electrical dyssynchrony compared to LV and BIV pacing. **A**: Representative ECG recordings from an instrumented rat during sinus rhythm (no pacing) and during RV, LV and BIV pacing. Arrows indicate the termination of the T wave in each trace. **B**: Summary of QT interval analysis in six instrumented rats. ** $P<0.01$. Horizontal lines above the bar graph indicate significant differences between pacing modes in the post-hoc analysis. **C**: Example of epicardial electrograms during RV pacing (left) and LV pacing (right). In each recording upper trace is a peripheral ECG signal (Lead I), middle trace is the epicardial electrogram and lower trace shows the time of cardiac pacing. Note that the epicardial activation in the RV electrode correlates with a late negative vector in the ECG signal. In contrast, the epicardial activation during RV pacing is correlated with a late positive vector in the ECG signal. Measurements of the time from end of stimulus artifact to the peaks of these late vectors in the ECG (dash vertical lines) indicate shorter activation time during LV pacing. Analysis of epicardial electrograms in an additional animal from group B demonstrated similar findings (not shown).

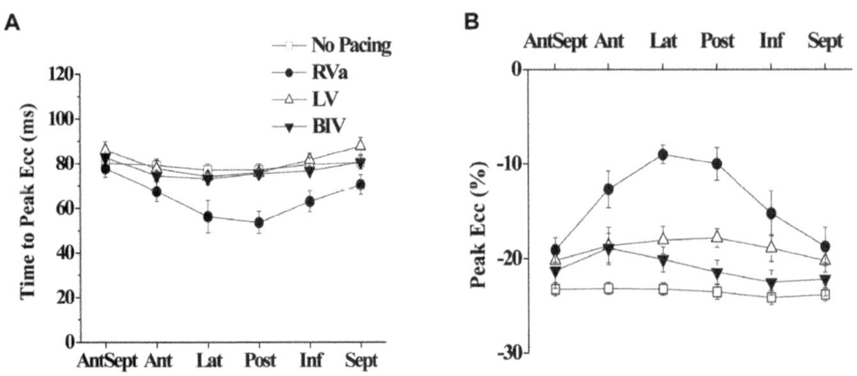

Figure 5. Segmental Ecc analysis during RV, LV and BIV pacing. Average segmental time to peak Ecc (**A**) and peak Ecc (**B**) in seven animals from group B subjected to no pacing, RV pacing, LV pacing and BIV pacing.

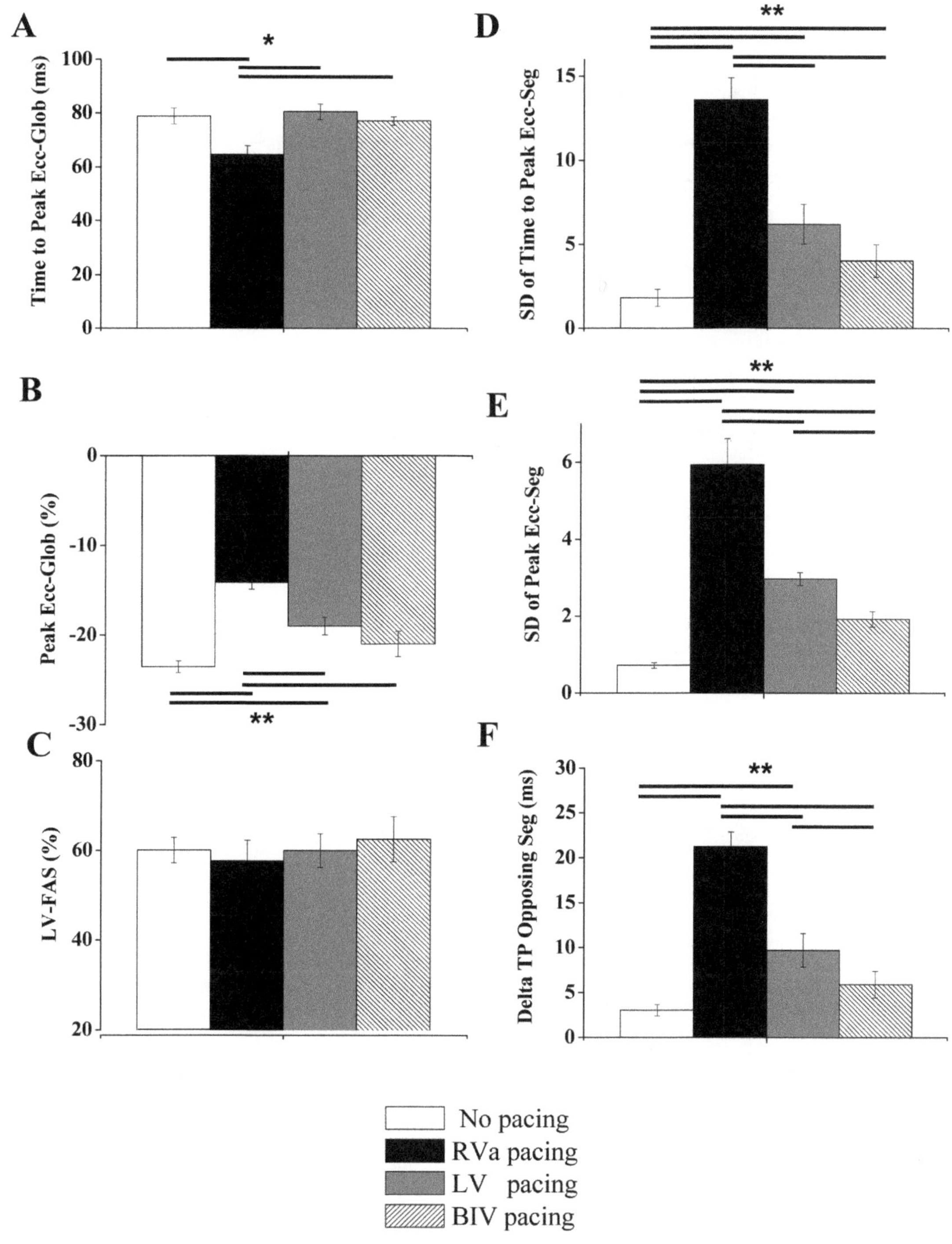

Figure 6. RV pacing induces mechanical dyssynchrony compared to LV and BIV pacing. Summary of echocardiographic parameters in six animals subjected to no pacing, RV, LV and BIV pacing. **A**: Average time to peak Ecc of all six segments (global). **B**: Average peak Ecc of all six segments (global) **C**: LV fractional area shortening **D**: Standard deviation of the time to peak Ecc of different segments. **E**: Standard deviation of the peak Ecc of different segments. **F**: Average time difference between the peak Ecc of opposing segments ('delta TP opposing segments', see Figure 3 for details). * P<0.05, ** P<0.01. Horizontal lines above\below the bar graphs indicate significant differences between pacing modes in the post-hoc analysis.

surprising that there were no significant effects of pacing on LV-FAS, while the effects of pacing site on segmental and global Ecc pattern were consistent and significant.

The main findings of our Ecc analysis indicate that while the rodent heart has some clear differences compared to the human heart in aspects such as action potential repolarization and calcium handling [22,23,25], its mechanical response to the effect of various pacing modes seems to have important similarities to the large mammalian heart. While previous studies in the mouse heart have already demonstrated negative effects of acute RV pacing on

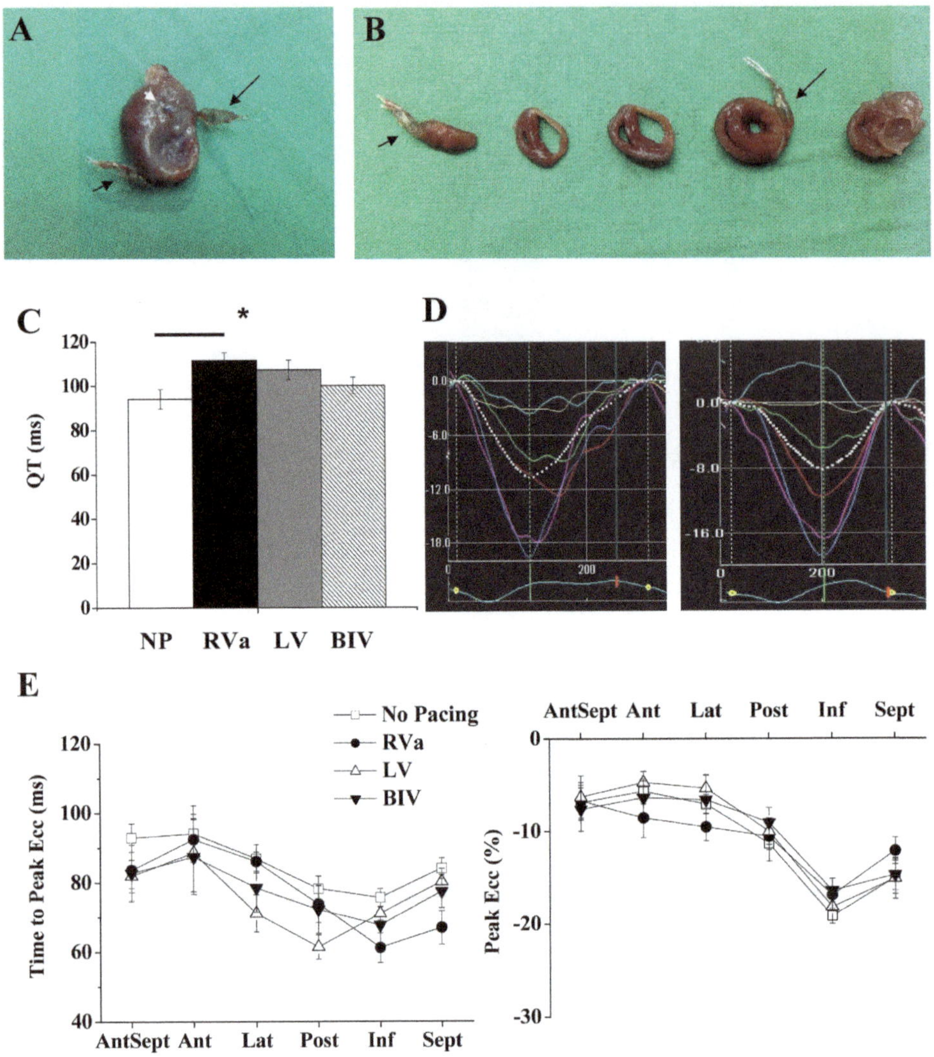

Figure 7. Combined model of pacing and ischemic heart failure. A: Anterior image of a heart subjected to electrodes implantation in combination with left coronary ligation. RV electrode and LV electrode are marked by short and long black arrows, respectively. White arrow; coronary artery ligation site. **B**: Transverse sections of the heart shown in A. Apical to basal sections are ordered from left to right. **C**: Summary of QT interval analysis in five instrumented rats with MI. * $P<0.01$. Horizontal line above the bar graph indicate significant difference in the post-hoc analysis. **D**: Representative strain waveforms of two instrumented rats with MI under control conditions. **E**: Average segmental time to peak Ecc (left) and peak Ecc (right) in five rats with ischemic heart failure subjected to no pacing, RV, LV and BIV pacing.

LV synchrony using M-mode echocardiography, [13,15] our study is the first to utilize speckled tracking analysis under various pacing modes in order to view the full segmental pattern during RA, RV, LV and BIV pacing. The results show clear beneficial effects of LV and to a greater extend BIV pacing on LV synchrony compared to RV pacing. In terms of electrical synchrony, we found it difficult to reliably measure the QRS duration during the different pacing modes due to the absence of apparent differentiation between the QRS complex and the T wave in the rat ECG. However, the effects of different pacing modes on the QT duration, which were consistent and significant (Figure 4 A,B), seem to reflect, at least partially, changes in QRS duration that are embedded in the QT interval. In addition, analysis of epicardial electrograms also supports longer activation time during RV pacing compared to LV pacing (Figure 4 C). Thus, LV and BIV pacing appear to induce beneficial effects on electrical synchrony compared with RV pacing in the rat heart. In terms of mechanical synchrony our results demonstrate that LV-only pacing has favorable outcome which is almost similar to the effect of BIV pacing. While many studies support the notion that LV-only pacing may have beneficial effects in HF patients [26], recent data in children with normal cardiac function and complete AV block demonstrated striking similarity to the results of our rat model in regard to LV-only pacing [27]. Moreover, LV-only pacing appears to be associated with good clinical outcome in this and other studies in the pediatric population [28,29]. It should be mentioned that the segmental findings of our study as well as the pediatric studies stated above appear to contrast the findings of [30], which demonstrated reduced Ecc near the LV pacing site compare to remote sites near the RV in the dog model of acute pacing. However, the segmental Ecc analysis in the above study was done by MRI using a much higher spatial resolution dividing the mid LV into 24 segments and 8 longitudinal segments. Thus the analysis focused on segments which are not in the same transverse plane and are much more refined to the actual vicinity of the pacing electrodes.

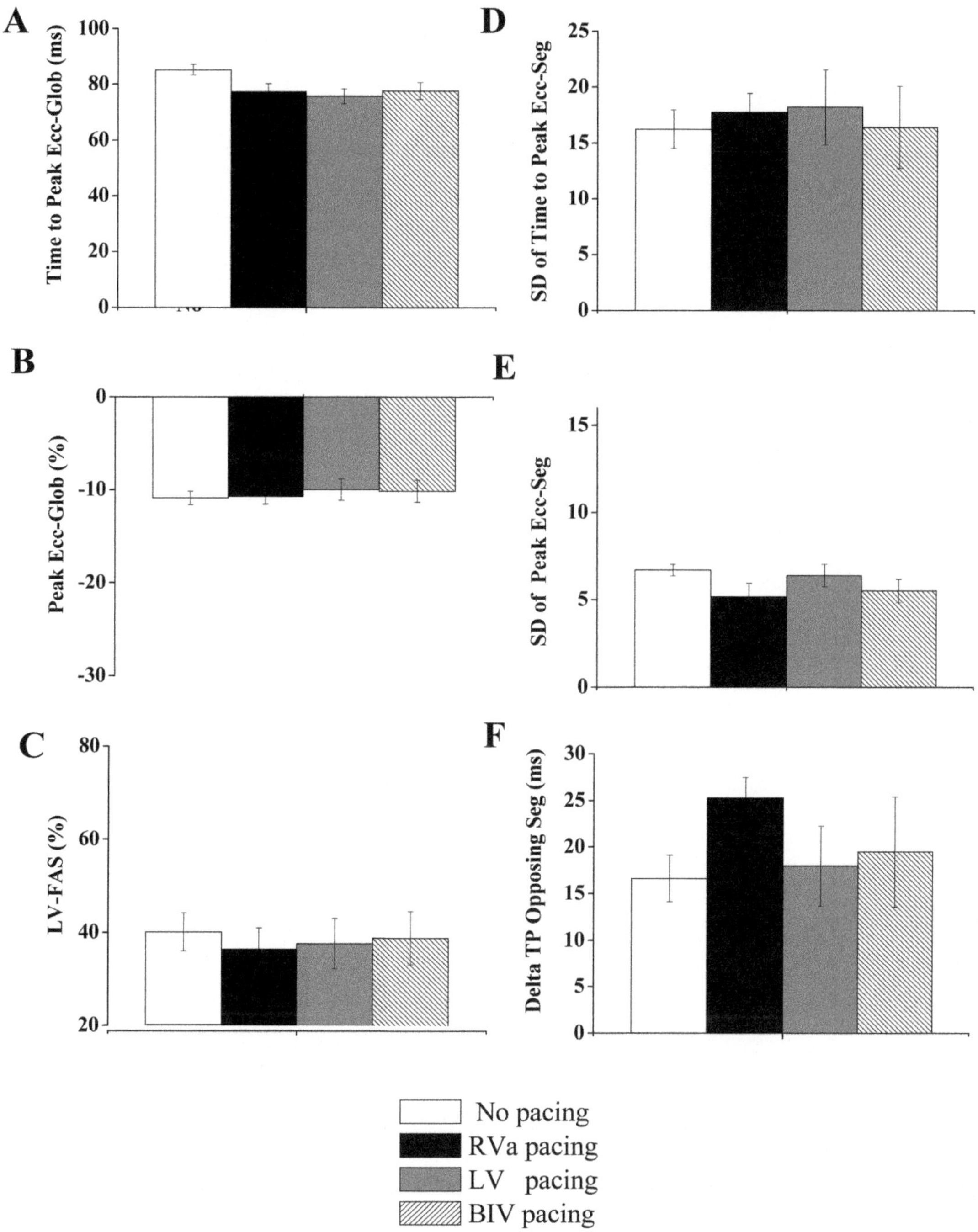

Figure 8. Attenuated effects of pacing in rats subjected to extensive MI. Summary of echocardiographic parameters in five rats with ischemic heart failure subjected to no pacing, RV pacing, LV pacing, and BIV pacing. **A**: Average time to peak Ecc of all six segments (global). **B**: Average peak Ecc of all six segments (global) **C**: LV fractional area shortening **D**: Standard deviation of the time to peak Ecc of different segments. **E**: Standard deviation of the peak Ecc of different segments. **F**: Average time difference between the peak Ecc of opposing segments ('delta TP opposing segments', see Figure 3 for details). Kruskal-Wallis test did not reveal a significant difference between the different pacing modes for any of the presented parameters.

The addition of MI-induced HF to the double site ventricular pacing model was performed as a proof of concept for the usefulness of our rat model in simulating a scenario that is clinically relevant. Our results indicate decreased beneficial effect of LV or BIV pacing in animals with extensive MI. These results are consistent with various clinical results indicating that the beneficial effect of CRT is highly dependent on the scar burden and is lost when the scar burden passes a certain limit [31,32]. A recent study in a dog model indicated, however, a clear beneficial effect of CRT in the setting of ~20% scar burden [33]. In this context, a limitation of our current analysis was the lack of a quantitative measurement of scar burden. However, based on the echocardiographic analysis of akinetic/dyskinetic segments, LV-FAS analysis (Figure 8C), and the macroscopic view of the MI in

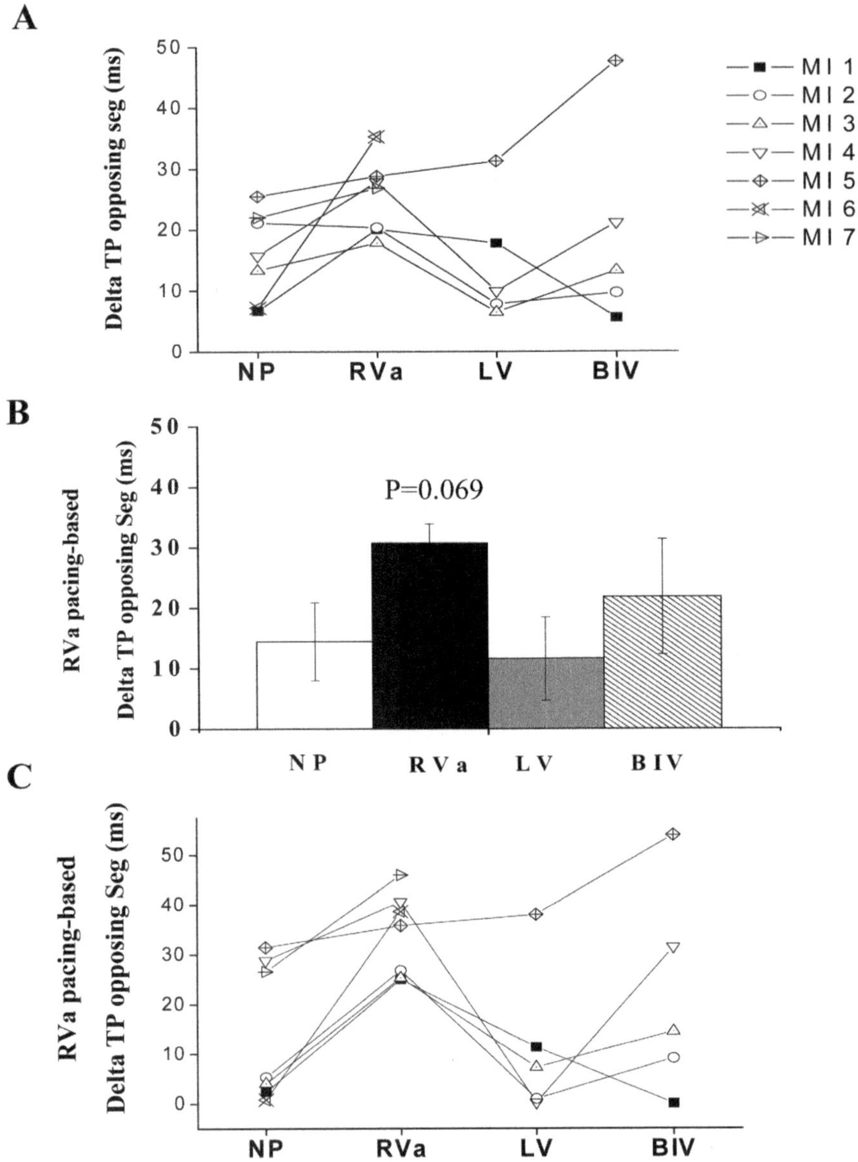

Figure 9. Individual variability in the effect of pacing in rats subjected to extensive MI. A: Average time difference between the peak Ecc of opposing segments in seven individual rats with MI (MI1 to MI7). Note the tendency of increased delta TP in all rats during RV pacing. **B**: Analysis of delta TP in each animal focused solely on the two opposing segments presenting maximal dyssynchrony during RV pacing. **C**: Delta TP focused on the two opposing segment presenting maximal dyssynchrony in seven individual rats with MI (as in Figure 9B).

the hearts (Figure 7A, B), it appears that the MIs of the present study were rather extensive in nature and were far beyond the 20% scar burden that was calculated in the dog model of Rademakers et al. [33]. Importantly, our initial analysis did not detect a marked deleterious effect of RV pacing in the MI animals when LV dyssynchrony parameters were compared to the no pacing mode (Figure 8). This phenomenon may be partially attributed to the nature the dyssynchrony parameters that were selected in our study, which may lose their sensitivity when high values are already present at the baseline. Nevertheless, it may also be possible that in the presence of an extensive MI, the effect of RV pacing on LV dyssynchrony is indeed small due to the high LV dyssynchrony that is already present at baseline. Looking specifically at the temporal synchrony of opposing segments, which appears to be specifically useful both clinically and experimentally [19,34], the picture that we obtained was somewhat different. Indeed, using this measure, we could identify a tendency of increased dyssynchrony during RV pacing in the majority of rats (Figure 9), a finding suggesting that this pacing still imposes a deleterious effect in the extensive MI setting but is harder to detect and analyze in this context. An examination of opposing segments also revealed marked variability in the response of individual rats with ischemic HF to the effect of LV and BIV pacing. While, in some animals, these modes of pacing seemed to be favorable compared to RV pacing, an opposite tendency was clearly noted in one out of the five fully analyzed rats. Clearly, more extensive work is required to further define the parameters that are responsible for the observed variability in the setting of MI. Quantitative analysis of scar burden and precise post mortem analysis of the location of LV pacing site in relation to the scar tissue, as well as invasive hemodynamic measurements during the different pacing modes, would all make a valuable contribution to further analysis in this complex setting.

The current rat model opens a window of opportunity for various studies regarding DHF and CRT using a rather simple and economically efficient model. The study might also pave the way to the application of double site pacing in genetically engineered mice models. New technical advances in the development of wireless pacing for mice, [35] imply that such studies may indeed become more feasible in the near future.

Limitations

There are several limitations to the present model. The absence of atrial sensing electrode and dependence on override pacing prevents atrioventricular synchrony. However, since the main comparisons of different ventricular pacing modes all rely on override pacing, this confounder should be equal in the different ventricular pacing modes. In addition, the pseudo LBBB pattern induced by RV pacing may not necessarily represent all the features of true LBBB. In this context, the epicardial location of our RV electrodes is also important to note, since this setting differs from the most common clinical RV pacing situation, where the RV lead is endocardial. Finally, the patterns of LV dyssynchrony observed in different animals are not completely identical, as can be appreciated by comparison of the segmental time to peak patterns in Figure 2 (group A) and Figure 5 (group B). The source of this variability between the groups was not clear to us. One of the things we suspect is that although the position of electrode implantation seems identical to the operator, the small size of the rat heart did not allow for detection of subtle differences in the position of the implantation, specifically in the anterior-posterior dimension. Such difference may affect the electrical activation sequence. Thus, if an electrode is positioned in a more anterior position close to the apex, the first LV segment that is activated is the inferior one as seen in the summary of animals in group A (Figure 2C). On the other hand, if the electrode is positioned in a more posterior location then the first LV segment that is activated is the posterior one as was dominantly observed in the animals of group B (Figure 5). This possibility implies that more attention to the exact location of the RV electrode should be used in future studies. Nevertheless, our current analysis also indicates that regardless of the exact segmental pattern of the time to peak strain, the variability of this parameter is remarkably larger during RV pacing compared to LV pacing and BIV pacing.

Conclusions

The present study shows the feasibility of an electrodes implantation procedure for double site epicardial pacing in rats, and the ability to combine this technique with conventional MI surgery. By the use of ECG recordings and speckle-tracking echocardiography we found that rodent pacing mimics important electromechanical features seen in large mammals and in people. Thus, this model may become a simple new tool to study the pathophysiology of ventricular dyssynchrony and CRT.

Supporting Information

Checklist S1 NC3Rs ARRIVE Guidelines Checklist.

Acknowledgments

The authors thank Prof. Amos Katz for important scientific insights. We also thank Yossi Tsadok and Dr. Noa Bachner-Hinenzon for technical assistance with the 2DS analysis.

Author Contributions

Conceived and designed the experiments: MM WM YE NLC. Performed the experiments: MM WM SE HG SD. Analyzed the data: MM WM SE SD. Contributed reagents/materials/analysis tools: MM WM HG. Wrote the paper: MM WM YE NLC.

References

1. Bader H, Garrigue S, Lafitte S, Reuter S, Jais P, et al. (2004) Intra-left ventricular electromechanical asynchrony. A new independent predictor of severe cardiac events in heart failure patients. J Am Coll Cardiol 43: 248–256.
2. Cho GY, Song JK, Park WJ, Han SW, Choi SH, et al. (2005) Mechanical dyssynchrony assessed by tissue Doppler imaging is a powerful predictor of mortality in congestive heart failure with normal QRS duration. J Am Coll Cardiol 46: 2237–2243.
3. Ludwig DR, Tanaka H, Friehling M, Gorcsan J, 3rd, Schwartzman D (2013) Further deterioration of LV ejection fraction and mechanical synchrony during RV apical pacing in patients with heart failure and LBBB. J Cardiovasc Transl Res 6: 425–429.
4. Rickard J, Cheng A, Spragg D, Cantillon D, Chung MK, et al. (2013) QRS narrowing is associated with reverse remodeling in patients with chronic right ventricular pacing upgraded to cardiac resynchronization therapy. Heart Rhythm 10: 55–60.
5. Tops LF, Schalij MJ, Bax JJ (2009) The Effects of Right Ventricular Apical Pacing on Ventricular Function and Dyssynchrony: Implications for Therapy. J Am Coll Cardiol 54: 764–776.
6. Bleeker GB, Bax JJ, Steendijk P, Schalij MJ, van der Wall EE (2006) Left ventricular dyssynchrony in patients with heart failure: pathophysiology, diagnosis and treatment. Nat Clin Pract Cardiovasc Med 3: 213–219.
7. Kashani A, Barold SS (2005) Significance of QRS complex duration in patients with heart failure. J Am Coll Cardiol 46: 2183–2192.
8. Leclercq C, Singh JP (2011) Cardiac resynchronization therapy: from treatment to prevention. Eur Heart J 32: 1580–1582.
9. Cho H, Barth AS, Tomaselli GF (2012) Basic science of cardiac resynchronization therapy: molecular and electrophysiological mechanisms. Circ Arrhythm Electrophysiol 5: 594–603.
10. Saba S, Mehdi H, Mathier MA, Islam MZ, Salama G, et al. (2010) Effect of Right Ventricular Versus Biventricular Pacing on Electrical Remodeling in the Normal Heart. Circ Arrhythm Electrophysiol 3: 79–87.
11. Chakir K, Daya SK, Tunin RS, Helm RH, Byrne MJ, et al. (2008) Reversal of global apoptosis and regional stress kinase activation by cardiac resynchronization. Circulation 117: 1369–1377. doi: 1310.1161/CIRCULATIONAHA.1107.706291. Epub 702008 Mar 706293.
12. Barth AS, Aiba T, Halperin V, DiSilvestre D, Chakir K, et al. (2009) Cardiac Resynchronization Therapy Corrects Dyssynchrony-Induced Regional Gene Expression Changes on a Genomic Level. Circ Cardiovasc Genet 2: 371–378.
13. Bilchick KC, Saha SK, Mikolajczyk E, Cope L, Ferguson WJ, et al. (2006) Differential regional gene expression from cardiac dyssynchrony induced by chronic right ventricular free wall pacing in the mouse. Physiol Genomics 26: 109–115.
14. Houser SR, Margulies KB, Murphy AM, Spinale FG, Francis GS, et al. (2012) Animal models of heart failure: a scientific statement from the American Heart Association. Circ Res 111: 131–150.
15. Kontogeorgis A, Kaba RA, Kang E, Feig JE, Gupta PP, et al. (2008) Short-term pacing in the mouse alters cardiac expression of connexin43. BMC Physiol 8:8: 10.1186/1472-6793-1188-1188.
16. Etzion Y, Mor M, Shalev A, Dror S, Etzion O, et al. (2008) New insights into the atrial electrophysiology of rodents using a novel modality: the miniature-bipolar hook electrode. Am J Physiol Heart Circ Physiol 295: H1460–1469 Epub 2008 Jul 1425.
17. Popovic ZB, Benejam C, Bian J, Mal N, Drinko J, et al. (2007) Speckle-tracking echocardiography correctly identifies segmental left ventricular dysfunction induced by scarring in a rat model of myocardial infarction. Am J Physiol Heart Circ Physiol 292: H2809–2816.
18. Bachner-Hinenzon N, Ertracht O, Leitman M, Vered Z, Shimoni S, et al. (2010) Layer-specific strain analysis by speckle tracking echocardiography reveals differences in left ventricular function between rats and humans. Am J Physiol Heart Circ Physiol 299: H664–672.
19. Bonios M, Chang CY, Pinheiro A, Dimaano VL, Higuchi T, et al. (2011) Cardiac resynchronization by cardiosphere-derived stem cell transplantation in an experimental model of myocardial infarction. J Am Soc Echocardiogr 24: 808–814.
20. Bachner-Hinenzon N, Ertracht O, Malka A, Leitman M, Vered Z, et al. (2012) Layer-specific strain analysis: investigation of regional deformations in a rat

model of acute versus chronic myocardial infarction. Am J Physiol Heart Circ Physiol 303: H549–558.

21. Rappaport D, Adam D, Lysyansky P, Riesner S (2006) Assessment of myocardial regional strain and strain rate by tissue tracking in B-mode echocardiograms. Ultrasound Med Biol 32: 1181–1192.
22. Salama G, London B (2007) Mouse models of long QT syndrome. J Physiol 578: 43–53.
23. Nerbonne JM (2004) Studying cardiac arrhythmias in the mouse–a reasonable model for probing mechanisms? Trends Cardiovasc Med 14: 83–93.
24. Dandel M, Hetzer R (2009) Echocardiographic strain and strain rate imaging–clinical applications. Int J Cardiol 132: 11–24.
25. Kaese S, Verheule S (2012) Cardiac electrophysiology in mice: a matter of size. Front Physiol 3: 345.
26. Strik M, van Deursen CJ, van Middendorp LB, van Hunnik A, Kuiper M, et al. (2013) Transseptal conduction as an important determinant for cardiac resynchronization therapy, as revealed by extensive electrical mapping in the dyssynchronous canine heart. Circ Arrhythm Electrophysiol 6: 682–689.
27. Tomaske M, Breithardt OA, Bauersfeld U (2009) Preserved cardiac synchrony and function with single-site left ventricular epicardial pacing during mid-term follow-up in paediatric patients. Europace 11: 1168–1176.
28. Tomaske M, Breithardt OA, Balmer C, Bauersfeld U (2009) Successful cardiac resynchronization with single-site left ventricular pacing in children. Int J Cardiol 136: 136–143.
29. Janousek J, van Geldorp IE, Krupickova S, Rosenthal E, Nugent K, et al. (2013) Permanent cardiac pacing in children: choosing the optimal pacing site: a multicenter study. Circulation 127: 613–623.
30. Prinzen FW, Hunter WC, Wyman BT, McVeigh ER (1999) Mapping of regional myocardial strain and work during ventricular pacing: experimental study using magnetic resonance imaging tagging. J Am Coll Cardiol 33: 1735–1742.
31. Adelstein EC, Tanaka H, Soman P, Miske G, Haberman SC, et al. (2011) Impact of scar burden by single-photon emission computed tomography myocardial perfusion imaging on patient outcomes following cardiac resynchronization therapy. Eur Heart J 32: 93–103.
32. Ypenburg C, Roes SD, Bleeker GB, Kaandorp TA, de Roos A, et al. (2007) Effect of total scar burden on contrast-enhanced magnetic resonance imaging on response to cardiac resynchronization therapy. Am J Cardiol 99: 657–660. Epub 2007 Jan 2004.
33. Rademakers LM, van Kerckhoven R, van Deursen CJ, Strik M, van Hunnik A, et al. (2010) Myocardial infarction does not preclude electrical and hemodynamic benefits of cardiac resynchronization therapy in dyssynchronous canine hearts. Circ Arrhythm Electrophysiol 3: 361–368.
34. Prinzen FW, Vernooy K, De Boeck BW, Delhaas T (2011) Mechano-energetics of the asynchronous and resynchronized heart. Heart Fail Rev 16: 215–224.
35. Laughner JI, Marrus SB, Zellmer ER, Weinheimer CJ, Macewan MR, et al. (2013) A fully implantable pacemaker for the mouse: from battery to wireless power. PLoS One 8: e76291.

Pyridostigmine Restores Cardiac Autonomic Balance after Small Myocardial Infarction in Mice

Marina T. Durand[1], Christiane Becari[1], Mauro de Oliveira[1], Jussara M. do Carmo[3], Carlos Alberto Aguiar Silva[1], Cibele M. Prado[2], Rubens Fazan Jr[1], Helio C. Salgado[1]*

1 Department of Physiology, School of Medicine of Ribeirão Preto, University of São Paulo, Ribeirão Preto, São Paulo, Brazil, **2** Department of Pathology, School of Medicine of Ribeirão Preto, University of São Paulo, Ribeirão Preto, São Paulo, Brazil, **3** Department of Physiology and Biophysics, University of Mississippi Medical Center, Jackson, Mississippi, United States of America

Abstract

The effect of pyridostigmine (PYR) - an acetylcholinesterase inhibitor - on hemodynamics and cardiac autonomic control, was never studied in conscious myocardial infarcted mice. Telemetry transmitters were implanted into the carotid artery under isoflurane anesthesia. Seven to ten days after recovery from the surgery, basal arterial pressure and heart rate were recorded, while parasympathetic and sympathetic tone (ΔHR) was evaluated by means of methyl atropine and propranolol. After the basal hemodynamic recording the mice were subjected to left coronary artery ligation for producing myocardial infarction (MI), or sham operation, and implantation of minipumps filled with PYR or saline. Separate groups of anesthetized (isoflurane) mice previously (4 weeks) subjected to MI, or sham coronary artery ligation, were submitted to cardiac function examination. The mice exhibited an infarct length of approximately 12%, no change in arterial pressure and increased heart rate only in the 1st week after MI. Vagal tone decreased in the 1st week, while the sympathetic tone was increased in the 1st and 4th week after MI. PYR prevented the increase in heart rate but did not affect the arterial pressure. Moreover, PYR prevented the increase in sympathetic tone throughout the 4 weeks. Concerning the parasympathetic tone, PYR not only impaired its attenuation in the 1st week, but enhanced it in the 4th week. MI decreased ejection fraction and increased diastolic and systolic volume. Therefore, the pharmacological increase of peripheral acetylcholine availability by means of PYR prevented tachycardia, increased parasympathetic and decreased sympathetic tone after MI in mice.

Editor: German E. Gonzalez, University of Buenos Aires, Faculty of Medicine, Cardiovascular Pathophysiology Institute, Argentina

Funding: Funding for this work came from Fapesp (2012/03349-1), NAP-NIC-USP (12.1.24345.01.0). The funders had no role in study design, data collection and analysis, decision to publish, or preparation of the manuscript.

Competing Interests: The authors have declared that no competing interests exist.

* Email: hcsalgado@fmrp.usp.br

Introduction

Myocardial infarction (MI) as a result of coronary artery occlusion is always accompanied by marked changes in cardiac autonomic control characterized by overall sympathetic activation and cardiac parasympathetic attenuation, contributing to progressive ventricular dysfunction [1,2]. While species such as dog, rabbit and rat have been studied exhaustively as models of autonomic dysfunction in heart failure, only recently the mouse has attracted much attention. This is because the mouse has been routinely genetically manipulated and is a reference in studies of the molecular factors involved in physiological functions and several diseases involving the cardiovascular system [3], for instance the MI. Moreover, the development of telemetric recording for mice allowed the evaluation of long term oscillations of arterial pressure (AP) and heart rate (HR), providing a reliable and powerful tool to exam the mechanisms of cardiovascular control in freely moving subjects for long periods [4,5].

Derangement of vagal control of the HR becomes apparent at early stage of left ventricular dysfunction [6,7] and is closely associated with poor long-term outcome and high mortality of patients following MI, or development of heart failure [8,9]. In addition, recent studies demonstrated that chronic disturbance of the cholinergic tone in genetically manipulated mice, i.e. acetylcholine receptor knockout or vesicular acetylcholine transporter knockdown, elicited a decrease in left ventricular performance associated with altered calcium handling and plastic alterations contributing to heart dysfunction [10,11]. Therefore, activation of parasympathetic function may have beneficial implications after acute cardiac ischemic injury or further development of heart failure [12,13]. Previous studies have demonstrated that chronic vagal stimulation improved ventricular performance, reduced cardiac remodeling and arrhythmias, and improved the cardiac autonomic control, lengthening long-term survival in experimental models of heart failure [14,15]. In patients with heart failure, vagus nerve stimulation carried out during a six-month period was associated with significant improvement in NYHA class, quality of life, 6-minute walk test, left ventricular ejection fraction and systolic volume [13]. Therefore, the increase in parasympathetic function seems to be a promising therapeutic alternative for preventing MI outcomes, by acting on the autonomic control of the heart and improving cardiac remodeling and function.

However, vagal nerve stimulation therapy is an invasive approach, whose feasibility is under active investigation [16,17]. Because the efferent vagal nerve activity is ultimately mediated by acetylcholine, modulation of this neurotransmitter, by means of pharmacological agents that augment the acetylcholine availability at the neuroeffector junction, should be considered a promising therapy for patients with MI and/or heart failure. Anticholinesterase agents have been used in experimental designs aiming to enhance the parasympathetic influences on the heart [18]. Pyridostigmine (PYR), a reversible anticholinesterase agent that does not cross the blood-brain barrier and acts particularly in the peripheral synaptic cleft, seems to be potentially useful in this context.

Previous studies have demonstrated that short-term administration of PYR may be potentially useful for cardiovascular protection because it shifts the autonomic balance toward parasympathetic predominance, resulting in beneficial effects on markers of cardiovascular risk and dysfunction [19–22]. PYR increased HR variability in normal rats [23], healthy humans [24] and patients with heart failure [25]. In humans, the acute administration of PYR produced bradycardia [26], increased the ventricular refractory period and displayed a potential anti-arrhythmic effect at higher HR [27]. In patients with coronary artery disease and heart failure, PYR prevented the myocardial dysfunction induced by mental stress [19], ameliorated the autonomic and hemodynamic profile during exercise [28–30], improved the HR recovery after exercise [31] and reduced ventricular arrhythmia density [25]. Moreover, our laboratory has observed a protective effect of PYR on cardiac autonomic control, intrinsic HR, baroreflex sensitivity, and cardiac function four [20] and six weeks [21] after the onset of heart failure in rats.

To our knowledge, the chronic effect of PYR administration has never hitherto been studied in mice with MI, a species amenable to genetic manipulation which has becoming a reference in studies of physiological functions and pathophysiology of many diseases, for instance MI. Therefore, the objective of the current study was to evaluate, by means of telemetry in conscious mice, whether the increase of parasympathetic function by with PYR administration improves the hemodynamics (AP and HR) and sympathovagal balance, one and four weeks after MI elicited by coronary artery ligation.

Methods

Animals

Experiments were carried out in male C57/BL6 mice, 10–15 weeks of age, averaging 25–30 g, supplied by the Animal Facility of the School of Medicine of Ribeirão Preto, University of São Paulo (Ribeirão Preto, SP, Brazil). The mice were fed a standard chow diet and tap water *ad libitum*, and were housed under controlled temperature (22°C) with a 12 h dark-light cycle. All procedures were approved by the Committee of Ethics in Animal Research of the Medical School of Ribeirão Preto, University of São Paulo (Ribeirão Preto, SP, Brazil) [Protocol # 203/2008].

Telemetry probe implantation

Mice were anesthetized with isoflurane (5% for induction and 2–2.5% for maintenance) diluted in 100% oxygen. The anesthetic mixture was provided via an isoflurane vaporizer (*Calibrated Vaporizer Takaoka, model ISOVAPOR 1224, K. Takaoka Ind. Com. Ltda., São Paulo-SP, Brazil*), which delivered the anesthetic mixture into a mask. Prior to implantation, the telemetry probes were carefully prepared with application of a biocompatible gel on the tip of the catheter, to prevent blood from entering the catheter lumen; following, the transmitter calibration was proceeded. Surgical procedures were performed under aseptic conditions and under magnification by a surgical microscope (*CM-A199 DFZ, DF Vasconcellos SA Optics and High Precision Mechanics, Valencia, RJ*). The animals were implanted with radio telemeter probes (*TA11PA-C10, Data Sciences International, St. Paul, MN*), as described by Butz and Davisson [5]. Briefly, after shaving the ventral neck region with a depilatory cream and disinfecting the skin, a midline incision was made and the left carotid artery was isolated by blunt dissection. After cranial permanent ligature and momentary caudal occlusion with a thread, the catheter of the radio telemeter was inserted into the carotid and the same thread was used to secure the catheter. Through the ventral neck incision, a subcutaneous pouch was formed for placement of the transmitter body along the animal's right flank. The skin was then closed with a 6-0 silk suture.

Myocardial infarction

MI was performed as described elsewhere [2]. Briefly, under the same anesthetic protocol described above, a ventral midline skin incision was made caudally to the larynx to access the trachea; then, a small incision was made in the trachea to introduce a 22G needle tip (*BD Angiocath Becton Dickinson Ind. Cir. Ltda., Juiz de Fora, MG, Brazil*) which was connected to a rodent ventilator (*Inspira Advanced Safety Single Animal Pressure/Volume Controlled Ventilator, Harvard Apparatus, Holliston, MA, USA*). The rodent ventilator acquired the anesthetic mixture from the isoflurane vaporizer. An 80-μL tidal volume was maintained at 70 cycles per minute. After the skin was shaved and disinfected, the 3rd intercostal space was opened, the heart was visualized and the pericardium was gently opened. The left anterior descending coronary artery was visualized and ligated with 8-0 polypropylene suture. The intercostal incision was closed with a 6-0 silk suture, and a 21G needle attached to a 3.0-mL syringe was introduced through the closed wound and the negative pressure of the thorax was reestablished avoiding damage to heart and lungs. Finally, the skin was closed with 6-0 silk suture. To prevent subsequent infection, 50 μL of a mixture of penicillin and streptomycin (*Pentabiótico Veterinário Pequeno Porte, Fort Dodge Saúde Animal, Campinas, SP, Brazil*) was administered intramuscularly. The infarct size was confirmed by postmortem examination. Control animals were submitted to sham surgery, in which all the steps, except the left anterior descending coronary artery ligation, were performed. All surgical procedures were carried out under microscope magnification (*CM-A199 DFZ, DF Vasconcellos SA Optics and High Precision Mechanics, Valencia, RJ*).

Implantation of mini pump for subcutaneous administration of pyridostigmine

Under the same anesthesia used to perform the MI an osmotic minipump (model 1004, volume of 0.11 μL/h over 28 days; *DURECT - ALZET Osmotic Pumps, Cupertino, CA, USA*) was implanted subcutaneously just below the scapular region. Following, the animal was released from the anesthesia and placed in an individual cage for recovery. The minipumps were prefilled with PYR (*Valeant Pharmaceuticals in Brazil Ltda, Campinas, SP, Brazil*), or vehicle (sterile NaCl 0.9%), and primed by incubation under isotonic saline solution at 37°C for 48 h, according to manufacturer's instructions. PYR was subcutaneously supplied at 3 mg/kg/day for four weeks.

Experimental Protocol 1

After the probe implantation, the animals were allowed to recover for 7 to 10 days before basal recordings. Basal AP and HR signals were sampled (2 kHz) continuously for two hours. After basal recording, the mice received methyl atropine (2 mg/kg, i.p.)

and propranolol (5 mg/kg, i.p.) separated by a 40 to 50 min interval. The AP and HR recording was maintained for at least 30 minutes after the blockade of the autonomic receptors. After 24 hours, the protocol was repeated with the autonomic blockers administered in reverse order, i.e. propranolol followed by methyl atropine. On the next day, a surgical procedure to produce MI and minipump implantation was carried out. The animals were randomly sorted to receive minipump filed with PYR (n = 7) or isotonic saline solution (n = 8). The protocol for data acquisition, as described above, was repeated one and four weeks after MI. The data from the telemetry device were collected by means of a receiver placed under the mouse cage (Dataquest, *Data Sciences International, Saint Paul, MN*).

Experimental Protocol 2

This protocol was carried out in separate groups of anesthetized mice previously (4 weeks) subjected to MI, or sham left anterior descending coronary artery ligation, and implanted with osmotic minipumps filed with PYR or saline, as described above. The mice were anesthetized by inhalation of isoflurane (5% for induction and 2–2.5% for maintenance). A microtip pressure-volume catheter (*SPR-839, Millar Instruments, Houston, TX, USA*) was inserted into the right carotid artery for measurement of the AP and then moved into the left ventricle as described elsewhere [32]. After stabilization, the signals were continuously recorded using the pressure-volume conductance system (*MPVS, Millar Instruments, Houston, TX, USA*) connected to a Power Lab/4SP (*ADI Instruments, Sydney, NSW, Australia*) feeding the digital signal to an IBM PC. The HR, left ventricular end-systolic pressure (LVESP), left ventricular end-diastolic pressure (LVEDP), maximal slope of the systolic pressure increment (+dP/dt) and diastolic pressure decrement (−dP/dt), end-systolic volume (ESV), end-diastolic volume (EDV), stroke volume (SV), ejection fraction (EF) and cardiac output (CO) were calculated using a cardiac pressure-volume analysis program (*PVAN Ultra 1.1, Millar Instruments, Houston, TX, USA*) as described elsewhere [32]. The CO was normalized to body weight [cardiac index (CI)]. The total peripheral resistance index (TPRI) was calculated by the following equation: TPRI = MAP/CI.

Morphological analysis

After the hemodynamic recordings, the animals were killed with an overdose of ketamine and xylazine (1:1; *Ketamina Agener União Saúde Animal, Embu-Guaçu, SP, Brazil; Dopaser Hertape Calier Saúde Animal S/A, Juatuba, MG, Brazil*) and the whole hearts were harvested, rinsed in 10% KCl solution for stopping the heart in diastole, and weighed. The hearts were cut transversely and fixed in phosphate-buffered 10% formalin for 24 to 48 hours. For histological processing the hearts were embedded into paraffin and each block was serially cut with 6 μm thickness. The sections were stained with picrosirius red or hematoxylin and eosin. For infarct size and volume fraction (%) of collagen analysis the hearts stained with picrosirius red were used. Assessment of the infarct size was performed according to Takagawa et al. [33]. Briefly, the infarct size (%) was calculated by dividing the infarct length - between the surfaces of the epicardium and endocardium - by the circumference of the left ventricle and multiplying by 100. To estimate the volume fraction (%) of collagen in picrosirius red-stained sections, quantitative examination of the surviving left ventricular was carried out on a medium-power light-microscopic field. For each heart, 15 fields per mice were randomly selected and the mean value was subsequently calculated. For morphometric analysis the hearts stained with hematoxylin and eosin were used and the minor diameter of myocytes in the surviving left ventricle was measured. Since the myocardial fiber has a tubular shape, the smallest axis is a measure perpendicular to the nucleus, no matter the myocardial fiber is sectioned in longitudinal, oblique or transversal manner. This is the right diameter of the structure [34]. Approximately 30 values were obtained per mice, and the mean value was calculated. The sections were analyzed using the video microscopy software Leica Qwin (*Leica Imaging Systems, Cambridge, UK*) and the public-domain software NIH ImageJ (*developed by U.S. National Institutes of Health and available at* http://rsb.info.nih.gov/nih-image/).

Data analysis

Pulsatile AP recordings were analyzed by customized computer software designed to detect inflection points of a periodic wave. Beat-by-beat time series of systolic AP were generated. Series of pulse intervals were obtained by measuring the time-interval between two consecutive systolic AP values.

Cardiac autonomic tone and intrinsic HR: Tonic sympathetic and vagal influences on the heart were assessed by HR changes induced by autonomic blockade produced by propranolol and methyl atropine, respectively. The difference between the HR measured at the end of the 40-min time-frame after propranolol administration and basal HR was considered the sympathetic tone. The difference between the HR measured at the end of the 40-min time-frame after methyl atropine administration and basal HR was considered the vagal tone. HR values obtained after the double autonomic receptor blockade provided the intrinsic HR, i.e. the HR remaining after the removal of adrenergic and cholinergic influence upon the heart.

Statistical Analysis

The data are expressed as the mean ± standard error of the mean (SEM). Comparisons of the general characteristics of the animals studied, morphological and cardiac function parameters were performed using two-way analysis of variance (ANOVA). For multiple comparisons of hemodynamic data over time (before, one week and four weeks), two-way ANOVA for repeated-measures analysis were performed. Data from cardiac sympathetic and vagal tone were compared among groups using one-way ANOVA followed by the Student-Newman-Keuls *post-hoc* comparisons. The level of significance was set as $p<0.05$.

Results

General characteristics of control and myocardial infarcted mice with or without pyridostigmine treatment

Representative heart sections of control and myocardial infarcted mice treated, or not, with PYR are shown in Figure 1. Remarkable scarring can be observed in the left ventricle of myocardial infarcted mice, while the control animals display normal left ventricular wall without damage to the myocardium.

The general characteristics of control and myocardial infarcted mice, with or without PYR treatment, are shown in Table 1. Body weight was similar in the four groups. However, heart weight and cardiac index were increased only in myocardial infarcted mice treated with PYR. The infarct size was similar between myocardial infarcted mice with and without PYR treatment. Nevertheless, Figure 2 shows that myocytes size and collagen were similar between groups.

Figure 3 shows that MI combined, or not, with PYR did not change the mean AP. Nevertheless, one week after MI it was observed an increase in HR which was back to normal levels - before - in the fourth week. Moreover, the increase in HR observed one week after the MI was prevented by PYR.

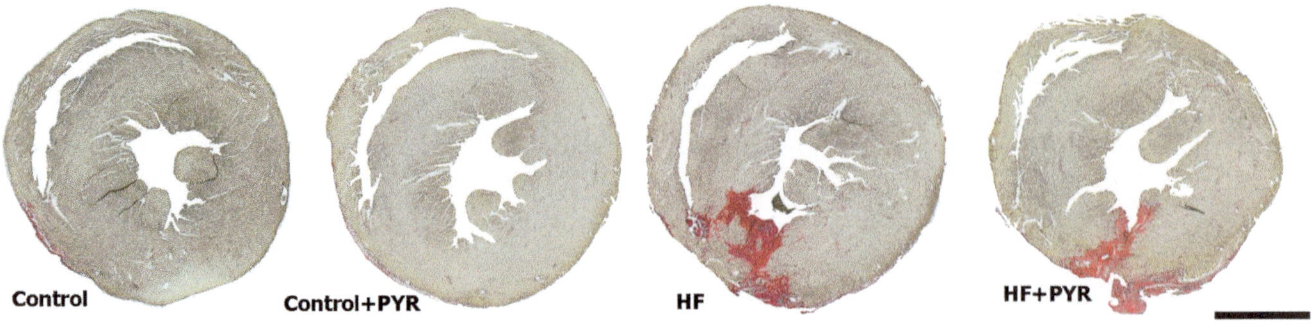

Figure 1. Cross sections of representative hearts, stained with picrosirius red, from control and mice with myocardial infarction (MI), treated, or not, with pyridostigmine (PYR). Bar = 1 mm.

Cardiac autonomic tone and intrinsic heart rate

Figure 4 (left upper panel) shows that one week after MI it is observed a significant decrease in vagal tone influence to the heart when compared with the observations before the ligation. However, this reduction in vagal tone was not maintained at four weeks after MI. In contrast, conscious mice showed significant increase in sympathetic tone in both one and four weeks after MI (Figure 4, left middle panel). PYR (Figure 4, right upper panel) not only prevented the decrease in vagal tone one week after MI but also increased this parameter in the fourth week as compared to observations from before MI. In addition, PYR also prevented the increase in sympathetic tone at one and four weeks after MI (Figure 4, right middle panel). The combined administration of methyl atropine and propranolol shows that neither MI (Figure 4, left lower panel) nor PYR (Figure 4, right lower panel) affected the intrinsic HR of the mice.

Hemodynamics and left ventricular function

In the groups used for cardiac function studies under isoflurane anesthesia, the infarct size in mice treated with PYR (11±1%) was the same as in those without PYR treatment (13±1%). Table 2 shows the hemodynamic parameters and the indices of systolic and diastolic function from P-V relations. The hemodynamic parameters, i.e. mean AP and HR were similar in the four groups studied. The parameters obtained from P-V analysis showed that mice with MI presented after four weeks a mild decrease in cardiac function, expressed by the increase in left ventricular end-systolic and end-diastolic volumes and lower ejection fraction. All other parameters expressing cardiac function were unaltered four weeks after MI. PYR did not affect the small alterations of cardiac function in myocardial infarcted mice.

Discussion

It was demonstrated that the increased availability of peripheral acetylcholine after blocking the acetylcholinesterase with PYR, prevented tachycardia, increased parasympathetic and decreased sympathetic tone after MI in mice.

The small infarct length (~12%) did not cause changes in AP but led to a rise in basal HR in the first week after MI. The literature does not have a consensus concerning the responses of AP and HR after MI. Overall, it has been shown that an infarct size of 20 to 30% in mice does not affect the HR [35–37], although the AP may be decreased [35,37] or unchanged [36]. Thus, it is possible that different methodological approaches for recording the AP (intra-arterial cannula, indirect measurement from tail cuff and telemetry), as well as different types of anesthesia and time frame after MI have significant influences on the AP and HR recorded. Nevertheless, hemodynamic long-term telemetric recording in conscious mice demonstrated that even a relatively

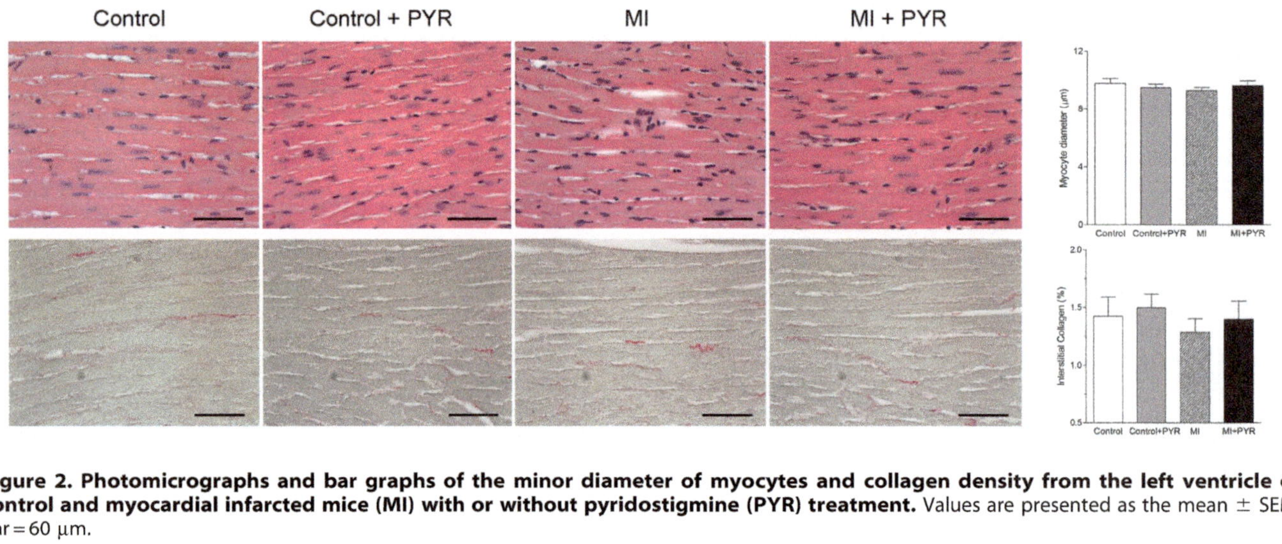

Figure 2. Photomicrographs and bar graphs of the minor diameter of myocytes and collagen density from the left ventricle of control and myocardial infarcted mice (MI) with or without pyridostigmine (PYR) treatment. Values are presented as the mean ± SEM. Bar = 60 µm.

Table 1. General characteristics of control and myocardial infarcted (MI) mice with or without pyridostigmine (PYR) treatment.

	Control (n = 6)	Control+PYR (n = 7)	MI (n = 13)	MI+PYR (n = 15)
Body weight (g)	29±1	30±1	30±0.5	31±1
Heart weight (mg)	119±3	118±4	124±3	135±3*#
Cardiac Weight Index (mg/g)	4.1±0.1	3.9±0.1	4.2±0.1	4.4±0.1*
Infarct size (% of left ventricle)	–	–	13±1	11±1

Values are presented as mean ± SEM;
*$p<0.05$ compared to control+PYR group.
#$p<0.05$ compared to MI group.

small MI caused tachycardia in the first week after the coronary artery ligation, which was prevented by PYR.

The extent of observed MI was enough to induce mild impairment in cardiac performance and significant changes in autonomic control of the heart. Apropos, in humans the median infarct size of silent MI involves 10% to 12% of the left ventricle, with a median left ventricular ejection fraction of 47% [38]. Of note, as observed in humans, the left ventricular function declines with the length of the infarcted area in mice [35]. Acute MI in mice has been thoroughly examined [1,2,33], but the characterization of the relationship between survival and extent of the infarcted area is considered a difficult task. Sallto-Tellez et al. [2] demonstrated that the histological changes found in myocardial infarcted mice are similar to those observed in humans, highlighting the importance of this model for translational studies.

Clinical and experimental studies have shown that MI followed by heart failure is combined with reduced cardiac vagal tone, which appears early in the development of this outcome, preceding sympathetic activation [8,39,40]. In patients and experimental models of heart failure, blockade of muscarinic receptor has a modest effect on HR compared to healthy subjects [20,21,39–41]. In the present study, the assessment of the cardiac autonomic balance showed reduced vagal tonic influence to the heart in the first week post MI, and increased cardiac sympathetic drive in the first and fourth week post MI. Thus, this autonomic imbalance may certainly be responsible for the increased HR observed one week after MI, because no alteration was observed in the intrinsic HR itself. At four weeks after MI, reduction of the vagal tone was not as evident as in the first week, which may explain the return of HR to baseline levels.

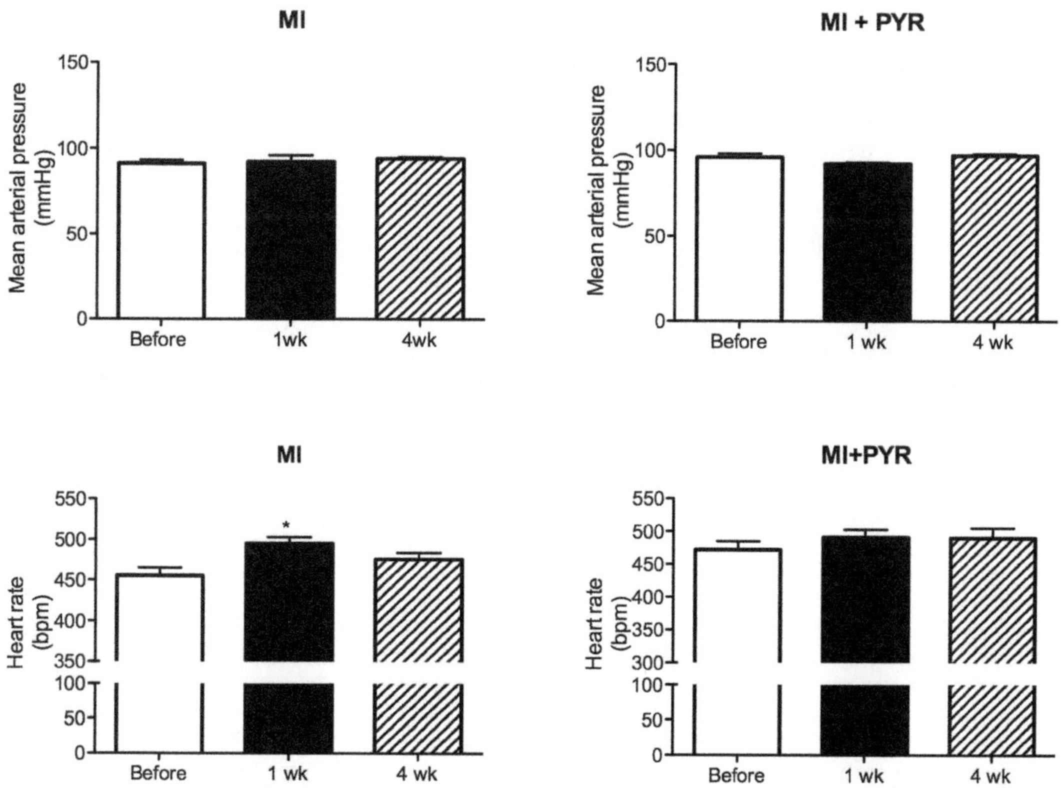

Figure 3. Mean arterial pressure and heart rate obtained before, one week (1 wk) and four weeks (4 wk) after myocardial infarction (MI) in mice treated with saline [n = 8] or pyridostigmine (PYR) [n = 7]. Values are presented as mean ± SEM. *$p<0.05$ compared to before.

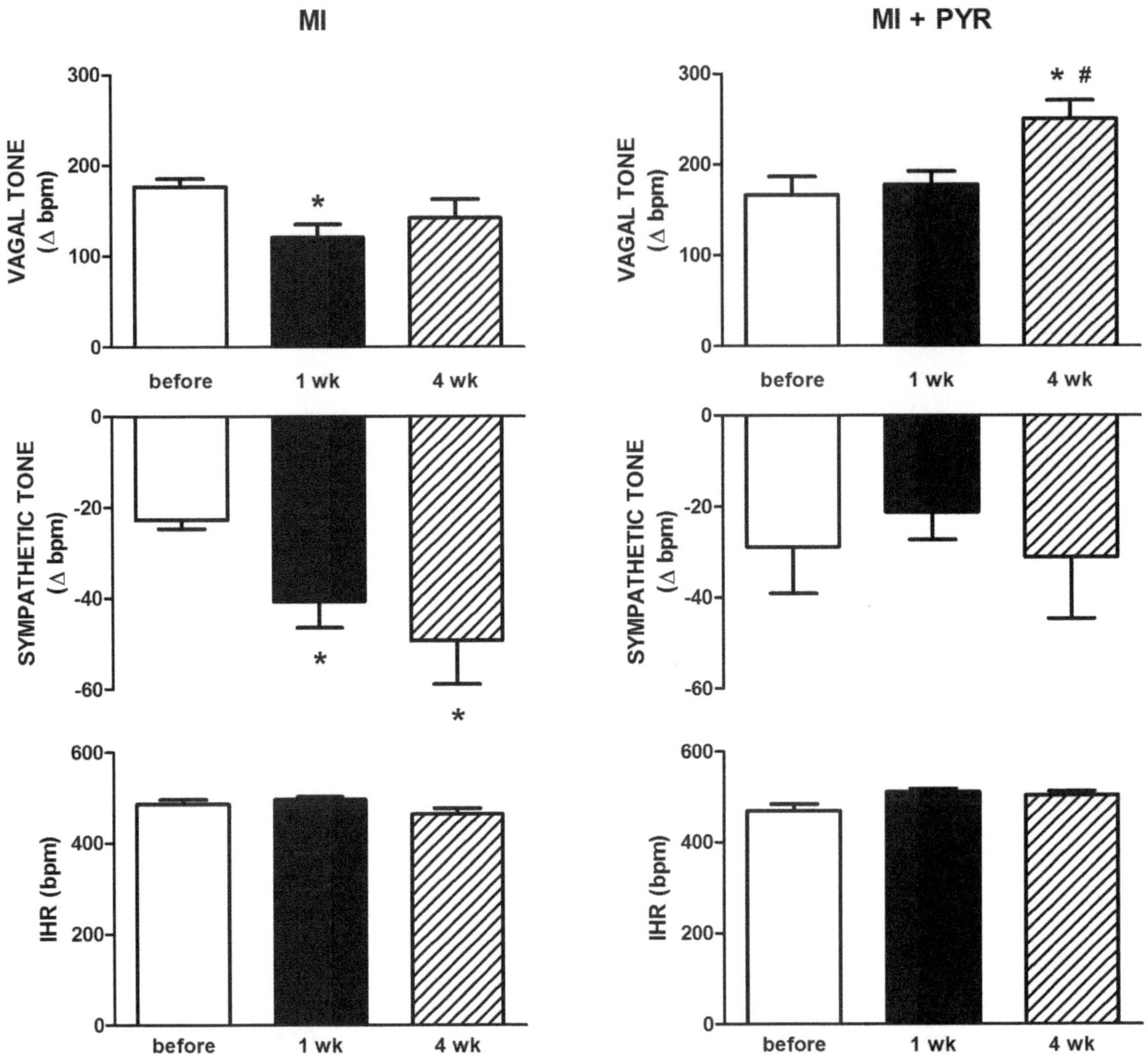

Figure 4. Tachycardic response caused by methyl atropine (Vagal Tone) [left and right upper panel], bradycardic response caused by propranolol (Sympathetic Tone) [left and right middle panel] and intrinsic heart rate (IHR) [left and right lower panel] before, one week (1 wk) and four weeks (4 wk) after MI with or without pyridostigmine (PYR) treatment. Values are presented as mean ± SEM. *$p<0.05$ compared to before; #$p<0.05$ compared to one week. MI: n = 8; MI+PYR: n = 7.

PYR was able to reduce the loss of vagal and the increase of the sympathetic cardiac tone at four weeks after MI. PYR has produced likewise a great increase in vagal tone at four weeks post MI, supporting the notion that the blockade of acetylcholinesterase was effective in preserving the cardiac autonomic balance in myocardial infarcted subjects. Previous studies have provided similar results, demonstrating that short- and long-term treatment with PYR reduced basal HR and prevented the reduction in the vagal tone and the increase of the sympathetic tone in the early and late phases of heart failure following MI in rats [20–22]. The increase in parasympathetic activity produced by PYR may be attributed to the potentiation of cholinergic neurotransmission. It has been shown that the same dose of PYR used in the present study (3 mg/kg) inhibited 85% of acetylcholinesterase activity one week after its administration, increasing the permanence of acetylcholine in the synaptic cleft [42].

The neural control of the heart is exerted by the tonic interaction between the sympathetic and parasympathetic arms of the autonomic nervous system [43]. Studies have demonstrated that acetylcholine released from vagal endings possess inhibitory effects on norepinephrine release from cardiac sympathetic nerves [44], suppressing the adrenergic signaling cascade in ventricular cardiac myocytes [45]. Acetylcholine can act on muscarinic receptors situated in sympathetic presynaptic nerve endings inhibiting the release of norepinephrine [46][47][48]. The interaction between the sympathetic and parasympathetic nervous system may also be partially modulated by second messengers in cardiac cells [9] where cholinergic stimulation may inhibit the increase of intracellular cAMP [49] inhibiting the adrenergic

Table 2. Hemodynamic parameters and indices of left ventricle function derived from pressure-volume recordings in isoflurane anesthetized control and myocardial infarcted (MI) mice with or without pyridostigmine (PYR) treatment.

	Control	Control+PYR	MI	MI+PYR
	(n = 6)	(n = 7)	(n = 5)	(n = 8)
MAP (mmHg)	81±3	79±3	74±4	85±3
HR (bpm)	492±14	457±33	503±29	527±16
+dP/dt (mmHg/s)	9393±631	8958±574	9285±487	8133±619
−dP/dt (mmHg/s)	−8845±864	−8677±1222	−9133±282	−6742±645#
LVEDP (mmHg)	3.5±1.3	5.7±2.0	5.0±1.3	7.6±2.6
ESV (μL)	11.6±0.9	15.1±3.7	24.1±2.5*	20.2±2.1
EDV (μL)	17.8±1.7	24.1±5.0	31.4±2.4*	29.5±3.7
SV (μL)	7.3±1.1	9.0±1.6	7.3±1.5	9.4±2.1
EF (%)	39±3	39±4	24±5*	29±5
CO (μL/min)	3583±579	3904±686	3785±904	4859±1084
CI (mL/min/kg)	106±18	117±20	115±27	147±34

Values are presented as the mean ± SEM.
*p<0.05 compared control group.
#p<0.05 compared to MI group.

signaling cascade [50]. It has been documented that on the sinoatrial node the parasympathetic modulation predominates over the sympathetic activity [50] [51]. This response is known as "accentuated antagonism" [50]. When a vagal electrical stimulation is applied simultaneously to a sympathetic electrical stimulus, there is a reduction in HR similar to that observed in the presence of vagal stimulation alone [52]. Thus, the results from the current study suggest that the parasympathetic improvement produced by PYR in MI mice was able to suppress the augmented sympathetic drive to the heart.

Left ventricle P-V measurements revealed only mild cardiac dysfunction, indicated by increased ventricular volumes and reduced ejection fraction. It has been reported that left ventricular function decreases proportionally with the MI size in mice [1,33]. Usually, animals with small MI size are excluded from published studies [53,54]. Nevertheless, in line with our findings, Ahn and co-workers [1] showed that even MI with relatively small size(< 20%) displayed significant reduction in ejection fraction. Nevertheless, the size of myocardial infarction in the present study did not affect important indices of ventricular function such as cardiac output (and cardiac index), left ventricular end-diastolic pressure and dP/dt. It is worth noting that Patten and colleagues [35] showed that only the volume and end-diastolic diameter of the left ventricle correlated significantly with the infarct size in mice. Therefore, the slight alterations of cardiac function might be attributed to the small infarct size (~12%) observed in the present study, while PYR was not able to affect these slight alterations.

Previous studies have shown that electrical stimulation of the vagus nerve improved cardiac function in rats [14] and dogs with heart failure [55]. Moreover, rodent studies using acetylcholinesterase blockers, e.g., PYR and donepezil, described an attenuation of the progression of both cardiac remodeling and cardiac dysfunction, as well as improvement of the long-term survival of animals with heart failure [14,20,56,57]. In addition, Lara and colleagues [11] observed, in mice with reduced expression of the vesicular acetylcholine transporter (VAChT KD), that increased cholinergic activity by means of PYR improved the ventricular dysfunction, indicating the protective role of parasympathetic function in the heart. Nevertheless, in the present study the increased vagal tonic influence to the heart induced by PYR, did not improve the slight cardiac dysfunction exhibited by myocardial infarcted mice.

Therefore, based in the findings of this study, it can be concluded that PYR administration initiated immediately after MI is an important pharmacological approach to protect the alterations in HR and cardiac autonomic imbalance induced by MI.

Supporting Information

Figure S1 Photomicrographs and bar graphs of the minor diameter of myocytes (yellow lines crossing perpendicular to the nuclei, in hematoxylin and eosin stain) and collagen density (in picrosirius red stain) from the left ventricle of control and myocardial infarcted mice (MI) with or without pyridostigmine (PYR) treatment. Values are presented as the mean ± SEM. Bar = 60 μm.

Author Contributions

Conceived and designed the experiments: HCS RF. Performed the experiments: MTD CB MO CAAS CMP JC. Analyzed the data: MTD CB JC. Contributed reagents/materials/analysis tools: HCS RF. Wrote the paper: MTD CB RF HCS.

References

1. Ahn D, Cheng L, Moon C, Spurgeon H, Lakatta EG, et al. (2004) Induction of myocardial infarcts of a predictable size and location by branch pattern probability-assisted coronary ligation in C57BL/6 mice. Am J Physiol Heart Circ Physiol 286: H1201–1207. doi:10.1152/ajpheart.00862.2003
2. Salto-Tellez M, Yung Lim S, El-Oakley RM, Tang TPL, ALmsherqi ZAM, et al. (2004) Myocardial infarction in the C57BL/6J mouse: a quantifiable and highly reproducible experimental model. Cardiovasc Pathol Off J Soc Cardiovasc Pathol 13: 91–97. doi:10.1016/S1054-8807(03)00129-7

3. Yutzey KE, Robbins J (2007) Principles of genetic murine models for cardiac disease. Circulation 115: 792–799. doi:10.1161/CIRCULATIONAHA.106.682534.
4. Carlson SH, Wyss JM (2000) Long-term telemetric recording of arterial pressure and heart rate in mice fed basal and high NaCl diets. Hypertension 35: E1–5.
5. Butz GM, Davisson RL (2001) Long-term telemetric measurement of cardiovascular parameters in awake mice: a physiological genomics tool. Physiol Genomics 5: 89–97.
6. Binkley PF, Nunziata E, Haas GJ, Nelson SD, Cody RJ (1991) Parasympathetic withdrawal is an integral component of autonomic imbalance in congestive heart failure: demonstration in human subjects and verification in a paced canine model of ventricular failure. J Am Coll Cardiol 18: 464–472.
7. Ishise H, Asanoi H, Ishizaka S, Joho S, Kameyama T, et al. (1998) Time course of sympathovagal imbalance and left ventricular dysfunction in conscious dogs with heart failure. J Appl Physiol Bethesda Md 1985 84: 1234–1241.
8. Bibevski S, Dunlap ME (2011) Evidence for impaired vagus nerve activity in heart failure. Heart Fail Rev 16: 129–135. doi:10.1007/s10741-010-9190-6.
9. Olshansky B, Sabbah HN, Hauptman PJ, Colucci WS (2008) Parasympathetic nervous system and heart failure: pathophysiology and potential implications for therapy. Circulation 118: 863–871. doi:10.1161/CIRCULATIONAHA.107.760405.
10. LaCroix C, Freeling J, Giles A, Wess J, Li Y-F (2008) Deficiency of M2 muscarinic acetylcholine receptors increases susceptibility of ventricular function to chronic adrenergic stress. Am J Physiol Heart Circ Physiol 294: H810–820. doi:10.1152/ajpheart.00724.2007.
11. Lara A, Damasceno DD, Pires R, Gros R, Gomes ER, et al. (2010) Dysautonomia due to reduced cholinergic neurotransmission causes cardiac remodeling and heart failure. Mol Cell Biol 30: 1746–1756. doi:10.1128/MCB.00996-09
12. Katare RG, Ando M, Kakinuma Y, Arikawa M, Yamasaki F, et al. (2010) Differential regulation of TNF receptors by vagal nerve stimulation protects heart against acute ischemic injury. J Mol Cell Cardiol 49: 234–244. doi:10.1016/j.yjmcc.2010.03.007
13. De Ferrari GM, Schwartz PJ (2011) Vagus nerve stimulation: from pre-clinical to clinical application: challenges and future directions. Heart Fail Rev 16: 195–203. doi:10.1007/s10741-010-9216-0
14. Li M, Zheng C, Sato T, Kawada T, Sugimachi M, et al. (2004) Vagal nerve stimulation markedly improves long-term survival after chronic heart failure in rats. Circulation 109: 120–124. doi:10.1161/01.CIR.0000105721.71640.DA.
15. Zheng C, Li M, Inagaki M, Kawada T, Sunagawa K, et al. (2005) Vagal stimulation markedly suppresses arrhythmias in conscious rats with chronic heart failure after myocardial infarction. Conf Proc Annu Int Conf IEEE Eng Med Biol Soc IEEE Eng Med Biol Soc Conf 7: 7072–7075. doi:10.1109/IEMBS.2005.1616135
16. Hauptman PJ, Schwartz PJ, Gold MR, Borggrefe M, Van Veldhuisen DJ, et al. (2012) Rationale and study design of the increase of vagal tone in heart failure study: INOVATE-HF. Am Heart J 163: 954–962.e1. doi:10.1016/j.ahj.2012.03.021
17. Schwartz PJ (2013) Vagal stimulation for heart diseases: from animals to men. An example of translational cardiology. Neth Heart J Mon J Neth Soc Cardiol Neth Heart Found 21: 82–84. doi:10.1007/s12471-012-0368-5
18. Desai MY, Watanabe MA, Laddu AA, Hauptman PJ (2011) Pharmacologic modulation of parasympathetic activity in heart failure. Heart Fail Rev 16: 179–193. doi:10.1007/s10741-010-9195-1
19. Nobrega ACL, Loures DL, Pontes PV, Sant'anna ID, Mesquita ET (2008) Cholinergic stimulation with pyridostigmine prevents the impairment in ventricular function during mental stress in coronary artery disease patients. Int J Cardiol 125: 418–421. doi:10.1016/j.ijcard.2007.01.043
20. Lataro RM, Silva CAA, Fazan R Jr, Rossi MA, Prado CM, et al. (2013) Increase in parasympathetic tone by pyridostigmine prevents ventricular dysfunction during the onset of heart failure. Am J Physiol Regul Integr Comp Physiol. doi:10.1152/ajpregu.00102.2013
21. Sabino JPJ, da Silva CAA, de Melo RF, Fazan R Jr, Salgado HC (2013) The treatment with pyridostigmine improves the cardiocirculatory function in rats with chronic heart failure. Auton Neurosci Basic Clin 173: 58–64. doi:10.1016/j.autneu.2012.11.007
22. De La Fuente RN, Rodrigues B, Moraes-Silva IC, Souza LE, Sirvente R, et al. (2013) Cholinergic stimulation with pyridostigmine improves autonomic function in infarcted rats. Clin Exp Pharmacol Physiol 40: 610–616. doi:10.1111/1440-1681.12121
23. Soares PP da S, da Nóbrega ACL, Ushizima MR, Irigoyen MCC (2004) Cholinergic stimulation with pyridostigmine increases heart rate variability and baroreflex sensitivity in rats. Auton Neurosci Basic Clin 113: 24–31. doi:10.1016/j.autneu.2004.05.002
24. Nóbrega AC, dos Reis AF, Moraes RS, Bastos BG, Ferlin EL, et al. (2001) Enhancement of heart rate variability by cholinergic stimulation with pyridostigmine in healthy subjects. Clin Auton Res Off J Clin Auton Res Soc 11: 11–17.
25. Behling A, Moraes RS, Rohde LE, Ferlin EL, Nóbrega ACL, et al. (2003) Cholinergic stimulation with pyridostigmine reduces ventricular arrhythmia and enhances heart rate variability in heart failure. Am Heart J 146: 494–500. doi:10.1016/S0002-8703(03)00319-3
26. Dewland TA, Androne AS, Lee FA, Lampert RJ, Katz SD (2007) Effect of acetylcholinesterase inhibition with pyridostigmine on cardiac parasympathetic function in sedentary adults and trained athletes. Am J Physiol Heart Circ Physiol 293: H86–92. doi:10.1152/ajpheart.01339.2006
27. Zimerman LI, Liberman A, Castro RRT, Ribeiro JP, Nóbrega ACL (2010) Acute electrophysiologic consequences of pyridostigmine inhibition of cholinesterase in humans. Braz J Med Biol Res Rev Bras Pesqui Médicas E Biológicas Soc Bras Biofísica Al 43: 211–216.
28. Castro RRT, Porphirio G, Serra SM, Nóbrega ACL (2004) Cholinergic stimulation with pyridostigmine protects against exercise induced myocardial ischaemia. Heart Br Card Soc 90: 1119–1123. doi:10.1136/hrt.2003.028167
29. Castro RRT, Serra SM, Porphirio G, Mendes FSNS, Oliveira LPJ, et al. (2006) Pyridostigmine reduces QTc interval during recovery from maximal exercise in ischemic heart disease. Int J Cardiol 107: 138–139. doi:10.1016/j.ijcard.2005.01.035
30. Serra SM, Costa RV, Teixeira De Castro RR, Xavier SS, Nóbrega ACLD (2009) Cholinergic stimulation improves autonomic and hemodynamic profile during dynamic exercise in patients with heart failure. J Card Fail 15: 124–129. doi:10.1016/j.cardfail.2008.10.018
31. Androne AS, Hryniewicz K, Goldsmith R, Arwady A, Katz SD (2003) Acetylcholinesterase inhibition with pyridostigmine improves heart rate recovery after maximal exercise in patients with chronic heart failure. Heart Br Card Soc 89: 854–858.
32. Pacher P, Nagayama T, Mukhopadhyay P, Bátkai S, Kass DA (2008) Measurement of cardiac function using pressure-volume conductance catheter technique in mice and rats. Nat Protoc 3: 1422–1434. doi:10.1038/nprot.2008.138
33. Takagawa J, Zhang Y, Wong ML, Sievers RE, Kapasi NK, et al. (2007) Myocardial infarct size measurement in the mouse chronic infarction model: comparison of area- and length-based approaches. J Appl Physiol Bethesda Md 1985 102: 2104–2111. doi:10.1152/japplphysiol.00033.2007
34. Higuchi ML, Moreira LF, Silvestre JM, Gutierrez PS, Savalli C, et al. (1999) Myocardial fiber diameter as a good indicator of outcome in Batista's operation. J Card Surg 14: 401–407.
35. Patten RD, Aronovitz MJ, Deras-Mejia L, Pandian NG, Hanak GG, et al. (1998) Ventricular remodeling in a mouse model of myocardial infarction. Am J Physiol 274: H1812–1820.
36. Bridgman P, Aronovitz MA, Kakkar R, Oliverio MI, Coffman TM, et al. (2005) Gender-specific patterns of left ventricular and myocyte remodeling following myocardial infarction in mice deficient in the angiotensin II type 1a receptor. Am J Physiol Heart Circ Physiol 289: H586–592. doi:10.1152/ajpheart.00474.2004
37. Infanger DW, Cao X, Butler SD, Burmeister MA, Zhou Y, et al. (2010) Silencing nox4 in the paraventricular nucleus improves myocardial infarction-induced cardiac dysfunction by attenuating sympathoexcitation and periinfarct apoptosis. Circ Res 106: 1763–1774. doi:10.1161/CIRCRESAHA.109.213025
38. Arenja N, Mueller C, Ehl NF, Brinkert M, Roost K, et al. (2013) Prevalence, extent, and independent predictors of silent myocardial infarction. Am J Med 126: 515–522. doi:10.1016/j.amjmed.2012.11.028
39. Porter TR, Eckberg DL, Fritsch JM, Rea RF, Beightol LA, et al. (1990) Autonomic pathophysiology in heart failure patients. Sympathetic-cholinergic interrelations. J Clin Invest 85: 1362–1371. doi:10.1172/JCI114580
40. Eckberg DL, Drabinsky M, Braunwald E (1971) Defective cardiac parasympathetic control in patients with heart disease. N Engl J Med 285: 877–883. doi:10.1056/NEJM197110142851602
41. Dunlap ME, Bibevski S, Rosenberry TL, Ernsberger P (2003) Mechanisms of altered vagal control in heart failure: influence of muscarinic receptors and acetylcholinesterase activity. Am J Physiol Heart Circ Physiol 285: H1632–1640. doi:10.1152/ajpheart.01051.2002
42. Bernatova I, Dubovicky M, Price WA, Grubbs RD, Lucot JB, et al. (2003) Effect of chronic pyridostigmine bromide treatment on cardiovascular and behavioral parameters in mice. Pharmacol Biochem Behav 74: 901–907.
43. Schwartz PJ, De Ferrari GM (2011) Sympathetic-parasympathetic interaction in health and disease: abnormalities and relevance in heart failure. Heart Fail Rev 16: 101–107. doi:10.1007/s10741-010-9179-1.
44. Manabe N, Foldes FF, Töröcsik A, Nagashima H, Goldiner PL, et al. (1991) Presynaptic interaction between vagal and sympathetic innervation in the heart: modulation of acetylcholine and noradrenaline release. J Auton Nerv Syst 32: 233–242.
45. Watanabe AM, Lindemann JP, Fleming JW (1984) Mechanisms of muscarinic modulation of protein phosphorylation in intact ventricles. Fed Proc 43: 2618–2623.
46. Azevedo ER, Parker JD (1999) Parasympathetic control of cardiac sympathetic activity: normal ventricular function versus congestive heart failure. Circulation 100: 274–279.
47. Manabe N, Foldes FF, Töröcsik A, Nagashima H, Goldiner PL, et al. (1991) Presynaptic interaction between vagal and sympathetic innervation in the heart: modulation of acetylcholine and noradrenaline release. J Auton Nerv Syst 32: 233–242.
48. Muscholl E (1980) Peripheral muscarinic control of norepinephrine release in the cardiovascular system. Am J Physiol 239: H713–720.
49. Watanabe AM, Lindemann JP, Fleming JW (1984) Mechanisms of muscarinic modulation of protein phosphorylation in intact ventricles. Fed Proc 43: 2618–2623.
50. Levy MN (1971) Sympathetic-parasympathetic interactions in the heart. Circ Res 29: 437–445.

51. Vanhoutte PM, Levy MN (1980) Prejunctional cholinergic modulation of adrenergic neurotransmission in the cardiovascular system. Am J Physiol 238: H275–281.
52. Levy MN, Zieske H (1969) Autonomic control of cardiac pacemaker activity and atrioventricular transmission. J Appl Physiol 27: 465–470.
53. Kumashiro H, Kusachi S, Moritani H, Ohnishi H, Nakahama M, et al. (1999) Establishment of a long-surviving murine model of myocardial infarction: qualitative and quantitative conventional microscopic findings during pathological evolution. Basic Res Cardiol 94: 78–84.
54. Sam F, Sawyer DB, Chang DL, Eberli FR, Ngoy S, et al. (2000) Progressive left ventricular remodeling and apoptosis late after myocardial infarction in mouse heart. Am J Physiol Heart Circ Physiol 279: H422–428.
55. Zhang Y, Popovic ZB, Bibevski S, Fakhry I, Sica DA, et al. (2009) Chronic vagus nerve stimulation improves autonomic control and attenuates systemic inflammation and heart failure progression in a canine high-rate pacing model. Circ Heart Fail 2: 692–699. doi:10.1161/CIRCHEARTFAILURE.109.873968
56. Handa T, Katare RG, Kakinuma Y, Arikawa M, Ando M, et al. (2009) Anti-Alzheimer's drug, donepezil, markedly improves long-term survival after chronic heart failure in mice. J Card Fail 15: 805–811. doi:10.1016/j.cardfail.2009.05.008
57. Okazaki Y, Zheng C, Li M, Sugimachi M (2010) Effect of the cholinesterase inhibitor donepezil on cardiac remodeling and autonomic balance in rats with heart failure. J Physiol Sci JPS 60: 67–74. doi:10.1007/s12576-009-0071-5

10

Plasma Cytokine Profile in Tropical Endomyocardial Fibrosis: Predominance of TNF-a, IL-4 and IL-10

Aline S. Bossa[1,2], Vera M. C. Salemi[3], Susan P. Ribeiro[2], Daniela S. Rosa[5], Ludmila Rodrigues Pinto Ferreira[1,2], Suzete C. Ferreira[3], Anna Shoko Nishiya[4], Charles Mady[3], Jorge Kalil[1,2], Edecio Cunha-Neto[1,2]*

1 Laboratory of Immunology, Heart Institute (InCor), University of São Paulo School of Medicine, São Paulo, Brazil, **2** Division of Clinical Immunology and Allergy, University of São Paulo School of Medicine, São Paulo, Brazil, **3** Cardiomyopathy Unit, Heart Institute (InCor), University of São Paulo School of Medicine, São Paulo, Brazil, **4** Pró-Sangue Foundation, São Paulo, Brazil; Institute for Investigation in Immunology (iii), INCT, São Paulo, Brazil, **5** Division of Immunology, Department of Microbiology, Immunology and Parasitology-Federal University of São Paulo-UNIFESP, São Paulo, Brazil

Abstract

Background: The participation of immune/inflammatory mechanisms in the pathogenesis of tropical endomyocardial fibrosis (EMF) has been suggested by the finding of early blood and myocardial eosinophilia. However, the inflammatory activation status of late-stage EMF patients is still unknown.

Methodology/Principal findings: We evaluated pro- and anti-inflammatory cytokine levels in plasma samples from late stage EMF patients. Cytokine levels of Tumor Necrosis Factor (TNF)-α, Interferon (IFN)-γ, Interleukin (IL)-2, IL-4, IL-6, and IL-10 were assayed in plasma samples from 27 EMF patients and compared with those of healthy control subjects. All EMF patients displayed detectable plasma levels of at least one of the cytokines tested. We found that TNF-α, IL-6, IL-4, and IL-10 were each detected in at least 74% of tested sera, and plasma levels of IL-10, IL-4, and TNF-α were significantly higher than those of controls. Plasma levels of such cytokines positively correlated with each other.

Conclusions/Significance: The mixed pro- and anti-inflammatory/Th2circulating cytokine profile in EMF is consistent with the presence of a persistent inflammatory stimulus. On the other hand, the detection of increased levels of TNF-α may be secondary to the cardiovascular involvement observed in these patients, whereas IL-4 and IL-10 may have been upregulated as a homeostatic mechanism to buffer both production and deleterious cardiovascular effects of pro-inflammatory cytokines. Further studies might establish whether these findings play a role in disease pathogenesis.

Editor: Naglaa H. Shoukry, University of Montreal Hospital Research Center (CRCHUM), Canada

Funding: This research was supported by the Brazilian Council for Scientific and Technological Development - CNPq and the São Paulo State Research Funding Agency - FAPESP. ASB is recipient of a São Paulo State Research Funding Agency - FAPESP fellowship. ECN and JK are recipients of Brazilian Council for Scientific and Technological Development - CNPq productivity awards. The funders had no role in study design, data collection and analysis, decision to publish, or preparation of the manuscript.

Competing Interests: The authors have declared that no competing interests exist.

* Email: edecunha@usp.br

Introduction

Tropical endomyocardial fibrosis (EMF) is a restrictive cardiomyopathy characterized by fibrous tissue deposition of the endomyocardium of one or both ventricles, associated with diastolic heart failure (HF), secondary valvular dysfunction, and atrial arrhythmias, such as atrial fibrillation (AF). The etiopathogenesis of EMF is still obscure [1]. Several factors involving immune mechanisms have been suggested to play a pathogenetic role, including infections, chronic helminthic infection-related hypereosinophilia, allergy, auto-immunity, and malnutrition. One of the major pathogenetic theories states that EMF could be considered a late effect of helminthic infection-induced eosinophil degranulation in the heart,due to its similarities with the eosinophilic endocarditis (EE) of Loeffler's syndrome [2–4]. At the late stage of the disease, the presence of a focal perivascular chronic inflammatory infiltrate deep within the endomyocardium, predominantly composed by lymphocytes and macrophages, with very rare eosinophils is consistent with a role of persistent immune-mediated inflammation [5]. Cytokines are key mediators of immunity, modulating the nature of the immune and inflammatory responses. Proinflammatory cytokines such as TNF-α and IL-6 have been found to be increased both in peripheral blood and heart tissue, in several cardiovascular (CV) diseases including HF [6–8] and have prognostic significance [9,10].

Direct pathogenic effects of TNF-α include progressive cardiomyocyte apoptosis, adverse ventricular remodelling, left ventricular (LV) wall thinning and dilation, which have been observed in mice overexpressing TNF-α [11]. Anti-inflammatory cytokines such as IL-4 and IL-10 are associated with helminthiasis and eosinophilia [12] and a limited number of studies have reported the detection ofsuch cytokines in CV disorders [13,14]. Several of the clinical features characteristic of EMF are associated themselves with increased levels of circulating cytokines [15]. Even though a persistent local inflammatory infiltrate is found in

Table 1. Demographic and echocardiographic data from EMF patients and healthy subjects.

Variable	EMF	HS
Gender (Male/Female)	3/24	12/26
Age (years - Male/Female)	34.6±15.5	33.9±12
Bilateral/RV/LV EMF (%)	49.5±13.3	53.9±12,9
Mitral regurgitation (%) *	30/26/44	NA
Tricuspid regurgitation (%)*	55.5%/26%/7.4%	NA
Diastolic dysfunction grade (%)**	37%/18.5%/7.4%	NA
Systolic dysfunction (%)	60,90%	NA
AF (%)	21.4	NA

NA – Not applicable; AF – Atrial Fibrillation; (Percentage of EMF patients with the conditionregistered in the medical records); Systolic dysfunction: Ejection Fraction < 55%; *Valvar regurgitation level: mild, moderate, and severe, respectively; Diastolic dysfunction: grades mild, moderate, and severe ** It was not possible to evaluate diastolic function in 4 patients, due to the presence of pacemaker or bioprosthetic heart valve.

late-stage EMF, it is yet unknown whether such patients display systemic inflammatory activation.In order to assess whether there is systemic inflammation in the late stages of EMF, we assessed the circulating levels of pro- and anti-inflammatory/Th2 cytokines in EMF patients and controls.

Methods

The protocol was approved by the Institutional Review Board of the University of São Paulo School of Medicine (Protocol number 0569/10), and written informed consent was obtained from all the subjects.

Patient selection

We evaluated cytokine plasma levels of 27 EMF outpatients (24 female, 34.6±15.5 years) followed at the Cardiomyopathy Unit of the Heart Institute (InCor), University of São Paulo Medical School between 2004 and 2012, and 38 healthy blood donors (26 female, 33.9±12.0 years) from Pró-Sangue Foundation, as control subjects. Patients had undergone bidimensional Doppler echocardiography and gadolinium-enhanced magnetic resonance imaging. The major inclusion criteria included clinical signs suggestive of diastolic HF, apical obliteration of one or both ventricles [16,17] and late gadolinium enhancement magnetic resonance imaging showing the typical pattern of fibrous tissue deposition [18]. There were no exclusion criteria.Nine (30%) patients hadbiventricular, seven (26%) right ventricular, and eleven (44%) left ventricular (LV) involvement. Patients came from lower socioeconomic strata, with poor housing and evidence of protein malnutrition during childhood. Twenty-one patients (78%) underwent surgical resection of endomyocardial fibrous tissue; gross anatomy and histopathology confirmed the diagnosis.

Sample collection and cytokine quantification

EDTA-anticoagulated peripheral blood samples were collected from the patients and from healthy controls. Plasma samples were stored at −80°C until cytokine assays were performed, using the Th1/Th2 II human bead array (BD Biosciences), according to the manufacturer's recommendations. Samples were analyzed with

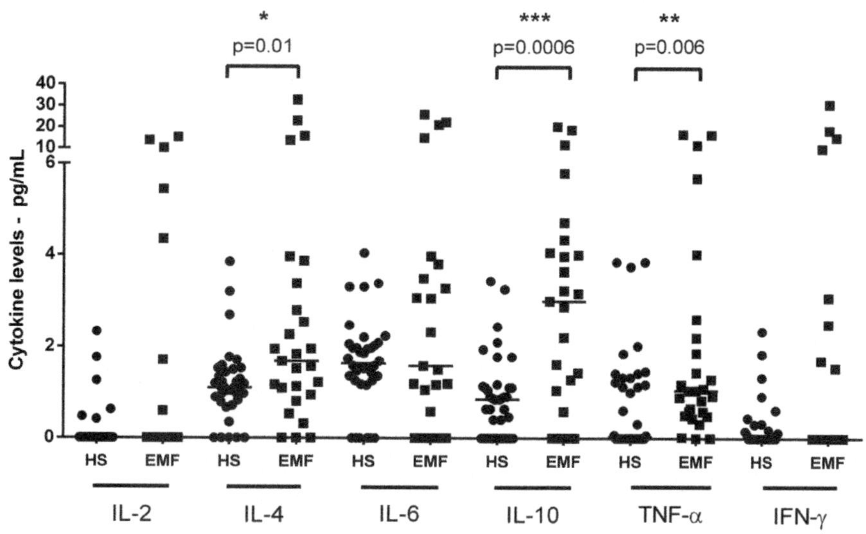

Figure 1. Cytokine plasma levels of endomyocardial fibrosis patients and healthy subjects. Dot plot represents cytokine levels (interleukin 2, 4, 6, 10, TNF-α and IFN-γ) from endomyocardial fibrosis patients (EMF) and healthy subjects (HS), evaluated by CBA. Horizontal lines indicate the median values. *Differences where *P*≤0.05 are indicated. (●Healthy Subjects; ■EMF patients).

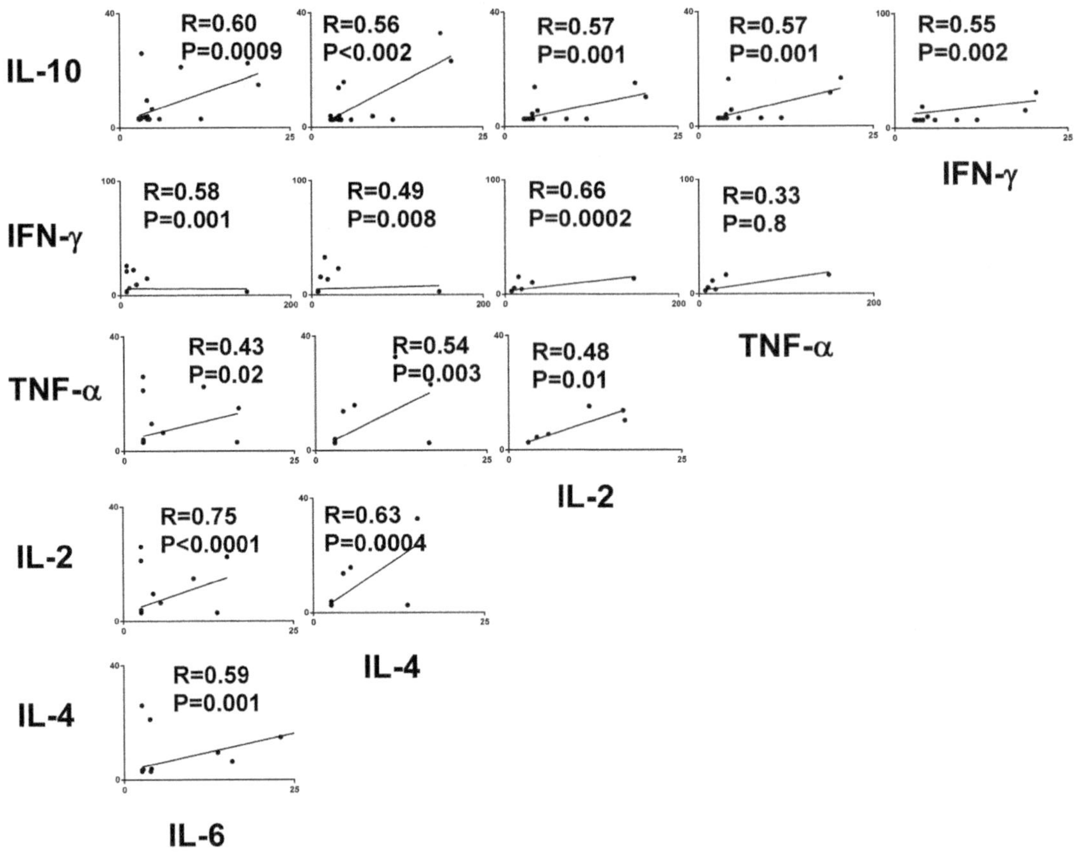

Figure 2. Correlation among cytokine plasma levels of endomyocardial fibrosis patients. Dot plots represent correlation between cytokine levels (interleukin 2, 4, 6, 10, TNF-α and IFN-γ) from endomyocardial fibrosis patients, evaluated by CBA.

the FACSCanto flow cytometer (BD Biosciences), and the FCAP Array software (BD Biosciences) was used for data analysis.

Statistical Methods

Cytokine levels were compared among EMF patients and subject controls by using the Mann-Whitney *U* test. Correlations of data were analyzed by the non-parametric Spearman test. All analysis was performed with Graph Pad Prism version 5 software (GraphPad Software, La Jolla, California, USA). A *P* value$<$0.05 was considered statistically significant.

Results

EMF and healthy subjects were age and sexmatched (Table 1). Plasma samples from all 27 EMF patients examined in this study showed detectable levels of at least one of the assayed cytokines. Increased levels of interleukin (IL)-4 (4.51±7.79 pg/mL), IL-10 (4.11±5.27 pg/mL), and tumor necrosis factor alpha (TNF-α) (2.77±4.64 pg/mL) were detected in a high proportion of EMF patients (88.8%, 92.6%, and 77.7%, respectively) compared with healthy control samples (1.22±0.87 pg/mL - $P = 0.001$, 0.99± 0.89 pg/mL- $P = 0.0001$ and 0.94±0.24 pg/mL - $P = 0.006$, respectively - Mann Whitney U Test) - (Figure 1 and 2). There was no significant difference in IL-6, IFN- γ and IL-2 levels compared with control samples. Interestingly, circulating IL-4 was present in 20/21 samples in which IL-10 was detectable. In addition, a positive correlation was observed between all cytokine levels in EMF patients, with the exception of TNF-α and IFN- γ ($P = 0.08$; Figure 2).

Discussion

Our study shows that EMF patient shave elevated plasma levels of pro- and anti-inflammatory cytokines, especially TNF-α, IL-4, and IL-10, which were significantly higher than those in healthy subjects. The correlation between levels of pro- and anti-inflammatory/Th2 cytokines may suggest that either the stimuli that induce both kinds of cytokines are the same, or that IL-10 and IL-4 may have a regulatory role and control the levels and deleterious effects of proinflammatory cytokines.

Multiple cardiovascular disorders are associated with increased levels of circulating pro-inflammatory cytokines, especially TNF-α and IL-6, which are related to a common cytokine profile found in acute and chronic HF patients independently of etiology [19,20]. Mann proposed that acute increased levels of IL-6, TNF-α and IL-1 could be an adaptive response for cardiac injury, with cardioprotective effects, whereas the chronic elevation of these mediators could be a maladaptive response and promote cardiac decompensation [21]. However, the underlying cause for the presence of the inflammatory response in different CV diseases is still under investigation [22]. It has been suggested that the predominant mechanism of upregulation of TNF-α production is secondary to advanced heart failure itself, such as low cardiac output and intestinal bacterial translocation [23].

In addition, a limited number of reports on HF have found increased plasma levels of the other cytokines detected in our study (IL-10, IL-4, and to a lesser extent IFN- γ and IL-2) [13,24–26]. It is thus possible that the triggers of cytokine production in EMF are similar to those found in HF with other causes, such as hypertensive or idiopathic dilated cardiomyopathy. On the other hand, our findings that late-stage EMF patients display increased IL-4 and IL-10 levels are also consistent with the observed early eosinophilia and helminthic infections in EMF, once this type of infection is usually associated with increased levels of these cytokines [27–30]. Whichever the stimulus for cytokine production may be, results suggest a possible relevance of a persisting Th2 (IL-4 and IL-10) cytokine-driven immune mechanism in the pathogenesis of EMF. Significantly, IL-10 is an anti-inflammatory cytokine that may reduce TNF-α production, which may be clinically significant in the pathogenesis of HF [31]. In our study, the almost universal co-detection of inflammatory and anti-inflammatory cytokines, as well as the correlation between their levels is consistent with such an antagonistic effect. On the other hand, along with its known anti-inflammatory effects, long-term overexpression of IL-10 has been associated with lung fibrosis [32].

Although blood eosinophilia (BE) has been reported in EMF cases [29], less than 40% of our patients displayed BE ($\geq$ 500 eosinophils/mm^3) during follow-up in the chronic phase of this disease. Our data are consistent with those reported by Patel and associates (1977) [33], who observed that the absolute BE in African EMF patients was similar to that of healthy control subjects. In a recent study from a similar cohort of patients in our Hospital, Iglezias et al. [5] found no eosinophils in the heart lesions of EMF patients. Together, these results suggest that neither blood nor endocardial eosinophilia are essential components of late-stage EMF. Our data are consistent with the hypothesis that early helminthic infestation could cause a waning eosinophilia that might be involved in initial heart damage in EMF pathogenesis, and along with a long-lasting Th2 response whose pathogenic or protective potential is yet unclear. However, we cannot exclude that the anti-inflamatory cytokine levels are raised as a homeostatic mechanism to buffer both production and effects of pro-inflammatory cytokines. Although persistent IL-10 production may lead to lung fibrosis [33], it is unknown whether the cytokine could accelerate fibrous tissue deposition in the endomyocardium of EMF patients. One limitation of this study is the lack of information about helminthic infection status in our patient group.

In summary, we have shown for the first time that late-stage EMF patients display detectable plasma levels of a mixed pro- and anti-inflammatory/Th2 cytokine profile, predominantly composed of TNF-α, IL-10 and IL-4 levels. The finding of such a mixed cytokine profile may either reflect the multiple cardiovascular disorders also experienced by EMF patients, or indicate a common persistent stimulus for production of both pro- and anti-inflammatory/Th2 cytokines. On the other hand, anti-inflammatory/Th2 cytokines IL-4 and IL-10 may either be upregulated by previous helminthic infection, or as a homeostatic mechanism to buffer both production and effects of pro-inflammatory cytokines. This antagonism is consistent with the almost universal co-detection of inflammatory and anti-inflammatory cytokines in EMF plasma samples, as well as the positive correlation between their plasma levels. Further studies may allow the identification of the stimulus for chronic cytokine production, and to establish whether cytokines play a role in pathogenesis or have a prognostic value for rates of disease progression or post-surgical follow-up.

Author Contributions

Conceived and designed the experiments: ASB VMCS ECN CM. Performed the experiments: ASB LRPF SPR ASN DSR SCF. Analyzed the data: ASB SPR ECN JK. Contributed reagents/materials/analysis tools: SPR LRPF ASN DSR ECN JK SCF. Wrote the paper: ASB VMCS ECN.

References

1. Davies JN (1948) Pathology of Central African Natives; Mulago Hospital post mortem studies. East Afr Med J 25: 454–467.
2. Roberts WC, Liegler DG, Carbone PP (1969) Endomyocardial disease and eosinophilia. A clinical and pathologic spectrum. Am J Med 46: 28–42.
3. Satoh M, Minami Y, Takahashi Y, Nakamura M (2008) Immune modulation: role of the inflammatory cytokine cascade in the failing human heart. Curr Heart Fail Rep 5: 69–74.
4. Brockington IF, Olsen EG (1972) Eosinophilia and endomyocardial fibrosis. Postgrad Med J 48: 740–741.
5. Iglezias SD, Benvenuti LA, Calabrese F, Salemi VM, Silva AM, et al. (2008) Endomyocardial fibrosis: pathological and molecular findings of surgically resected ventricular endomyocardium. Virchows Arch 453: 233–241.
6. Torre-Amione G, Kapadia S, Benedict C, Oral H, Young JB, et al. (1996) Proinflammatory cytokine levels in patients with depressed left ventricular ejection fraction: a report from the Studies of Left ventricular Dysfunction (SOLVD). J Am Coll Cardiol 27: 1201–1206.
7. Mocelin AO, Issa VS, Bacal F, Guimarães GV, Cunha E, et al. (2005) The influence of aetiology on inflammatory and neurohumoral activation in patients with severe heart failure: a prospective study comparing Chagas' heart disease and idiopathic dilated cardiomyopathy. Eur J Heart Fail 7: 869–73.
8. Ferreira RC, Ianni BM, Abel LC, Buck P, Mady C, et al. (2003) Increased plasma levels of tumor necrosis factor-alpha in asymptomatic/"indeterminate" and Chagas disease cardiomyopathy patients. Mem Inst Oswaldo Cruz 98: 407–11.
9. Rauchhaus M, Doehner W, Francis DP, Davos C, Kemp M, et al. (2000) Plasma cytokine parameters and mortality in patients with chronic heart failure. Circulation 102: 3060–3067.
10. Oru's J, Roig E, Perez-Villa F, Paré C, Azqueta M, et al. (2000) Prognostic value of serum cytokines in patients with congestive heart failure. J Heart LungTransplant 19: 419–425.
11. Haudek SB, Taffet GE, Schneider MD, Mann DL (2007) TNF provokes cardiomyocyte apoptosis and cardiac remodeling through activation of multiple cell death pathways. J Clin Invest 117: 2692–2701.
12. MacDonald AS, Araujo MI, Pearce EJ (2002) Immunology of parasitic helminth infections. Infect Immun 70: 427–33.
13. Sato Y, Takatsu Y, Kataoka K, Yamada T, Taniguchi R, et al. (1999) Serial circulating concentrations of C-reactive protein, interleukin (IL)-4, and IL-6 in patients with acute left heart decompensation. Clin Cardiol 22: 811–3.
14. Amir O, Rogowski O, David M, Lahat N, Wolff R, et al. (2010) Circulating interleukin-10: association with higher mortality in systolic heart failure patients with elevated tumor necrosis factor-alpha. Isr Med Assoc J 12: 158–162.
15. Sliwa K, Mocumbi AO (2010) Forgotten cardiovascular diseases in Africa. Clin Res Cardiol 99: 65–74.
16. Salemi VM, Leite JJ, Picard MH, Oliveira LM, Reis SF, et al. (2009) Echocardiographic predictors of functional capacity in endomyocardial fibrosis patients. Eur J Echocardiogr 10: 400–405.
17. Salemi VM, Picard MH, Mady C (2004) Assessment of diastolic function in endomyocardial fibrosis: value of flow propagation velocity. Artif Organs 28: 343–346.
18. Salemi VM, Rochitte CE, Shiozaki AA, Andrade JM, Parga JR, et al. (2011) Late gadolinium enhancement magnetic resonance imaging in the diagnosis and prognosis of endomyocardial fibrosis patients. Circ Cardiovasc Imaging 4: 304–311.
19. Anker SD, von Haehling S (2004) Inflammatory mediators in chronic heart failure: an overview. Heart 90: 464–470.
20. Aukrust P, Gullestad L, Ueland T, Damås JK, Yndestad A (2005) Inflammatory and anti-inflammatory cytokines in chronic heart failure: potential therapeutic implications. Ann Med 37: 74–85.
21. Mann DL (2003) Stress-activated cytokines and the heart: from adaptation to maladaptation. Annu Rev Physiol 65: 81–101.
22. Mehra VC, Ramgolam VS, Bender JR (2005) Cytokines and cardiovascular disease. J Leukoc Biol 78: 805–818.
23. Muller-Werdan U, Engelmann H, Werdan K (1998) Cardiodepression by tumor necrosis factor-alpha. Eur Cytokine Netw 9: 689–691.
24. Sato Y, Takatsu Y, Kataoka K, Yamada T, Taniguchi R, et al. (1999) Serial circulating concentrations of C-reactive protein, interleukin (IL)-4, and IL-6 in patients with acute left heart decompensation. Clin Cardiol 22: 811–813.
25. Gage JR, Fonarow G, Hamilton M, Widawski M, Martínez-Maza O, et al. (2004) Beta blocker and angiotensin-converting enzyme inhibitor therapy is associated with decreased Th1/Th2 cytokine ratios and inflammatory cytokine production in patients with chronic heart failure. Neuroimmunomodulation.11: 173–180.
26. Guinjoan SM, Vigo DE, Castro MN, Tateosian N, Chuluyan E, et al. (2009) Mood, Th-1/Th-2 cytokine profile, and autonomic activity in older adults with acute/decompensated heart failure: preliminary observations. World J Biol Psychiatry 10: 913–918.

27. Yu L, Sun X, Yang F, Yang J, Shen J, et al. (2012) Inflammatory cytokines IFN-γ, IL-4, IL-13 and TNF-α alterations in schistosomiasis: a meta-analysis. Parasitol Res 110: 1547–52.
28. Ive FA, Willis AJ, Ikeme AC, Brockington IF (1967) Endomyocardial fibrosis and filariasis. Q J Med 36: 495–516.
29. Andy JJ, Ogunowo PO, Akpan NA, Odigwe CO, Ekanem IA, et al. (1988) Helminth associated hypereosinophilia and tropical endomyocardial fibrosis (EMF) in Nigeria. Acta Trop 69: 127–140.
30. Schopf LR, Hoffmann KF, Cheever AW, Urban JF, Wynn TA (2002) IL-10 is critical for host resistance and survival during gastrointestinal helminth infection. J Immunol. 168: 2383–2392.
31. Yamaoka M, Yamaguchi S, Okuyama M, Tomoike H (1999) Anti-inflammatory cytokine profile in human heart failure: behavior of interleukin-10 in association with tumor necrosis factor-alpha. Jpn Circ J 63: 951–956.
32. Sun L, Louie MC, Vannella KM, Wilke CA, LeVine AM, et al. (2011) New concepts of IL-10-induced lung fibrosis: fibrocyte recruitment and M2 activation in a CCL2/CCR2 axis. Am J Physiol Lung Cell Mol Physiol. 300(3):L341–53.
33. Patel AK, D'Arbela PG, Somers K (1977) Endomyocardial fibrosis and eosinophilia. Br Heart JMar 39: 238–241.

11

Action Potential-Evoked Calcium Release Is Impaired in Single Skeletal Muscle Fibers from Heart Failure Patients

Marino DiFranco[1], Marbella Quiñonez[1], Perry Shieh[2], Gregg C. Fonarow[3], Daniel Cruz[3], Mario C. Deng[3], Julio L. Vergara[1], Holly R. Middlekauff[1,3]*

1 Department of Physiology, David Geffen School of Medicine, University of California Los Angeles, Los Angeles, California, United States of America, **2** Department of Neurology, David Geffen School of Medicine, University of California Los Angeles, Los Angeles, California, United States of America, **3** Division of Cardiology, Department of Medicine, David Geffen School of Medicine, University of California Los Angeles, Los Angeles, California, United States of America

Abstract

Background: Exercise intolerance in chronic heart failure (HF) has been attributed to abnormalities of the skeletal muscles. Muscle function depends on intact excitation-contraction coupling (ECC), but ECC studies in HF models have been inconclusive, due to deficiencies in the animal models and tools used to measure calcium (Ca^{2+}) release, mandating investigations in skeletal muscle from HF patients. The purpose of this study was to test the hypothesis that Ca^{2+} release is significantly impaired in the skeletal muscle of HF patients in whom exercise capacity is severely diminished compared to age-matched healthy volunteers.

Methods and Findings: Using state-of-the-art electrophysiological and optical techniques in single muscle fibers from biopsies of the locomotive *vastus lateralis* muscle, we measured the action potential (AP)-evoked Ca^{2+} release in 4 HF patients and 4 age-matched healthy controls. The mean peak Ca^{2+} release flux in fibers obtained from HF patients (10 ± 1.2 μM/ms) was markedly (2.6-fold) and significantly ($p<0.05$) smaller than in fibers from healthy volunteers (28 ± 3.3 μM/ms). This impairment in AP-evoked Ca^{2+} release was ubiquitous and was not explained by differences in the excitability mechanisms since single APs were indistinguishable between HF patients and healthy volunteers.

Conclusions: These findings prove the feasibility of performing electrophysiological experiments in single fibers from human skeletal muscle, and offer a new approach for investigations of myopathies due to HF and other diseases. Importantly, we have demonstrated that one step in the ECC process, AP-evoked Ca^{2+} release, is impaired in single muscle fibers in HF patients.

Editor: Nicole Beard, University of Canberra, Australia

Funding: Research reported in this publication was supported by the National Institute of Arthritis and Musculoskeletal and Skin Diseases of the National Institutes of Health under award numbers AR047664, AR54816, and AR041802; the Clinical and Translational Science Institute Grant #UL1TR000124; and funds from the UCLA Department of Medicine and Dean's Office. The funders had no role in study design, data collection and analysis, decision to publish, or preparation of the manuscript.

Competing Interests: The authors have declared that no competing interests exist.

* Email: hmiddlekauff@mednet.ucla.edu

Introduction

Chronic heart failure (HF) patients with systolic dysfunction have benefited from advances in pharmacological and device therapies that have reduced mortality [1]. Nonetheless, residual poor exercise tolerance characterized by skeletal muscle weakness and early fatigue contribute to ongoing suffering and morbidity, leading to 3.5 million hospitalizations per year, 11 million outpatient doctor visits/year, and skyrocketing medical costs [2]. It is a fact that a large proportion of HF patients would trade increased length of life for increased quality of life [3], which in HF patients is directly linked to exercise capacity [4]. Surprisingly, exercise dysfunction in HF patients is not directly related to severity of left ventricular dysfunction, intra-cardiac hemodynamics at rest or during exercise, or inadequate skeletal muscle blood flow [5–8]. Instead, exercise dysfunction is directly related to abnormalities of the skeletal muscles themselves; in fact a skeletal myopathy has been described which includes a fiber shift from type I aerobic fibers to type II anaerobic fibers and decreased mitochondrial volume and metabolic function [8–11].

Skeletal muscle function depends critically on both intact energy metabolism and on the robustness of the sequence of events linking the electrical with the mechanical activation of the muscle fibers (the so-called excitation-contraction coupling [ECC] process). The role of metabolic deficiencies in skeletal muscle function in HF patients on optimal medical therapy has recently been questioned [12–14]. We have recently reported marked abnormalities of several key proteins participating in the ECC process in humans with HF [15]; however, it remains unknown whether these abnormalities in protein content are accompanied by functional abnormalities in calcium (Ca^{2+}) cycling in humans with HF. The integrity of important steps in the ECC chain of events, such as the Ca^{2+} release from the sarcoplasmic reticulum (SR), is a decisive factor for normal exercise ability; ECC impairments are expected to critically contribute to muscle weakness and poor exercise tolerance [8,14–16].

Animal models of HF have been used to investigate ECC abnormalities that may recapitulate the skeletal myopathy seen in HF patients [17–22]. However, these animal studies have intrinsic limitations in that they provide inconsistent information depending on the HF model and they do not fully reproduce the HF phenotype of decreased exercise tolerance [23]. Furthermore, to date, tools capable of measuring the rapid physiological Ca^{2+} release in skeletal muscle fibers have not been utilized in animal models. Altogether, the findings from animal studies are inconclusive and contradictory [18–22]. We chose to bypass the animal models and procure biopsies of the *vastus lateralis* (VL) muscles directly from HF patients and healthy age-matched volunteers, and used state-of-the-art electrophysiological and optical techniques to test our hypothesis that the ECC process is significantly impaired in the locomotive skeletal muscle of HF patients compared to healthy volunteers. Our approach puts special emphasis on the fibers' ability to generate Ca^{2+} transients in response to action potential (AP) stimulation and, by using low affinity Ca^{2+} indicators in conjunction with high internal EGTA concentrations [17–20], allows for a direct comparison of their physiological robustness.

Methods

Ethics Statement

The study was approved by the University of California Los Angeles (UCLA) Human Subjects Protection Committee, and the participants gave their written informed consent.

Study Population

Advanced HF patients, New York Heart Association Class II–III meeting the following eligibility criteria were recruited from the Ahmanson-UCLA Cardiomyopathy Center: 1) age 21–65 years, 2) Left ventricular ejection fraction <35%, 3) HF duration > 1 year, 4) not involved in a formal exercise training program, 5) on stable, guideline appropriate HF medications, and not taking warfarin or non-warfarin oral anticoagulants. Age and gender-matched healthy, non-smoking controls, without chronic illnesses and taking no daily medications, who drank <2 drinks/day, and who did not participate in regular exercise (30 minutes most days), served as controls.

Skeletal muscle biopsy

The procedure was performed at the UCLA Out-Patient Surgery Center under local anesthesia. An incision was made in the lateral aspect of the thigh, at about 20 cm proximal to the patella, and a sample of vastus lateralis (VL) muscle measuring 40 mm in length, 8 mm in width and 5 mm in depth was obtained. The biopsy was transported to the lab in ice-cold oxygenated Tyrode solution, where it was pinned in a Sylgard bottomed Petri dish containing oxygenated Tyrode solution and divided into 10–12 bundles (~2 mm in diameter), as delimited by the perimysium. Bundle pulling was kept at a minimum at all times during dissection. When kept in oxygenated Tyrode solution at room temperature, bundles remained viable for >10 hours. Although not studied systematically, viability was found to be longer the greater the biopsy length. In many cases, bundles 40 mm in length contracted upon stimulation with 10 Hz trains after 1.5 hours from biopsy.

Muscle fiber dissection

A bundle was pinned down at slack length in a dish containing Tyrode, which was subsequently slowly exchanged by relaxing solution (see Solutions). In this solution, fibers became electrically and mechanically inactivated, thus preventing contractures during dissection and increasing the rate of success of intact fiber isolation. A peripheral smaller bundle comprised of ~20 fibers was dissected aside using small Vannas scissors and #5 tweezers. The tissue was divided progressively into smaller bundles until a single fiber of about 20 mm in length was obtained. For this finer dissection, #5 tweezers and retina surgical scissors (gauge 25, Alcon) were used. Fiber stretching was avoided at all times. Only fiber segments crystalline in appearance, devoid of contractured regions, freely flexible, and exhibiting a sharp banding pattern were used for electrophysiological experiments. The degree of difficulty of dissection of fibers from HF biopsies was not significantly different from that of control biopsies.

Fiber mounting and stimulation

Fibers were mounted in an inverted double-gap grease chamber, under stereoscopic microscope observation, as previously described [24,25] but with modifications. Fibers (~8 mm in length) were transferred to the chamber previously flooded with relaxing solution using a heat polished glass capillary connected to a 100 µl pippetor via a Tygon tubing. To avoid adhesion of the fiber to the capillary, it was rinsed in relaxing solution containing 3 mg/ml serum bovine albumin prior to fiber transfer. Using #5 tweezers the fiber was placed across the chamber's gaps, where pre-seals (a shallow layer of grease) had been constructed. Each end of the fiber was secured to the coverslip at the chamber's lateral compartments with grease, and straightened and stretched by ~ 40–50% the slack length by gently pulling the ends embedded in grease. The grease seals were then constructed at the chamber's gaps (Figure 1 in [24]), and the excess solution was removed to render each of the 3 compartments electrically independent. The central pool of the experimental chamber was 300±45 µm (n = 25). The segments of the fiber at the lateral compartments were permeabilized with saponine (10 µg/ml in internal solution, 30 sec). After washing out saponine, internal solution containing the Ca^{2+} sensor was added to the lateral compartments. Finally, the chamber was placed on the stage of the microscope and connected to the perfusion system and the electrical amplifier. Fibers requiring more than −70 nA to be repolarized to −90 mV were discarded. Recordings were started 15–20 min after adding the Ca^{2+} sensor to the lateral pools. The circuit used to stimulate the fibers and to record the membrane potential and currents has been previously described [25]. One cut end of the fiber was connected to a current source, the other was connected to a high impedance amplifier, and the central segment of the fiber was held at virtual ground. APs were elicited by current pulses (0.2 ms, 10–15% above threshold) applied at one cut end. Membrane potential was measured as the difference between the potential at the other cut end (i.e. the myoplasm) and the central pool (i.e. the extracellular milieu).

Ca^{2+} transients

AP evoked Ca^{2+} concentration changes were measured using the low affinity dye OregonGreenBapta488-5N (OGB-5N) [26–29]. OGB5N was added to the internal solution bathing both cut ends of the fibers at a final concentration of 250µM. Large concentrations of EGTA semi-saturated with Ca^{2+} were added to the internal solution with two purposes in mind: a) to prevent fiber movements that would distort optical recordings and potentially dislodge the grease seals; and, b) to allow for the calculation of

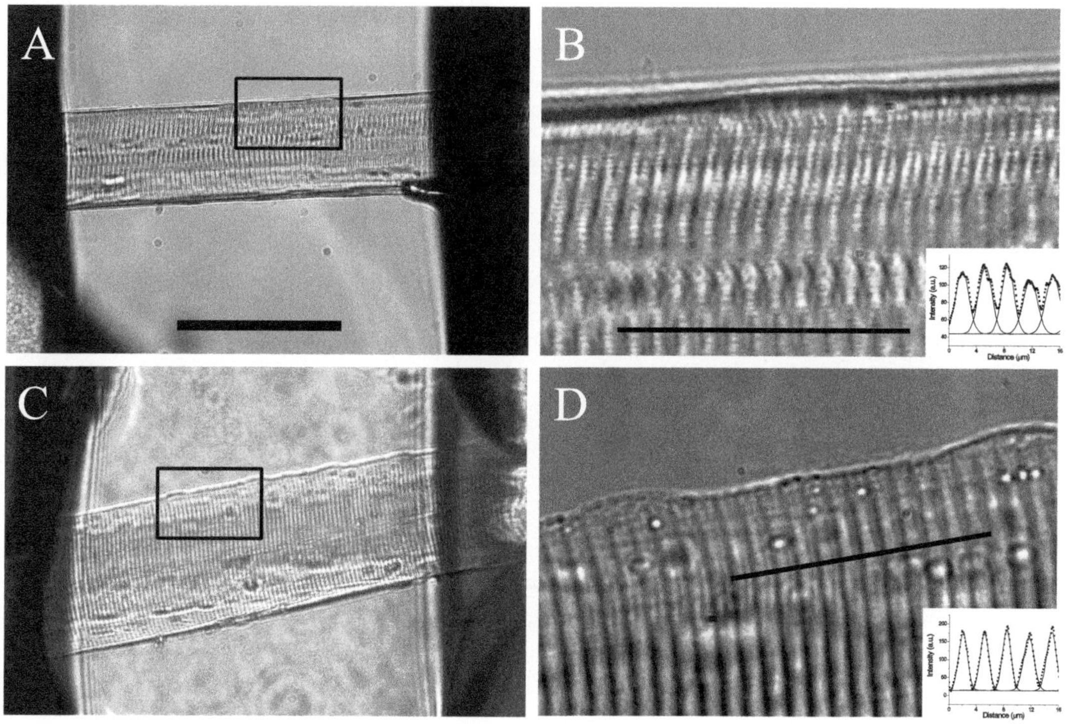

Figure 1. Isolated fibers mounted in the inverted double grease-gap chamber. Panel A: Image of a VL fiber from a healthy volunteer obtained with a 20× objective. The inner part of the grease seals delimiting the experimental pool can be seen at both sides of the image. Panel B: The area delimited by the square in A was imaged with a 100× immersion objective. A sharp banding pattern and smooth border can be seen. Panels C and D shows a VL fiber from a HF patient at the same magnifications as in A and B, respectively. The diameter and sarcomere length were 62.0 and 3.0 µm for the fiber in A, and 80 and 2.8 µm for the fiber in B, respectively. The insets in panels B and D show intensity profiles measured across ~4 sarcomeres. The profiles span ~16 mm along the directions indicated by the lines superimposed in the corresponding images. The dots and lines represent the intensity values and Gaussian fits to the data, respectively. The scale in A corresponds to 100 µm in A and C, and 20 µm in B and D.

peak Ca^{2+} flux from OGB-5N Ca^{2+} transients using a single compartment model that is extensively described elsewhere [27,28,30]. Two mixtures were used: 30:15 and 20:10 EGTA:Ca. The large [EGTA] used are expected to equalize the resting myoplasmic free [Ca] to ~80 nM in all experiments. The Ca^{2+} dependent fluorescence transients (referred to simply as Ca^{2+} transients) are reported as $\Delta F/F$ transients (dimensionless). These transients are used to calculate Ca^{2+} flux transients (µM/ms).

The optical setup was similar to that described elsewhere [28,29]. Briefly, it consisted of an inverted microscope (Olympus IX71) equipped with a standard epifluorescence attachment, a 480-40/510/540-30 nm cube combination, and a 100× 1.4 NA oil immersion objective. The light was focused to a spot with a diameter similar to that of fibers (40–50 µm). In order to reduce stray fluorescence from the grease, the illumination spot was place at the center of the experimental pool. To remove contributions from stray fluorescence to the OGB5N fluorescence, the fluorescence from areas outside the fiber was recorded and subtracted from every Ca^{2+} transient before calculating $\Delta F/F$ transients.

Solutions

The composition of solutions (mM) was:

Tyrode: 150 NaCl, 4KCl, $1MgCl_2$, $2CaCl_2$, 10 glucose, 10 MOPS.

Relaxing solution: 120 K_2SO_4, 10 MOPS, 1 $MgCl_2$, 1 $CaCl_2$, 10 glucose.

Internal solution: 92 K-Aspartate, 20 MOPS, 1 $MgCl_2$, 5 reduced Glutathione, 5 ATP-TRIS, 5 Creatine Phosphate-Na_2, 20 EGTA, 10 $Ca(OH)_2$.

All solutions were adjusted to ph = 7.4 and had 300±5 mOsmol/kg H_2O.

Signal conditioning and statistical analysis

Voltage, current and optical signals were filtered at 10, 5 and 2 kHz (8 pole low-pass-filter; Frequency Devices), respectively, and acquired at 10µs/point. Optical and electrical data from control and HF fibers were compared using the Student's t test. Significance was set at $p<0.05$.

Results

Study population characteristics

Four HF patients at an advanced stage, and four healthy age-matched human volunteers participated in these studies. The major features of the cohorts are presented in Table 1. Importantly, HF patients and healthy volunteers did not differ in age, sex, or body mass index. In addition, HF patients had severe exercise limitation as measured by peak oxygen consumption of 13.1±1.0 ml/kg/min (compared with that of untrained healthy adult values, always >28 ml/kg/min).

Fibers dissected from VL muscle biopsies of healthy volunteers and HF patients appear similarly intact under the light microscope

In contrast to previous reports in rat muscles [19], we found that dissecting single fibers from VL muscle biopsies was not more cumbersome when they were obtained from HF patients

Table 1. Study Population Characteristics.

	Subjects	
	Heart Failure Patients	**Healthy Volunteers**
Number of Subjects	4	4
Age (years)	57.3±2.1	52.8±2.4
BMI[a] (kg/m^2)	29.2±1.6	30.8±2.9
Female	1	1
Druation of HF (years)	8.5±2.2	
Peak VO$_2$ (ml/kg/min)	13.1±1.0	
LVEF[c](%)	26.0±4.0	
Diabetes mellitus	2	
Hypertension	2	
Etiology of HF		
• CAD[d]	2	
• Idiopathic	2	
• Familial	0	
Medications		
• Beta-blockers	4	
• ACEI[e]	2	
• ARB[f]	1	
• Statin	4	
• Aldosterone antagonist	2	
• Aspirin	3	
• Clopidogrel	0	
• Furosemide	3	
• Digoxin	1	
• Amiodarone	1	

[a]body mass index, [b]peak oxygen consumption, [c]left ventricular ejection fraction, [d]coronary artery disease, [e]angiotensin inhibitor, [f]angiotensin receptor blocker. Values are mean±SEM.

compared to healthy volunteers. Moreover, as illustrated in Figure 1, bright-field images demonstrate that there are no obvious differences in appearance between fibers obtained from healthy volunteers (Figures 1A and B) and HF patients (Figures 1C and D) as they are mounted in the experimental chamber. Specifically, both sets of fibers have comparable diameters. The average diameters (mean±SD) were 75.2±17.2 μm [n = 10; minimum 58.8 μm, maximum = 113.1 μm) for fibers from healthy volunteers, and 75.5±16.4 μm (n = 5; minimum 51.8 μm, maximum = 103.0 μm) for fibers from HF patients. In addition, the fibers exhibited equally sharp sarcomere banding with no indications of contractures or vacuolation suggestive of obvious structural damages. Further, the sets of fibers from HF patients and controls had comparable sarcomere lengths, 3.31±0.34 μm, (range 2.64–3.71 μm) versus 3.21±0.33 μm, (range 2.76–3.69 μm), respectively, confirming that they did not undergo gross contractures. It should be noted that the mean sarcomere length is larger than typical slack sarcomere length (~2.2 μm) because during the mounting process, fibers are slightly stretched (see methods). Even in a more advanced inspection of the structural integrity of the transverse tubular system in live fibers stained with the fluorescence dye di-8-ANEPPS fibers [31], there were no detectable alterations in either set of fibers (see Figure S1).

Fibers dissected from VL muscle biopsies of healthy volunteers and HF patients are comparably healthy in electrical terms

Additional direct evidence for the fibers' intactness was obtained by measuring their spontaneous repolarization after exchanging the high K relaxing solution with Tyrode in the central compartment of the experimental chamber. Isolated fibers from both healthy volunteers and HF patients repolarized spontaneously to a similar membrane potential (−13.6±3.42 mV [n = 8] and −16.5±5.1 mV [n = 10] respectively), and required almost identical holding currents in order to maintain them at a resting potential of −90 mV (−59.2±18.3 nA [n = 8] and −60.8 ±28.5 nA [n = 10] respectively), and V_r changed only slightly throughout the typical 30 min of electrophysiological experimentation. Interestingly, these values are comparable to those previously measured in frog fibers mounted in a similar experimental chamber [24,25], which are known to be resilient to mechanical dissection. We also determined that all fibers responded to pulses of increasing amplitude with a sharp threshold, separating electrotonic from all-or-none responses (i.e. APs). Examples of such responses obtained from a healthy volunteer and a HF patient are shown in Figures 2A and 2B, respectively. When relatively small current pulses (sub-threshold) are applied, similar graded electrotonic responses are elicited in both preparations, which peak at about −50 mV. By increasing the pulse amplitude by 10–15%, comparable all-or-none responses are evoked, which take off from about −40 mV. Threshold potentials were found between these two values. Although the threshold for HF fibers is slightly more depolarized (~3 mV) than healthy fibers, the mean values (±SD) calculated from 10 healthy fibers (−48.3±6.5 mV) and 10 HF fibers (−45.3±4.1 mV) were not significantly different (inset of Figure 2A).

AP-evoked Ca^{2+} release is impaired in isolated fibers from HF patients

Secure that fibers dissected from biopsies of both HF patients and healthy volunteers were equally intact for study in isolation, we proceeded to investigate their respective ability to release Ca^{2+} in response to AP stimulation. A smaller population of fibers was used for this purpose (5 fibers from healthy volunteers and 9 fibers from HF patients). The fibers were allowed to equilibrate with internal solutions containing high [EGTA] and free Ca^{2+} concentration [Ca^{2+}] close to the physiological value ~0.1 μM [26,28]. Figure 3B shows an example of a Ca^{2+} transient recorded in a fiber from a healthy volunteer and equilibrated with internal solution containing 30:15 EGTA:Ca (see Solutions). In response to the AP (Figure 3A), a fast fluorescence transient (Ca^{2+} transient) was elicited that reached a peak ΔF/F of ~0.24. Interestingly, knowing the concentration and Ca^{2+} binding properties of the Ca^{2+} indicator (OGB-5N) and EGTA, we were able to estimate with accuracy the Ca^{2+} release flux (in μM/ms) responsible for this fluorescence transient [26,28–30,32]. The resulting flux record is shown in the inset of Figure 3B; the peak value, representing the maximal rate of Ca^{2+} release, was ~29 μM/ms. In comparison, Ca^{2+} transients recorded from a muscle fiber dissected from a HF patient's VL biopsy under the same conditions as those used for the fiber from the healthy volunteer were ~3-fold smaller amplitude (peak ΔF/F~0.09, Figure 3D). The calculated Ca^{2+} release flux (compare insets of Figures 3B and 3D) was also markedly reduced, ~3-fold (from ~29 to ~10 μM/ms).

This impairment in AP-evoked Ca^{2+} transients was observed in every HF fiber studied, regardless of the EGTA:Ca ratio used to equilibrate control fibers. In order to compare reliably the Ca^{2+} release strength in all fibers studied, we calculated the Ca^{2+} fluxes underlying Ca^{2+} transients recorded at either 30:15 or 20:10 (EGTA:Ca) conditions. As demonstrated in Figure 4A, the mean Ca^{2+} fluxes determined in fibers from healthy volunteers equilibrated with 30:15 (n = 2) and 20:10 (n = 3) EGTA mixtures were comparable to each other. Since the mean flux from fibers was independent of the EGTA:Ca ratio, the data from healthy volunteers was pooled. The results demonstrate that the mean peak Ca^{2+} release flux in fibers obtained from HF patients equilibrated with a 30:15 EGTA:Ca mixture (10±1.2 μM/ms; 4 biopsies, 9 fibers) is substantially (2.6-fold) and significantly ($p < 0.05$) smaller than that in fibers from healthy volunteers (28±3.3 μM/ms; 4 biopsies, 5 fibers). We then compared the frequency distribution of peak Ca^{2+} fluxes from healthy volunteers and HF patients (Figure 4B). The values for AP-evoked Ca^{2+} release fluxes in fibers from healthy volunteers are widely distributed between values as high as ~40 μM/ms to low values of ~18 μM/ms. In contrast, those of fibers from HF patients span a much narrower, left-shifted range of lower values, between ~17 and ~5 μM/ms. AP-evoked Ca^{2+} release fluxes were smaller in all the fibers isolated from HF patients, compared to those from healthy volunteers. Our results demonstrate for the first time that a key step in the ECC process, that is, Ca^{2+} release from the SR, is severely impaired in skeletal muscle fibers of HF patients compared to age-matched healthy volunteers. These findings are consistent with, and expand on, our previous report that the expression of key proteins involved in ECC are reduced in HF fibers [15], to demonstrate that the deficiency in the expression of those proteins has devastating functional implications for HF patients.

Properties of the AP in fibers isolated from biopsies of healthy volunteers and HF patients

Since the AP is the physiological trigger of the ECC process, one potential mechanism underlying the severe reduction in the Ca^{2+} release fluxes observed in fibers from HF patients could be that their AP properties are significantly altered. To our knowledge, there is no published information about the electrical activity of human VL muscle fibers; consequently, we compared the amplitude, full duration at half-maximum (FDHM), time to peak

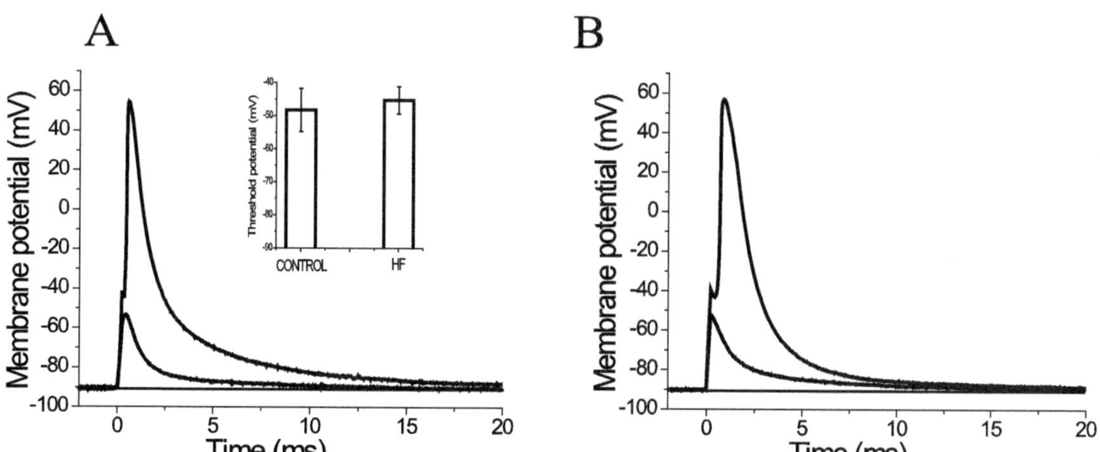

Figure 2. Fibers from healthy volunteers and HF patients have similar thresholds. Panels A and B show electrotonic responses (small depolarizations elicited by sub-threshold current pulses) and actions potentials (large autoregenerative depolarization elicited by suprathreshold current pulses) in a fiber from a healthy volunteer (A) and a HF patient (B). The inset in panel A shows the mean (±SD) threshold potentials for a population of fibers from healthy volunteers (n = 10 fibers) and HF patients (n = 10 fibers).

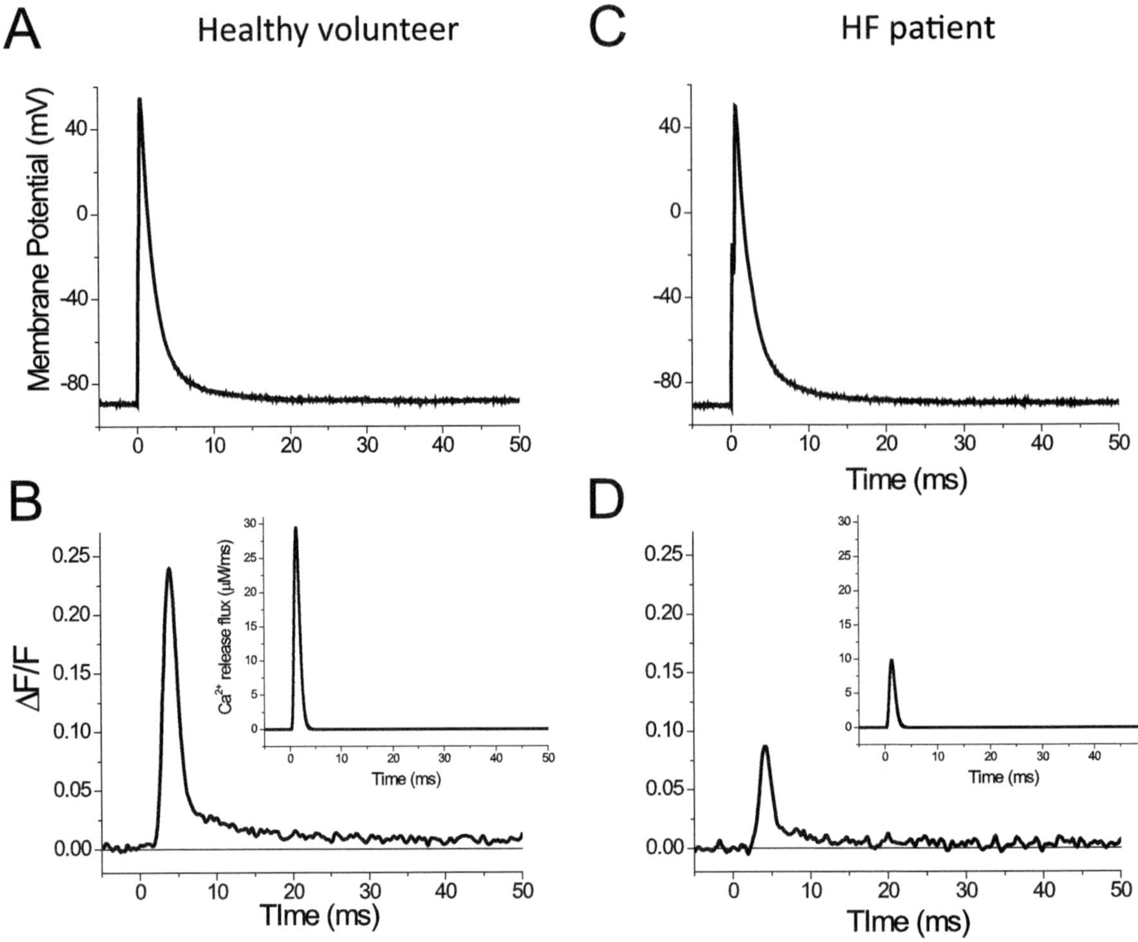

Figure 3. AP evoked Ca^{2+} transients in fibers dissected from a healthy volunteer and a HF patient. Figures A and C are the APs and panels B and D are the corresponding Ca^{2+} transients. The insets in B and D are Ca^{2+} release fluxes (in μM/ms) calculated from the corresponding optical records. The fibers were equilibrated with an internal solution containing 30:15 EGTA:Ca^{2+}.

(TTP), and maximal rate of depolarization ($[dV/dt]_{max}$) of APs recorded in fibers isolated from the skeletal muscle biopsies of HF patients and healthy volunteers (see Table 2). The APs of fibers dissected from biopsies of healthy volunteers and HF patients have almost identical amplitudes and durations. Since the resting potential was kept at −90 mV in both groups of fibers, their APs have similar overshoots (to ~+54 mV). Interestingly, the maximum depolarization rate was significantly faster in fibers from HF patients compared to healthy volunteers ($p<0.05$). Potential implications of this faster depolarization will be addressed in the Discussion.

Discussion

Using state-of-the-art electrophysiological and optical techniques, we have performed studies in single fibers procured from the *vastus lateralis* muscle of advanced HF patients and healthy volunteers, and have demonstrated for the first time that one critical step of the ECC process, specifically, the AP-evoked Ca^{2+} release, is impaired in this locomotive muscle of HF patients. As will be discussed in detail below, these findings are transformative because: 1) they circumvent the inherent limitations of studying ECC in models of HF by utilizing actual tissue obtained directly from patients afflicted with the HF condition; 2) they confirm the feasibility of performing electrophysiological experiments characterizing individual steps of the ECC process in single fibers from human skeletal muscle according to fiber type; and critically, 3) they offer new approaches to investigate other myopathic conditions that may also involve impairments in the ECC process, such as chronic obstructive pulmonary disease and chronic renal disease [33,34].

Inherent limitations in animal models and the need for human studies

Animal models of HF, including the infarct model and the sympathetic hyperactivity-induced model, are critical to our further investigations and improved understanding of human diseases, but have inherent limitations [17–23]. In the rat infarct model, the left coronary artery is ligated, which results in infarction of ~35% of cardiac tissue and elevated left ventricular end-diastolic pressures, mimicking human HF. However, despite significant cardiac damage and dysfunction, HF rats demonstrate no decline in locomotive activity when quantified by the photocell activation technique [23]. That is, the phenotypic expression of decreased exercise tolerance and early fatigue is absent in this model, thereby raising the question of its validity to study exercise dysfunction in patients with HF who suffer from profound exercise limitation. The sympathetic hyperactivity-induced HF model is a

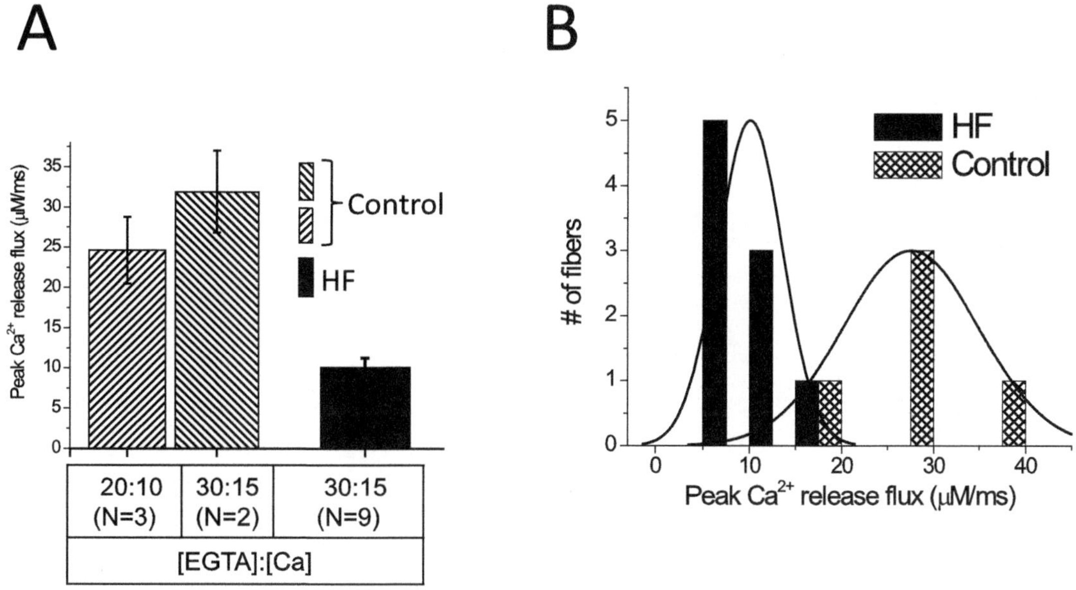

Figure 4. Average values and frequency distribution of peak Ca^{2+} release flux values in fibers from healthy volunteers and HF patients. Panel A shows the mean (±SD) of peak Ca^{2+} flux in fibers of healthy volunteers (hatched) and of HF patients (black) equilibrated with internal solution containing either 30:15 or 20:10 EGTA:Ca. Panel B shows the frequency distribution of peak Ca^{2+} release fluxes from all fibers in panel A. The binning width was 2.5 µM/ms and the lines correspond to fits of the data to standard normal distributions.

congenic α_{2A}/α_{2C} adrenoceptor knockout mouse that leads to sympathetic hyperactivity-induced HF and quantified exercise dysfunction [18]. However, since α_{2A}/α_{2C} adrenoceptors are absent in all tissues, including the skeletal muscle, it is difficult to know whether muscle changes are due to HF, or to the genetic modification. In fact, in this model, the sympathetic hyperactivity leads to early skeletal muscle changes attributable to relatively increased β_2-adrenoceptor activity [17]. These limitations, as well as species' variations in Ca^{2+} cycling proteins and muscle fiber type composition, generally confound data interpretation and detract from these models. As noted earlier, some [18,19,21,35], but not all studies in animal models [20], have uncovered definite, but variable, abnormalities in the ECC process. These intriguing findings in imperfect animal models mandate further investigations in skeletal muscle from HF patients.

Physiological Ca^{2+} release in normal human skeletal fibers

To our knowledge there are no previous studies of the Ca^{2+} release evoked by AP stimulation in human skeletal muscle fibers in health or disease. Two reports of the Ca^{2+} release flux in healthy human fibers performed under voltage-clamp conditions have been published [36,37]. Interestingly, though it would be expected that under these conditions maximal Ca^{2+} fluxes would be recorded, the values calculated in these reports were significantly smaller than ours, by a factor of at least 2-fold. Differences in the fibers' integrity, the use of Ca^{2+} sensors, and calculation methodologies may partially explain these differences. In one study, percutaneous needle biopsies were obtained, yielding only short muscle segments [36]. It is possible that the short length of these fibers adversely affected their functional performance; in our experience electrophysiological integrity of the fibers increases with increasing biopsy length. In the other study [37], a very low

Table 2. Properties of action potentials recorded in fibers from healthy volunteers and HF patients.

	Subjects	
	Heart Failure Patients	**Healthy Volunteers**
Number of Subjects	4	4
Number of fibers	10	10
AP amplitude (mV)	143.5±3.2	144.1±3.9
FDHM[a] (ms)	2.19±0.16	2.18±0.16
TTP[b] (ms)	0.68±0.16	0.62±0.09
dV/dt (m/s)	791.3±83.0*	647.5±57.7*
Threshold (mV)	−45.3±4.1	−48.3±6.5

For all fibers, the resting potential was maintained at −90 mV. [a]Full-duration-at-half-maximum, [b]time to peak. Values given as Mean±SEM. * HF vs healthy volunteer, $p<0.05$.

rate of success per biopsy was reported, again raising the question of the fibers' integrity. In general, the recording of normal electrical activity and larger Ca^{2+} release fluxes suggests that our fibers were possibly in better physiological condition throughout the experimentation.

Reduced Ca^{2+} release in fibers from HF patients

The most important and novel finding in our study is that the ECC process, specifically AP-evoked Ca^{2+} release, is impaired in fibers from the VL muscle of HF patients compared to those of healthy volunteers. We have previously reported a reduced expression of sarcoplasmic reticulum Ca^{2+}-ATPase (SERCA2a) and dihydropyridine receptor (DHPR) in homogenates of VL muscle from HF patients compared to healthy volunteers, whereas SERCA1a and ryanodine receptor (RyR1) levels were not different [15]. The simplest predictions from those biochemical data would be that SR Ca^{2+} content is reduced in fibers from HF patients compared to those from healthy volunteers, and/or that there are orphaned RyR1s. Either alteration could result in a significant reduction of Ca^{2+} fluxes potentially leading to reduced exercise performance and increased fatigability characteristic of HF patients. Diminished peak Ca^{2+} release was present in response to single APs; a finding that would be expected to result in smaller peak twitch and tetanic tension (i.e. muscle weakness and premature fatigability). Further investigations are necessary to identify the exact step(s) in the ECC process that lead to this marked impairment in AP-evoked Ca^{2+} release in HF patients. Comparisons of the physiological trigger for Ca^{2+} release (the AP which initiates the ECC process) in healthy volunteers and HF patients were performed and essentially eliminated this as a potential cause (see discussion below).

Electrical activity

The amplitude and duration of the transverse tubular system depolarization are key factors in determining the features of Ca^{2+} release. Our measurements demonstrate that the Ca^{2+} release in fibers from HF patients are triggered by unaltered APs. The constancy and similarity of AP amplitude in fibers from both healthy volunteers and HF patients is remarkable; since the "resting" potential is kept close to -90 mV in both fiber groups, this result implies that the AP overshoot was also similar between (i.e. circa +54 mV).

The maximum depolarization rates of the AP in control and HF fibers are similar to that found in frog fibers using a similar method [24]; nevertheless, we found that the rate of depolarization is larger in HF fibers. There may be a number of physiological reasons for this difference, including differences in ionic channel endowment. It has been recently reported that the expression of the adult isoform of the Na^{+} channels (NaV1.4) is significantly increased in *soleus muscles* of rat models of muscle disuse, a condition to which HF patients may be prone [38,39]. In fact, an important controversy in the HF literature is whether the skeletal myopathy in HF stems from simple disuse or from the HF condition characterized by neurohumoral activation and inflammation [39]. The increased expression of NaV1.4 might partially explain why paradoxically the weaker fibers of HF patients are electrically more rapid than those of healthy volunteers, lending support to the disuse position. Other possibilities, such as differences in specific capacitance, and/or fine geometry of the transverse tubular system (diameter and luminal resistance of the tubules) may also explain our findings, thus warranting further investigations on this topic.

Ca^{2+} release results may be ubiquitous

Both the kinetics and magnitude of the Ca^{2+} transients have been reported to differ between fast and slow muscle fibers, and to correlate with the myosin heavy chain (MHC) type expressed; specifically, Ca^{2+} release rates are larger in type II than in type I fibers [40]. Exercise fatigue in HF patients has been suggested to result from fiber type transformation [10,13,41]; arguably, a decreased proportion of slow, aerobic, type I fibers with respect to the number of fast, anaerobic, fatigable, type IIx fibers in the locomotion muscles, such as the VL, might explain the fatigability phenotype. However, an increased proportion of type II fibers in which the ECC process is intact in HF patients would be expected to produce more powerful and quicker muscles; of course, this not the case. In our prior report in HF patients [15], we confirmed the previously reported fiber type shift [10,13,41]. We also reported the novel finding that SERCA2a and DHPR protein levels were decreased in homogenates of VL muscle in HF patients compared to healthy volunteers, whereas SERCA1a and ryanodine receptor (RyR1) levels were not different. Although the observed fiber shift could explain the decrease in SERCA2a, which is present only in type I fibers, it cannot explain either the decrease in DHPR level, since DHPR/RyR1 density is greater in type II than type I fibers in rodents [42,43], or the constancy of the SERCA1a and RyR content.

Interestingly, we found a narrow, left-shifted distribution of peak Ca^{2+} fluxes in HF patients, without overlap with the peak Ca^{2+} fluxes in healthy volunteers, consistent with a ubiquitous abnormality affecting the ECC process in every fiber type (I and II) of VL muscles. In other words, the level of Ca^{2+} release from HF fibers with the greatest Ca^{2+} flux, (presumably type II fibers, also expected in larger proportions in the biopsies of HF patients), was even lower than the level of Ca^{2+} release from healthy fibers with the lowest Ca^{2+} flux, presumably type I fibers. A simple fiber-type shift (i.e. from type I to type II) should have resulted in an overall right-shifted distribution of HF fibers, not seen in Figure 4B; that is, a fiber shift would have been expected to produce a larger proportion of the HF fiber population displaying larger Ca^{2+} release.

In summary, our results strongly support the hypothesis that fibers from HF patients have marked and ubiquitous impairments in ECC, specifically AP-evoked Ca^{2+} release that affects all the fibers, independent of their type, in VL muscles.

Limitations

The use of humans, in place of animals, for investigation, has its own limitations, which we acknowledge here: First, patients are on medications including statins, which, for ethical reasons, cannot be interrupted, and these medications may have systemic effects. Nonetheless, it is well established that despite optimal medical therapy HF patients have severe exercise limitations. We would argue that it is precisely these individuals who need to be studied, since despite the best medical therapy, their exercise capacity continues to be impaired. It is worth noting that no patient was diagnosed with a statin myopathy. Secondly, patients have diverse etiologies of HF, however, the severity of exercise dysfunction, and the characteristics of the skeletal myopathy, including the fiber type transformation, are known to be independent of the specific etiology of the HF [44,45]. Finally, since the experiments in fibers from both HF patients and healthy volunteers were performed at room temperature, the absolute values of the Ca^{2+} release fluxes reported here are possibly smaller than those that could be obtained at normal body temperatures. Though future experimentation will take this into account, the observed impairments in Ca^{2+} release of fibers from HF patients are likely to represent a general limitation rather than an experimental peculiarity linked to the choice of temperature.

Conclusion

We report for the first time in single fibers from HF patients compared to healthy volunteers, that AP-evoked Ca^{2+} release is significantly diminished in fibers obtained from the locomotive VL muscle in HF patients. This diminished Ca^{2+} release is not attributable to significant alterations in the AP of fibers from HF patients compared to fibers from healthy volunteers, since the electrical activity in both groups is virtually identical. Our previous findings of diminished DHPR and SERCA2 expression are suggestive of decreased SR Ca^{2+} content, and/or orphaned RyR1; the relative contributions of these abnormalities and others in the ECC process await further investigation. This decrease in Ca^{2+} flux was present in every fiber tested, consistent with a ubiquitous abnormality involving the ECC process in every fiber type in the VL muscle of HF patients, and unlikely to be attributable to a simple fiber type shift. Finally, using this approach, Ca^{2+} fluxes in individual fibers can be compared between muscles of locomotion, vulnerable to disuse, and compared to fibers in non-locomotive muscles, such as the deltoid, to assess if abnormalities of the ECC process are a systemic problem, attributable to systemic neurohumoral activation and inflammation, or a localized problem, more easily explained by disuse. The impact of exercise training on the impairment of ECC and Ca^{2+} release has widespread clinical relevance, both in understanding the role of disuse in this impairment, as well as an important therapeutic approach, and warrants further study.

Supporting Information

Figure S1 The transverse tubular system in live fibers from control and HF individuals. Muscle bundles dissected from biopsies obtained from control individuals (A) and HF patients (B) were stretched to a sarcomere length similar to that in the electrophysiological experiments and pinned down on a Sylgard bottomed dish. The fibers were stained with di-8-ANEPPS and imaged using a two-photon laser scanning microscope (Biorad Radiance 2000). The dye was excited with a 920 nm laser beam, and the emission was collected using a dichroic/band-pass combination of 506 nm/620–650 nm. It can be seen in the optical section in A that, as previously described for other mammalian fibers, di-8-ANEPPS clearly demonstrate the regular double row pattern of the transverse tubular system. The surface membrane can also be seen at the right upper part of the image. The image in B demonstrate that the transverse tubular system of fibers from HF patients is indistinguishable from that of control fibers. The scale represent 15 μm in both images.

Acknowledgments

We thank Dr. Thomas O'Dell (Department of Physiology, UCLA) for the use of his chemiluminescence detection instrument, and Mr. R. Serrano (Staff Research Assistant, Department of Physiology, UCLA) for technical support during the course of the experimentation. We are especially grateful to the generous HF patients of the Ahmanson-UCLA Cardiomyopathy Center, without whom this research would not be possible.

Author Contributions

Conceived and designed the experiments: HRM JLV MD MQ. Performed the experiments: MD MQ. Analyzed the data: HRM MD JLV MQ. Contributed reagents/materials/analysis tools: HRM GCF DC MCD MD MQ JLV PS. Wrote the paper: HRM MD GCF DC MCD JLV MQ PS.

References

1. Yancy CW, Jessup M, Bozkurt B, Butler J, Casey DE Jr, et al. (2013) 2013 ACCF/AHA Guideline for the Management of Heart Failure: Executive Summary: A Report of the American College of Cardiology Foundation/ American Heart Association Task Force on Practice Guidelines. Circulation 128: 1810–1852.
2. Go AS, Mozaffarian D, Roger VL, Benjamin EJ, Berry JD, et al. (2013) Heart disease and stroke statistics–2013 update: a report from the American Heart Association. Circulation 127: e6–e245.
3. Stevenson LW, Hellkamp AS, Leier CV, Sopko G, Koelling T, et al. (2008) Changing preferences for survival after hospitalization with advanced heart failure. J Am Coll Cardiol 52: 1702–1708.
4. Dracup K, Walden JA, Stevenson LW, Brecht ML (1992) Quality of life in patients with advanced heart failure. J Heart Lung Transplant 11: 273–279.
5. Franciosa JA, Park M, Barry Levine T (1981) Lack of correlation between exercise capacity and indexes of resting left ventricular performance in heart failure. The American Journal of Cardiology 47: 33–39.
6. Higginbotham MB, Morris KG, Conn EH, Coleman RE, Cobb FR (1983) Determinants of variable exercise performance among patients with severe left ventricular dysfunction. The American Journal of Cardiology 51: 52–60.
7. Maskin CS, Forman R, Sonnenblick EH, Frishman WH, LeJemtel TH (1983) Failure of dobutamine to increase exercise capacity despite hemodynamic improvement in severe chronic heart failure. The American Journal of Cardiology 51: 177–182.
8. Middlekauff HR (2010) Making the Case for Skeletal Myopathy as the Major Limitation of Exercise Capacity in Heart Failure. Circulation: Heart Failure 3: 537–546.
9. Drexler H, Riede U, Munzel T, Konig H, Funke E, et al. (1992) Alterations of skeletal muscle in chronic heart failure. Circulation 85: 1751–1759.
10. Sullivan MJ, Green HJ, Cobb FR (1990) Skeletal muscle biochemistry and histology in ambulatory patients with long-term heart failure. Circulation 81: 518–527.
11. Wilson JR, Rayos G, Yeoh TK, Gothard P (1995) Dissociation between peak exercise oxygen consumption and hemodynamic dysfunction in potential heart transplant candidates. J Am Coll Cardiol 26: 429–435.
12. Mettauer B, Zoll J, Sanchez H, Lampert E, Ribera F, et al. (2001) Oxidative capacity of skeletal muscle in heart failure patients versus sedentary or active control subjects. Journal of the American College of Cardiology 38: 947–954.
13. Williams AD, Selig S, Hare DL, Hayes A, Krum H, et al. (2004) Reduced exercise tolerance in CHF may be related to factors other than impaired skeletal muscle oxidative capacity. J Card Fail 10: 141–148.
14. Middlekauff HR, Verity MA, Horwich TB, Fonarow GC, Hamilton MA, et al. (2013) Intact skeletal muscle mitochondrial enzyme activity but diminished exercise capacity in advanced heart failure patients on optimal medical and device therapy. Clin Res Cardiol 102: 547–554.
15. Middlekauff HR, Vigna C, Verity MA, Fonarow GC, Horwich TB, et al. (2012) Abnormalities of calcium handling proteins in skeletal muscle mirror those of the heart in humans with heart failure: a shared mechanism? J Card Fail 18: 724–733.
16. Rullman E, Andersson DC, Melin M, Reiken S, Mancini DM, et al. (2013) Modifications of skeletal muscle ryanodine receptor type 1 and exercise intolerance in heart failure. J Heart Lung Transplant 32: 925–929.
17. Bacurau AV, Jardim MA, Ferreira JC, Bechara LR, Bueno CR Jr, et al. (2009) Sympathetic hyperactivity differentially affects skeletal muscle mass in developing heart failure: role of exercise training. J Appl Physiol (1985) 106: 1631–1640.
18. Bueno CR Jr, Ferreira JC, Pereira MG, Bacurau AV, Brum PC (2010) Aerobic exercise training improves skeletal muscle function and Ca2+ handling-related protein expression in sympathetic hyperactivity-induced heart failure. J Appl Physiol (1985) 109: 702–709.
19. Lunde PK, Dahlstedt AJ, Bruton JD, Lannergren J, Thoren P, et al. (2001) Contraction and intracellular Ca(2+) handling in isolated skeletal muscle of rats with congestive heart failure. Circ Res 88: 1299–1305.
20. Lunde PK, Sejersted OM, Thorud HM, Tonnessen T, Henriksen UL, et al. (2006) Effects of congestive heart failure on Ca2+ handling in skeletal muscle during fatigue. Circ Res 98: 1514–1519.
21. Perreault CL, Gonzalez-Serratos H, Litwin SE, Sun X, Franzini-Armstrong C, et al. (1993) Alterations in contractility and intracellular Ca2+ transients in isolated bundles of skeletal muscle fibers from rats with chronic heart failure. Circ Res 73: 405–412.

22. Shah KR, Ganguly PK, Netticadan T, Arneja AS, Dhalla NS (2004) Changes in skeletal muscle SR Ca2+ pump in congestive heart failure due to myocardial infarction are prevented by angiotensin II blockade. Can J Physiol Pharmacol 82: 438–447.
23. Simonini A, Long CS, Dudley GA, Yue P, McElhinny J, et al. (1996) Heart failure in rats causes changes in skeletal muscle morphology and gene expression that are not explained by reduced activity. Circ Res 79: 128–136.
24. DiFranco M, Quinonez M, DiGregorio DA, Kim AM, Pacheco R, et al. (1999) Inverted double-gap isolation chamber for high-resolution calcium fluorimetry in skeletal muscle fibers. Pflugers Arch 438: 412–418.
25. Quinonez M, DiFranco M (2000) Novel inverted triple grease-gap isolation chamber for electrophysiological and calcium release studies in skeletal muscle fibers. Jpn J Physiol 50: 457–462.
26. Woods CE, Novo D, DiFranco M, Capote J, Vergara JL (2005) Propagation in the transverse tubular system and voltage dependence of calcium release in normal and mdx mouse muscle fibres. J Physiol 568: 867–880.
27. Woods CE, Novo D, DiFranco M, Vergara JL (2004) The action potential-evoked sarcoplasmic reticulum calcium release is impaired in mdx mouse muscle fibres. J Physiol 557: 59–75.
28. Capote J, DiFranco M, Vergara JL (2010) Excitation-contraction coupling alterations in mdx and utrophin/dystrophin double knockout mice: a comparative study. Am J Physiol Cell Physiol 298: C1077–1086.
29. DiFranco M, Woods CE, Capote J, Vergara JL (2008) Dystrophic skeletal muscle fibers display alterations at the level of calcium microdomains. Proc Natl Acad Sci U S A 105: 14698–14703.
30. Song LS, Sham JS, Stern MD, Lakatta EG, Cheng H (1998) Direct measurement of SR release flux by tracking 'Ca2+ spikes' in rat cardiac myocytes. J Physiol 512 (Pt 3): 677–691.
31. DiFranco M, Capote J, Vergara JL (2005) Optical imaging and functional characterization of the transverse tubular system of mammalian muscle fibers using the potentiometric indicator di-8-ANEPPS. J Membr Biol 208: 141–153.
32. DiFranco M, Novo D, Vergara JL (2002) Characterization of the calcium release domains during excitation-contraction coupling in skeletal muscle fibres. Pflugers Arch 443: 508–519.
33. Troosters T, Gosselink R, Decramer M (2004) Chronic obstructive pulmonary disease and chronic heart failure: two muscle diseases? J Cardiopulm Rehabil 24: 137–145.
34. Adams GR, Vaziri ND (2006) Skeletal muscle dysfunction in chronic renal failure: effects of exercise. Am J Physiol Renal Physiol 290: F753–761.
35. Ward CW, Reiken S, Marks AR, Marty I, Vassort G, et al. (2003) Defects in ryanodine receptor calcium release in skeletal muscle from post-myocardial infarct rats. FASEB J 17: 1517–1519.
36. Delbono O, O'Rourke KS, Ettinger WH (1995) Excitation-calcium release uncoupling in aged single human skeletal muscle fibers. J Membr Biol 148: 211–222.
37. Struk A, Lehmann-Horn F, Melzer W (1998) Voltage-dependent calcium release in human malignant hyperthermia muscle fibers. Biophys J 75: 2402–2410.
38. Desaphy JF, Pierno S, Leoty C, George AL Jr, De Luca A, et al. (2001) Skeletal muscle disuse induces fibre type-dependent enhancement of Na(+) channel expression. Brain 124: 1100–1113.
39. Rehn TA, Munkvik M, Lunde PK, Sjaastad I, Sejersted OM (2012) Intrinsic skeletal muscle alterations in chronic heart failure patients: a disease-specific myopathy or a result of deconditioning? Heart Fail Rev 17: 421–436.
40. Baylor SM, Hollingworth S (2012) Intracellular calcium movements during excitation-contraction coupling in mammalian slow-twitch and fast-twitch muscle fibers. J Gen Physiol 139: 261–272.
41. Schaufelberger M, Eriksson BO, Grimby G, Held P, Swedberg K (1997) Skeletal muscle alterations in patients with chronic heart failure. Eur Heart J 18: 971–980.
42. Ferguson DG, Franzini-Armstrong C (1988) The Ca2+ ATPase content of slow and fast twitch fibers of guinea pig. Muscle Nerve 11: 561–570.
43. Lamb GD, Walsh T (1987) Calcium currents, charge movement and dihydropyridine binding in fast- and slow-twitch muscles of rat and rabbit. J Physiol 393: 595–617.
44. Mancini DM, Coyle E, Coggan A, Beltz J, Ferraro N, et al. (1989) Contribution of intrinsic skeletal muscle changes to 31P NMR skeletal muscle metabolic abnormalities in patients with chronic heart failure. Circulation 80: 1338–1346.
45. Whellan DJ, Nigam A, Arnold M, Starr AZ, Hill J, et al. (2011) Benefit of exercise therapy for systolic heart failure in relation to disease severity and etiology-findings from the Heart Failure and A Controlled Trial Investigating Outcomes of Exercise Training study. Am Heart J 162: 1003–1010.

12

Impact of Body Mass Index on Plasma N-Terminal ProB-Type Natriuretic Peptides in Chinese Atrial Fibrillation Patients without Heart Failure

Li-hui Zheng, Ling-min Wu, Yan Yao*, Wen-sheng Chen, Jing-ru Bao, Wen Huang, Rui Shi, Kui-jun Zhang, Shu Zhang

State Key Laboratory of Cardiovascular Disease, Clinical EP Lab & Arrhythmia Center, Fuwai Hospital, National Center for Cardiovascular Diseases, Chinese Academy of Medical Sciences and Peking Union Medical College, Beijing, China

Abstract

Background: An inverse relationship between body mass index (BMI) and circulating levels of N-terminal proB-type natriuretic peptide (NT-proBNP) has been demonstrated in subjects with and without heart failure. Obesity also has been linked with increased incidence of atrial fibrillation (AF), but its influence on NT-proBNP concentrations in AF patients remains unclear. This study aimed to investigate the effect of BMI on NT-proBNP levels in AF patients without heart failure.

Methods: A total of 239 consecutive patients with AF undergoing catheter ablation were evaluated. Levels of NT-proBNP and clinical characteristics were compared in overweight or obese (BMI≥25 kg/m^2) and normal weight (BMI<25 kg/m^2) patients.

Results: Of 239 patients, 129 (54%) were overweight or obese. Overweight or obese patients were younger, more likely to have a history of nonparoxysmal AF, hypertension, and diabetes mellitus. Levels of NT-proBNP were significantly lower in overweight or obese than in normal weight subjects ($P<0.05$). The relationship of obesity and decreased NT-proBNP levels persisted in subgroup of hypertension, both gender and both age levels (≥65 yrs and <65 yrs).Multivariate linear regression identified BMI as an independent negative correlate of LogNT-proBNP level.

Conclusions: An inverse relationship between BMI and plasma NT-proBNP concentrations have been demonstrated in AF patients without heart failure. Overweight or obese patients with AF appear to have lower NT-proBNP levels than normal weight patients.

Editor: Marta Letizia Hribal, University of Catanzaro Magna Graecia, Italy

Funding: The authors have no support or funding to report.

Competing Interests: The authors have declared that no competing interests exist.

* Email: ianyao@263.net.cn

Introduction

B-type natriuretic peptide (BNP) is synthesized as preproBNP in response to the stretch and pressure overload of the cardiac myocyte. After enzymatic cleavage, it is released into the circulation system in equimolar proportions as the hormonally active BNP and the inactive N-terminal fragment (N-terminal-pro-B-type natriuretic peptide, NT-proBNP).The expression of NT-proBNP is affected by several variations, such as age, gender, hypertension, renal function and thyroid function [1].

Several recent reports suggest that obesity, as indexed by elevated body mass index (BMI), may also affect NT-proBNP levels, with lower circulating levels in those with higher BMI in subjects with acute or chronic heart failure [2,3], significant coronary artery disease or acute myocardial infarction [4,5] and healthy general populations [6]. However, isolated study showed that obesity is not statistically associated with NT-proBNP in asymptomatic patients with hypertension [7].

Atrial fibrillation (AF) is the most common cardiac arrhythmia in the clinical practice. NT-proBNP levels are increased in AF [8], and have proven their potential utility in the risk stratification, prognostication, and therapeutic decision-making in AF [9–11]. However, the effect of obesity on NT-proBNP in AF patients has yet to be clarified. We aimed to explore this relationship in the present study. Because AF has been linked with congestive heart failure, we hypothesized that a similar relationship might exist in AF.

Methods

Patients

Two hundred and thirty-nine consecutive patients with AF undergoing radiofrequency catheter ablation in our institution between January 2007 and January 2009 were included in this study. Exclusion criteria included chronic heart failure or left ventricular ejection fraction (LVEF) ≤50%, cardiomyopathy, valvular heart disease, hepatic or renal failure, acute coronary

Table 1. Characteristics of patients with body mass index (BMI)≥25 or <25 kg/m².

	Overweight or obese: BMI≥25 kg/m² (n = 129)	Normal weight: BMI<25 kg/m² (n = 110)	P value
BMI(kg/m²)	26.9±1.9	22.0±1.6	<0.05
Age (yrs)	55±12	58±9	<0.05
Men (%)	94/129(72.9%)	85/110(77.3%)	NS
AF duration (yrs)	6.4±7.1	6.7±5.6	NS
Nonparoxysmal AF	50/129(38.8%)	29/110(26.4%)	<0.05
Smoking	50/129(38.8%)	41/110(37.2%)	NS
Diabetes mellitus(%)	20/129(15.5%)	7/110(6.4%)	<0.05
Hypertension(%)	76/129(58.9%)	45/110(40.9%)	<0.05
CHD(%)	6/129(4.7%)	5/110(4.5%)	NS
Serum creatinine (umol/L)	81±15	81±13	NS
Systolic blood pressure (mmHg)	130±16	126±15	NS
Diastolic blood pressure (mmHg)	79±13	77±11	NS
Heart rate (bpm)	79±18	76±15	NS
LAD (mm)	43±7	41±8	<0.05
LVEDD (mm)	50±4	49±5	<0.05
LVEF (%)	62±7	62±7	NS
Medications			
Warfarin(%)	6/129(4.7%)	4/110(3.6%)	NS
Aspirin(%)	24/129(18.6%)	21/110(19.1%)	NS
ACEI/ARB(%)	47/129(36.4%)	24/110(21.8%)	<0.05
Statin(%)	9/129(7.0%)	6/110(5.5%)	NS
CCB(%)	16/129(12.4%)	5/110(4.5%)	<0.05
βblocker(%)	42/129(32.6%)	33/110(30%)	NS
Profenanone(%)	19/129(14.7%)	17/110(15.5%)	NS
Amiodarone(%)	23/129(17.8%)	18/110(16.4%)	NS
NT-proBNP(fmol/ml)	437(324–550)	501(447–638)	<0.05
Log NT-proBNP	2.62±0.18	2.75±0.15	<0.001

CHD = Coronary heart disease; LAD = Left atrial diameter; LVEDD = Left ventricular end diastolic diameter; LVEF = Left ventricular ejection fraction; ACEI = Angiotensin-converting enzyme inhibitor; ARB = Angiotensin receptor blocker; CCB = Calcium channel blocker; NT-proBNP = N-terminal proB-type natriuretic peptide; NS = No significant.

syndrome, acute pulmonary embolism, chronic obstructive pulmonary disease, rheumatic heart disease, and thyroid dysfunction. Informed written consent was obtained from all patients, and this study was approved by the Ethics Committee of Fuwai Hospital and clinical investigations are conducted according to the principles expressed in the Declaration of Helsinki.

Clinical characteristics

Patients were interviewed and records were reviewed to determine past medical history, medications, and pertinent laboratory values. Left atrial diameter (LAD), left ventricular end diastolic diameter (LVEDD), and LVEF was determined within 3 days before the ablation procedure by echocardiography. Blood pressure and heart rate were measured in the morning upon admission, prior to the procedure. The BMI was calculated as body weight (kg) divided by the square of the height (m) at the time of the admission.

According to the World Health Organization/National Institutes of Health classification scheme, BMI groups were divided into 2 categories: overweight or obesity (BMI≥25 kg/m²) and normal weight (BMI<25 kg/m²) [12].

Measurement of NT-proBNP concentrations

Venous blood samples were collected from the antecubital vein in the morning upon admission, prior to the procedure. For each NT-proBNP measurement, 5 ml of whole blood was collected into tubes containing potassium EDTA (1 mg/ml blood) as anticoagulant to produce plasma. Specimens were centrifuged at 3000 r/min within 1 hour of collection. The resulting serum or plasma was aliquoted into respective storage vials and then frozen and maintained at −70°C until analysis. All testing and system operation were in accordance with manufacturer's recommendations. The serum specimen was used for NT-proBNP measurements using the assay kits (BIOMEDICA Medizinpordukte GmbH & Co KG, Wein, Australia). Assays were performed in a single run and normalized to a standard curve. Inter-assay coefficients of variation for NT-proBNP were <9%.

Statistical analysis

All statistical analyses were performed in SPSS 13.0 (SPSS, Inc., Chicago, Illinois). Continuous data are presented as mean ± SD or median plus interquartile ranges, as appropriate. Because of the large range in NT-proBNP, analysis and results of its log are also

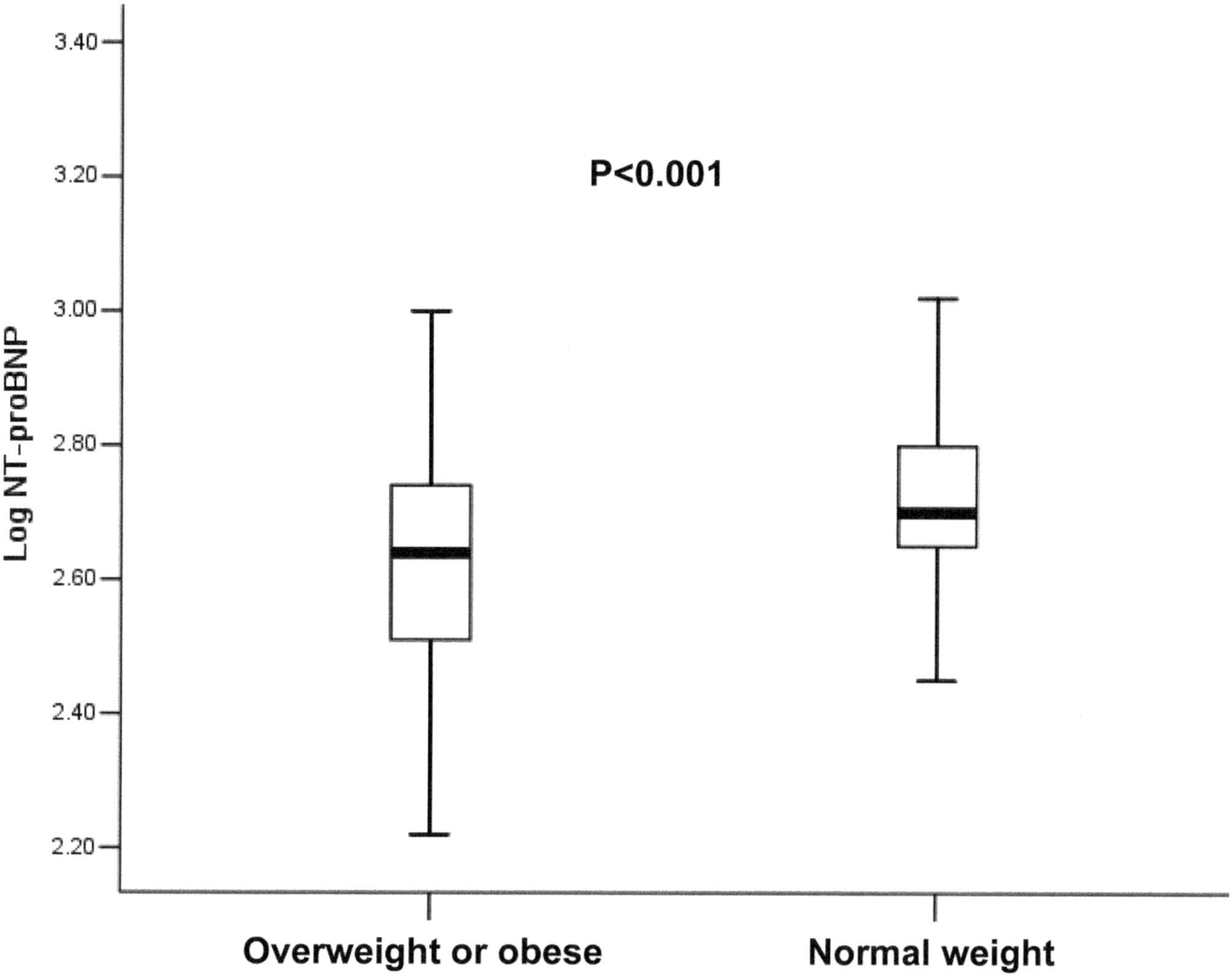

Figure 1. Comparison of LogNT-proBNP between overweight or obese patients and normal weight patients. Box plots of log of circulating N-terminal proB-type natriuretic peptide (NT-proBNP) levels showing medians with interquartile ranges. Overweight or obese patients have lower levels of Log NT-proBNP (2.62±0.18) compared with that of normal weight patients (2.75±0.15) with atrial fibrillation ($P<0.001$).

reported. Categorical variables were compared using the Pearson's χ^2 test. With continuous variables, group mean values were compared using the Student *t* test or analysis of variants, as appropriate. If the data distribution did not follow the normality assumption, the Wilcoxon rank-sum test was used. $P<0.05$ is considered statistically significant.

Further linear regression was performed to determine the independent relationship of BMI and LogNT-proBNP. In addition to BMI, the following covariates were also analyzed by multivariate linear regression: age, gender, AF duration, nonparoxysmal AF, smoking, diabetes mellitus, hypertension, coronary heart disease, serum creatinine, systolic blood pressure, diastolic blood pressure, LAD, LVEDD, LVEF, heart rate, using of warfarin, aspirin, angiotensin-converting enzyme inhibitor (ACEI)/angiotensin receptor blocker (ARB), statin, calcium channel block,β-blocker, propafenone, and amiodarone. The models were fit by a stepwise backward-selection algorithm, where all variables were entered into the original model and then variables with probability values of >0.05 were removed.

Results

Patients

The study included 239 consecutive patients (age 56±11 yrs; 75% men) with AF. Of these, the mean LVEF was 62±7%, the mean LAD was 41±8 mm, and the mean LVEDD was 50±4 mm. The mean serum creatinine was 81±14 umol/L. Of these, 121 (50.6%) had hypertension, 27 (11.3%) had diabetes mellitus, and 11(4.6%) had a history of coronary heart disease. The total population's BMI was 24.7±3.0 kg/m^2, 129 (54%) were overweight or obese (≥25 kg/m^2), and 110 (46%) normal weight (<25 kg/m^2). Overweight or obese patients were younger, and more likely to have a history of nonparoxysmal AF, hypertension, and diabetes mellitus (Table 1).

Comparison of NT-proBNP levels in overweight or obese and normal weight patients

Levels of NT-proBNP were significantly lower in overweight or obese patients than in normal weight patients (Table 1) (Figure 1). The median NT-proBNP in overweight or obese patients were

Table 2. Relationships of BMI and NT-proBNP levels in the subgroups.

	Overweight or obese: BMI≥25 kg/m² (fmol/ml)	Normal weight: BMI<25 kg/m² (fmol/ml)	P value
Male (n = 179)			
NT-proBNP	431(316–552)	489(436–638)	<0.001
Log NT-proBNP	2.69±0.18	2.74±0.15	<0.001
Female(n = 60)			
NT-proBNP	436(346–549)	513(468–686)	0.004
Log NT-proBNP	2.63±0.19	2.77±0.16	0.003
Age<65 yrs(n = 188)			
NT-proBNP	417(314–537)	495(437–603)	<0.001
Log NT-proBNP	2.60±0.17	2.72±0.13	0.005
Age≥65 yrs(n = 51)			
NT-proBNP	490(363–661)	795(490–1097)	0.003
Log NT-proBNP	2.69±0.20	2.88±0.18	0.001
Hypertension(n = 121)			
NT-proBNP	437(306–543)	490(447–617)	0.001
Log NT-proBNP	2.62±0.19	2.75±0.15	<0.001

NT-proBNP = N-terminal proB-type natriuretic peptide; BMI = body mass index.

437 fmol/ml, compared to 501 fmol/ml in the normal weight patients. The higher concentrations occurred despite similar LVEF and higher LVEDD and LAD.

To further evaluate the influence of age and its possible interaction with NT-proBNP levels in the context of obesity, we divided the cohort into elderly (≥65 yrs) and nonelderly (<65 yrs), and found that the relationship of obesity and decreased NT-proBNP levels persisted in both nonelderly and elderly ($P<0.05$), respectively. Similarly, the relationship of obesity and decreased NT-BNP concentrations persisted in patients with hypertension ($P<0.001$), and over the different gender ($P<0.05$), respectively (Table 2).

An inverse relationship between the LogNT-proBNP and BMI was found in the total study population ($r = -0.306$, $P<0.001$) (Figure 2), and for the two BMI groups, respectively (normal weight $r = -0.276$, $P<0.001$; overweigh or obese $r = -0.273$, $P<0.001$) and for both genders, respectively (male $r = -0.275$, $P<0.001$; female $r = -0.381$; $P<0.001$).

Multivariate predictors of NT-proBNP levels

Multivariate regressions analysis revealed BMI as an independent negative correlate of LogNT-BNP level ($t = -10.063$, $P<0.001$). Other independent factors included age ($t = 3.415$, $P = 0.001$),using of ACEI/ARB ($t = -2.080$, $P = 0.039$), and LAD ($t = 7.098$, $P<0.001$). Particularly, we did not find any significant independent influence of hypertension and diabetes mellitus on NT-proBNP levels (Table 3).

Discussion

Major Findings

This study demonstrates an inverse relationship between higher BMI and lower NT-proBNP levels in AF patients; overweight or obese patients with AF have lower NT-proBNP levels compared to normal weight AF subjects. The validity of this observation is supported by its consistency in subgroup of hypertension, both gender and both age levels (≥65 yrs and <65 yrs).

Average level and distribution of BMI

In this study, the average level (around 24.7 kg/m^2) and distribution of BMI was comparable with other Asian studies [4,13], but it was much lower in comparison with the western populations (around 28 kg/m^2) [2,3,5,7]. Of this study populations, 46% was normal weight (BMI<25 kg/m^2), 51% overweight (BMI = 25–29.9 kg/m^2), and 3% obese (BMI≥30 kg/m^2). Therefore, in the present study, the actual obese patients were rare, and we divided the study patients into overweight or obese group and normal weight group. The difference of average level and distribution of BMI may be due to an ethnic difference.

AF and NT-proBNP

Recently, the relationship between AF and NT-proBNP has been intensely studied. NT-proBNP is increased in AF [8]. In a community-based population, increased NT-proBNP levels at baseline independently predicted newly detected AF [8]. Deftereos et al demonstrated that NT-proBNP levels could predict the presence of left atrial thrombus in AF patients of unknown onset and no heart failure [10]. Furthermore, baseline NT-proBNP levels could predict risk of new-onset AF after cardiac surgery [11] or non-cardiac surgery [14], and predict AF recurrence after successful electrical cardioversion [15] or catheter ablation [9]. Thus, NT-proBNP has proven their diagnostic usefulness in the risk stratification, prognostication, and guiding therapy in patients with AF.

Obesity and NT-proBNP

Many studies have evaluated the relationship between plasma NT-proBNP and obesity. An inverse relationship between BMI and NT-proBNP levels has been demonstrated in subjects with acute or chronic heart failure [2,3], significant coronary artery disease or acute myocardial infarction [4,5] and healthy general populations in Framingham Heart study [6]. However, in asymptomatic patients with essential hypertension, with or without left ventricular hypertrophy, the inverse association was not observed [7]. In addition, two recent studies showed that NT-proBNP is closely associated with lean mass than with fat mass [6],

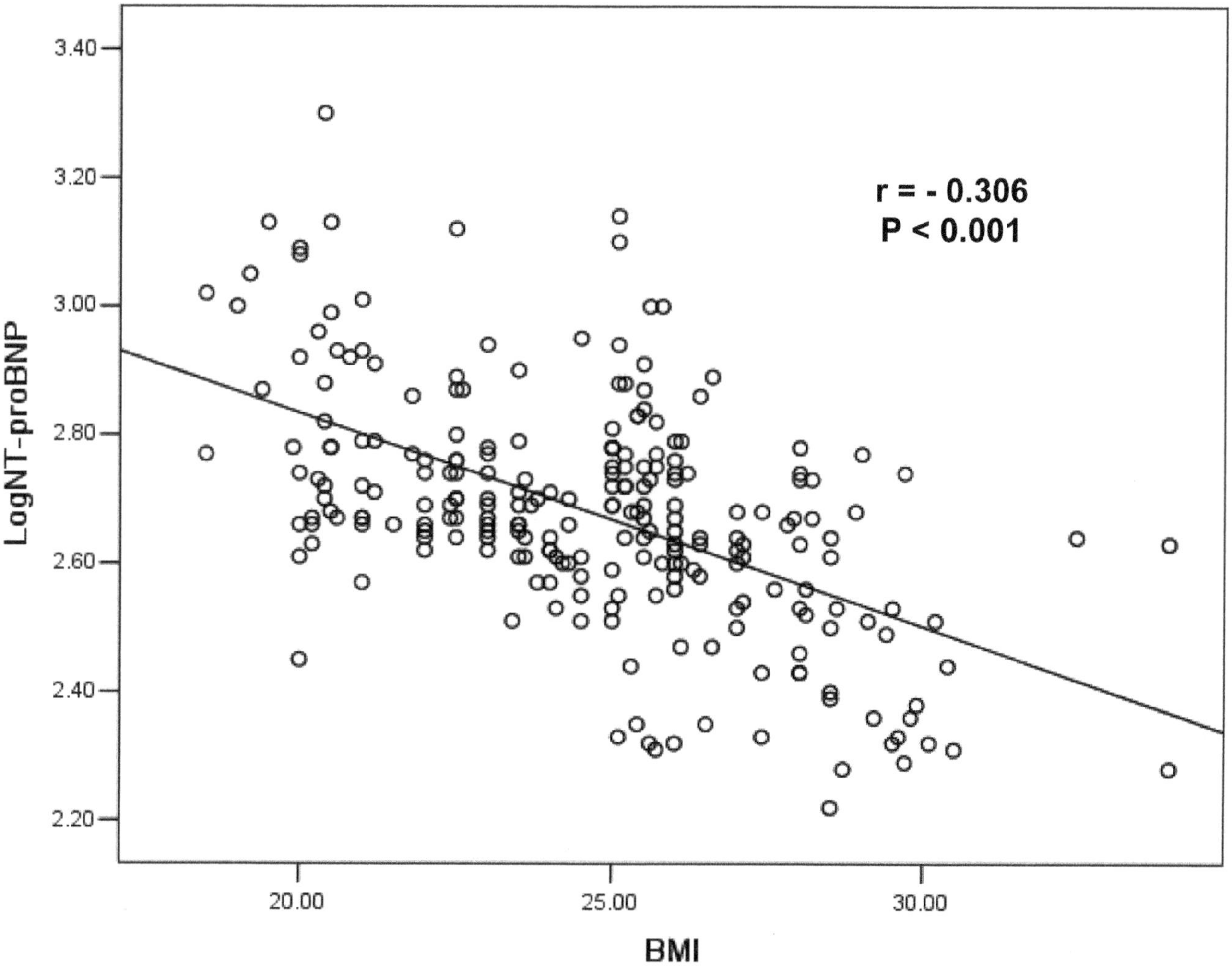

Figure 2. Inverse relationship between LogNT-proBNP and BMI in atrial fibrillation. This figure depicts the raw data demonstrating a significant inverse correlation between log of circulating N-terminal proB-type natriuretic peptide (NT-proBNP) levels and body mass index (BMI) in patients with atrial fibrillation ($r = -0.306$, $P < 0.001$).

and is related with visceral adipose tissue than subcutaneous adipose tissue [16]. Nevertheless, the relationship between plasma NT-proBNP levels and BMI in AF patients has not been analyzed. In one study from the Framingham Heart study [17], Wang et al reported that higher BMI was associated with decreased BNP and N-terminal proatrial natriuretic peptides (NT-proANP) levels. In that study, only a small number of AF patients were included, and accounted for 0.5%, 1% and 2% of the normal, overweight and obese group. Furthermore, the BNP levels of AF patients were not compared among different BMI groups.

In this study, although the patient average BMI level was much lower than the general western populations, the association between higher BMI and lower NT-proBNP levels were observed in AF patients. Furthermore, the validity of our findings is supported by its consistency across both genders, by the adjustment methods with numerous covariates. The present results therefore extend previous studies from heart failure, coronary artery disease to atrial fibrillation, at least in selected patients.

The exact mechanisms for the inverse relationship between NT-proBNP levels and BMI remain uncertain. Natriuretic peptide clearance receptors (NPR-C) are abundant in adipose tissue, and it is suggested that lipolysis is driven partly by natriuretic peptides, leading to the lower levels of natriuretic peptides in obese individuals [18]. However, the structure of NT-proBNP is distinct from natriuretic peptides and thus unlikely to be cleared via NPR-C, suggesting that the inverse relationship may be due to non-clearance mechanisms. A previous study reported that NT-proBNP decreased with increasing BMI in a manner nearly parallel to the decrease of BNP [3]. In addition, in the Framingham Heart study, NT-proANP levels were also lower in the obese subjects [17]. Because both NT-proANP and NT-proBNP are not cleared by NPR-C in adipose tissue, thus, decreased release or impaired synthesis of natriuretic peptides from the heart may at least partly underlie the possible mechanism. In addition, natriuretic peptides itself may exert potential lipolytic effects in human adipose tissue, leading to lipolysis and weight loss [19]. Further studies are required to explore the associated mechanisms.

Pathophysiological implications

Several studies have demonstrated that obesity is a major risk factor for the development of AF [20,21]. The potential mechanism may be that eccentric and concentric left ventricular hypertrophy with resultant progressive atrial enlargement [22,23]. The elevated circulating volume and enhanced neurohormonal activation (obliged by a larger body mass) may also contribute to

Table 3. Multivariate linear regression results for detecting independent factors on log-transformed plasma NT-proBNP in AF patients.

Variable	t	P value
Age	3.415	0.001
Gender	1.763	0.079
AF duration	0.721	0.471
Nonparoxysmal AF	0.026	0.979
Smoking	1.559	0.120
Diabetes mellitus	0.987	0.325
Hypertension	0.221	0.826
CHD	0.062	0.951
Serum creatinine	0.810	0.419
Systolic blood pressure	−0.149	0.881
Diastolic blood pressure	1.546	0.124
LAD	7.098	0.000
LVEDD	0.938	0.349
LVEF	−0.423	0.672
Heart rate	−0.358	0.720
Warfarin	0.234	0.815
Aspirin	−0.785	0.433
ACEI/ARB	−2.080	0.039
Statin	1.045	0.297
CCB	1.801	0.069
βblocker	0.916	0.361
Profenanone	0.290	0.772
Amiodarone	1.132	0.259
BMI	−10.063	0.000

NT-proBNP = N-terminal proB-type natriuretic peptide; AF = Atrial fibrillation; CHD = Coronary heart disease; LAD = Left atrial diameter; LVEDD = Left ventricular end diastolic diameter; LVEF = Left ventricular ejection fraction; ACEI = Angiotensin-converting enzyme inhibitor; ARB = Angiotensin receptor blocker; CCB = Calcium channel blocker; BMI = body mass index.

the left atrium dilation and electrical instability [21,24]. Although the exact significance of decreased NT-proBNP levels in overweight or obese state of AF patients are not yet understood, it at least raises the possibility that there may be lesser natriuretic-mediated vasodilation and antagonism of the rennin-angiotensin system, or loss of natriuretic ability in overweight or obese patients, which may also play a role in the development of the AF in overweight or obese patients.

Study limitations

The present study has several limitations. First, this study included Chinese populations, which may be different with those from western countries. As discussed previously, the average level and distribution of BMI in the present study was much lower than that reported in previous western studies. In addition, the use of warfarin for stroke prevention among AF patients was low in this study, although it is similar to other Chinese study [25]. This may reflect the current medical system pattern in China. Thus, our results must be extended to other populations with caution.

Second, this study involved a population of patients referred for catheter ablation of AF.Thus, due to the patients not eligible for ablation have been excluded, therefore, the conclusions may be possibly not extrapolated to the general population of patients with AF.However, with the increasing numbers of patients receiving ablation, we believe that the results of this study remains valuable, at least in selected patients, which could be millions.

Third, the usual dosage of NT-proBNP is based on pg/ml. In this study, the plasma NT-proBNP level was quantitatively determined using competitive enzyme immunoassay from BIOMEDICA; results are given in fmol/ml. In order to convert the results of NT-proBNP from fmol/ml to pg/ml, results should be multiplied by 8.457 [26]. However, we think that the results using fmol/ml did not affect our conclusions between BMI and NT-proBNP.

Conclusions

In the present study, we demonstrated an inverse association between higher BMI and lower NT-proBNP levels in AF patients. Overweigh or obese patients have reduced levels of NT-proBNP compared to lean patients. In the clinical practice, it should be considered the effect of the obesity on the NT-proBNP levels for the AF patients.

Author Contributions

Conceived and designed the experiments: LHZ LMW YY. Performed the experiments: LHZ LMW. Analyzed the data: LHZ RS WH. Contributed reagents/materials/analysis tools: LMW. Wrote the paper: LHZ. Acquisition of data: WSC JRB. Final review and correction of the version to be published: YY KJZ SZ.

References

1. Raymond I, Groenning BA, Hildebrandt PR, Nilsson JC, Baumann M, et al. (2003) The influence of age, sex and other variables on the plasma level of N-terminal pro brain natriuretic peptide in a large sample of the general population. Heart 89: 745–751.
2. Rivera M, Cortés R, Salvador A, Bertomeu V, de Burgos FG, et al. (2005) Obese subjects with heart failure have lower N-terminal pro-brain natriuretic peptide plasma levels irrespective of aetiology. Eur J Heart Fail 7: 1168–1170.
3. Krauser DG, Lloyd-Jones DM, Chae CU, Cameron R, Anwaruddin S, et al. (2005) Effect of body mass index on natriuretic peptide levels in patients with acute congestive heart failure: a ProBNP Investigation of Dyspnea in the Emergency Department (PRIDE) substudy. Am Heart J 149: 744–750.
4. Hong SN, Ahn Y, Yoon NS, Moon JY, Kim KH, et al. (2008) N-terminal pro-B-type natriuretic peptide level is depressed in patients with significant coronary artery disease who have high body mass index. Int Heart J 49: 403–412.
5. Lorgis L, Cottin Y, Danchin N, Mock L, Sicard P, et al. (2011) Impact of obesity on the prognostic value of the N-terminal pro-B-type natriuretic peptide (NT-proBNP) in patients with acute myocardial infarction. Heart 97: 551–956.
6. Das SR, Drazner MH, Dries DL, Vega GL, Stanek HG, et al. (2005) Impact of body mass and body composition on circulating levels of natriuretic peptides: results from the Dallas Heart Study. Circulation 112: 2163–2168.
7. Cortés R, Otero MR, Morillas P, Roselló-Lletí E, Grigorian L, et al. (2008) Obese and nonobese patients with essential hypertension show similar N-terminal proBNP plasma levels. Am J Hypertens 21: 820–825.
8. Patton KK, Ellinor PT, Heckbert SR, Christenson RH, DeFilippi C, et al. (2009) N-terminal pro-B-type natriuretic peptide is a major predictor of the development of atrial fibrillation: the Cardiovascular Health Study. Circulation 120: 1768–1774.
9. den Uijl DW, Delgado V, Tops LF, Ng AC, Boersma E, et al. (2011) Natriuretic peptide levels predict recurrence of atrial fibrillation after radiofrequency catheter ablation. Am Heart J 161: 197–203.
10. Deftereos S, Giannopoulos G, Kossyvakis C, Raisakis K, Kaoukis A, et al. (2011) Estimation of atrial fibrillation recency of onset and safety of cardioversion using NTproBNP levels in patients with unknown time of onset. Heart 97: 914–917.
11. Gibson PH, Croal BL, Cuthbertson BH, Rae D, McNeilly JD, et al. (2009) Use of preoperative natriuretic peptides and echocardiographic parameters in predicting new-onset atrial fibrillation after coronary artery bypass grafting: a prospective comparative study. Am Heart J 158: 244–251.
12. National Heart, Lung, and Blood Institute Expert Panel (1998) Clinical Guidelines on the Identification, Evaluation, and Treatment of Overweight and Obesity in Adults: Evidence Report. Bethesda, Md: National Heart, Lung, and Blood Institute; June.
13. Sugisawa T, Kishimoto I, Kokubo Y, Makino H, Miyamoto Y, et al. (2010) Association of plasma B-type natriuretic peptide levels with obesity in a general urban Japanese population: the Suita Study. Endocr J 57: 727–733.
14. Karthikeyan G, Moncur RA, Levine O, Heels-Ansdell D, Chan MT, et al. (2009) Is a pre-operative brain natriuretic peptide or N-terminal pro-B-type natriuretic peptide measurement an independent predictor of adverse cardio-vascular outcomes within 30 days of noncardiac surgery? A systematic review and meta-analysis of observational studies. J Am Coll Cardiol 54: 1599–1606.
15. Mollmann H, Weber M, Elsasser A, Nef H, Dill T, et al. (2008) NT-ProBNP predicts rhythm stability after cardioversion of lone atrial fibrillation. Circ J 72: 921–925.
16. Malavazos AE, Morricone L, Marocchi A, Ermetici F, Ambrosi B, et al. (2006) N-terminal pro-B-type natriuretic peptide and echocardiographic abnormalities in severely obese patients: correlation with visceral fat. Clin Chem 52: 1211–1213.
17. Wang TJ, Larson MG, Levy D, Benjamin EJ, Leip EP, et al. (2004) Impact of obesity on plasma natriuretic peptide levels. Circulation 109: 594–600.
18. Sengenès C, Berlan M, De Glisezinski I, Lafontan M, Galitzky J (2000) Natriuretic peptides: a new lipolytic pathway in human adipocytes. FASEB J 14: 1345–1351.
19. Sarzani R, Dessì-Fulgheri P, Paci VM, Espinosa E, Rappelli A (1996) Expression of natriuretic peptide receptors in human adipose and other tissues. J Endocrinol Invest 19: 581–585.
20. Benjamin EJ, Levy D, Vaziri SM, D'Agostino RB, Belanger AJ, et al. (1994) Independent risk factors for atrial fibrillation in a population-based cohort. The Framingham Heart Study. JAMA 271: 840–844.
21. Wang TJ, Parise H, Levy D, D'Agostino RB Sr, Wolf PA, et al. (2004) Obesity and the risk of new-onset atrial fibrillation. JAMA 292: 2471–2477.
22. Hense HW, Gneiting B, Muscholl M, Broeckel U, Kuch B, et al. (1998) The associations of body size and body composition with left ventricular mass: impacts for indexation in adults. J Am Coll Cardiol 32: 451–457.
23. de Simone G, Daniels SR, Devereux RB, Meyer RA, Roman MJ, et al. (1992) Left ventricular mass and body size in normotensive children and adults: assessment of allometric relations and impact of overweight. J Am Coll Cardiol 20: 1251–1260.
24. Abed HS, Samuel CS, Lau DH, Kelly DJ, Royce SG, et al. (2013) Obesity results in progressive atrial structural and electrical remodeling: implications for atrial fibrillation. Heart Rhythm 10: 90–100.
25. Zhou ZQ, Hu DY, Chen J, Zhang RH, Li KB, et al. (2003) An epidemiological survey of atrial fibrillation in China. Chin J Intern Med (Chin) 43: 491–494.
26. Rutten FH, Gramer MJM, Zuithoff NPA, Lammers JWJ, Verweij W, et al. (2007) Comparison of B-type natriuretic peptide assays for identifying heart failure in stable elderly patients with a clinical diagnosis of chronic obstructive pulmonary disease. Eur J Heart Fail 9: 651–659.

Empiric Potassium Supplementation and Increased Survival in Users of Loop Diuretics

Charles E. Leonard[1,2]*, Hanieh Razzaghi[1,2], Cristin P. Freeman[1,2], Jason A. Roy[1,2], Craig W. Newcomb[1], Sean Hennessy[1,2,3]

1 Center for Clinical Epidemiology & Biostatistics, Department of Biostatistics & Epidemiology, Perelman School of Medicine at the University of Pennsylvania, Philadelphia, Pennsylvania, United States of America, **2** Center for Pharmacoepidemiology Research and Training, Perelman School of Medicine at the University of Pennsylvania, Philadelphia, Pennsylvania, United States of America, **3** Department of Pharmacology, Perelman School of Medicine at the University of Pennsylvania, Philadelphia, Pennsylvania, United States of America

Abstract

Background: The effectiveness of the clinical strategy of empiric potassium supplementation in reducing the frequency of adverse clinical outcomes in patients receiving loop diuretics is unknown. We sought to examine the association between empiric potassium supplementation and 1) all-cause death and 2) outpatient-originating sudden cardiac death (SD) and ventricular arrhythmia (VA) among new starters of loop diuretics, stratified on initial loop diuretic dose.

Methods: We conducted a one-to-one propensity score-matched cohort study using 1999–2007 US Medicaid claims from five states. Empiric potassium supplementation was defined as a potassium prescription on the day of or the day after the initial loop diuretic prescription. Death, the primary outcome, was ascertained from the Social Security Administration Death Master File; SD/VA, the secondary outcome, from incident, first-listed emergency department or principal inpatient SD/VA discharge diagnoses (positive predictive value = 85%).

Results: We identified 654,060 persons who met eligibility criteria and initiated therapy with a loop diuretic, 27% of whom received empiric potassium supplementation (N = 179,436) and 73% of whom did not (N = 474,624). The matched hazard ratio for empiric potassium supplementation was 0.93 (95% confidence interval, 0.89–0.98, $p = 0.003$) for all-cause death. Stratifying on initial furosemide dose, hazard ratios for empiric potassium supplementation with furosemide <40 and ≥ 40 milligrams/day were 0.93 (0.86–1.00, $p = 0.050$) and 0.84 (0.79–0.89, $p < 0.0001$). The matched hazard ratio for empiric potassium supplementation was 1.02 (0.83–1.24, $p = 0.879$) for SD/VA.

Conclusions: Empiric potassium supplementation upon initiation of a loop diuretic appears to be associated with improved survival, with a greater apparent benefit seen with higher diuretic dose. If confirmed, these findings support the use of empiric potassium supplementation upon initiation of a loop diuretic.

Editor: Yan Gong, University of Florida, United States of America

Funding: This study was supported by RC1AG035751 and R01AG025152 from the US Department of Health & Human Services (DHHS) National Institute on Aging, R01DK102694 from the US DHHS National Institute of Diabetes and Kidney Diseases, and UL1TR000003 from the US DHHS National Center for Advancing Translational Sciences. The National Institutes of Health had no role in the design and conduct of the study; management, analysis, and interpretation of the data; preparation, review, or approval of the manuscript; or decision to submit the manuscript for publication.

Competing Interests: The following Coauthors report no conflicts of interest: Leonard, Razzaghi, Roy, and Newcomb. Coauthors Freeman and Hennessy receive research support from AstraZeneca and Bristol-Myers Squibb, although unrelated to this topic. Dr. Hennessy has consulted for Bristol-Myers Squibb, AstraZeneca, Amgen, Millennium, and CSL Behring, all unrelated to this topic.

* Email: celeonar@upenn.edu

Introduction

Furosemide was introduced in the 1960s and is very widely used to treat heart failure and edema [1,2]. Furosemide and other loop diuretics cause urinary potassium loss [3], which can lead to potassium depletion and might be expected to increase mortality by mechanisms including ventricular ectopy [4,5]. On this basis, among others, the 2000 National Council on Potassium in Clinical Practice recommended that potassium supplementation be routinely considered in persons with hypertension receiving a non-potassium sparing diuretic, and in persons with heart failure even if normokalemic [6]. However, no studies have examined the efficacy or effectiveness of empiric potassium supplementation (defined as preventive/prophylactic supplementation, in contrast to repletion reactive to serum potassium laboratory results) on reducing the risk of adverse clinical outcomes in users of loop diuretics. As a result of this evidence gap, a 2012 evidence review recommended against the routine use of empiric potassium supplementation in patients receiving loop diuretics [7], despite the aforementioned practice guidelines. A randomized trial addressing this important question seems unlikely. To provide evidence to help inform this common clinical decision, we sought to examine the effectiveness of empiric potassium supplementation in reducing all-cause mortality in a cohort of new users of loop diuretics. Recognizing that the effects of empiric potassium supplementation might vary by diuretic dose [7], we wished to examine the effect stratified on diuretic dose. We secondarily examined the effectiveness of empiric potassium supplementation in reducing a composite endpoint of sudden cardiac death/ ventricular arrhythmia (SD/VA) to look for mechanistic evidence.

Methods

Ethics statement

This observational study was approved by the University of Pennsylvania's institutional review board.

Overview and study population

We performed a propensity score-matched cohort study of new users of loop diuretics. Our cohort consisted of person-time exposed to a new course of a loop diuretic (bumetanide, ethacrynic acid, furosemide, or torsemide). Data for this study included that of the Medicaid programs of California, Florida, New York, Ohio, and Pennsylvania from 1999–2007 [8]. These states comprise about 38% of the United States Medicaid population [9], with the nine-year dataset recording the experience of over 48 million cumulative enrollees and 108 million person-years (p-y) of observation. Because up to 27% of Medicaid beneficiaries (varying by state and year) were co-enrolled in Medicare (i.e., dually enrolled) [10–12], we also obtained Medicare claims (including Part D data from 2006 onward) to ascertain a more complete picture of enrollees' healthcare. We linked these data to the Social Security Administration Death Master File to ascertain deaths.

Defining the study cohort: identification of incident loop diuretic courses

We defined new users of loop diuretics as those with at least a 12-month baseline period of Medicaid enrollment before the first loop diuretic prescription was filled. Beneficiaries meeting any of the following criteria were excluded: a) incident loop prescription was a liquid dosage form, as their inability to swallow a solid dosage form may have been indicative of functional impairments that are not reliably captured in administrative data; b) use of another diuretic class during the baseline period except for thiazide or thiazide-related agent use (hereafter simply referred to as thiazide), as we wished not to exclude those who had progressed from a thiazide to a loop; c) prescription for a potassium supplement in the baseline period; d) cancer diagnosis in the baseline period; e) occurrence of an outcome of interest in the baseline period; or f) age <18 or ≥95 years. The beginning of the course was defined by the fill date of the beneficiary's first loop diuretic prescription. The end of the course was defined by the first occurrence of the following: a) an outcome of interest; b) death, for the study of SD/VA; c) a cancer diagnosis; d) a switch to another class of diuretics; e) a >60-day gap between consecutive loop diuretic prescriptions; or f) the end of follow-up time in the database. Incident courses ≤2 days in length were excluded, as this was the time period over which exposure to empiric potassium supplementation was assessed (see below) and therefore such courses provided no follow-up time. For the 96% of subjects whose initial loop diuretic was furosemide, we stratified the death analyses by initial furosemide dose, expressed as <40 mg/day vs. ≥40 mg/day.

Ascertainment of exposure and covariates

The exposure of interest was empiric potassium supplementation, defined as filling a prescription for potassium (as a solid bicarbonate, chloride, citrate, or gluconate salt—and excluding from study persons having received a liquid preparation based on the aforementioned rationale) on the same day as or on the day following the initial loop diuretic prescription. We did not examine potassium dispensed ≥2 days following initiation of loop diuretic therapy because such potassium prescriptions were likely to represent responses to clinical or laboratory signs of hypokalemia (i.e., reactive supplementation) rather than clinical decisions to supplement empirically. Those without empiric potassium supplementation served as the reference group.

We measured three types of potential confounders: 1) demographics—age, sex, race, state of residence, calendar year, dual-eligibility status, and nursing home residence status; 2) diseases, measured as ever prior to the initial loop course—such as chronic illnesses (e.g., diabetes mellitus, chronic kidney disease), potential risk factors for death or SD/VA (e.g., heart failure), labeled and off-labeled indications for diuretics or potassium supplementation (e.g., ascites, metabolic alkalosis), and contraindications for receiving potassium supplementation (e.g., acidosis); and 3) drug markers of chronic disease, measured as ever prior to the initial loop course (e.g., insulin as a marker for diabetes mellitus). Table 1 lists all measured covariates.

For the overall group of loop diuretic users, and for furosemide users stratified by initial furosemide dose, we performed propensity score matching using one-to-one, nearest neighbor matching (caliper width = 10% of the standard deviation of the logit of the propensity score [13]) without replacement. Propensity scores were calculated by logistic regression using the variables listed in Table 1. Age was modeled using splines [14].

Study Outcomes

The primary outcome was all-cause death. The secondary outcome was outpatient-originating SD/VA resulting in emergency department or hospital presentation. The rationale for considering SD/VA as a composite outcome is that sudden cardiac death is often due to undocumented ventricular arrhythmia [15]. Incident SD/VA outcomes were identified in emergency department and inpatient claims having one of the following International Classification of Diseases (ICD-9) discharge diagnoses in a first-listed or principal position: paroxysmal ventricular tachycardia (427.1), ventricular fibrillation and flutter (427.4), ventricular fibrillation (427.41), ventricular flutter (427.42), cardiac arrest (427.5), sudden death (798), instantaneous death (798.1), or death occurring in <24 hours from onset of symptoms, not otherwise explained (798.2). This algorithm has a positive predictive value of 85% for identifying outpatient-originating SD/VA not due to extrinsic causes [16,17].

Statistical analyses

We first compared baseline characteristics of the cohorts before and after propensity score matching. We evaluated baseline differences by calculating standardized mean differences, using a threshold of 0.10 to indicate potential imbalance [18]. We next calculated incidence rates (with 95% confidence intervals [CIs]) for each outcome, stratified by empiric potassium use. We then plotted time-to-event curves by furosemide dose. Finally, we fitted stratified Cox proportional hazards models, which account for matching, to obtain estimated hazard ratios (HRs) for the associations between empiric potassium supplementation and the outcome within furosemide dose strata. Sub-analyses stratified by furosemide dose examined potential effect modification by: age; history of arrhythmia/conduction disorder in the 12 months prior to the loop course; history of kidney disease (an algorithm for which has an expected sensitivity of ~80% [19]) in the 12 months prior to the loop course; potassium laboratory monitoring within

Table 1. Baseline characteristics of beneficiaries in the primary outcome (all-cause death) cohort, before and after propensity score matching.

	OVERALL LOOP DIURETIC COHORT						FUROSEMIDE <40 MG/DAY COHORT						FUROSEMIDE ≥40 MG/DAY COHORT					
	Before PS Matching			After 1-to-1 PS Matching			Before PS Matching			After 1-to-1 PS Matching			Before PS Matching			After 1-to-1 PS Matching		
Covariate	K^+ = YES	K^+ = NO	SDiff	K^+ = YES	K^+ = NO	SDiff	K^+ = YES	K^+ = NO	SDiff	K^+ = YES	K^+ = NO	SDiff	K^+ = YES	K^+ = NO	SDiff	K^+ = YES	K^+ = NO	SDiff
	n = 179,436	n = 474,624		n = 179,425	n = 179,425		n = 71,631	n = 243,436		n = 71,631	n = 71,631		n = 101,704	n = 210,460		n = 100,869	n = 100,869	
DEMOGRAPHICS																		
Age, in years		0.05		<0.01		0.09		<0.01		0.03		<0.01						
18–44	14.3%	15.5%	—	14.3%	14.1%	—	14.4%	16.4%	—	14.4%	14.6%	—	14.3%	14.6%	—	14.3%	13.9%	—
45–54	14.1%	14.4%	—	14.1%	14.2%	—	13.0%	13.8%	—	13.0%	12.8%	—	14.9%	15.1%	—	14.9%	14.9%	—
55–64	15.0%	15.6%	—	15.0%	14.9%	—	13.5%	14.4%	—	13.5%	13.4%	—	16.2%	17.0%	—	16.2%	16.2%	—
65–74	20.6%	20.7%	—	20.6%	20.6%	—	19.9%	20.1%	—	19.9%	19.9%	—	21.2%	21.2%	—	21.2%	21.4%	—
75–84	22.3%	21.3%	—	22.3%	22.4%	—	23.4%	21.6%	—	23.4%	23.5%	—	21.4%	20.7%	—	21.4%	21.6%	—
85–94	13.7%	12.6%	—	13.7%	13.8%	—	15.8%	13.7%	—	15.8%	15.7%	—	12.0%	11.3%	—	12.0%	12.0%	—
Sex, female	71.0%	70.0%	0.03	71.0%	71.2%	<0.01	73.8%	72.9%	0.02	73.8%	73.7%	<0.01	68.8%	66.2%	0.06	68.8%	68.9%	<0.01
Race																		
white	54.6%	49.6%	0.10	54.6%	54.8%	<0.01	54.3%	49.5%	0.10	54.3%	54.3%	<0.01	54.2%	48.6%	0.11	54.0%	54.2%	<0.01
black	15.6%	17.5%	0.05	15.6%	15.4%	<0.01	13.2%	15.6%	0.06	13.2%	13.3%	<0.01	17.3%	19.9%	0.07	17.4%	17.2%	<0.01
hispanic	15.4%	18.1%	0.07	15.4%	15.4%	<0.01	16.1%	18.6%	0.07	16.1%	16.1%	<0.01	15.1%	17.8%	0.07	15.1%	15.0%	<0.01
other/unknown	14.4%	14.8%	0.01	14.4%	14.5%	<0.01	16.3%	16.4%	<0.01	16.3%	16.3%	<0.01	13.5%	13.7%	<0.01	13.5%	13.6%	<0.01
Medicaid-Medicare dual eligibility status, yes	69.9%	67.4%	0.05	69.9%	70.0%	<0.01	70.7%	66.2%	0.10	70.7%	70.7%	<0.01	68.9%	68.0%	0.02	68.9%	69.0%	<0.01
Nursing home residence status, yes	15.4%	14.6%	0.02	15.4%	15.4%	<0.01	16.8%	15.1%	0.05	16.8%	17.0%	<0.01	13.9%	13.7%	<0.01	13.9%	14.0%	<0.01
COHORT-DEFINING CHARACTERISTICS																		
Cohort-initiating loop: bumetanide*	1.8%	2.1%	—	1.8%	2.3%	—	0.0%	0.0%	—	0.0%	0.0%	—	0.0%	0.0%	—	0.0%	0.0%	—
Cohort-initiating loop: ethacrynic acid*	0.0%	0.1%	—	0.0%	0.1%	—	0.0%	0.0%	—	0.0%	0.0%	—	0.0%	0.0%	—	0.0%	0.0%	—
Cohort-initiating loop: furosemide*	96.6%	95.7%	—	96.6%	95.3%	—	100%	100%	—	100%	100%	—	100%	100%	—	100%	100%	—
Starting dose < 40 mg/day*	41.5%	53.8%	—	41.3%	54.5%	—	100%	100%	—	100%	100%	—	—	—	—	—	—	—
Starting dose = 40 mg/day*	47.0%	35.4%	—	47.2%	35.1%	—	—	—	—	—	—	—	80.5%	76.7%	—	80.4%	80.4%	—
Starting dose > 40 mg/day*	11.5%	10.8%	—	11.4%	10.3%	—	—	—	—	—	—	—	19.5%	23.3%	—	19.6%	19.6%	—
Cohort-initiating loop: torsemide*	1.6%	2.2%	—	1.6%	2.3%	—	0.0%	0.0%	—	0.0%	0.0%	—	0.0%	0.0%	—	0.0%	0.0%	—

Table 1. Cont.

	OVERALL LOOP DIURETIC COHORT						FUROSEMIDE <40 MG/DAY COHORT						FUROSEMIDE ≥40 MG/DAY COHORT					
	Before PS Matching			After 1-to-1 PS Matching			Before PS Matching			After 1-to-1 PS Matching			Before PS Matching			After 1-to-1 PS Matching		
Covariate	K^+=YES	K^+=NO	SDiff	K^+=YES	K^+=NO	SDiff	K^+=YES	K^+=NO	SDiff	K^+=YES	K^+=NO	SDiff	K^+=YES	K^+=NO	SDiff	K^+=YES	K^+=NO	SDiff
	n = 179,436	n = 474,624		n = 179,425	n = 179,425		n = 71,631	n = 243,436		n = 71,631	n = 71,631		n = 101,704	n = 210,460		n = 100,869	n = 100,869	
EXPOSURE-DEFINING AND RELATED CHARACTERISTICS																		
K^+ at any time during follow-up*	100%	13.5%	—	100%	15.7%	—	100%	11.6%	—	100%	13.6%	—	100%	15.7%	—	100%	18.2%	—
K^+ during the entirety of follow-up*	46.3%	0%	—	46.3%	0%	—	49.0%	0.0%	—	49.0%	0%	—	44.7%	0%	—	44.7%	0%	—
Proportion of days on K^+ (mean, standard deviation)*	0.849 (0.23)	0.067 (0.20)	—	0.849 (0.23)	0.079 (0.21)	—	0.858 (0.23)	0.056 (0.18)	—	0.858 (0.23)	0.067 (0.20)	—	0.842 (0.23)	0.079 (0.21)	—	0.841 (0.23)	0.093 (0.23)	—
Proportion of days on K^+ (median, IQR)*	0.98 (0.77–1.00)	0.00 (0.00–0.00)	—	0.98 (0.77–1.00)	0.00 (0.00–0.00)	—	0.99 (0.80–1.00)	0.00 (0.00–0.00)	—	0.99 (0.80–1.00)	0.00 (0.00–0.00)	—	0.97 (0.75–1.00)	0.00 (0.00–0.00)	—	0.97 (0.75–1.00)	0.00 (0.00–0.00)	—
Lab monitoring of K^+ in first 30 days of loop prescription*	35.9%	32.2%	—	34.6%	31.3%	—	35.0%	30.6%	—	36.6%	33.7%	—	35.5%	32.1%	—	35.5%	31.4%	—
DISEASES, EVER PRIOR TO INITIAL LOOP COURSE																		
Acidosis	2.1%	2.5%	0.03	2.1%	2.0%	<0.01	1.9%	2.0%	<0.01	1.9%	1.8%	<0·01	2.2%	3.2%	0.06	2.2%	2.1%	<0.01
Alcohol abuse**	6.3%	6.6%	0.01	6.3%	6.2%	<0.01	5.9%	6.6%	0.03	5.9%	5.8%	<0.01	6.6%	6.8%	0.01	6.5%	6.4%	<0.01
Alkalosis, metabolic	0.5%	0.5%	<0.01	0.5%	0.5%	<0.01	0.5%	0.4%	<0.01	0.5%	0.5%	<0.01	0.5%	0.6%	0.01	0.5%	0.5%	<0.01
Amyloidosis	0.1%	0.1%	<0.01	0.1%	0.1%	<0.01	0.1%	0.1%	<0.01	0.1%	0.1%	<0.01	0.1%	0.1%	0.02	0.1%	0.1%	<0.01
Anemia	43.2%	43.1%	<0.01	43.2%	43.0%	<0.01	44.5%	42.2%	0.05	44.5%	44.3%	<0.01	42.2%	43.9%	0.03	42.1%	41.8%	<0.01
Arrhythmia/ conduction disorder	36.0%	33.1%	0.06	36.0%	36.0%	<0.01	35.0%	31.6%	0.07	35.0%	34.9%	<0.01	36.4%	34.6%	0.04	36.3%	36.2%	<0.01
Ascites	1.6%	2.1%	0.03	1.6%	1.6%	<0.01	1.5%	1.6%	0.01	1.5%	1.5%	<0.01	1.8%	2.6%	0.05	1.8%	1.8%	<0.01
Asthma/COPD	44.9%	39.7%	0.11	44.9%	44.8%	<0.01	44.0%	39.4%	0.09	44.0%	43.9%	<0·01	45.4%	39.9%	0.11	45.2%	44.9%	<0.01
Cerebrovascular disease	30.8%	28.8%	0.04	30.8%	30.8%	<0.01	31.7%	28.7%	0.06	31.7%	31.5%	<0.01	29.9%	28.6%	0.03	29.7%	29.7%	<0.01
Coronary artery disease	48.8%	45.2%	0.07	48.8%	48.8%	<0.01	47.0%	42.9%	0.08	47.0%	46.8%	<0.01	49.8%	47.4%	0.05	49.5%	49.2%	<0.01
Corticoadrenal insufficiency	0.9%	1.0%	0.01	0.9%	0.9%	<0.01	1.0%	1.1%	<0.01	1.0%	1.0%	<0.01	0.9%	1.0%	0.01	0.9%	0.9%	<0.01
Cushing's syndrome	0.2%	0.2%	<0.01	0.2%	0.2%	<0.01	0.2%	0.2%	<0.01	0.2%	0.2%	<0.01	0.2%	0.2%	<0.01	0.2%	0.2%	<0.01
Diabetes insipidus	0.1%	0.2%	<0.01	0.1%	0.1%	<0.01	0.1%	0.2%	0.01	0.1%	0.1%	<0.01	0.1%	0.2%	<0.01	0.1%	0.1%	<0.01
Diabetes mellitus	45.3%	47.6%	0.05	45.3%	45.2%	<0.01	42.7%	44.7%	0.04	42.7%	42.4%	<0.01	46.9%	50.7%	0.08	47.0%	46.9%	<0.01
Edema	27.0%	25.2%	0.04	27.0%	27.1%	<0.01	27.6%	24.5%	0.07	27.6%	27.5%	<0.01	26.2%	25.4%	0.02	26.1%	26.0%	<0.01

Table 1. Cont.

	OVERALL LOOP DIURETIC COHORT						FUROSEMIDE <40 MG/DAY COHORT						FUROSEMIDE ≥40 MG/DAY COHORT					
	Before PS Matching			After 1-to-1 PS Matching			Before PS Matching			After 1-to-1 PS Matching			Before PS Matching			After 1-to-1 PS Matching		
Covariate	K^+ = YES	K^+ = NO	SDiff	K^+ = YES	K^+ = NO	SDiff	K^+ = YES	K^+ = NO	SDiff	K^+ = YES	K^+ = NO	SDiff	K^+ = YES	K^+ = NO	SDiff	K^+ = YES	K^+ = NO	SDiff
	n = 179,436	n = 474,624		n = 179,425	n = 179,425		n = 71,631	n = 243,436		n = 71,631	n = 71,631		n = 101,704	n = 210,460		n = 100,869	n = 100,869	
Glaucoma	14.3%	14.9%	0.02	14.3%	14.3%	<0.01	14.9%	15.4%	0.01	14.9%	14.7%	<0.01	13.8%	14.2%	0.01	13.8%	13.8%	<0.01
Heart failure/ cardiomyopathy	42.2%	39.2%	0.06	42.2%	42.2%	<0.01	37.6%	33.8%	0.08	37.6%	37.3%	<0.01	45.2%	45.1%	<0.01	45.1%	44.7%	<0.01
HIV/AIDS	1.8%	3.1%	0.08	1.8%	1.7%	<0.01	1.8%	3.3%	0.09	1.8%	1.7%	<0.01	1.7%	3.1%	0.09	1.8%	1.7%	<0.01
Hypercholesterolemia	52.9%	50.5%	0.05	52.9%	52.8%	<0.01	53.1%	50.9%	0.04	53.1%	52.7%	<0.01	52.7%	49.8%	0.06	52.5%	52.3%	<0.01
Hyperkalemia	3.9%	7.1%	0.13	3.9%	3.8%	<0.01	3.6%	5.5%	0.09	3.6%	3.5%	<0.01	4.1%	8.7%	0.18	4.1%	3.7%	0.02
Hyperosmolality	1.4%	1.6%	0.02	1.4%	1.3%	<0.01	1.5%	1.5%	<0.01	1.5%	1.5%	<0.01	1.2%	1.6%	0.03	1.3%	1.3%	<0.01
Hypertension	75.3%	74.9%	<0.01	75.3%	75.2%	<0.01	74.0%	73.1%	0.02	74.0%	73.7%	<0.01	76.0%	76.6%	0.01	75.9%	75.6%	<0.01
Hyperthyroidism	5.5%	5.2%	0.01	5.5%	5.5%	<0.01	5.9%	5.5%	0.02	5.9%	5.8%	<0.01	5.2%	4.9%	0.02	5.2%	5.2%	<0.01
Hypokalemia	10.4%	8.3%	0.07	10.4%	10.2%	<0.01	10.3%	7.7%	0.09	10.3%	10.0%	<0.01	10.3%	8.8%	0.05	10.1%	10.0%	<0.01
Hypothyroidism	25.1%	22.6%	0.06	25.1%	25.2%	<0.01	26.3%	23.3%	0.07	26.3%	26.1%	<0.01	24.3%	21.5%	0.07	24.2%	24.1%	<0.01
Kidney disease	24.3%	30.0%	0.13	24.3%	24.1%	<0.01	23.7%	26.3%	0.06	23.7%	23.5%	<0.01	24.5%	33.8%	0.20	24.6%	24.4%	<0.01
Liver disease	17.0%	17.6%	0.02	17.0%	16.9%	<0.01	17.4%	17.3%	<0.01	17.4%	17.2%	<0.01	16.8%	18.0%	0.03	16.8%	16.6%	<0.01
Mg^{2+} metabolism disorder	1.8%	1.8%	<0.01	1.8%	1.7%	<0.01	1.7%	1.6%	0.01	1.7%	1.7%	<0.01	1.7%	2.1%	0.02	1.7%	1.7%	<0.01
Nocturia	2.1%	2.0%	0.01	2.1%	2.2%	<0.01	2.3%	2.2%	0.01	2.3%	2.3%	<0.01	2.0%	1.8%	0.02	2.0%	1.9%	<0.01
Obesity**	18.0%	16.1%	0.05	18.0%	17.9%	<0.01	15.6%	15.3%	<0.01	15.6%	15.6%	<0.01	19.6%	16.9%	0.07	19.4%	19.3%	<0.01
Pulmonary circulation	7.8%	7.0%	0.03	7.8%	7.7%	<0.01	7.0%	6.0%	0.04	7.0%	6.9%	<0.01	8.2%	8.0%	<0.01	8.1%	8.1%	<0.01
Pulmonary congestion and hypostasis/pulmonary edema	11.5%	10.3%	0.04	11.5%	11.5%	<0.01	10.6%	8.8%	0.06	10.6%	10.5%	<0.01	12.0%	12.0%	<0.01	11.9%	11.8%	<0.01
Pyloric stenosis	0.2%	0.2%	<0.01	0.2%	0.2%	<0.01	0.2%	0.2%	<0.01	0.2%	0.2%	<0.01	0.2%	0.2%	<0.01	0.2%	0.2%	<0.01
Rheumatoid arthritis and other inflammatory polyarthropathies	27.8%	25.6%	0.05	27.8%	27.8%	<0.01	28.6%	26.8%	0.04	28.6%	28.3%	<0.01	27.5%	24.2%	0.07	27.3%	27.3%	<0.01
Sickle cell disease	0.2%	0.2%	0.01	0.2%	0.2%	<0.01	0.2%	0.3%	0.02	0.2%	0.2%	<0.01	0.2%	0.2%	0.02	0.2%	0.2%	<0.01
Smoking, tobacco**	15.0%	12.4%	0.08	15.0%	14.9%	<0.01	14.6%	12.3%	0.07	14.6%	14.8%	<0.01	15.4%	12.6%	0.08	15.2%	14.8%	<0.01
Substance abuse**	5.6%	6.2%	0.03	5.6%	5.5%	<0.01	5.4%	6.2%	0.03	5.4%	5.4%	<0.01	5.8%	6.3%	0.02	5.8%	5.6%	<0.01
Systemic lupus erythematosus	1.3%	1.3%	<0.01	1.3%	1.3%	<0.01	1.2%	1.3%	<0.01	1.2%	1.2%	<0.01	1.3%	1.4%	<0.01	1.3%	1.2%	<0.01
Uropathy, obstructive	0.1%	0.1%	<0.01	0.1%	0.1%	<0.01	0.1%	0.1%	<0.01	0.1%	0.1%	<0.01	0.1%	0.1%	<0.01	0.1%	0.1%	<0.01
Valvular heart disease	28.5%	24.4%	0.09	28.4%	28.4%	<0.01	27.4%	22.9%	0.10	27.4%	27.4%	<0.01	28.9%	25.8%	0.07	28.6%	28.4%	<0.01
DRUGS MARKER OF CHRONIC DISEASE, EVER PRIOR TO INITIAL LOOP COURSE																		

Table 1. Cont.

	OVERALL LOOP DIURETIC COHORT						FUROSEMIDE <40 MG/DAY COHORT						FUROSEMIDE ≥40 MG/DAY COHORT					
	Before PS Matching			After 1-to-1 PS Matching			Before PS Matching			After 1-to-1 PS Matching			Before PS Matching			After 1-to-1 PS Matching		
Covariate	K^+=YES	K^+=NO	SDiff	K^+=YES	K^+=NO	SDiff	K^+=YES	K^+=NO	SDiff	K^+=YES	K^+=NO	SDiff	K^+=YES	K^+=NO	SDiff	K^+=YES	K^+=NO	SDiff
	n = 179,436	n = 474,624		n = 179,425	n = 179,425		n = 71,631	n = 243,436		n = 71,631	n = 71,631		n = 101,704	n = 210,460		n = 100,869	n = 100,869	
ACEIs/ATIIRBs	43.4%	47.1%	0.07	43.4%	43.4%	<0.01	43.0%	47.0%	0.08	43.0%	42.9%	<0.01	44.2%	47.7%	0.07	44.2%	44.0%	<0.01
Adrenergic bronchodilators	33.6%	30.5%	0.07	33.6%	33.4%	<0.01	34.8%	32.6%	0.05	34.8%	34.8%	<0.01	33.1%	28.4%	0.10	32.8%	32.5%	<0.01
Anorexiants/ antiobesity agents	0.4%	0.3%	0.02	0.4%	0.4%	<0.01	0.3%	0.3%	0.01	0.3%	0.3%	<0.01	0.4%	0.2%	0.03	0.4%	0.4%	<0.01
Antiadrenergic agents	6.6%	7.5%	0.04	6.6%	6.5%	<0.01	6.4%	6.8%	0.02	6.4%	6.2%	<0.01	6.8%	8.5%	0.06	6.9%	6.7%	<0.01
Antiarrhythmics, type I, except lidocaine and phenytoin	0.7%	0.6%	0.02	0.7%	0.7%	<0.01	0.8%	0.6%	0.02	0.8%	0.8%	<0.01	0.7%	0.6%	0.01	0.7%	0.7%	<0.01
Antiarrhythmics, type III	2.0%	1.8%	0.02	2.0%	2.1%	<0.01	2.0%	1.7%	0.02	2.0%	2.0%	<0.01	2.1%	1.9%	0.01	2.1%	2.1%	<0.01
Antidiabetics	27.5%	30.9%	0.07	27.5%	27.6%	<0.01	25.7%	29.3%	0.08	25.7%	25.6%	<0.01	28.9%	33.0%	0.09	29.0%	29.0%	<0.01
Antiglaucoma agents, ophthalmic	7.2%	7.6%	0.01	7.2%	7.2%	<0.01	7.7%	8.0%	<0.01	7.7%	7.6%	<0.01	6.8%	7.1%	0.01	6.9%	6.7%	<0.01
Antiglaucoma agents, oral	0.5%	0.6%	<0.01	0.5%	0.5%	<0.01	0.5%	0.6%	<0.01	0.5%	0.5%	<0.01	0.5%	0.5%	<0.01	0.5%	0.5%	<0.01
Antihyperlipidemics	34.6%	35.1%	0.01	34.6%	34.5%	<0.01	35.4%	36.4%	0.02	35.4%	35.2%	<0.01	34.3%	33.9%	<0.01	34.2%	34.1%	<0.01
Antiretrovirals	0.8%	1.3%	0.05	0.8%	0.7%	<0.01	0.8%	1.3%	0.05	0.8%	0.7%	<0.01	0.8%	1.3%	0.05	0.8%	0.7%	<0.01
Beta blockers, systemic	30.4%	31.5%	0.02	30.4%	30.3%	<0.01	31.5%	32.3%	0.02	31.5%	31.5%	<0.01	29.9%	30.9%	0.02	29.9%	29.7%	<0.01
Bisphosphonates	11.0%	9.9%	0.04	11.0%	10.9%	<0.01	13.4%	11.7%	0.05	13.4%	13.2%	<0.01	9.3%	7.8%	0.05	9.3%	9.2%	<0.01
Calcium channel blockers, non-verapamil	31.9%	33.7%	0.04	31.9%	31.6%	<0.01	32.2%	33.5%	0.03	32.2%	31.9%	<0.01	32.0%	34.3%	0.05	32.0%	31.5%	0.01
Calcium channel blocker, verapamil	4.9%	4.6%	0.02	4.9%	4.9%	<0.01	4.8%	4.6%	0.01	4.8%	4.7%	<0.01	5.0%	4.5%	0.02	4.9%	4.9%	<0.01
Corticosteroids, inhaled	15.8%	14.1%	0.05	15.8%	15.7%	<0.01	16.4%	15.2%	0.03	16.4%	16.3%	<0.01	15.5%	13.0%	0.07	15.4%	15.2%	<0.01
Corticosteroids, oral	22.2%	20.1%	0.05	22.2%	22.0%	<0.01	23.4%	21.7%	0.04	23.4%	23.3%	<0.01	21.5%	18.3%	0.08	21.3%	20.9%	<0.01
Digoxin	7.1%	6.4%	0.03	7.1%	7.1%	<0.01	7.3%	6.2%	0.05	7.3%	7.3%	<0.01	7.0%	6.8%	0.01	7.0%	7.0%	<0.01
Diuretics, thiazides*	32.6%	31.0%	—	32.6%	30.1%	—	32.3%	31.7%	—	32.3%	30.5%	—	33.1%	30.2%	—	33.1%	30.2%	—
Immunosuppressives	0.4%	1.1%	0.07	0.4%	0.4%	0.01	0.4%	0.8%	0.05	0.4%	0.4%	<0.01	0.4%	1.4%	0.09	0.4%	0.4%	<0.01
Nitrates	19.9%	18.2%	0.05	19.9%	19.9%	<0.01	20.1%	18.4%	0.04	20.1%	20.0%	<0.01	20.0%	18.0%	0.05	19.8%	19.8%	<0.01
Thyroid hormones	11.3%	10.8%	0.02	11.3%	11.3%	<0.01	12.3%	11.5%	0.03	12.3%	12.3%	<0.01	10.7%	9.9%	0.03	10.6%	10.6%	<0.01
Vasodilators, non-nitrates	0.9%	1.6%	0.06	0.9%	0.9%	<0.01	0.8%	1.1%	0.03	0.8%	0.8%	<0.01	1.0%	2.2%	0.09	1.0%	0.9%	0.01

Table 1. Cont.

Covariate	OVERALL LOOP DIURETIC COHORT						FUROSEMIDE <40 MG/DAY COHORT						FUROSEMIDE ≥40 MG/DAY COHORT					
	Before PS Matching			After 1-to-1 PS Matching			Before PS Matching			After 1-to-1 PS Matching			Before PS Matching			After 1-to-1 PS Matching		
	K^+ = YES	K^+ = NO	SDiff	K^+ = YES	K^+ = NO	SDiff	K^+ = YES	K^+ = NO	SDiff	K^+ = YES	K^+ = NO	SDiff	K^+ = YES	K^+ = NO	SDiff	K^+ = YES	K^+ = NO	SDiff
	n = 179,436	n = 474,624		n = 179,425	n = 179,425		n = 71,631	n = 243,436		n = 71,631	n = 71,631		n = 101,704	n = 210,460		n = 100,869	n = 100,869	
Warfarin	8.2%	7.8%	0.01	8.2%	8.2%	<0.01	8.1%	7.6%	0.02	8.1%	8.1%	<0.01	8.2%	8.0%	<0.01	8.2%	8.2%	<0.01
Xanthine derivatives	4.9%	3.9%	0.05	4.9%	4.8%	<0.01	4.9%	4.1%	0.04	4.9%	4.9%	<0.01	4.9%	3.7%	0.06	4.8%	4.7%	<0.01

* not included in the propensity score.
** health-related behavior or state ascertained via diagnostic codes alone.
PS: propensity score; K^+: empiric potassium supplementation; SDiff: standardized difference; IQR = interquartile range; COPD: chronic obstructive pulmonary disease; HIV: human immunodeficiency virus; AIDS: acquired immunodeficiency syndrome; Mg^{2+}: magnesium; ACEIs: angiotensin-converting enzyme inhibitors; ATIIRBs: angiotensin-II receptor blocker.

30 days following the loop course; and initial empiric potassium dose. The potassium laboratory monitoring subgroup analysis excluded deaths occurring in the first 30 days in order to minimize immortal time bias. Analyses were conducted using SAS v9.3 (SAS Institute Inc.: Cary, NC).

Results

Cohort composition

We identified 654,060 persons who met eligibility criteria and initiated therapy with a loop diuretic (Table 1). Greater than 70% were female and about 50% were white; the mean age of these individuals was about 65 years. Within this cohort, 27% received empiric potassium supplementation (N = 179,436) and 73% did not (N = 474,624). The proportions of persons receiving empiric potassium supplementation differed between users of furosemide <40 mg/day and ≥40 mg/day, at 23% and 33% respectively. The proportion of follow-up days covered by an active potassium prescription was 0.849 in the empiric supplementation group and 0.079 in the reference group.

When comparing users of loop diuretics at any dose by exposure status, only three measured baseline factors were potentially unevenly distributed—prior history of: asthma/chronic obstructive pulmonary disease; hyperkalemia; and kidney disease. We found an acceptable match for all but 11 potassium-exposed persons (N = 179,425) and therefore the underlying study cohort consisted of 358,850 loop users—164,833 in the furosemide < 40 mg/day cohort and 179,439 in the furosemide ≥40 mg/day cohort. After propensity score matching, all of the standardized mean differences were <0.02 (Table 1), suggesting that propensity score matching resulted in very similar distributions of measured covariates by exposure group.

Primary outcome: all-cause death

In the overall loop user cohort, we identified 31,653 deaths for a mortality rate of 90.7 per 1,000 p-y (95% CI: 89.7 to 91.7). Mortality rates were 88.5 (95% CI: 87.0 to 89.9) and 91.6 (95% CI: 90.2 to 93.1) per 1,000 p-y in furosemide <40 mg/day and ≥40 mg/day cohorts respectively. The overall crude and matched HRs for empiric potassium supplementation and all-cause death were 1.02 (95% CI: 0.99 to 1.06, $p = 0.189$) and 0.93 (95% CI: 0.89 to 0.98, $p = 0.003$), respectively. Among those whose initial furosemide dose was <40 mg/day, the crude and matched HRs for empiric potassium supplementation were 1.12 (95% CI: 1.07 to 1.18, $p < 0.0001$) and 0.93 (95% CI: 0.86 to 1.00, $p = 0.050$), respectively. Among those whose initial furosemide dose was ≥40 mg/day, the crude and matched HRs for empiric potassium were 0.93 (95% CI: 0.89 to 0.97, $p = 0.002$) and 0.84 (95% CI: 0.79 to 0.89, $p < 0.0001$), respectively. The time-to-event curves, in the matched cohorts, for receiving potassium supplementation vs. not in those whose initial furosemide dose was ≥40 mg/day began to diverge during the first year; see Figure 1.

To further examine whether the apparent benefit of potassium increased monotonically with furosemide dose, we separately calculated matched HRs for empiric potassium in those whose initial furosemide dose was exactly 40 mg/day and >40 mg/day, yielding matched HRs of 0.84 (95% CI: 0.78 to 0.90, $p < 0.0001$) and 0.83 (95% CI: 0.74 to 0.93, $p = 0.001$) respectively. Thus, monotonicity was observed across three levels (<40, = 40, and > 40 mg) of daily furosemide dose.

Figure 2 shows the results of subgroup analyses stratified on initial furosemide dose. Of note, for the subgroup analyses of age, arrhythmia/conduction disorder, kidney disease, and potassium

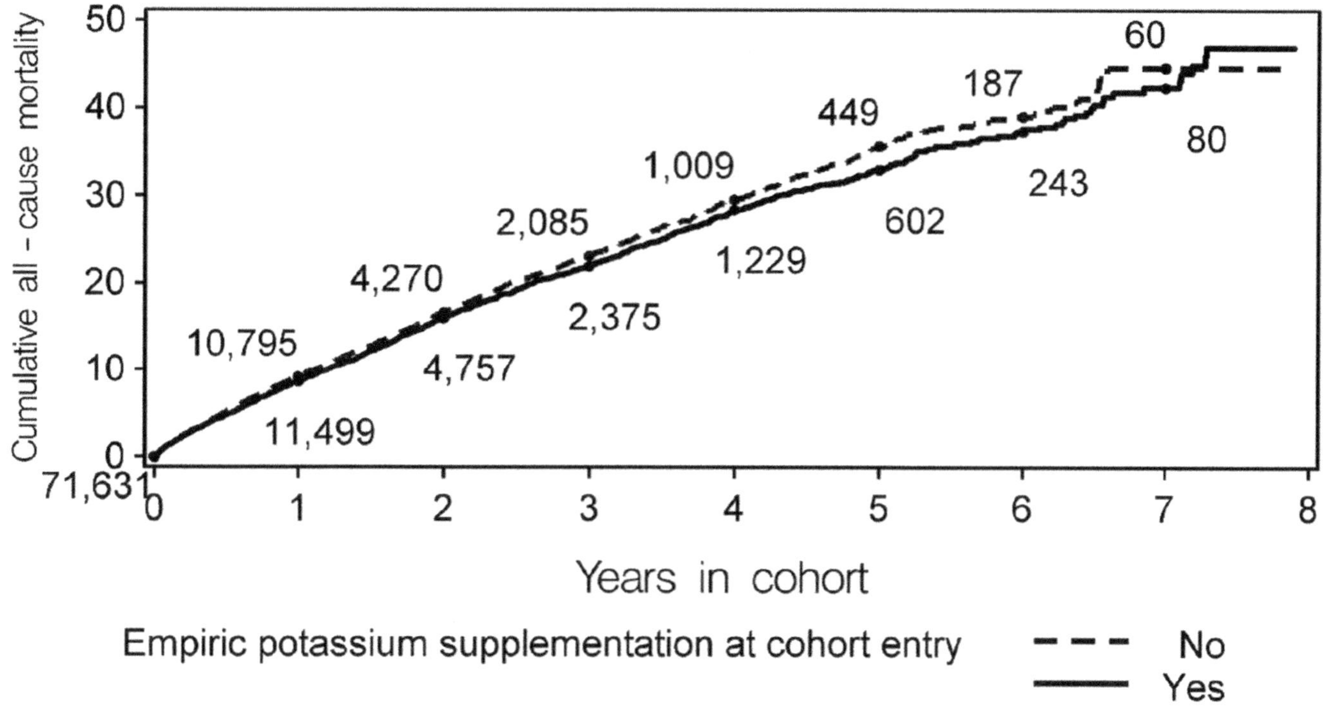

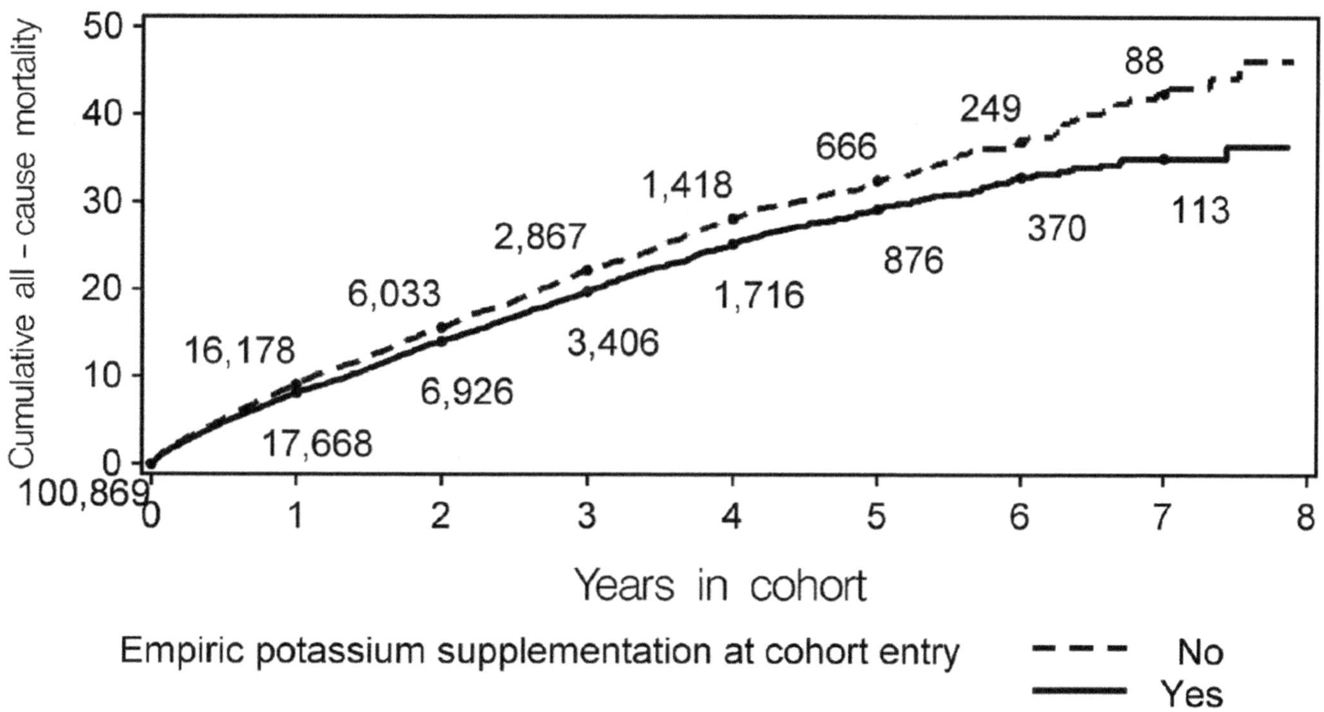

Figure 1. Time-to-death curves for empiric potassium supplementation among furosemide initiators, stratified by initial furosemide dose. Figure 1a. Initial furosemide dose <40 mg/day (N = 71,631 in each of the empiric potassium exposed and unexposed groups). Figure 1b. Initial furosemide dose ≥40 mg/day (N = 100,869 in each of the empiric potassium exposed and unexposed groups).

laboratory monitoring, all of the standardized mean differences for covariates by exposure status were <0.10 after propensity score matching (data not shown). For the subgroup analysis examining potassium dose, while the vast majority of post-propensity score matching standardized mean differences were <0.10, the maximum was 0.20 (see Appendix S1).

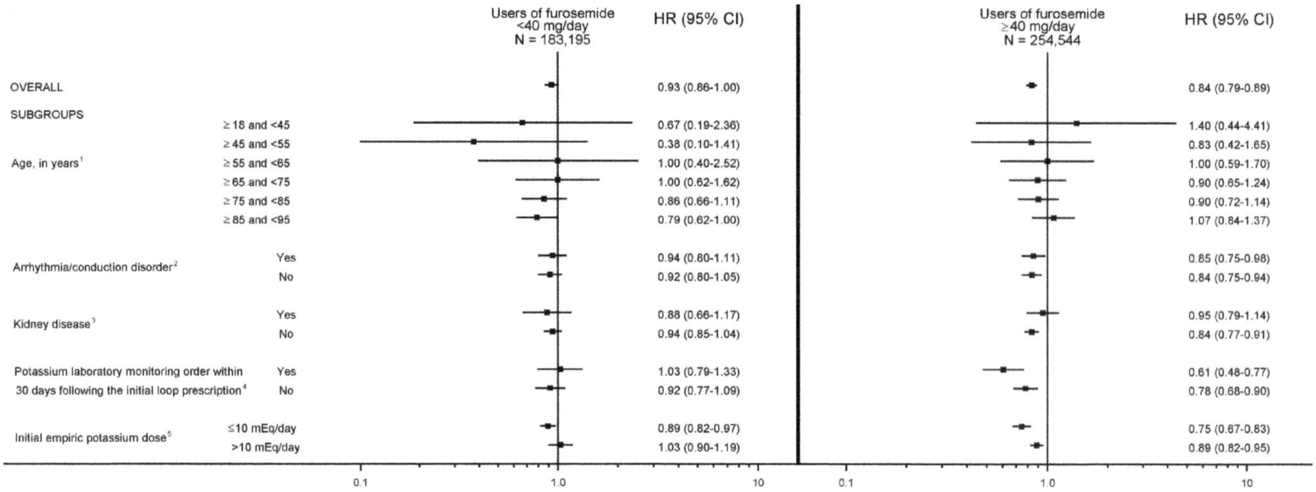

Figure 2. Risk of death for empiric potassium supplementation vs. no empiric potassium supplementation among furosemide initiators: propensity score-matched analyses examining patient subgroups. HR = hazard ratio; CI = confidence interval. p-values for the difference in effect estimates within stratum, in users of furosemide <40 mg/day and in users of furosemide ≥40 mg/day. 1, p = 0.86 and p = 0.24, respectively. 2, p = 0.75 and p = 0.81, respectively. 3, p = 0.66 and p = 0.49, respectively. 4, p = 0.74 and p = 0.37, respectively. 5, p = 0.08 and p<0.01, respectively.

A statistically significant difference in the association between empiric potassium supplementation and death was observed in the underlying cohort of furosemide ≥40 mg/day users within the following subgroup: initial empiric potassium dose ≤10 mEq/day vs. >10 mEq/day (HRs = 0.75 vs. 0.89, p-value for difference < 0.01).

Secondary outcome: sudden cardiac death/ventricular arrhythmia

Among 629,949 incident courses of loop diuretic use, we identified 1,470 incident occurrences of SD/VA for an incidence rate of 4.5 per 1,000 p-y (95% CI: 4.2 to 4.7) within the overall loop user cohort. The overall crude and matched HRs for empiric potassium supplementation and SD/VA were 1.13 (95% CI: 1.01 to 1.26, p = 0.030) and 1.02 (95% CI: 0.83 to 1.24, p = 0.879), respectively.

Discussion

In new initiators of loop diuretics, empiric potassium supplementation was associated with a reduction in all-cause mortality. The relative reduction was 7% and at the threshold for statistical significance (p = 0.05) in those whose initial furosemide dose was <40 mg/day, and 16% and statistically significant in those whose initial furosemide dose was ≥40 mg/day. Monotonicity was observed across three levels of furosemide dose, and the apparent benefit of potassium in persons receiving ≥40 mg/day of furosemide was observable within the first year. Taken together, these results suggest that empiric potassium supplementation may be associated with improved survival in those receiving a loop diuretic, and that the degree of benefit increases with diuretic dose. Given that mortality was about 9% per year in this cohort, the magnitude of the absolute benefit is substantial, especially in those receiving higher doses of furosemide. The estimated number of patients needed to be empirically-supplemented with potassium (i.e., number needed to treat) [20] to prevent one death within the first year after initiating furosemide <40 mg/day, = 40 mg/day, and >40 mg/day is 164, 72, and 67, respectively.

In a subgroup analysis of persons with no history of kidney disease receiving ≥40 mg/day of furosemide, empiric potassium supplementation was associated with a 16% reduction in death, an association not evident among persons with existing kidney disease. The latter is not surprising, given that persons with renal impairment may be at increased risk for hyperkalemia, which may negate potassium's otherwise beneficial effect [21,22]. Further, a 25% reduction in mortality among users of furosemide ≥40 mg/day was limited to persons receiving empiric potassium doses of ≤ 10 mEq/day. Whether this is indicative of the optimal dosage range of empiric potassium supplementation or due to confounding (i.e., because propensity score matching was not designed to balance covariates between potassium dose strata) deserves further elucidation.

To our knowledge, this is the first study designed to examine the association between empiric potassium supplementation and rates of clinical outcomes in new initiators of loop diuretics. Earlier studies have found no effect of potassium supplementation on the risk of either laboratory-defined hypokalemia or clinical outcomes [23–25], but these studies examined either thiazide users alone or included together with users of loop diuretics. An additional study examined clinical outcomes associated with baseline potassium use in patients with heart failure [26], but included patients receiving and not receiving diuretics, did not begin follow-up with the initiation of a diuretic, and did not stratify on diuretic dose.

Given that one major mechanism by which potassium may improve survival is reduction in the risk of serious ventricular arrhythmia caused by potassium depletion, it was surprising that potassium did not appear to reduce the risk of SD/VA. However, our finding is consistent with a retrospective analysis of trial data [27] in which potassium supplementation did not affect the incidence of arrhythmic death (p = 0.4) among persons with left ventricular dysfunction [28].

Strengths of this study include its large sample size, unambiguous primary outcome measure, similarity of compared groups even before matching, restriction to new starters of loop diuretics, examination of empiric rather than reactive potassium supplementation, and stratification by furosemide dose.

This study has limitations. First, because of the design, the effect of reactive potassium supplementation was not examined. Second, despite our demonstration of covariate balance between the exposure groups both pre- and post-propensity score adjustment, there exists the potential for residual confounding by unmeasured or poorly-measured variables and/or behaviors. In particular, it is possible that persons with mild renal insufficiency may be channeled away from potassium supplementation and may be at higher risk for death than baseline. Arguing against this possibility are findings that mild-to-moderate renal insufficiency may not be an independent risk factor for death [29,30]. Regardless, we controlled for the presence of diagnosed chronic kidney disease, codes for which may have a sensitivity as high as 80% [19]. Third, we were unable to capture magnesium supplement exposures due to their typical use over-the-counter. An additional limitation includes the potential insensitivity of the SD/VA diagnoses and wide confidence intervals in subgroup analyses.

In conclusion, this study provides evidence that the strategy of initiating potassium supplementation together with loop diuretic therapy appears to be associated with increased survival, and that the degree of benefit increases with increasing diuretic dose. Because of the importance of this question, these results deserve to be replicated.

Supporting Information

Appendix S1 Baseline characteristics of beneficiaries in the subgroup analysis examining potassium supplementation dose and all-cause death, before and after propensity score matching on potassium exposure status.

Acknowledgments

Hanieh Razzaghi and Cristin P. Freeman contributed to this research while employed by the University of Pennsylvania; they have since left the institution. The authors wish to thank Brian L. Strom (Rutgers, The State University of New Jersey), Geralyn Barosso (University of Minnesota), Qing Liu (University of Pennsylvania), Daohang Sha (University of Pennsylvania), and Qufei Wu (University of Pennsylvania) for their assistance and guidance. A portion of the research described herein was presented, in abstract form, at the 27th International Conference on Pharmacoepidemiology & Therapeutic Risk Management; August 17, 2011; Chicago, Illinois, United States.

Author Contributions

Conceived and designed the experiments: CL JR SH. Performed the experiments: CL HR CF JR CN SH. Analyzed the data: CL JR CN SH. Contributed reagents/materials/analysis tools: JR CN. Wrote the paper: CL HR CF JR CN SH.

References

1. Sica DA, Carter B, Cushman W, Hamm L (2011) Thiazide and loop diuretics. J Clin Hypertens (Greenwich) 13(9):639–643. PubMed: 21896142.
2. van Kraaij DJ, Jansen RW, Gribnau FW, Hoefnagels WH (1998) Loop diuretics in patients aged 75 years or older: general practitioners' assessment of indications and possibilities for withdrawal. Eur J Clin Pharmacol 54(4):323–327. PubMed: 9696957.
3. Sica DA (2004) Diuretic-related side effects: Development and treatment. J Clin Hypertens (Greenwich) 6(9):532–540. PubMed: 15365284.
4. MacMahon S, Collins G, Rautaharju P, Cutler J, Neaton J, et al. (1989) Electrocardiographic left ventricular hypertrophy and effects of antihypertensive drug therapy in hypertensive participants in the Multiple Risk Factor Intervention Trial. Am J Cardiol 63(3):202–210. PubMed: 2521269.
5. Holland OB, Nixon JV, Kuhnert L (1981) Diuretic-induced ventricular ectopic activity. Am J Med 70(4):762–768. PubMed: 7211912.
6. Cohn JN, Kowey PR, Whelton PK, Prisant LM (2000) New guidelines for potassium replacement in clinical practice: A contemporary review by the national council on potassium in clinical practice. Arch Intern Med 160(16):2429–2436. PubMed: 10979053.
7. Rose BD (2012) Diuretic-induced hypokalemia. UpToDate Topic 2355: Version 4.0. http://web.archive.org/web/20120927044502/http://www.uptodate.com/contents/diuretic-induced-hypokalemia. Literature review current through: 10/2012. Last updated: 05/10/2010. Last accessed: 04/03/2014.
8. Hennessy S, Carson JL, Ray WA, Strom BL (2005) Medicaid databases. In: Strom BL, ed. Pharmacoepidemiology. 4th ed. Sussex: John Wiley.
9. Kaiser Family Foundation (2011) Medicaid enrollment: June 2010 data snapshot. Publication #8050-03. kaiserfamilyfoundation.files.wordpress.com/2013/01/8050-03.pdf. Last accessed: 04/02/2014.
10. Holahan J, Ghosh A (2005) Dual eligibles: Medicaid enrollment and spending for Medicare beneficiaries in 2003. Kaiser Family Foundation. Publication #7346: 1–24. http://www.kff.org/medicaid/7346.cfm. Last accessed: 04/02/2014.
11. Holahan J, Miller DM, Rousseau D (2009) Dual eligibles: Medicaid enrollment and spending for Medicare beneficiaries in 2005. Kaiser Family Foundation. Publication #7846: 1–17. http://web.archive.org/web/20110608201215/http://www.kff.org/medicaid/upload/7846.pdf. Last accessed: 04/03/2014.
12. Rousseau D, Clemans-Cope L, Lawton E, Langston J, Connolly J, et al. (2010) Dual eligibles: Medicaid enrollment and spending for Medicare beneficiaries in 2007. Kaiser Family Foundation. Publication #7846-02: 1–17. http://www.ncbi.nlm.nih.gov/nlmcatalog/101560987. Last accessed: 04/02/2014.
13. Austin PC (2011) Optimal caliper widths for propensity-score matching when estimating differences in means and differences in proportions in observational studies. Pharm Stat 10(2):150–161. PubMed: 20925139.
14. Ruppert D, Wand M, Carroll R (2003) Semiparametric Regression. Cambridge: The Press Syndicate of the University of Cambridge.
15. Abildstrom SZ, Køber L, Torp-Pedersen C (1999) Epidemiology of arrhythmic and sudden death in the chronic phase of ischemic heart disease. Card Electrophysiol Rev 3(3):177–179. doi: 10.1023/A:1009971104937.
16. Hennessy S, Leonard CE, Freeman CP, Deo R, Newcomb C, et al. (2010) Validation of diagnostic codes for outpatient-originating sudden cardiac death and ventricular arrhythmia in Medicaid and Medicare claims data. Pharmacoepidemiol Drug Saf 19(6):555–562. PubMed: 19844945.
17. Leonard CE, Freeman CP, Deo R, Newcomb C, Kimmel SE, et al. (2010) Response to commentary entitled "commentary on the validation studies of sudden cardiac death and ventricular arrhythmia by Hennessy et al. and Chung et al.". Pharmacoepidemiol Drug Saf 19(6):576–576. In PubMed: 20087851.
18. Normand ST, Landrum MB, Guadagnoli E, Ayanian JZ, Ryan TJ, et al. (2001) Validating recommendations for coronary angiography following acute myocardial infarction in the elderly: a matched analysis using propensity scores. J Clin Epidemiol 54(4):387–398. PubMed: 11297888.
19. Grams ME, Plantinga LC, Hedgeman E, Saran R, Myers GL, et al. (2011) Validation of CKD and related conditions in existing data sets: A systematic review. Am J Kidney Dis 57(1):44–54. PubMed: 20692079.
20. Altman DG, Andersen PK (1999) Calculating the number needed to treat for trials where the outcome is time to an event. BMJ 319(7223):1492–1495. PubMed: 10582940.
21. Henz S, Maeder MT, Huber S, Schmid M, Loher M, et al. (2008) Influence of drugs and comorbidity on serum potassium in 15 000 consecutive hospital admissions. Nephrol Dial Transplant 23(12):3939–3945. PubMed: 18614817.
22. Ahmed MI, Ekundayo OJ, Mujib M, Campbell RC, Sanders PW, et al. (2010) Mild hyperkalemia and outcomes in chronic heart failure: a propensity matched study. Int J Cardiol 144(3):383–388. PubMed: 19500863.
23. Green DM, Ropper AH, Kronmal RA, Psaty BM, Burke GL, et al. (2002) Serum potassium level and dietary potassium intake as risk factors for stroke. Neurology 59(3):314–320. PubMed: 12177362.
24. Siscovick DS, Raghunathan TE, Psaty BM, Koepsell TD, Wicklund KG, et al. (1994) Diuretic therapy for hypertension and the risk of primary cardiac arrest. N Engl J Med 330(26):1852–1857. PubMed: 8196728.
25. Siegel D, Hulley SB, Black DM, Cheitlin MD, Sebastian A, et al. (1992) Diuretics, serum and intracellular electrolyte levels, and ventricular arrhythmias in hypertensive men. JAMA 267(8):1083–1089. PubMed: 1735925.
26. Ekundayo OJ, Adamopoulos C, Ahmed MI, Pitt B, Young JB, et al. (2010) Oral potassium supplement use and outcomes in chronic heart failure: A propensity-matched study. Int J Cardiol 141(2):167–174. PubMed: 19135741.
27. The SOLVD Investigators (1990) Studies of left ventricular dysfunction (SOLVD)–rationale, design, and methods: 2 trials that evaluate the effect of enalapril in patients with reduced ejection fraction. Am J Cardiol 66(3):315–322. PubMed: 2195865.
28. Cooper HA, Dries DA, Davis CE, Shen YL, Domanski MJ (1999) Diuretics and risk of arrhythmic death in patients with left ventricular dysfunction. Circulation 100(12):1311–1315. PubMed: 10491376.
29. Garg AX, Clark WF, Haynes RB, House AA (2002) Moderate renal insufficiency and the risk of cardiovascular mortality: results from the NHANES I. Kidney Int 61(4):1486–1494. PubMed: 11918756.
30. Culleton BF, Larson MG, Wilson PW, Evans JC, Parfrey PS, et al. (1999) Cardiovascular disease and mortality in a community-based cohort with mild renal insufficiency. Kidney Int 56(6):2214–2219. PubMed: 10594797.

14

Cholinergic Signaling Exerts Protective Effects in Models of Sympathetic Hyperactivity-Induced Cardiac Dysfunction

Mariana Gavioli[1], Aline Lara[1], Pedro W. M. Almeida[1], Augusto Martins Lima[1,4], Denis D. Damasceno[1], Cibele Rocha-Resende[1], Marina Ladeira[1], Rodrigo R. Resende[2], Patricia M. Martinelli[3], Marcos Barrouin Melo[1,4], Patricia C. Brum[5], Marco Antonio Peliky Fontes[1,4], Robson A. Souza Santos[1,4], Marco A. M. Prado[6], Silvia Guatimosim[1,4]*

1 Department of Physiology and Biophysics, Institute of Biological Sciences, Universidade Federal de Minas Gerais, Belo Horizonte, Brazil, **2** Department of Biochemistry, Institute of Biological Sciences, Universidade Federal de Minas Gerais, Belo Horizonte, Brazil, **3** Department of Morphology, Institute of Biological Sciences, Universidade Federal de Minas Gerais, Belo Horizonte, Brazil, **4** National Institute of Science and Technology in Nanobiopharmaceutics, Universidade Federal de Minas Gerais, Belo Horizonte, MG, Brazil, **5** School of Physical Education and Sport, Universidade de São Paulo, São Paulo, Brazil, **6** Robarts Research Institute, University of Western Ontario, Department of Physiology and Pharmacology, Department of Anatomy & Cell Biology, Schulich School of Medicine & Dentistry, University of Western Ontario, London, Canada

Abstract

Cholinergic control of the heart is exerted by two distinct branches; the autonomic component represented by the parasympathetic nervous system, and the recently described non-neuronal cardiomyocyte cholinergic machinery. Previous evidence has shown that reduced cholinergic function leads to deleterious effects on the myocardium. Yet, whether conditions of increased cholinergic signaling can offset the pathological remodeling induced by sympathetic hyperactivity, and its consequences for these two cholinergic axes are unknown. Here, we investigated two models of sympathetic hyperactivity: i) the chronic beta-adrenergic receptor stimulation evoked by isoproterenol (ISO), and ii) the α_{2A}/α_{2C}-adrenergic receptor knockout (KO) mice that lack pre-synaptic adrenergic receptors. In both models, cholinergic signaling was increased by administration of the cholinesterase inhibitor, pyridostigmine. First, we observed that isoproterenol produces an autonomic imbalance characterized by increased sympathetic and reduced parasympathetic tone. Under this condition transcripts for cholinergic proteins were upregulated in ventricular myocytes, indicating that non-neuronal cholinergic machinery is activated during adrenergic overdrive. Pyridostigmine treatment prevented the effects of ISO on autonomic function and on the ventricular cholinergic machinery, and inhibited cardiac remodeling. α_{2A}/α_{2C}-KO mice presented reduced ventricular contraction when compared to wild-type mice, and this dysfunction was also reversed by cholinesterase inhibition. Thus, the cardiac parasympathetic system and non-neuronal cardiomyocyte cholinergic machinery are modulated in opposite directions under conditions of increased sympathetic drive or ACh availability. Moreover, our data support the idea that pyridostigmine by restoring ACh availability is beneficial in heart disease.

Editor: Andrea Barbuti, University of Milan, Italy

Funding: This work was supported by grants from NIH R03TW008425 from the Fogarty International Center (Guatimosim S), Conselho Nacional de Desenvolvimento Científico e Tecnológico (CNPq), Fundação de Amparo à Pesquisa do Estado de Minas Gerais, PRONEX (APQ-04334-10) and National Institute of Science and Technology in Nanobiopharmaceutics. MAMP is supported by the Heart and Stroke Foundation of Ontario (Grant-in aid NA6656). Gavioli, M is recipient of CNPq PhD fellowship at the Post-graduation Program in Biological Science: Physiology and Pharmacology at UFMG. The funders had no role in the study design, data collection and analysis, decision to publish, or preparation of the manuscript.

Competing Interests: The authors have declared that no competing interests exist.

* Email: guatimosim@icb.ufmg.br

Introduction

A substantial amount of data suggests that sympathetic regulation of heart function, via adrenergic receptors, contributes to cardiac remodeling and provides a major pathway for intervention in heart failure (HF) [1], [2], [3]. In contrast, the precise mechanisms required for long-term cholinergic regulation of heart function are only now started to be dissected. Acetylcholine (ACh) is synthesized in the cytoplasm by choline acetyltransferase (ChAT) and stored within vesicles for release. Activity-coupled transport of ACh to synaptic vesicles in nerve-endings is mediated by the vesicular ACh transporter (VAChT) [4], [5]. All ACh released is degraded by cholinesterases mainly, acetylcholinesterase (AChE), to form choline and acetate. Choline is then transported into the cell by the high affinity choline-transporter (CHT1). Cardiac regulation by the parasympathetic nervous system is mediated primarily by ACh binding to the M_2 muscarinic ACh receptor (M_2-AChR). Previous studies demonstrated that M_2-AChR knockout (KO) mice exhibited increased susceptibility to cardiac stress [6], suggesting a protective role for the parasympathetic nervous system in the heart. In line with this finding, vagal stimulation has been shown to be of benefit in heart failure [7]. Mice with reduced expression of the VAChT (VAChT knockdown homozygous mice, VAChT KD^{HOM} mice) [5] have been generated and were pivotal in demonstrating a role for VAChT in sustaining cholinergic tone *in vivo*. These mutant mice express only 30% of the normal level of VAChT, and present a number of cholinergic deficits. Our previous publication has shown that chronic decrease of cholinergic tone in VAChT KD^{HOM} mice evoked significant cardiac remodeling characterized by depressed contractile function, calcium (Ca^{2+}) signaling dysfunction and altered gene expression in cardiomyocytes [8]. Importantly, these changes were reversed by chronic administration of pyridostigmine, a cholinesterase inhibitor, indicating an important relationship between ACh availability and proper heart function. Altogether, these results support the broad theme that reduced cholinergic function can lead to deleterious effects on the myocardium, and support the notion that increased parasympathetic tone can exert protective effects. In fact, infusion with the cholinesterase inhibitor, neostigmine or with a muscarine receptor agonist, pilocarpine significantly reduced cardiac hypertrophy, reduced TNF alpha levels, elevated interleukin-10 in heart tissues, and improved ventricular function in rats with transverse aortic constriction [9]. Similar cardioprotective effects were observed when another cholinesterase inhibitor, donepezil, was administered to a rat model of myocardial infarction [10] and to a murine model of volume-overloaded congestive heart failure [11]. In addition, previous data from Kanazawa *et al.* [12] have provided evidence that cholinergic transdifferentiation of sympathetic neurons takes place during heart failure and this plays a protective role in the pathogenesis of heart disease. Finally, recent epidemiological data indicate that the use of cholinesterase inhibitors in Alzheimer's disease associates with 34% reduced risk of myocardial infarction and death [13].

Recently, an intrinsic cardiomyocyte cholinergic system has been described [14], [15], [16] supporting the assumption of local ACh release by ventricular myocytes in the heart. Our group has investigated the importance of this local cholinergic machinery, and presented evidence that ACh released by cardiomyocytes is capable of offsetting the deleterious effects of hyperadrenergic stimulation *in vitro* [16]. In addition, removal of VAChT or ChAT exclusively from cardiomyocytes leads to increased levels of oxidative stress and cardiac hypertrophy [17]. Thus, these data bring into perspective another level of cholinergic control of cardiac function that goes beyond the cardiac parasympathetic system, and it is intrinsic to ventricular myocytes. Yet, whether this machinery is regulated *in vivo*, and its relationship with parasympathetic activity is unknown.

In this study, our goal was twofold: (i) to assess the consequences of increased adrenergic and cholinergic signaling for the heart and its influence on autonomic function and in the expression levels of cholinergic and adrenergic components in ventricular myocytes, and (ii) to investigate whether activation of cholinergic signaling is capable of offsetting the deleterious effects of increased sympathetic drive *in vivo*. Here, we show that upregulation of non-neuronal cholinergic machinery in the heart is observed under conditions of increased sympathetic drive and reduced parasympathetic tone. When ACh availability is increased by pyridostigmine administration cardiac pathological remodeling is prevented and ventricular function is restored in two animal models of sympathetic hyperactivity. Thus, our data indicate that cholinergic signaling might be an important target in heart failure.

Methods

Animal models and drug administration

34 Male Wistar rats (250 g) were used in this study. Cardiac hypertrophy was induced by daily intraperitoneal injection of (±) isoproterenol hydrochloride for seven days (4.5 mg/kg body weight) to rats [18]. Isoproterenol was used as a non-specific β-adrenergic agonist (ISO; Sigma, St. Louis, MO, USA). Two distinct doses of Pyridostigmine bromide (0.2 mg/kg body weight or 0.5 mg/kg body weight) were used in this study. The drug was administered twice daily by intraperitoneal injection and treatment started concomitantly with ISO injection. Another group of rats received pyridostigmine alone (0.5 mg/kg body weight). Control animals were saline-injected.

A cohort of 10 male wild-type (control WT group) and 26 congenic α2A/α2C-adrenergic receptor knockout (KO) mice in a C57BL6/J genetic background were studied from 5 to 7 months of age. At this age, these mice display advanced stage cardiomyopathy as previously described [19]. α2A/α2C-KO mice were randomly assigned to receive daily pyridostigmine (3 mg/kg/day) for 28 days. Pyridostigmine was delivered via subcutaneously implanted osmotic mini-pumps.

Ethics statement

Animals were maintained at the Universidade Federal de Minas Gerais (UFMG), Brazil. This study was approved by the Institutional Animal Care and Use Committee at Universidade Federal de Minas Gerais.

Vagal and sympathetic function evaluation

The autonomic function and the intrinsic heart rate were evaluated by autonomic blockade using intravenous injections of methylatropine (3 mg/Kg, Sigma) or propranolol (4 mg/Kg, Sigma) at a maximal volume of 0.2 ml per injection after 20 min of baseline conditions. The experiments were performed in two consecutive days. On the first day, methylatropine was the first drug injected and after 15 min propranolol injection was performed. In the second day, to obtain the reverse sequence of the blockade, propranolol was the first drug administered. After 15 min, methylatropine was injected intravenously. The intrinsic HR was evaluated after the injection of methylatropine and propranolol. Using the maximum change of each drug, the sympathetic tone was calculated, on the first day, as the difference between the tachycardia evoked by methylatropine and the intrinsic HR. In the second day, the vagal tone was calculated as the difference between the intrinsic HR and the bradycardic response induced by propranolol [20], [21].

Echocardiography

Animals were anaesthetized using a nose cone with isoflurane at 5% for one minute and the maintenance dose was 1.25%. The anterior chest was shaved, and the animals were placed in supine position on an imaging stage equipped with built-in electrocardiographic electrodes for continuous heart rate monitoring and a proper heating pad to avoid hypothermia. *In vivo* cardiac function was assessed noninvasively using a high-frequency, high-resolution echocardiographic system consisting of a VEVO 2100 ultrasound machine equipped with a 30–40 MHz bifrequencial transducer (Visual Sonics, Toronto, Canada). High-resolution images were obtained as previously described [22], [23], [24].

Langendorff-perfused hearts

Briefly, after removal the hearts were perfused with a Krebs-Ringer solution, which was delivered at 37°C in the presence of continuous gassing with 5% CO_2 to yield a physiological pH of 7.4. Hearts were perfused with this solution for 50 min, as previously described [25], [26].

Cardiomyocyte isolation and Ca^{2+} recording

Adult ventricular myocytes were freshly isolated and stored in DMEM media (Sigma), until they were used (within 4 h), as previously described [27]. Intracellular Ca^{2+} ($Ca^{2+}{}_i$) imaging experiments were performed in Fluo-4 AM (6 µmol/L; Invitrogen, Eugene, OR) loaded-cardiomyocytes for 25 min which were subsequently washed with an extracellular solution that contained 1.8 mmol/L Ca^{2+} to remove the excess dye. Cells were electrically stimulated at 1 Hz to produce steady-state conditions. The confocal line-scan imaging was performed by a Zeiss LSM 510META confocal microscope. For isoproterenol response cardiomyocytes were perfused with Normal Tyrode control solution (in mmol/L, solution 1): NaCl (140), KCl (4), $MgCl_2$ (1), $CaCl_2$ (1.8), Glucose (10), and HEPES (5); pH = 7.4 adjusted with NaOH. Ca^{2+} transients were first recorded in cardiomyocytes superfused with solution 1, followed by isoproterenol stimulation of cells produced by the addition of 50 nmol/L isoproterenol to solution 1. The myocytes were field-stimulated at 1 Hz and the data plotted as the percentage increase in Ca^{2+} transient fluorescence in the presence of isoproterenol relative to the Ca^{2+} transient obtained in non-stimulated cells.

Neonatal rat cardiomyocyte culture

Neonatal rat cardiomyocytes were cultured as previously described [28]. Briefly, cardiac cells were plated in dishes containing M199 medium supplemented with 100 units/mL penicillin, 100 µg/mL streptomycin, 10% Fetal Bovine Serum and 2 mmol/L L-glutamine. To prevent growth of fibroblasts, medium was supplemented with 20 µg/mL cytosine-D-arabinofuranoside (ARA-c) for 48 hours. For siRNA studies, neonatal cardiomyocyte cultures at day 4 were transfected with 100 nM of siRNA. The cells were incubated at 37°C in an atmosphere of 5% CO_2 for 30 h and then exposed to isoproterenol (10 µmol/L) for another 24 h prior to use. The cells were then used for qPCR analyses. The siRNA for AChE was prepared as previously described [16].

Quantitative real time PCR

For RNA purifications, tissues were grounded in a potter and pestle with liquid nitrogen and total RNA was extracted using TRIzol® (Invitrogen). For quantitative PCR (qPCR), total RNA was treated with DNase I (Ambion, Austin, TX, USA) and first strand cDNA was synthesized using High Capacity cDNA Transcription Kit (Applied Biosystems, CA, USA) according to the manufacturer's instructions. After reverse transcription, the cDNA was subjected to qPCR on a 7500 Real Time PCR System (Applied Biosystems, CA, USA) using Power SYBR Green PCR Master Mix (Applied Biosystems, CA, USA), as previously described [8].

Cardiac morphometry

Heart hypertrophy was evaluated by morphometry (n = 5 per group). The rats were anesthetized with 10% ketamine/2% xylazine (4:3, 0.1 mL/100 g, i.p.) and heart beat was stopped in diastole using 10% KCl (i.v.). Hearts were immersed in 4% paraformaldehyde in 0.1 M phosphate buffer, pH 7.4 for 24 hours at room temperature. The tissues were dehydrated by sequential washes with 70, 80, 90 and 100% ethanol and embedded in paraffin. Transversal sections (5 µm) were cut starting from base area of the heart at intervals of 40 µm and stained with hematoxylin-eosin for cell morphometry. Tissue sections (2 for each animal) were examined with Axioplan 2 Zeiss microscope, and analyzed with ImageJ software. Only digitized images of cardiomyocytes cut longitudinally with nuclei and cellular limits visible were used for analysis (an average of 40 cardiomyocytes for each animal). The diameter of each myocyte was measured across the region corresponding to the nucleus.

Western blot

40–60 µg of protein were separated by SDS-PAGE 10% gels. Antibodies and their sources are as follows: anti-SERCA2 (1:1000 ABR), and anti-GAPDH (1:4000 Santa Cruz Biotechnology). Immunodetection was carried out using enhanced chemiluminescence (Amersham Biosciences). Protein levels were expressed as a ratio of optical densities. GAPDH was used as a control for any variations in protein loading.

Statistical analysis

All data are expressed as means ± SEM, and the number of cells or experiments is shown as *n*. Significant differences between groups were determined with a Student's *t*-test or ANOVA followed by the Newman-Keuls *post hoc* test. Values of $p<0.05$ were considered to be statistically significant.

Results

Cholinergic signaling in the heart depends on the parasympathetic nervous system as well as on the recently described cardiomyocyte cholinergic machinery [14], [15], [16]. Firstly, we assessed whether cholinergic activity at the parasympathetic nerve endings was modulated in rats with increased sympathetic drive. To assess the activity of the cardiac autonomic nervous system, we monitored changes in heart rate (HR) under the inhibition of parasympathetic and/or sympathetic nervous tone in control and isoproterenol (ISO)-treated rats. Fig. 1 shows HR responses to intravenous injections of methylatropine and propranolol used to calculate the cardiac sympathetic and vagal tone. As shown in Fig. 1A, ISO administration to rats for seven days produces an autonomic imbalance characterized by increased cardiac sympathetic tone when compared with control group ($p<0.05$). In contrast, cardiac vagal tone tended to be lower in ISO rats when compared to control (Fig. 1B). When cholinergic signaling was increased by administration of the cholinesterase inhibitor pyridostigmine to rats opposite results were observed. Pyridostigmine-treated rats displayed reduced sympathetic and increased parasympathetic tone, respectively. In order to assess the consequences of increased cholinergic function to the diseased heart we treated rats simultaneously with ISO and pyridostigmine. Two distinct doses of pyridostigmine were used in this study (0.2 mg/kg body weight or 0.5 mg/kg body weight), as shown in Fig. 1A–B. Pyridostigmine administration to ISO rats prevented changes in parasympathetic and sympathetic tone, with significant results observed at the higher dose. Altogether, our data show that both ISO and pyridostigmine are capable of modulating cardiac sympathetic and parasympathetic tone in opposite ways, and that increased ACh availability induced by pyridostigmine administration to rats is capable of overcoming isoproterenol induced changes in autonomic function.

To investigate whether the non-neuronal cardiomyocyte cholinergic machinery is modulated *in vivo* in ISO rats, we isolated ventricular myocytes and investigated expression levels of cholinergic components. mRNA levels of VAChT, ChAT and M_2 muscarinic receptors were upregulated in cardiac cells isolated from ISO-treated rats (Fig. 2A–C). In contrast, lower levels of

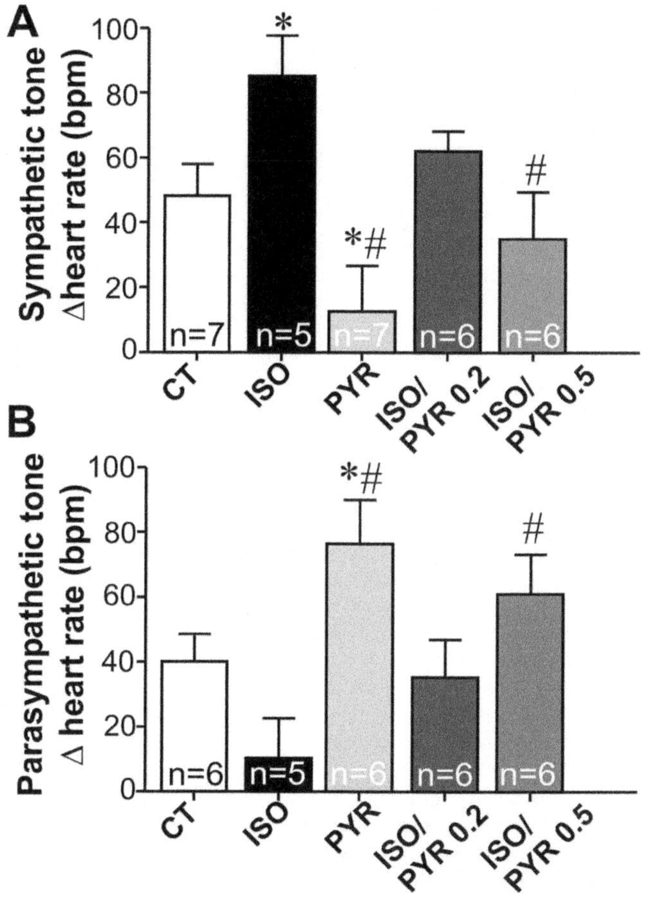

Figure 1. Cholinesterase inhibition alters the activity of the cardiac autonomic system evoked by isoproterenol. Changes in heart rate (HR) under the inhibition of parasympathetic and/or sympathetic nervous system were monitored in rats injected with methylatropine and propranolol for further calculation of sympathetic and vagal tone, as described in Methods. Two different doses of pyridostigmine were combined with isoproterenol in this study (0.2 mg/kg body weight or 0.5 mg/kg body weight). **A–B.** ISO administration to rats for seven days resulted in increased sympathetic tone when compared with control group. Vagal tone was lower in isoproterenol treated rats when compared to control rats. The higher dose of pyridostigmine was more efficient in preventing the isoproterenol-induced changes in heart rate. Rats treated with pyridostigmine alone (0.5 mg/kg body weight) presented reduced sympathetic and increased parasympathetic tone, respectively. n = number of rats. *$p<0.05$ when compared to control group and #$p<0.05$ when compared to the ISO-treated rat using Student's *t* test.

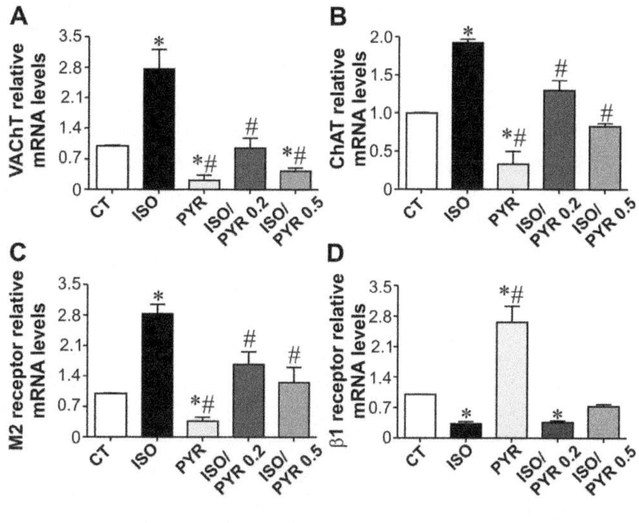

Figure 2. Opposite modulation of cardiomyocyte cholinergic machinery by isoproterenol and pyridostigmine. A–C. qPCR experiments show that cardiomyocytes from ISO-rats present upregulation of VAChT, ChAT and M_2 muscarinic receptor mRNA levels. Cholinesterase inhibition prevented these effects. Lower levels of VAChT, ChAT and M_2 ACh muscarinic receptor transcripts were observed in cardiomyocytes from pyridostigmine treated rats. **D.** Downregulation of β1-AR transcript is observed in ventricular myocytes from ISO-rats, while pyridostigmine-treated rats presented opposite results. Cholinesterase therapy partially reversed the effect of ISO on β1-AR transcripts. n = 4–6 cardiomyocyte preparations from each group. *$p<0.05$ when compared to control group and #$p<0.05$ when compared to the ISO-treated rat.

VAChT, ChAT and M_2 mRNA were found in rats with increased ACh availability due to cholinesterase inhibition. As shown in Fig. 2A–C, both doses of pyridostigmine used in this study were efficient in preventing the upregulation of the cholinergic machinery induced by isoproterenol. Taken together, these data indicate that reprogramming of cardiomyocyte cholinergic machinery is under opposing modulation by isoproterenol and pyridostigmine. Moreover, our finding that cardiomyocyte cholinergic proteins are modulated *in vivo* is potentially important since it suggests that this intrinsic ACh synthesis site can be activated directly in the ventricles under hyperadrenergic conditions, and this occurs in parallel with a reduction in parasympathetic tone. In order to extend these findings and to better understand under what conditions this intrinsic cholinergic system is modulated, we next performed studies in isolated cardiac cells and assessed the expression levels of VAChT mRNA in response to increased adrenergic and cholinergic stimulation. In order to deplete endogenous acetylcholinesterase and simulate conditions of increased cholinergic signaling in rat cardiomyocytes, we used specific siRNA targeting AChE. In rat cardiomyocytes, VAChT mRNA was upregulated by isoproterenol, while cells treated with an AChE-siRNA presented significantly decreased VAChT mRNA levels (Fig.S1). Importantly, AChE silencing partially abolished the effect of isoproterenol on VAChT expression levels. Thus these data further support our *in vivo* findings and confirm the hypothesis that non-neuronal cholinergic signaling is under differential modulation by adrenergic and cholinergic signals.

We also assessed expression levels of β1-adrenergic receptor in ventricular myocytes from ISO and pyridostigmine-treated rats. As shown in Fig. 2D, 7-day ISO injection to rats led to a significant β1-adrenergic receptor downregulation. In contrast, ventricular myocytes from pyridostigmine treated rats presented a robust increase in β1-AR transcript levels. Administration of pyridostigmine to ISO-rats attenuated the ISO-induced-β1-AR downregulation. Collectively, our data from Fig. 2 suggest that cholinergic signaling is activated in ventricular myocytes under conditions of increased adrenergic drive, while expression of β1 receptors is downregulated. Interestingly, both effects were prevented when ACh availability was increased upon pyridostigmine treatment.

To investigate the functional consequences of these changes in cholinergic signaling for the heart, we performed morphometric and echocardiographic analyses. Morphometric analyses of fiber diameter revealed a significant increase in cardiomyocyte hypertrophy in ISO rats (Fig. 3A–B). Pyridostigmine alone, had no effect on cardiomyocyte size (data not shown), but when combined with isoproterenol the drug was capable of preventing ISO-induced

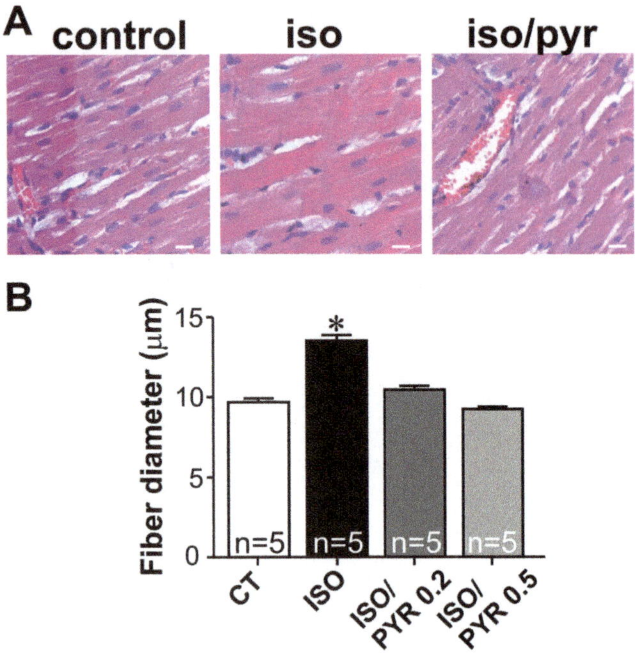

Figure 3. Cholinesterase inhibition prevents isoproterenol induced-hypertrophy. A. Representative images. **B.** Morphometry analyses showing the increase in fiber diameter in rats subjected to seven day ISO administration. Cholinesterase inhibition prevented the ISO-induced cardiomyocyte hyperthophy. n = number of hearts analysed. *$p<0.05$ when compared to other groups. Scale bar = 10 μm.

hypertrophy. Since the higher pyridostigmine dose was more effective in preventing autonomic imbalance and cardiomyocyte hypertrophy, we performed all the remaining experiments in ISO rats treated with the higher dose of pyridostigmine. Real-time experiments supported the morphometry data since transcript levels of hypertrophic markers atrial natriuretic peptide (ANP) and β-myosin heavy chain (β-MHC) were upregulated in cardiomyocytes from ISO-rats (Fig. 4A), an effect that was attenuated in cardiomyocytes from ISO-rats treated concomitantly with pyridostigmine. Interestingly, pyridostigmine treatment alone significantly decreased fetal gene expression when compared to control. Table 1 shows that after seven days of ISO administration to rats there was a significant increase in ejection fraction (EF) and fractional shortening (FS) indicating that at this stage ventricular function was still preserved. Interestingly, concomitant treatment with pyridostigmine produced a similar increase in EF and FS. In spite of enhanced ejection fraction, pronounced cardiac remodeling was observed in ISO-rats. As shown in Table 1, ISO injection led to significant thickening of the left ventricular posterior wall and septum both in systole and diastole with most of these changes significantly attenuated by pyridostigmine. In addition, the left ventricular internal dimension at diastole was significantly reduced in ISO-rats. This alteration was accompanied by a decrease in end-diastolic volume. As shown in Table 1, both changes were prevented by pyridostigmine. Except for an increase in chamber dimension at diastole, pyridostigmine treatment had no effect on cardiac parameters. Thus, these functional data clearly indicate that increased cholinergic signaling induced by cholinesterase inhibition significantly attenuated isoproterenol-induced pathological remodeling.

To further assess the consequences of cholinergic signaling activation by pyridostigmine in the diseased heart we used the Langendorff-isolated heart preparation. As shown in Fig. 4B, a marked decrease in systolic tension was observed in hearts from the ISO group. This finding contrasted with echocardiography data where heart function was increased, indicating that *in vivo* compensatory mechanisms were contributing to preserve cardiac function in ISO rats. Combined administration of ISO and pyridostigmine resulted in significant improvement of cardiac systolic tension when compared to hearts from ISO-rats. Pyridostigmine, alone had no effect on systolic tension (data not shown). To further investigate the underlying cellular basis for the effects of pyridostigmine on ISO-injected rats, we examined intracellular Ca^{2+} in freshly isolated Fluo-4AM loaded ventricular myocytes. Figure 4C shows representative profiles of intracellular Ca^{2+} transient recorded in Fluo-4AM loaded ventricular myocytes. As shown in Figure 4D, ventricular myocytes from ISO rats present a significant reduction of the peak calcium transient ($p< 0.05$). The impaired Ca^{2+} handling observed in cells from ISO rats corroborates data obtained by the Langendorff technique. In contrast, the amplitude of the $[Ca^{2+}]_i$ transient in cardiomyocytes from rats treated with a combination of pyridostigmine and ISO was not statistically different from that obtained in control cardiomyocytes. The reduced amplitude of the $[Ca^{2+}]_i$ transient in ISO-cardiomyocytes is consistent with the decreased expression of the sarcoplasmic reticulum Ca^{2+} pump (SERCA2), therefore we examined SERCA2 levels in these hearts. As shown in Fig. 4E, SERCA2 expression levels were significantly reduced in cardiomyocytes from ISO-treated rats relative to controls. In contrast, cardiomyocytes from rats treated with a combination of pyridostigmine and ISO, presented normal levels of SERCA2.

Since pyridostigmine administration prevented the ISO-induced β-1 receptor downregulation, we addressed the functionality of these receptors by assessing the percentage increase in Ca^{2+} transient amplitude upon ISO stimulation. Upon reaching steady state in our normal Tyrode control solution, perfusion of myocytes with a sub-maximal dose of ISO (50 nmol/L) produced a large increase in Ca^{2+} transient amplitude in cells from control rats. This effect is shown in Fig. 4F, which shows the % Δ in response to ISO. As expected, perfusion with ISO had a less pronounced effect on the Ca^{2+} transient amplitude in myocytes from ISO-rats, indicating impaired β-adrenergic responsiveness of cells from this group. In contrast, cardiomyocytes from rats treated with a combination of ISO and pyridostigmine presented normal response to ISO stimulation, comparable to that observed in cells from control rats. Thus, pyridostigmine treatment restores the functionality of β-adrenergic receptors in ISO-myocytes corroborating our real time PCR data. Taking together, our data show that increased cholinergic signaling induced by pyridostigmine is capable of preventing deleterious effects of increased sympathetic drive.

To investigate whether increased cholinergic signaling would also revert pre-existing sympathetic hyperactivity-induced heart failure, we treated α_{2A}/α_{2C}-KO mice with pyridostigmine. Mice lacking both α_{2A}-and α_{2C}- adrenergic receptors (α_{2A}/α_{2C}-KO) develop sympathetic hyperactivity-induced heart failure [19], [29]. The first signs of heart failure are observed at age of 5 months. Fig. 5A–B shows that α_{2A}/α_{2C}-KO mice present reduced left ventricular ejection fraction and fractional shortening as assessed by echocardiography, and administration of pyridostigmine for 28 days significantly increased these parameters towards control levels. These data confirm our previous finding that baseline fractional shortening was significantly reduced in α_{2A}/α_{2C}-KO mice, when compared with control mice [19]. To further assess directly the heart dysfunction in α_{2A}/α_{2C}-KO mice we used the Langendorff-isolated heart preparation. In agreement with the

Table 1. Echocardiographic parameters.

Parameter	CT (n = 8)	ISO (n = 8)	ISO+PYR (n = 9)	PYR (n = 4)
Cardiac output (mL/min)	65.09±3.03	48.74±6.11*	71.22±2.31&	76.64±3.84&
LV internal dimension (diastole, mm)	6.87±0.18	5.92±0.18*	6.83±0.15&	7.63±0.22*& #
LV internal dimension (systole, mm)	4.08±0.10	3.24±0.20*	3.48±±0.13*	4.28±0.39&#
LV posterior wall (systole, mm)	2.29±0.08	3.27±0.19*	2.85±0.15*	2.60±0.17&
LV posterior wall (diastole, mm)	1.43±0.05	2.19±0.14*	1.81±0.10&	1.54±0.17&
interventricular septal dimension (systole, mm)	1.90±0.10	2.67±0.13*	2.36±0.07*&	1.90±0.13&#
interventricular septal dimension (diastole, mm)	1.05±0.04	1.57±0.07*	1.29±0.04*&	1.18±0.06&
LV ejection fraction (%)	72.21±1.74	78.94±1.28*	79.1±1.73*	73.72±3.32
LV fractional shortening (%)	41.3±1.73	47.5±1.31*	51.0±1.57*	44.34±2.97
LV systolic volume (µL)	178.2±8.98	134.2±15.92*	200.0±5.33&	215.8±13.73&
End diastolic LV volume (µL)	246.2±9.12	169.9±19.35*	253.0±4.85&	293.8±19.06&
End systolic LV volume (µL)	68.04±4.37	35.63±4.15*	52.98±4.58*&	77.97±11.69&#
Heart rate (bpm)	367.0±11.11	361.5±5.79	356.4±8.61	356.1±5.56

Echocardiographic measurements of cardiac parameters in rats following isoproterenol injection for 7 days. Pyridostigmine treatment of ISO-rats attenuated the development of cardiac remodeling induced by isoproterenol. n = number of rats analysed in each experimental group.
* = $p<0.05$ versus CT,
& = $p<0.05$ versus ISO,
# = $p<0.05$ versus ISO+PYR.

results obtained with echocardiography studies, isolated hearts from α_{2A}/α_{2C}-KO mice had significantly decreased systolic tension when compared to WT hearts (Fig. 5C). Pyridostigmine treatment reversed the decreased systolic tension observed in α_{2A}/α_{2C}-KO hearts. Similarly, a contractile dysfunction was observed in freshly isolated adult ventricular myocytes from α_{2A}/α_{2C}-KO mice, which demonstrated reduced fractional shortening when compared to cardiomyocytes from WT mice (Fig. 5D). Cholinesterase inhibition of α_{2A}/α_{2C}-KO mice reversed this change thus confirming that increased cholinergic signaling protects against chronic adrenergic stimulation.

Discussion

Here, we show that both cholinergic axes, the cardiac parasympathetic system and non-neuronal cardiomyocyte cholinergic machinery are modulated in opposite directions under conditions of increased sympathetic drive or of increased ACh availability. As such, in a model of increased adrenergic stimulation, parasympathetic tone is reduced while a significant induction of VAChT, ChAT and M_2-receptors is observed in ventricular myocytes, thus uncovering a new site of ACh synthesis in the ventricles *in vivo*. When ACh availability increases, for example by administration of pyridostigmine, this effect is suppressed. In the presence of pyridostigmine, normal parasympathetic response is restored and pathological remodeling induced by increased sympathetic drive is prevented. Thus, our findings indicate that therapies aimed at enhancing cholinergic activity might be an important target in heart failure.

Modulation of cardiomyocyte cholinergic machinery *in vivo*

We have previously shown that ventricular myocytes express cholinergic components ChAT, VAChT, CHT1 and muscarinic receptor type 2 and release ACh [16], [17]. Here, we show that this intrinsic cholinergic machinery is upregulated *in vivo* and *in vitro* by isoproterenol, suggesting that under this condition ACh release by cardiomyocytes is increased. These data corroborate our previous finding that isoproterenol treatment *in vitro* leads to a significant increase in expression levels of cholinergic components in neonatal cardiomyocytes [16]. A possibility raised by these findings is that ACh released by cardiomyocytes acts as a feedback signal to counteract excessive adrenergic stimulation thus exerting protective effects. Evidence supporting this hypothesis comes from the fact that when ACh synthesis by cardiomyocytes is blocked, for example in vesamicol treated myocytes isoproterenol treatment leads to a greater increase in cell surface area when compared with cells treated with isoproterenol alone [16]. Therefore, in the absence of VAChT the extent of cardiac hypertrophy induced by isoproterenol is increased corroborating the fact that cardiomyocyte cholinergic machinery exerts protective effects. In addition, mice with targeted deletion of VAChT in cardiomyocytes present cardiac dysfunction, increased ROS levels, and cardiomyocyte hypertrophy [17]. Similar findings were also observed in another genetic mouse model with ablation of ChAT (the enzyme responsible for ACh synthesis) in cardiomyocytes [17]. Along these lines, Kakinuma *et al.* have demonstrated that increased expression of ChAT in cardiomyocytes turns the heart more resistant to injury caused by ischemia and reperfusion [30]. Taking all these into consideration, it appears that under stress conditions the cardiomyocyte cholinergic machinery is activated and this may contribute to cardiac protection. When ACh availability is restored, for example during cholinesterase therapy, upregulation of cardiomyocyte cholinergic machinery is no longer required. This assumption is further supported by our finding that pyridostigmine administration *in vivo* leads to a significant reduction in VAChT, ChAT, and M_2 expression, and by our *in vitro* data showing that cardiomyocytes transfected with AChE siRNA

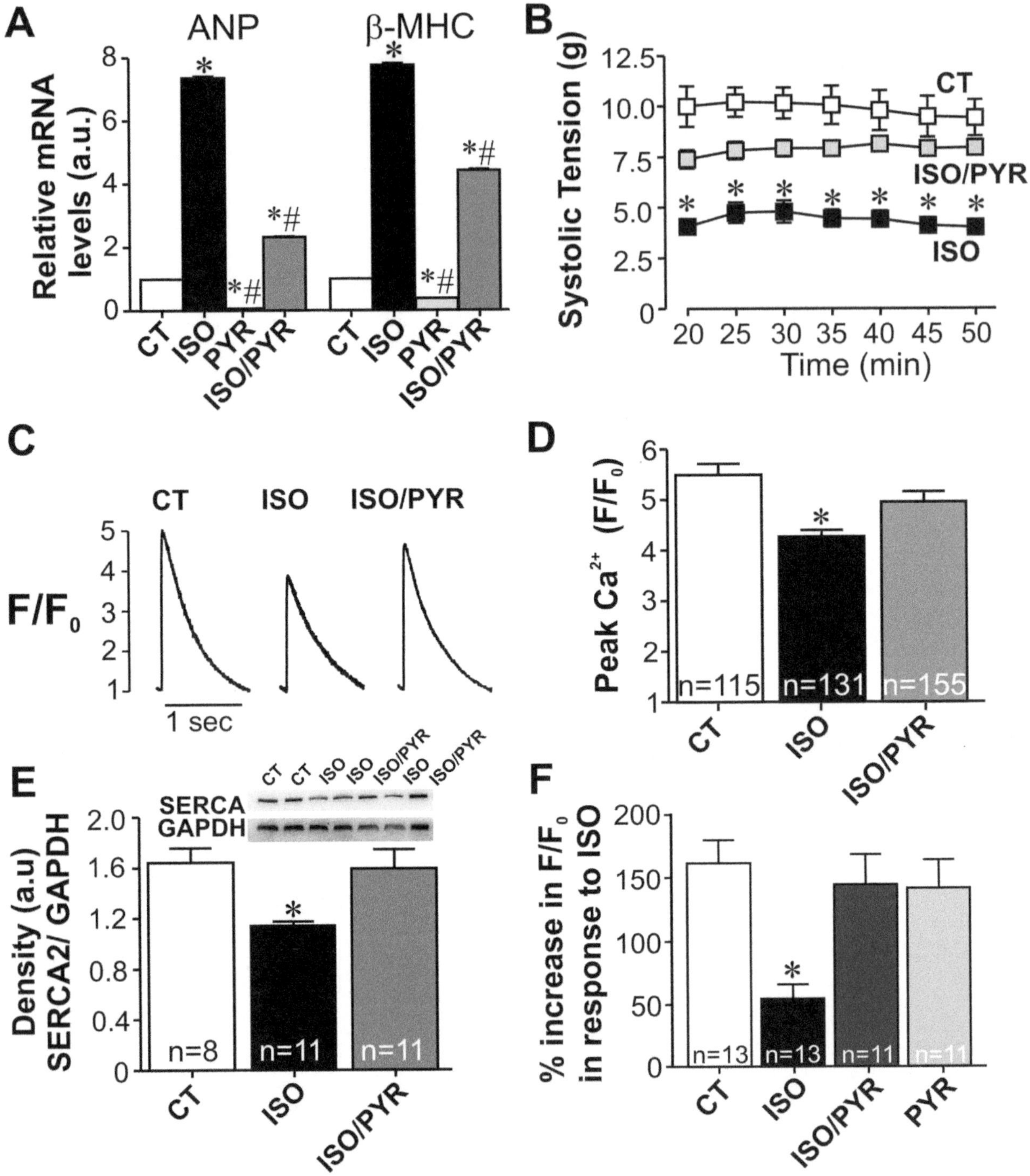

Figure 4. Increased cholinergic signaling functionally prevents ISO-induced pathological remodeling. A. Differential effects of isoproterenol and pyridostigmine on transcripts for ANP and β-MHC were detected by real-time PCR in cardiomyocytes from each experimental group. Administration of pyridostigmine prevents the upregulation of hypertrophic markers in cardiomyocytes from ISO-rats. n = 4–6 cardiomyocyte preparations from each group. *$p<0.05$ when compared to control group and #$p<0.05$ when compared to the ISO-treated rat. **B.** Pyridostigmine treatment restored systolic tension in ISO-treated rats back to control levels. n = 7 hearts per group. **C.** Representative profile of the Ca^{2+} transient. **D.** Bar graph shows averaged-peak Ca^{2+} transient. Significant reduction in peak Ca^{2+} transient is observed in cardiomyocytes from ISO-rats. Anticholinesterase therapy significantly prevented intracellular Ca^{2+} dysfunction in cardiomyocytes from ISO-rats. n = number of ventricular myocytes analysed. **E.** Top, representative western-blot. Bottom, averaged-densitometry. Pyridostigmine-treatment prevents SERCA2 downregulation in ISO cardiomyocytes. **F.** % Increase in cytosolic Ca^{2+} concentration ($[Ca^{2+}]_i$) above basal level measured 2 minutes after stimulation with 50nmol/L isoproterenol. β-adrenergic stimulation increased Ca^{2+} transient amplitude in cardiomyocyters from saline-treated group more than in cells from ISO-rats. Cardiomyocytes from ISO/PYR rats presented a similar increase in $[Ca^{2+}]_i$ transient amplitude in response to acute ISO perfusion as control cells. * = $p<0.05$ when compared to other experimental groups. n = number of cells analysed from 4 different animals in each group.

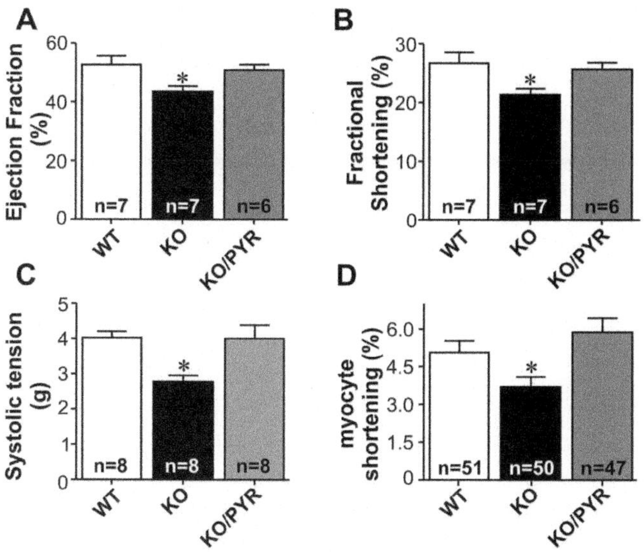

Figure 5. Increased cholinergic signaling improves cardiac function in mice with sympathetic hyperactivity-induced heart failure. A–B. Percentage increase in left ventricular ejection fraction and fractional shortening measured by echocardiography. Systolic tension (**C**) and cardiomyocyte shortening (**D**) measurements were performed in WT and α_{2A}/α_{2C}-KO mice treated or not with pyridostigmine. Cholinesterase inhibition therapy restored cardiac function and and cellular contractile function of α_{2A}/α_{2C}-KO mice to control levels. *$p<0.05$ when compared to WT and α_{2A}/α_{2C}-KO/PYR.

present significant reduction in VAChT mRNA. It is worth noting the fact that this cardiomyocyte intrinsic cholinergic machinery is subjected to opposing modulation by isoproterenol and pyridostigmine, suggesting that cardiac cells may represent another level of cholinergic control of heart function, that goes beyond the parasympathetic autonomic system.

Cardioprotective effects of cholinesterase inhibition

The present results with pyridostigmine are consistent with the idea that enhancing ACh signaling may limit adverse remodeling and cardiac deterioration by controlling cardiac gene expression, preventing cardiomyocyte hypertrophy, and therefore preserving Ca^{2+} cycling and contractile function. Taken together, these results provide the cellular basis to attempt to improve cholinergic neurotransmission and restore parasympathetic-sympathetic balance to influence the outcome of heart failure in clinical settings.

Previous data in the literature have shown that treatment with pyridostigmine improves cardiocirculatory parameters in rats with chronic heart failure due to coronary artery ligation [31], [32]. Here, we extended these findings by showing the mechanisms involved in the protective effects of cholinesterase inhibition therapy. Accordingly, pyridostigmine improves cardiac function by preventing the increase in sympathetic activity, hypertrophic growth, and by improving calcium dynamics. The signaling pathways mediating these effects, however, have yet to be elucidated. In addition, we found that pyridostigmine can reverse pre-existing pathological remodeling in a model of hyperadrenergic induced heart failure, indicating that increased ACh availability is associated to cardioprotection. Overall, these findings are consistent with a recent study using a cohort of 7073 subjects showing that the use of cholinesterase inhibitor was associated with a reduced risk of myocardial infarction and death [13].

Importantly, beneficial effects of cholinesterase inhibition are not restricted to the synaptic cleft but also observed locally in ventricular myocytes. Ventricular myocytes are known to express AChE [16], and its inhibition leads to a local increase in cardiomyocyte derived-ACh [17]. In cardiac cells, ACh acting through M_2 receptors activates nitric oxide synthesis exerting anti-hypertrophic effects [16]. In addition, we have demonstrated that neonatal rat cardiomyocytes transfected with siRNA directed to AChE presented reduced expression levels of ANP and β-MHC, and were protected from hypertrophic effects of isoproterenol [16].

Taking together, our data suggest that the cardiomyocyte cholinergic machinery plays a role as an adaptative defense mechanism activated under conditions of increased sympathetic drive. Increased cholinergic tone induced by pyridostigmine is important to restore the balance of the autonomic nervous system and prevent cardiovascular dysfunction in two models of sympathetic hyperactivity. Overall our data support the fact that therapies aimed at enhancing cholinergic signaling in the synaptic cleft and locally in the heart might be an important target in heart failure.

Supporting Information

Figure S1 Adrenergic and cholinergic signals regulate VAChT mRNA levels in neonatal cardiomyocytes. siRNA targeting AChE significantly reduces mRNA expression levels of VAChT. Isoproterenol treatment significantly increases VAChT mRNA levels in neonatal cardiomyocytes, an effect that is significantly attenuated in cells transfected with siRNA targeting AChE. $n = 4$ samples from each group. *$p<0.05$ when compared to control group and #$p<0.05$ when compared to the ISO-treated cardiomyocytes.

Author Contributions

Conceived and designed the experiments: SG MAMP RASS MAPF PCB. Performed the experiments: MG PWMA AL CRR DDD AML PMM MBM RRR ML. Analyzed the data: MG PWMA AL CRR DDD AML PMM MBM RRR ML MAPF SG. Contributed reagents/materials/analysis tools: RASS MAPF PCB RRR MAMP SG PMM. Wrote the paper: SG MAMP MG.

References

1. Packer M, Coats AJ, Fowler MB, Katus HA, Krum H, et al. (2001) Effect of carvedilol on survival in severe chronic heart failure. N Engl J Med 344: 1651–1658.
2. Packer M, Fowler MB, Roecker EB, Coats AJ, Katus HA, et al. (2002) Effect of carvedilol on the morbidity of patients with severe chronic heart failure: results of the carvedilol prospective randomized cumulative survival (COPERNICUS) study. Circulation 106: 2194–2199.
3. Rockman HA, Koch WJ, Lefkowitz RJ (2002) Seven-transmembrane-spanning receptors and heart function. Nature 415: 206–212.
4. de Castro BM, Pereira GS, Magalhaes V, Rossato JI, De J, X, et al. (2009) Reduced expression of the vesicular acetylcholine transporter causes learning deficits in mice. Genes Brain Behav 8: 23–35.
5. Prado VF, Martins-Silva C, de Castro BM, Lima RF, Barros DM, et al. (2006) Mice deficient for the vesicular acetylcholine transporter are myasthenic and have deficits in object and social recognition. Neuron 51: 601–612.
6. LaCroix C, Freeling J, Giles A, Wess J, Li YF (2008) Deficiency of M2 muscarinic acetylcholine receptors increases susceptibility of ventricular function to chronic adrenergic stress. Am J Physiol Heart Circ Physiol 294: H810–H820.

7. Li M, Zheng C, Sato T, Kawada T, Sugimachi M, et al. (2004) Vagal nerve stimulation markedly improves long-term survival after chronic heart failure in rats. Circulation 109: 120–124.
8. Lara A, Damasceno DD, Pires R, Gros R, Gomes ER, et al. (2010) Dysautonomia due to reduced cholinergic neurotransmission causes cardiac remodeling and heart failure. Mol Cell Biol 30: 1746–1756.
9. Freeling J, Wattier K, LaCroix C, Li YF (2008) Neostigmine and pilocarpine attenuated tumour necrosis factor alpha expression and cardiac hypertrophy in the heart with pressure overload. Exp Physiol 93: 75–82.
10. Okazaki Y, Zheng C, Li M, Sugimachi M (2010) Effect of the cholinesterase inhibitor donepezil on cardiac remodeling and autonomic balance in rats with heart failure. J Physiol Sci 60: 67–74.
11. Handa T, Katare RG, Kakinuma Y, Arikawa M, Ando M, et al. (2009) Anti-Alzheimer's drug, donepezil, markedly improves long-term survival after chronic heart failure in mice. J Card Fail 15: 805–811.
12. Kanazawa H, Ieda M, Kimura K, Arai T, Kawaguchi-Manabe H, et al. (2010) Heart failure causes cholinergic transdifferentiation of cardiac sympathetic nerves via gp130-signaling cytokines in rodents. J Clin Invest 120: 408–421.
13. Nordstrom P, Religa D, Wimo A, Winblad B, Eriksdotter M (2013) The use of cholinesterase inhibitors and the risk of myocardial infarction and death: a nationwide cohort study in subjects with Alzheimer's disease. Eur Heart J 34: 2585–2591.
14. Kakinuma Y, Akiyama T, Sato T (2009) Cholinoceptive and cholinergic properties of cardiomyocytes involving an amplification mechanism for vagal efferent effects in sparsely innervated ventricular myocardium. FEBS J 276: 5111–5125.
15. Rana OR, Schauerte P, Kluttig R, Schroder JW, Koenen RR, et al. (2010) Acetylcholine as an age-dependent non-neuronal source in the heart. Auton Neurosci 156: 82–89.
16. Rocha-Resende C, Roy A, Resende R, Ladeira MS, Lara A, et al. (2012) Non-neuronal cholinergic machinery present in cardiomyocytes offsets hypertrophic signals. J Mol Cell Cardiol 53: 206–216.
17. Roy A, Fields WC, Rocha-Resende C, Resende RR, Guatimosim S, et al. (2013) Cardiomyocyte-secreted acetylcholine is required for maintenance of homeostasis in the heart. FASEB J 27: 5072–5082.
18. Oliveira EM and Krieger JE (2005) Chronic beta-adrenoceptor stimulation and cardiac hypertrophy with no induction of circulating renin. Eur J Pharmacol 520: 135–141.
19. Bartholomeu JB, Vanzelli AS, Rolim NP, Ferreira JC, Bechara LR, et al. (2008) Intracellular mechanisms of specific beta-adrenoceptor antagonists involved in improved cardiac function and survival in a genetic model of heart failure. J Mol Cell Cardiol 45: 240–249.
20. De AK, Wichi RB, Jesus WR, Moreira ED, Morris M, et al. (2004) Exercise training changes autonomic cardiovascular balance in mice. J Appl Physiol 96: 2174–2178.
21. Negrao CE, Moreira ED, Brum PC, Denadai ML, Krieger EM (1992) Vagal and sympathetic control of heart rate during exercise by sedentary and exercise-trained rats. Braz J Med Biol Res 25: 1045–1052.
22. Marques FD, Ferreira AJ, Sinisterra RD, Jacoby BA, Sousa FB, et al. (2011) An oral formulation of angiotensin-(1–7) produces cardioprotective effects in infarcted and isoproterenol-treated rats. Hypertension 57: 477–483.
23. Marques FD, Melo MB, Souza LE, Irigoyen MC, Sinisterra RD, et al. (2012) Beneficial effects of long-term administration of an oral formulation of Angiotensin-(1–7) in infarcted rats. Int J Hypertens 2012: 795452.
24. Gava E, de Castro CH, Ferreira AJ, Colleta H, Melo MB, et al. (2012) Angiotensin-(1–7) receptor Mas is an essential modulator of extracellular matrix protein expression in the heart. Regul Pept 175: 30–42.
25. Castro CH, Santos RA, Ferreira AJ, Bader M, Alenina N, et al. (2005) Evidence for a functional interaction of the angiotensin-(1–7) receptor Mas with AT1 and AT2 receptors in the mouse heart. Hypertension 46: 937–942.
26. Ferreira AJ, Oliveira TL, Castro MC, Almeida AP, Castro CH, et al. (2007) Isoproterenol-induced impairment of heart function and remodeling are attenuated by the nonpeptide angiotensin-(1-7) analogue AVE 0991. Life Sci 81: 916–923.
27. Guatimosim S, Sobie EA, dos Santos CJ, Martin LA, Lederer WJ (2001) Molecular identification of a TTX-sensitive Ca(2+) current. Am J Physiol Cell Physiol 280: C1327–C1339.
28. Guatimosim S, Amaya MJ, Guerra MT, Aguiar CJ, Goes AM, et al. (2008) Nuclear Ca2+ regulates cardiomyocyte function. Cell Calcium 44: 230–242.
29. Rolim NP, Medeiros A, Rosa KT, Mattos KC, Irigoyen MC, et al. (2007) Exercise training improves the net balance of cardiac Ca2+ handling protein expression in heart failure. Physiol Genomics 29: 246–252.
30. Kakinuma Y, Tsuda M, Okazaki K, Akiyama T, Arikawa M, et al. (2013) Heart-specific overexpression of choline acetyltransferase gene protects murine heart against ischemia through hypoxia-inducible factor-1alpha-related defense mechanisms. J Am Heart Assoc 2: e004887.
31. Sabino JP, da Silva CA, de Melo RF, Fazan R, Jr., Salgado HC (2013) The treatment with pyridostigmine improves the cardiocirculatory function in rats with chronic heart failure. Auton Neurosci 173: 58–64.
32. Lataro RM, Silva CA, Fazan R, Jr., Rossi MA, Prado CM, et al. (2013) Increase in parasympathetic tone by pyridostigmine prevents ventricular dysfunction during the onset of heart failure. Am J Physiol Regul Integr Comp Physiol 305: R908–R916.

15

Electrophysiological and Structural Remodeling in Heart Failure Modulate Arrhythmogenesis. 2D Simulation Study

Juan F. Gomez, Karen Cardona, Laura Martinez, Javier Saiz, Beatriz Trenor*

Instituto de Investigación en Ingeniería Biomédica, UniversitatPolitècnica de València, Valencia, Spain

Abstract

Background: Heart failure is operationally defined as the inability of the heart to maintain blood flow to meet the needs of the body and it is the final common pathway of various cardiac pathologies. Electrophysiological remodeling, intercellular uncoupling and a pro-fibrotic response have been identified as major arrhythmogenic factors in heart failure.

Objective: In this study we investigate vulnerability to reentry under heart failure conditions by incorporating established electrophysiological and anatomical remodeling using computer simulations.

Methods: The electrical activity of human transmural ventricular tissue (5 cm×5 cm) was simulated using the human ventricular action potential model Grandi et al. under control and heart failure conditions. The MacCannell et al. model was used to model fibroblast electrical activity, and their electrotonic interactions with myocytes. Selected degrees of diffuse fibrosis and variations in intercellular coupling were considered and the vulnerable window (VW) for reentry was evaluated following cross-field stimulation.

Results: No reentry was observed in normal conditions or in the presence of HF ionic remodeling. However, defined amount of fibrosis and/or cellular uncoupling were sufficient to elicit reentrant activity. Under conditions where reentry was generated, HF electrophysiological remodeling did not alter the width of the VW. However, intermediate fibrosis and cellular uncoupling significantly widened the VW. In addition, biphasic behavior was observed, as very high fibrotic content or very low tissue conductivity hampered the development of reentry. Detailed phase analysis of reentry dynamics revealed an increase of phase singularities with progressive fibrotic components.

Conclusion: Structural remodeling is a key factor in the genesis of vulnerability to reentry. A range of intermediate levels of fibrosis and intercellular uncoupling can combine to favor reentrant activity.

Editor: Alexander V. Panfilov, Gent University, Belgium

Funding: This work was partially supported by (i) the "VI Plan Nacional de Investigación Científica, Desarrollo e Innovación Tecnológica" from the Ministerio de Economía y Competitividad of Spain (grant number TIN2012-37546-C03-01) and the European Commission (European Regional Development Funds – ERDF - FEDER), (ii) by the Dirección General de Política Científica de la Generalitat Valenciana (grant number GV/2013/119), and by (iii), Programa Prometeo (PROMETEO/ 2012/030) de la Conselleria d'Educació Formació I Ocupació, Generalitat Valenciana. The funders had no role in study design, data collection and analysis, decision to publish, or preparation of the manuscript.

Competing Interests: The authors have declared that no competing interests exist.

* Email: btrenor@gbio.i3bh.es

Introduction

Ventricular arrhythmias in patients with congestive heart failure (HF), contribute to the high incidence of sudden cardiac death associated with HF [1,2]. The mechanisms of the arrhythmias occurring in the setting of HF are not fully understood. After-depolarization-induced trigger activity has a high tendency to develop in the failing myocardium. However, conditions favoring reentrant arrhythmias have also been described in failing hearts [2]. Reentrant activity is generated by wave interaction with anatomical or functional obstacles combined with specific excitability conditions [3]. In diseased hearts, preexisting electro anatomic tissue heterogeneity is amplified considerably, increasing vulnerability to reentrant arrhythmias [3,4].

In the case of HF, electrical and structural changes significantly increase the occurrence of reentry. The failing heart phenotype is characterized by distinct alterations in selected ion channels, changes in intracellular calcium cycling, alterations in cell-cell coupling proteins, enhanced interstitial fibrosis, and cellular hypertrophy [5–7]. Experimental studies in animal models provide evidence for enhanced repolarization gradients in the setting of the failing heart [8,9] and these can promote reentrant arrhythmias. However, recent studies performed using explanted failing human hearts [6,10,11] provide little evidence for these enhanced repolarization gradients. These controversial results were theoretically approached in our accompanying paper [12], showing that heterogeneous ionic remodeling modulates repolarization gradients. These repolarization gradients can also be enhanced by structural remodeling, for example fibrosis and/or cellular uncoupling [13], which simultaneously alter conduction properties [11,14,15], increasing the likelihood of reentry. The lack of detailed functional and structural information limits the utility of experimental studies for identifying the precise role of HF remodeling on propagation disorders of the cardiac electrical activity. Computational approach can provide a powerful tool for the analysis of the contributions of different components of a disease. Simulations of reentrant rhythms in the human heart with emphasis on electrophysiological remodeling in HF have been published by Moreno et al. [16] focussing on the effect of drugs. Zlochiver et al. [17] evaluated the current density threshold for cardiac resynchronization treatment, and Turner et al. [18] analyzed electrogram fractionation. Recent studies have simulated the effects of fibrosis on reentry in ventricle [4,17,19–23] and atrium [24,25]. However, no simulation studies combining electrophysiological HF remodeling, fibrosis and intercellular uncoupling to analyze the vulnerability to reentry in the failing human heart have been performed (see Figure S1, Figure S2, Figure S3, and Figure S4 in File S1). Furthermore, the analysis of the reentry dynamics under these pathological conditions has not been addressed. We have evaluated whether phase analysis could reveal how heterogeneities caused by electrophysiological and structural remodeling may lead to reentrant waves. Indeed, phase analysis provides a useful tool to follow the electrical propagation activity of the spiral wave and to analyze the arrhythmogenic substrate under such pathophysiological settings. Several studies have used phase maps to follow the trajectory of reentrant activity experimentally [26,27] and theoretically [28,29] but none of these have focused on considered conditions of heart failure remodeling in conjunction with fibrosis.

In the present study the electrical activity of a transmural two-dimensional human ventricular tissue was simulated using a human action potential (AP) model [30,31] modified to replicate a HF phenotype. The influence of HF-induced electrophysiological and structural remodeling on vulnerability for reentrant arrhythmia occurrence was studied, and the dynamics of reentrant circuits under such pathological conditions were analyzed.

Methods

Tansmural failing tissue

The electrical activity of a two dimensional (2D) cardiac tissue of 5 cm×5 cm was simulated. Anisotropy was modeled by considering that transverse conductivity was lower than longitudinal conductivity (anisotropy conductance ratio $\frac{\sigma_x}{\sigma_y} = 4$), and the longitudinal direction of cellular fibers was horizontal. Half of the tissue corresponded to endocardial cells and the other half to epicardial cells. This domain was discretized with 250000 square elements ($\Delta x = 0.01$ cm) which resulted in a total of 251001 nodes within the tissue. Temporal resolution (Δt) was fixed to 0.002 ms to ensure numerical convergence ($\Delta t < \Delta x^2/2D$). Human myocyte electrical activity was simulated using a modified version of Grandi et al. model (GPB) [30], in which a late sodium current (I_{NaL}) was added [31]. In order to assess the influence of HF-induced electrophysiological remodeling, our HF model [31] was implemented, as described in the accompanying paper [12]. Thereafter, structural remodeling was also considered by adding 'fibrosis' and/or intercellular uncoupling within this tissue. The electrical activity of fibroblasts was simulated using the 'active' formulation of MacCannell et al. [32].

The diffusion coefficient (D) in normal conditions (NC) for myocytes was set to $D_M = 0.0013$ cm^2/ms resulting in a conduction velocity (CV) of 50 cm/s which agreed with experimental measurements of transmural conduction [33]. To simulate cell-to-cell uncoupling in heart failure, D was reduced in accordance with experimental data [34]. A 50% reduction was applied between failing myocytes (D_{LOW}) and a three-fold reduction was used between fibroblasts [35,36] and for the myocyte-fibroblast interaction (D_{Fib}). A wide range of fibroblast-myocyte gap-junctional conductance has been reported in experimental [35,37,38] and simulation studies [4,32,36,39,40]. Selected values within these ranges were used.

Fibroblast distribution was organized randomly, by assigning a probabilistic function. Random arrays were generated with different probabilities of assigning the fibroblast ionic model to the nodes. Four configurations of the same random condition were made. These gave rise to different levels of fibrosis quantified as the percentage of nodes executing the fibroblast model (P_f). Tissue configurations were denoted as "minimal fibrosis" ($P_f = 4\%$), "mild fibrosis 1" ($P_f = 14.5\%$), "mild fibrosis 2" ($P_f = 28\%$), and "high fibrosis" ($P_f = 40\%$). These values of P_f are similar to the ones considered in [20] and would correspond to fibrotic areas within experimental ranges [41].

As stated above, the mesh was discretized in square elements of 100 μm×100 μm. One element was composed of four nodes (separated in 100 μm), as shown in Figure 1. Each node executed either the fibroblast ionic model or the myocyte AP model. The value of the diffusion coefficient of a myocyte (D_M) was assigned to an element composed of 4 nodes executing the myocyte AP model. If one or more nodes of an element executed the fibroblast ionic

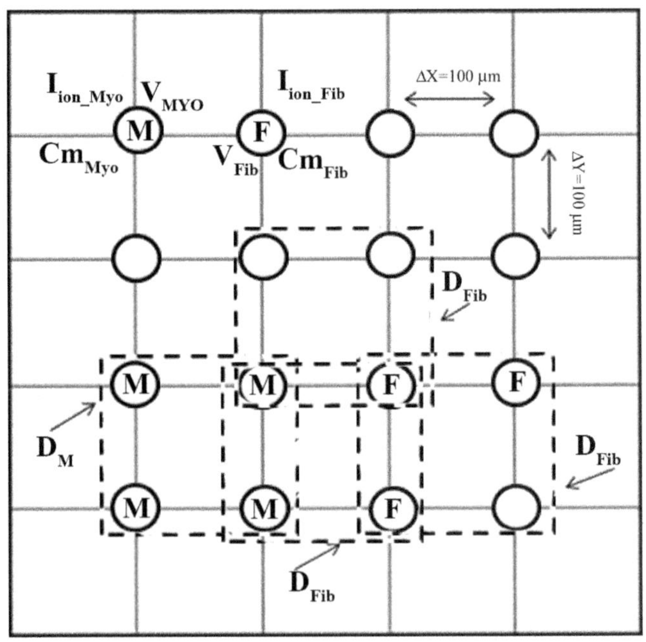

Figure 1. Illustration of the configuration of our virtual human ventricular mesh of interconnected myocytes and fibroblasts. V is the membrane voltage computed for each node, i.e. V_{MYO} for myocytes and V_{Fib} for fibroblasts. C_m is the cell capacitance, i.e. C_{mMyo} for myocytes and C_{mFib} for fibroblasts. D is the diffusion coefficient, i.e. D_M between myocytes in normal conditions ($D_M = 0.0013$ cm^2/ms), and D_{Fib} between a myocyte and a fibroblast, assigned to each element in the discretized domain. I_{ion} is the total transmembrane ionic current, i.e. I_{MYO} for myocytes and I_{Fib} for fibroblasts. 'M' and 'F' correspond to the 'myocyte' and 'fibroblast' model respectively that are computed in each node.

model, then the diffusion coefficient of a fibroblast (D_{Fib}), was assigned to this element.

Stimulation Protocol

After achieving steady-state conditions, five stimuli adjusted to 2 times the excitation threshold in amplitude and 2 ms in duration were applied at the endocardial end of the tissue with a basic cycle length (BCL) of 1000 ms. Electrophysiological properties were measured for the last AP.

To generate spiral wave in 2D simulations, we applied the cross-field stimulation protocol [42]. Once the tissue was stabilized, five stimuli were applied at the endocardial end of the tissue to get an entire wavefront throughout the tissue. After allowing the excitation wave-tail corresponding to the last stimulus to reach the middle part of the tissue, a second S2 stimulation was applied at the endocardial left bottom corner of the tissue (2.5 cm high × 1.25 cm wide). This triggered a meandering activation wave (due to wavefront/wave-tail interaction) leading to the formation of a spiral wave. The vulnerable window (VW), an indicator for vulnerability to reentry, was defined as the value of the coupling intervals (CIs) for S2 that led to reentry (at least two spiral wave rotations).

Spiral Wave Dynamics

To analyze the dynamics of the spiral waves, the dominant spiral wave period was calculated and phase analyses were performed.

Using the information of the AP upstroke in all points of the sheet, histograms of cycle lengths values measured to the nearest 1 ms were developed during the simulation and were used to calculate the dominant spiral wave period as in [43].

Phase analysis of the membrane potential signal (V_m) represents a useful method to identify and quantify spatiotemporal organization of reentry dynamics. The phase tracks the progression of a defined region of the myocardium through the action potential and has been demonstrated to be an effective parameter in analyzing spatiotemporal changes. Points around which the phase progresses through a complete cycle from $-\pi$ to π are of special interest. At these points, the phase becomes indeterminate and the activation wave fronts hinge on these points and rotate around them in an organized fashion. These points in the phase map are called phase singularity points (PS). PSs share location with anatomic heterogeneities, and their spatial meandering is modulated by these heterogeneities. PS also correlate with the location of wave breaks [44] in myopathic human hearts. At a phase singularity point the following condition is met:

$$\oint \nabla\theta \cdot dr = \pm 2\pi \tag{1}$$

where θ is the instantaneous phase. The integral is computed along the closed curve surrounding the anatomical or functional defect.

To obtain phase maps an algorithm in MATLAB calculated the Hilbert Transform (HT) of the membrane potential (V_m) signal in every node of the discretized domain to avoid the results dependence with the chosen time delay [26], and the 'instantaneous phase' was calculated in each node as follows:

$$\theta = \tan^{-1}\frac{HT(V_m)}{V_m} \tag{2}$$

Phase maps were codified between [−π, π] as in [45]. In our discretized mesh domain PS was defined as a singular point around which the condition of equation (3) was met.

$$||\Delta\theta_1 + \Delta\theta_2 + \Delta\theta_3 + \Delta\theta_4| - 2\pi| < 0.001 \tag{3}$$

where $\Delta\theta_1$ is the phase difference between nodes B and A, $\Delta\theta_2$ is the phase difference between nodes C and B, $\Delta\theta_3$ is the phase difference between nodes D and C, $\Delta\theta_4$ is the phase difference between nodes A and D [45], as depicted in Figure 2.

Computational methods

ELVIRA software was used in our simulations, which is based on a pseudo-adaptive finite element method in space and time to solve reaction–diffusion equations with highly nonlinear reactive terms [46]. The scheme accounts for the anisotropy of the media and incorporates an adaptive time step algorithm to integrate the stiff reactive term associated with the ionic currents. The solution of the monodomain equation (4) is computed using the technique of operator splitting.

$$\nabla(\tilde{D}\nabla V_m) = \frac{dV_m}{dt} + \frac{I_{ion}}{C_m} + \frac{I_{stm}}{C_m} \tag{4}$$

$$n\cdot(D\nabla V_m) = 0 \tag{5}$$

Where V_m is membrane potential in (V), $\tilde{D} = \frac{\tilde{\sigma}}{S_V C_m}$ in (m^2/s) is the diffusion conductivity tensor, $\tilde{\sigma}$ is the conductivity tensor in (S.m), S_V is the surface to volume ratio of the cell in (m^{-1}), C_m in (F) is the membrane capacity, I_{ion} is the ionic total current in (A), and I_{stm} in (A) is the stimulus current. Equation (4) has boundary conditions (5). Further information will be found in [46]. Tissue mesh representation is shown in Figure 1.

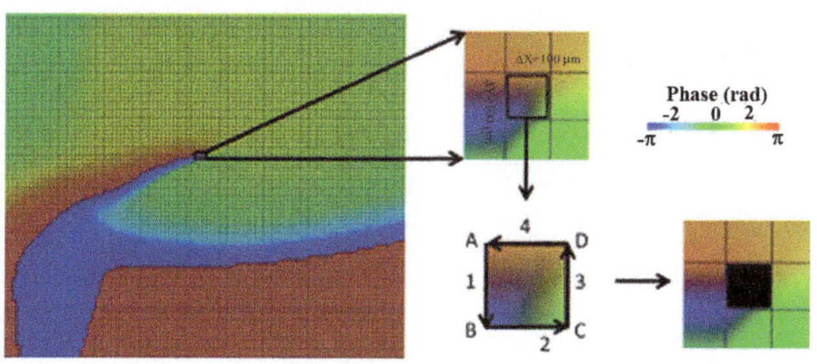

Figure 2. Illustration of phase map analysis. Instantaneous phase of the membrane potential (V_m) signal at the different nodes of the tissue is computed. A phase singularity in an element is operationally defined as all phases being detected within the element (see Methods section for details).

Results

Effects of heart failure remodeling on reentry generation

To simulate reentrant activity, cross-field stimulation was applied to the transmural tissue composed of endocardial and epicardial cells, as described in the Methods section. Reentrant activity or unidirectional block was not observed, either in normal conditions or under HF ionic remodeling conditions. In both situations repolarization time was too large to enable propagation and the wave front was blocked after premature stimulation. If the premature stimulus S2 was applied with a longer coupling interval (S1–S2), complete propagation of S2 was achieved. It is to be noted that the size of the tissue, 5 cm×5 cm in the present simulations, is an important factor for the generation of spiral waves [47], and bigger tissues might lead to the generation of reentry for the above conditions. However, because of the high computational cost of a larger tissue, simulations were performed for the described size.

Fibrosis (14.5%) was then added to NC configuration and reentrant activity was observed (see Figure 3, panel A). The spatiotemporal evolution of the reentrant wave is shown in Video S1. A set of simulations varying the coupling interval was performed to determine the vulnerable window for reentry (VW). This was approximately 20 ms. When the HF model was studied with the same amount of fibrosis, reentrant activity was also observed (see Figure 3, panel B). The VW was as wide as that in NC, but the limits of the VW were delayed (corresponding to bigger coupling intervals).

These results suggest that HF electrical remodeling does not alter the width of the VW, and for this reason the likelihood of reentrant activity is unchanged. However, fibrosis seems to be an important determining factor for reentry generation.

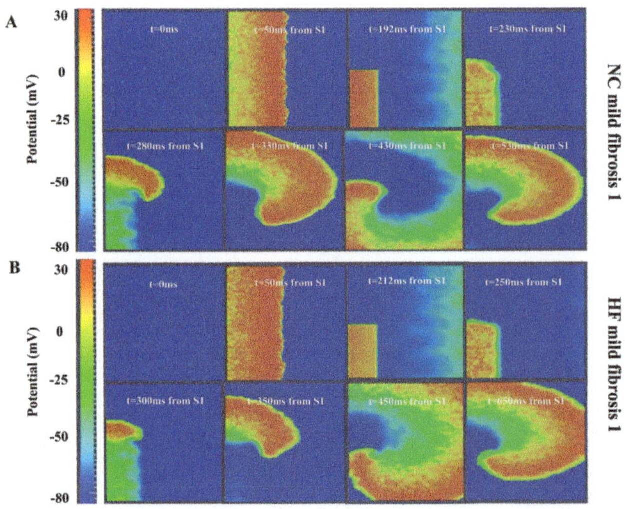

Figure 3. Reentrant activity intransmural fibrotic human ventricular tissue. A. Voltage snapshots in the transmural tissue under normal conditions (NC) and following introduction of 14.5% random fibrosis (mildfibrosis1). B. Voltage snapshots in the transmural tissue assuming heart failure (HF) induced electrophysiological remodeling together with 14.5% random fibrosis (mildfibrosis1). In both panels a cross-field protocol S1–S2 was applied to initiate conduction (see Methods section for details). For full spatiotemporal evolution of panel A see **Video S1**.

Effects of fibrosis on reentry generation

In order to understand the role of fibrosis in reentry generation several degrees of fibrosis were considered. Figure 4 panel A shows the initial membrane potential for different densities of fibroblasts in the failing tissue. Due to the depolarized resting potential of fibroblasts, spontaneous activity appeared in different zones of the ventricular tissue even when the percentage of fibrosis was relatively small (mild fibrosis 2), as shown in Figure 4 panel B (ectopic activity shown in Video S2). After cross-field stimulation, as described above, the presence of intermediate fibrosis ('mild fibrosis 1', 14.5% of fibrotic content) led to reentrant activity in both normal and HF conditions. A more detailed analysis of how fibrosis density can affect the probability of reentry was carried out in HF conditions, (when fibrosis is known to develop). Indeed, the quantity of fibrosis significantly alters the electrical properties of the tissue, as we have shown in the accompanying paper [12]. When 'low fibrosis' (4%) configuration was considered, we could not induce reentrant activity, regardless of the CI. Thus, there was no VW. As described in the previous section, with an intermediate level of fibrosis (14.5%) a VW of around 20 ms was obtained (see Table 1). Indeed, when enough fibrosis is present, the APD and effective refractory period of the myocardial cells are shortened [12], so that when the premature stimulation was applied, part of the ventricular tissue had recovered enough to be excited and a spiral reentry was generated (see Figure 3 panel B). Similar results were obtained using 'mild-fibrosis 2' (28%) configuration, and an example of reentry is shown in Figure 4 panel C. Under these conditions, the VW was even longer, around 33 ms. When the 'high fibrosis' (40%) configuration was evaluated (see Figure 4 panel D), a spiral wave front could be observed. However, in this case, the depolarizing wave front reached very low potentials, leading to electrotonic voltage changes (the spatiotemporal evolution of the wave is shown in Video S3), and could not be considered as reentrant activity, as will be demonstrated later in the phase maps analysis. Thus, intermediate fibrosis increases the VW and very high fibrosis avoids reentry generation, as summarized in Table 1. Several random realizations were simulated for each degree of fibrosis (see Table S1 in File S1) and similar results were obtained for the widths of the vulnerable windows corresponding to the same amount of fibrosis.

In the cases where spiral waves were obtained the dominant period was measured, as shown in Figure 5 and indicated in Table 1. For a reentrant wave generated after an S2 stimulus applied at an instant of time within the vulnerable window (S2 applied at t = 210 ms for mild fibrosis 1 and t = 170 ms for mild fibrosis 2) the dominant spiral wave periods were 240 ms and 250 ms for mild fibrosis 1 and 2, respectively. Thus, the rotation frequency of the spiral wave slightly decreased with increased fibrosis.

Intercellular uncoupling effects on reentry generation

The structural remodeling of HF includes not only fibrosis but also intercellular uncoupling. To understand the role of this uncoupling in the generation of reentry, simulations were performed using NC tissue with reduced electrical conductivity (DLOW). Under normal coupling conditions, reentry was not obtained (see Figure 6 panel A) for the selected size of the tissue. Thus, the conductivity was gradually reduced until reentrant activity developed (see Figure 6 panel B), which would be formally equivalent to increase the size of the tissue. This required a ten-fold reduction of the diffusion coefficient (the spatiotemporal evolution of the reentrant wave is shown in Video S4). Normal CV was 50 cm/s [33], and was reduced down to 18 cm/s, for the low

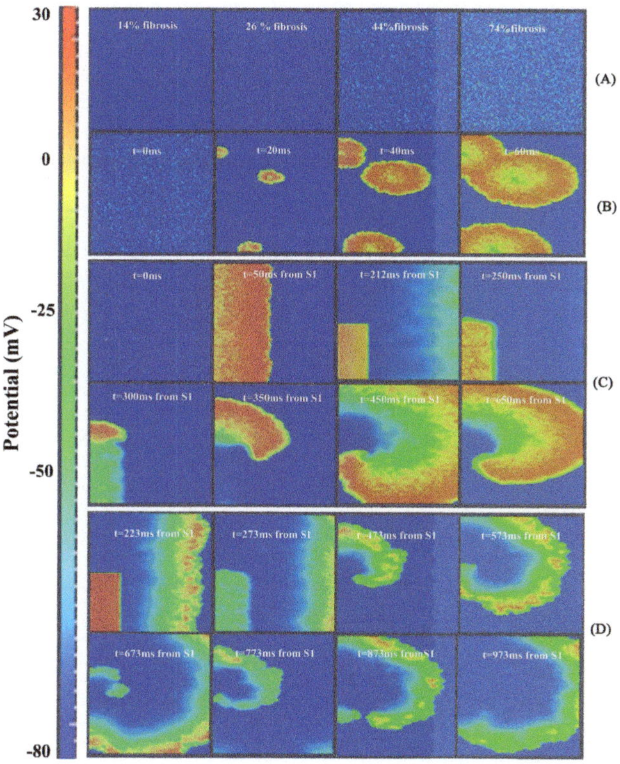

Figure 4. Illustration of the effect of fibrosis in human ventricular tissue. A. Voltage snapshots corresponding to initial conditions, different fibrotic tissue configurations. B. Spontaneous electrical activity in 'mildfibrosis 2'. C. Voltage snapshots of transmural tissue assuming heart failure conditions together with 28% of random fibrosis ('mildfibrosis 1'). In the first two frames, propagation of the action potential due to the S1 stimulus is observed and note also that propagation of the action potential elucidated by the S2 stimulus is observed after the third frame. D. Voltage snapshots of transmural tissue assuming heart failure conditions together with 40% of random fibrosis ('high fibrosis'). S1–S2 cross-field protocol was also used to stimulate the tissue, but in this case only the propagation of stimulus S2 is shown. For full spatiotemporal evolution of panel B see **Video S2**. For full spatiotemporal evolution of panel D see **Video S3**.

conductivity conditions. This could also be estimated by the proportionality between CV and $\sqrt{D}$.

Although intercellular uncoupling led to reentry in normal conditions, we also investigated this effect in failing tissues with defined levels of fibrosis. To determine how the VW was modified by intercellular uncoupling, 'mild-fibrosis 2' configuration was adopted and different levels of uncoupling were employed in the simulations. Under such conditions with normal cellular coupling, the VW was 30 ms (see Table 1). When intercellular uncoupling was increased (two-fold decrease of the diffusion coefficient), VW was increased to 42 ms. A ten-fold reduction of conductivity yielded a VW of 112 ms. For very low diffusion coefficients (one hundred-fold reduction), cellular uncoupling was high enough to block the electrical propagation. Thus, as shown in Figure 7, an intermediate level of cellular uncoupling favors reentry generation.

Analysis of reentry generation in HF with fibrosis using phase maps

To more completely understand the dynamics of reentry in the presence of fibrosis, we employed phase maps, to illustrate and analyze the spatiotemporal organization of reentry dynamics. Figure 8 depicts the evolution of the spiral wave for the selected fibrotic conditions with electrical HF-induced ionic remodeling. When no fibroblasts were present ("without fibrosis" configuration), concentrated phase singularities were detected, revealing clearly the trajectory of the rotor tip. This trajectory can be observed in red color in the last snapshot of panel A. In this setting, reentry developed when intercellular uncoupling was increased. The corresponding spatiotemporal evolution of the instantaneous phase is shown in Video S5. As the fibrotic content of the tissue increased ('mild fibrosis 2'), under HF electrophysiological remodeling conditions and normal intercellular coupling, the phase singularities were transient and sparse throughout the ventricular tissue. The trajectory of the rotor tip could also be identified (red color in the last snapshot of panel B), although it was less concentrated than in the absence of fibrosis, due to the fibroblast –induced electrical heterogeneities. In this last snapshot all transient phase singularities throughout the simulation time are also shown in black. The corresponding spatiotemporal evolution of the instantaneous phase is shown in Video S6. When a high level of fibrosis was introduced ('high fibrosis' configuration), with HF electrophysiological remodeling and normal intercellular coupling, multiple phase singularities appeared during the entire simulation. However, PSs did not follow a specific trajectory. In this case, a rotor tip could not be defined. The phase maps show (in red and blue colors) the phases of the small depolarization, showing only electrotonic interactions, as opposed to AP propagation. The corresponding spatiotemporal evolution of the instantaneous phase is shown in Video S7.

Discussion

This computational study focussed on the vulnerability to reentry and the dynamics of spiral waves in a virtual failing human ventricular tissue, with transmural heterogeneity, electrophysio-

Table 1. Vulnerable window analysis.

Simulation	Vulnerable window for reentry (ms)	Limits of the VW (ms)	Rotation Period (ms)
HF 4% fibrosis	0	-	0
HF 14.5% fibrosis	20	[204;224]	240
HF 28% fibrosis	33	[170;203]	250
HF 40% fibrosis	0	-	0

Vulnerable window for reentry under conditions of heart failure (HF) induced ionic remodeling with different amounts of diffuse fibrosis. The first column shows the width of the vulnerable window, the second column shows the limits of the vulnerable windows, i.e. the first and last instants of time at which S2 is applied to generate reentry, the third column shows the rotation period of the spiral waves taken from Figure 5.

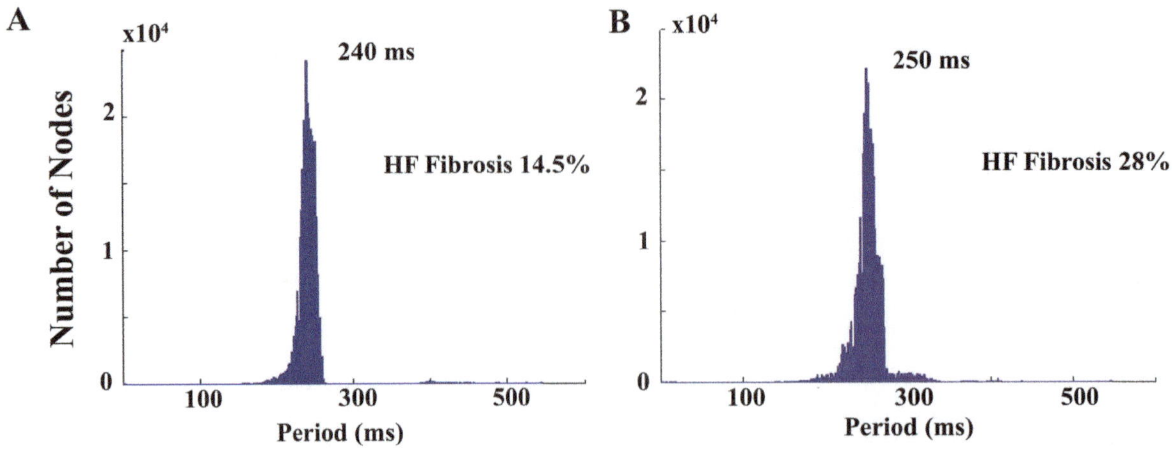

Figure 5. Spiral waves periods. Using the information of the AP upstroke in all points of the sheet, histograms of cycle lengths values measured to the nearest 1 ms were developed during the simulation as in [43]. The reentrant waves generated after an S2 stimulus applied at an instant of time situated in the center of the vulnerable window (S2 applied at t = 210 ms for mild fibrosis 1 and t = 170 ms for mild fibrosis 2) were considered to build the histograms. The dominant spiral wave periods were 240 ms and 250 ms for mild fibrosis 1 and 2, respectively.

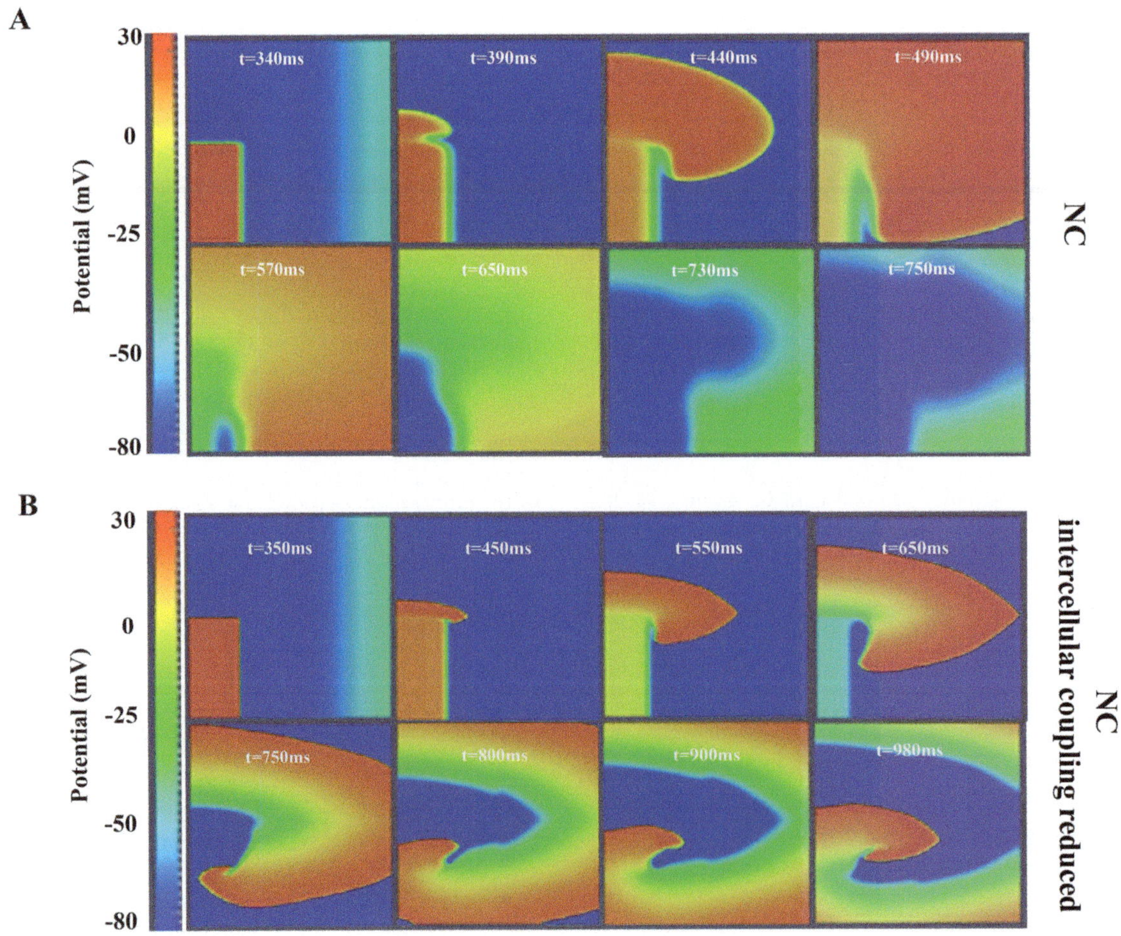

Figure 6. Effects of cell-to-cell uncoupling on reentry generation. A. Voltage snapshots in the transmural human ventricular tissue under normal conditions (NC). B. Voltage snapshots in the transmural tissue NC with a marked decrease in intercellular coupling (conductivity was reduced ten-fold). S1–S2 cross-field protocol was used to stimulate the tissue. Only the response to S2 stimulus is shown. For full spatiotemporal evolution of panel B see **Video S4**.

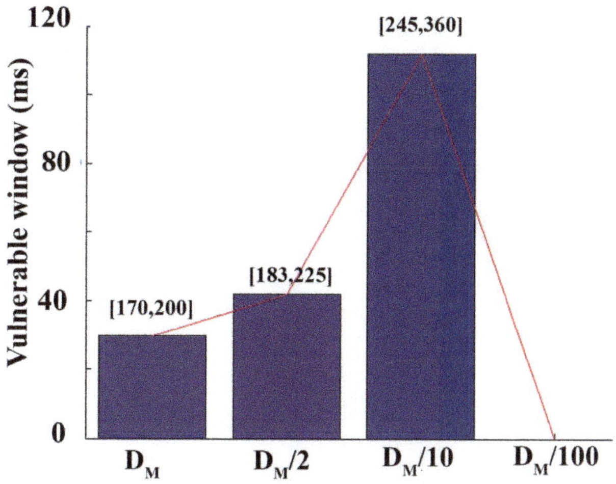

Figure 7. Summary of the computed vulnerable window corresponding to selected reductions inintercellular coupling. Vulnerable window for reentry in ms versus diffusion coefficient in 'mild fibrosis 2' configuration (HF ionic remodeling and 28% of fibrosis).

logical remodeling, cellular uncoupling and fibrosis. It was designed to assess the contributions of each component of heart failure, i.e. ionic remodeling, intercellular uncoupling and fibrosis, to arrhythmogenesis. The principal findings and insights from our work are (i) demonstration that HF electrophysiological remodeling delays the limits of the vulnerable window for reentry but does not alter the width of the VW, so that the likelihood of reentrant activity is not enhanced; (ii) confirmation that fibrosis is determinant for reentry generation; intermediate fibrotic levels increase the VW and favor reentry generation, while high levels hamper it; (iii) evidence that intermediate intercellular uncoupling enhances the VW; (iv) understanding how the active interaction between fibroblasts and failing myocytes increases the presence of phase singularities in ventricular tissues and alters the spiral wave dynamics in reentrant circuits.

Contribution of electrical remodeling on reentry generation

Patients with severe heart failure are at high risk of sudden cardiac death. In the majority of these patients, sudden cardiac death is due to ventricular tachyarrhythmias (VT). Alterations of the electric properties of single myocytes in heart failure may favor the occurrence of VT in these patients by inducing early or delayed afterdepolarizations (EADs or DADs) [5]. In failing hearts with a healed infarct, VT is caused by reentrant excitation within the network of surviving myocardial fibers in the infarct. In non-ischemic cardiomyopathies, both in humans and in animal models, VT is predominantly due to non-reentrant mechanisms, most likely triggered activity caused by DADs [2,48]. The generation of EADs and DADs in failing human hearts has also been simulated in computational studies [31,49] using Grandi et al. AP model [30]. Electrophysiological remodeling in failing hearts not only facilitates triggered activity but it also results in an arrhytmogenic substrate, as shown in the accompanying paper [12]. Both effects are necessary to reentry generation. One of the aims of the present study was to evaluate how HF electrophysiological remodeling affects the probability of reentry generation. Our results suggest that HF electrical remodeling (alone) does not alter the width of the VW with respect to normal conditions, although the limits of the VW are delayed. Indeed, repolarization is delayed in HF and premature stimulation can lead to reentry if applied at later instants of time Moreno et al. [16] evaluated the effects of drugs on reentry generation in a virtual human ventricular tissue with HF-induced electrophysiological remodeling and observed also that conduction block occurred at slower frequencies with HF remodeling, thus delaying the limits of the vulnerable window for reentry generation. This was due to the alteration of cell excitability caused by prolongation of APD in HF. Other computational studies introducing HF electrophysiological remodeling in 2D tissues [17,18] have been performed but none of these studies focused on the effect of electrical remodeling on vulnerability to reentry, as illustrated in the present study.

Contribution of structural remodeling on reentry generation

Structural remodeling in the failing heart, i.e. fibrosis and intercellular uncoupling, is an important factor favoring the formation of reentrant waves. Fibrosis is thought to contribute to the deterioration of LV function (impairing the mechanical properties of the left ventricle during diastole) and electrical activity (facilitating arrhythmogenesis) [50,51]. As shown in the accompanying paper [12], fibrosis decreased conduction velocity in accordance with other studies [4,11]. Videos S1, S2 and S3 and Figures 3 and 4 show a discontinuous wavefront in the presence of fibrosis as in [20]. Experimentally, Glukhov et al. [11] optically mapped the coronary perfused left ventricular wedge preparations from human hearts with end-stage nonischemic cardiomyopathy and reported nonuniform propagation discontinuities and wave breaks conditioned by strands of increased interstitial fibrosis. It is also known that the excitability of the tissue is altered in the presence of fibroblasts and spontaneous depolarizations were observed in our simulations (see Figure 4). As shown experimentally by Miragoli et al. [52] in tissue cultures, myocytes coupled to fibroblasts might exhibit spontaneous depolarizations, depending on the density of fibrosis and heterocellular coupling conductance (see [53] for review). Similarly, in their simulation study, Greisas and Zlochiver [42] obtained spontaneous excitations. These spontaneous excitations are the result of the myocyte membrane depolarization up to the threshold imposed by the coupled fibroblasts, which exhibit a less negative resting potential. Dispersion of repolarization is also enhanced by structural remodeling [12], setting the substrate for reentry. The alteration of the electrical properties of the tissue in the presence of fibrosis might lead to a higher probability of reentry generation. Indeed, our results suggest that intermediate fibrosis increases the VW and that very high fibrosis hampers reentry generation. A similar biphasic behavior was observed in the computational work of McDowell et al. [21] who simulated reentry in a virtual infarcted rabbit heart for different degrees of fibrosis. Xie et al. [4] also demonstrated that functional fibroblast-myocyte coupling facilitates induction of reentry in a virtual heterogeneous cardiac tissue. Majumder et al. [20] added several levels of diffuse fibrosis with passive interaction with myocytes, in a two dimensional transmural tissue. They reported a variety of non-equilibrium states which led to conduction block and spiral waves; they did not consider the possibility of active interaction between both kind of cells as we did in the present study.

Our results also highlighted the fact that an intermediate level of cellular uncoupling favors reentry generation. This was also reported by Ramirez et al. in the setting of myocardial ischemia (phase 1b) with different intercellular uncouling degrees. Wiegerink et al. [14] also related the increase of intercellular coupling to arrhtyhmia inducibility in a rabbit experimental model of HF.

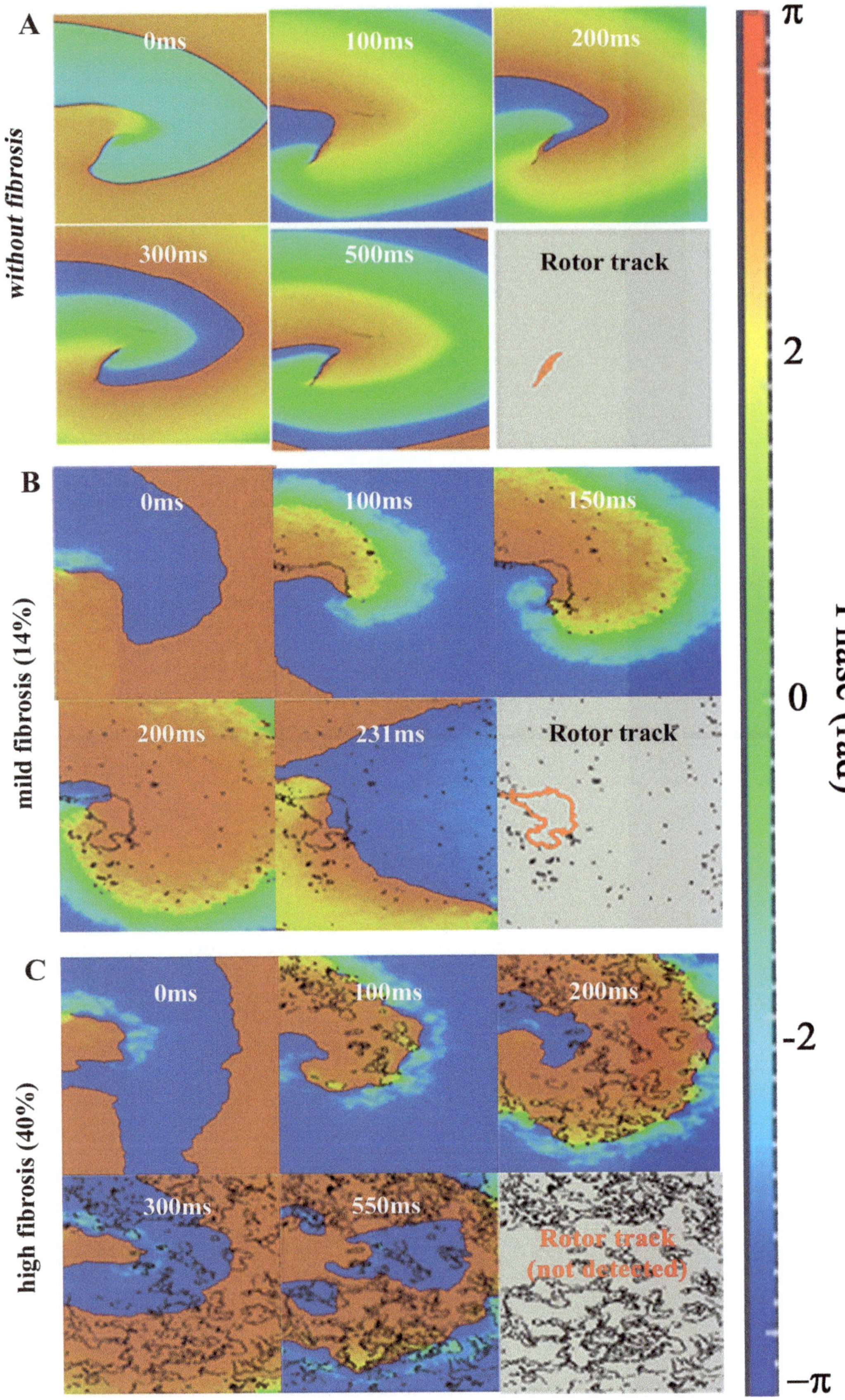
A
without fibrosis
0ms
100ms
200ms
300ms
500ms
Rotor track
B
mild fibrosis (14%)
0ms
100ms
150ms
200ms
231ms
Rotor track
C
high fibrosis (40%)
0ms
100ms
200ms
300ms
550ms
Rotor track
(not detected)
π
2
0
-2
−π
Phase (rad)

Figure 8. Phase map analysis of evoked rhythm disturbances on the failing human ventricular tissue. Phase maps in electrically remodeled failing tissues assuming selected levels of fibrotic content. In the first case (panel A), 'without fibrosis', the intercellular coupling is increased ten-fold. The 'mild fibrosis' (panel B) and 'high fibrosis' (panel C) cases assume normal intercellular coupling conditions. All transient phase singularities are indicated in black, and the tip of the trajectory is indicated in red in the last snapshot of each panel. For full spatiotemporal evolution of panels A, B, and C, see **Videos S5, S6,** and **S7,** respectively.

Thus, structural remodeling strongly modulates the substrate for arrhythmogenesis, as was demonstrated in the accompanying paper [12], and seems to be a determinant factor in reentry generation according to our present results. Although the relationship between the type of reentry and tissue architecture has not been identified, it is likely that in hearts with diffuse fibrosis one or more rotors may maintain the arrhythmia [54] whereby the tissue discontinuities may function as (temporary) anchoring points for the mother rotor [55]. The analysis of the reentrant waves dynamics with structural remodeling deserves in fact special attention.

Reentrant wave dynamics in the failing heart

During reentry, electrical activity propagates within a defined closed path, thus forming a spiral wave of activation in two dimensions and a scroll wave in three dimensions (3D) [47]. Spiral and scroll waves are active sources of excitation, which organize the spatiotemporal pattern of excitation of the myocardium during arrhythmia. 2D spiral waves are characterized by a wave break at the core of the spiral (spiral wave tip). Gray et al. [56] developed the technique we used in the present study based on phase plane analysis to investigate the dynamics of spiral rotors. They identified phase singularities, and their characterization allowed the tracking of the spiral and its tip dynamics in space, over time [57] and the systematic study of initiation, maintenance and termination of rotors. Wave break and formation of a PS is an essential condition for a rotor to exist. The formation of PS is necessary, although not sufficient, for sustained rotation. In addition, a new excitation wave must be generated. Furthermore, a PS must last over time (at least one rotation period) to form a rotor.

In the present work phase maps analysis was used to assess for the first time the influence of fibrotic content under failing conditions on reentry generation. Our simulation results showed that in the absence of fibrosis the induced reentrant waves presented concentrated and regular rotors; when intermediate levels of fibrosis were considered, the tip of the reentry meandered within a larger area and the vulnerable window was wider. The compactness of the tip trajectory prevents a single spiral from splitting into multiple spirals [19]. Thus, the extent of the fibrosis is a key factor in determining the dynamics of reentrant waves under failing conditions. In the case of a high level of fibrosis only electrotonic cell-cell communication was found, the density of PSs was very high but no tip trajectory could be identified. The amount of PSs in this case gave evidence of the heterogeneous nature of the tissue. The ability to correlate PSs with anatomy provides the potential to investigate the relationship between PSs and structural heterogeneities.

Others have employed phase map analysis to follow the trajectory of the spiral tip and the rotor dynamics during tachycardia or fibrillation [26,27]. However, little research has been done on the relationship between fibrosis, phase singularities and spiral wave dynamics. Recently Majumder et al. [20] and Nayak et al. [19] performed a dynamical analysis of simulated spiral waves in the presence of fibrosis. However, their study was focussed on the tip trajectory and the non-equilibrium states. A phase analysis was not performed. To our knowledge, the only study analyzing the relationship between simulated fibrosis and phase maps was done by Zlochiver et al. [58]. They demonstrated also that the amount of PSs increased with fibrotic content. However, in their work fibroblasts were considered as passive elements and no heart failure ionic remodeling was considered. In this way, our simulation work complements the above mentioned studies and brings new insights into the effects of heart failure induced electrophysiological and structural remodeling on spiral wave dynamics.

To further characterize the dynamics of spiral waves the spiral wave rotation period was calculated under different conditions of fibrosis (see Figure 5 and table 1) and the rotation frequency slightly decreased with the increase of fibrosis. Zlochiver et al. [58] also observed a decrease in the rotor frequency when the amount of fibrosis was increased. Tanaka et al. [25] reported as well a decrease in the dominant frequency in atrial fibrillation in failing sheep atria and related it to the presence of fibrosis. In a recent study, Greisas et al. [42] calculated the rotation period of the spiral wave, however they used the information of the AP in only one site of the tissue to calculate the period of the rotation wave and found a biphasic behavior: the rotation frequency increased and then decreased when fibrosis was increased.

Limitations of the study

This study provides novel mechanistic insights into reentry generation in the human failing human heart. We acknowledge, however, that our work has some significant limitations. Firstly, our anatomical description of the cardiac tissue does not include accurate fiber orientation or electrophysiological heterogeneities, as more detailed 3D ventricular models can provide. However, anisotropic conduction was considered in our 2D tissue simulations. Secondly, only the active model of fibroblasts (including ionic currents) was considered as in [21,32,39,59], while others have considered a passive interaction between myocytes and fibroblasts [4,19,20,58]. Although functional coupling between myocytes and fibroblasts has been identified in cultured preparations [60] and ionic currents have been identified in fibroblasts [38], no experiments have reported the presence of active fibroblasts in human. Furthermore, due to the irregular shape of coupled fibroblasts, these are difficult to identify [61]. Thus, modeling and simulation work provides a helpful tool to reproduce this hypothetical scenario. It is also to be noted that a smaller spatial discretization as in [4], would allow a more realistic definition of the size of fibroblasts, taking into account that a fibroblast is more than four times smaller than a myocyte. However, this would increase significantly the computational cost. In any case, in our simulations the ionic models consider the difference of capacity between a fibroblast and a myocyte, scaling accordingly the ionic currents. Finally, with regard to the random introduction of fibroblasts in the tissue, an increase in the number of random configurations for each level of fibrosis would allow to perform a statistical analysis of the effects of fibrosis. Because of the high computational cost this would suppose, we only simulated four different configurations for each case, and it can be stated that the results were very similar.

Conclusions and clinical implications

In summary, this study shows that electrophysiological and structural remodeling in failing hearts exert an essential influence on reentry generation and dynamics. Electrical coupling of cardiomyocytes with fibroblasts cells alters the anisotropic action potential propagation in the human failing heart in a fashion that significantly depends on the density of fibrotic content and on the degree of intercellular coupling. This raises the possibility that pharmaceutical treatment with eg. rotigaptide, (which increases intercellular coupling), might affect reentrant activity. Phase maps analysis provides a powerful tool to explore abnormal conduction patterns in the setting of ventricular fibrosis. Identifying and studying the different organizational manifestations of phase distribution during arrhythmias in the presence of fibrosis provides one means for objective characterization of arrhythmias. Our findings also may be relevant to ablative procedures, which might have improved success when the targets for ablation enclose the boundaries of tip meandering, as revealed by the phase analysis. Indeed, understanding the relationship between VT organizing centers and fibrosis has important implications for VT ablation since it could provide guidance in determining the optimal targets of VT ablation, as demonstrated by Ashikaga et al. 2013 [62] in their simulation study. They accurately identified optimal targets of ablation in patient-specific heart models and carried out effectively non-invasive ablation. This computational method prior to the clinical procedure supposes a potential translational effort in developing simulation predictions for the optimal targets of VT ablation. Similarly, ablation in zones of complex fractionated electrograms, which are related to the presence of fibrosis [63], and surrounded by phase singularities, has been shown to be effective in simulation studies [64]. Thus, phase maps analysis related to fibrosis seems to be a potent tool prior to the clinical ablation procedures.

Supporting Information

File S1

Video S1 Spiral-wave dynamics in our 2D model of heart failure (HF) in human ventricular myocyte-fibroblast tissue. This movie shows the evolution of membrane potential (V_m) in our 2D failing tissue with a fibrotic content of 14.5% (mild fibrosis 1 configuration). The S1–S2 cross-field stimulation protocol was applied (see Methods section for details). Evolution of a spiral wave is shown. 15 frames per second (fps) are used and the movie shows 900 ms of simulation. These results are also shown in Figure 3 panel A.

Video S2 Ectopic activity in our 2D failing myocyte-fibroblast tissue. This movie shows the evolution of membrane potential (V_m) in our 2D failing tissue with a fibrotic content of 28% (mild fibrosis 2 configuration). The differences in resting potential between fibroblasts and myocytes are responsible for the electrotonic interactions between these groups of cells. When the density of fibroblasts is quite high, V_m of the adjacent myocytes is depolarized to the action potential (AP) threshold. 15 frames per second (fps) are used and the movie shows 300 ms of simulation. These results are also shown in Figure 4 panel B.

Video S3 Non reentrant activity our 2D failing myocyte-fibroblast tissue. This movie shows the evolution of membrane potential (V_m) in our 2D heart failure (HF) tissue with a fibrotic content of 40% (high fibrosis configuration). The S1–S2 cross-field stimulation protocol was applied (see Methods section for details) and the evolution of electrotonic change in the membrane potential profile is shown. 15 frames per second (fps) are used and the movie shows 800 ms of simulation. These results are also shown in Figure 4 panel D.

Video S4 Spiral-wave dynamics under conditions of selected levels of intercellular uncoupling. This movie shows the evolution of membrane potential (V_m) in our 2D tissue under non electrical remodeling conditions (GPB model) but with structural remodeling included (intercellular resistance ten-fold reduced). S1–S2 cross-field stimulation protocol was applied (see Methods section for details) and the evolution of a spiral wave is shown. 15 frames per second (fps) are used and the movie shows 650 ms of simulation. These results are also shown in Figure 5 panel B.

Video S5 Phase spatiotemporal evolution without fibrosis. This movie shows the evolution of the membrane potential (V_m) (left movie) and the instantaneous phase (right movie) in our 2D tissue with heart failure induced electrical remodeling and intercellular uncoupling (diffusion coefficient was reduced 10 fold). The S1–S2 cross-field stimulation protocol was applied (see Methods section for details). All transient phase singularities are indicated in black; these are maintained in the video to observe their trajectory. 15 frames per second (fps) are used and the movie shows 260 ms of simulation. These results are also shown in Figure 7 panel A.

Video S6 Phase spatiotemporal evolution with mild fibrosis. This movie shows the evolution of the membrane potential (V_m) (left movie) and the instantaneous phase (right movie) in our 2D tissue with heart failure induced electrical remodeling and mild fibrosis. The S1–S2 cross-field stimulation protocol was applied (see Methods section for details). All transient phase singularities are indicated in black; these are maintained in the video to observe their trajectory. 15 frames per second (fps) are used and the movie shows 140 ms of simulation. These results are also shown in Figure 7 panel B.

Video S7 Phase spatiotemporal evolution with high fibrosis. This movie shows the evolution of the membrane potential (V_m) (left movie) and the instantaneous phase (right movie) in our 2D tissue with heart failure induced electrical remodeling and high fibrosis. The S1–S2 cross-field stimulation protocol was applied (see Methods section for details). All transient phase singularities are indicated in black; these are maintained in the video to observe their trajectory. 15 frames per second (fps) are used and the movie shows 425 ms of simulation. These results are also shown in Figure 7 panel C.

Author Contributions

Conceived and designed the experiments: BT JFG. Performed the experiments: JFG. Analyzed the data: JFG LM KC. Contributed reagents/materials/analysis tools: JFG LM. Wrote the paper: BT JFG JS.

References

1. Tomaselli GF, Zipes DP (2004) What causes sudden death in heart failure? Circ Res 95: 754–763.
2. Janse MJ (2004) Electrophysiological changes in heart failure and their relationship to arrhythmogenesis. Cardiovasc Res 61: 208–217.
3. Wit AL, Coromilas J (1993) Role of alterations in refractoriness and conduction in the genesis of reentrant arrhythmias. Implications for antiarrhythmic effects of class III drugs. Am J Cardiol 72: 3F–12F.
4. Xie Y, Garfinkel A, Camelliti P, Kohl P, Weiss JN, et al. (2009) Effects of fibroblast-myocyte coupling on cardiac conduction and vulnerability to reentry: A computational study. Heart Rhythm 6: 1641–1649.
5. Coronel R, Wilders R, Verkerk AO, Wiegerinck RF, Benoist D, et al. (2013) Electrophysiological changes in heart failure and their implications for arrhythmogenesis. Biochim Biophys Acta 1832: 2432–2441.
6. Lou Q, Fedorov VV, Glukhov AV, Moazami N, Fast VG, et al. (2011) Transmural heterogeneity and remodeling of ventricular excitation-contraction coupling in human heart failure. Circulation 123: 1881–1890.
7. Tomaselli GF, Marban E (1999) Electrophysiological remodeling in hypertrophy and heart failure. Cardiovasc Res 42: 270–283.
8. Akar FG, Rosenbaum DS (2003) Transmural electrophysiological heterogeneities underlying arrhythmogenesis in heart failure. Circ Res 93: 638–645.
9. Shi C, Wang X, Dong F, Wang Y, Hui J, et al. (2013) Temporal alterations and cellular mechanisms of transmural repolarization during progression of mouse cardiac hypertrophy and failure. Acta Physiol (Oxf) 208: 95–110.
10. Glukhov AV, Fedorov VV, Lou Q, Ravikumar VK, Kalish PW, et al. (2010) Transmural dispersion of repolarization in failing and nonfailing human ventricle. Circ Res 106: 981–991.
11. Glukhov AV, Fedorov VV, Kalish PW, Ravikumar VK, Lou Q, et al. (2012) Conduction remodeling in human end-stage nonischemic left ventricular cardiomyopathy. Circulation 125: 1835–1847.
12. Gomez JF, Cardona K, Romero L, Rajamani S, Belardinelli L, et al. (2013) Electrophysiological and structural remodeling in heart failure modulate arrhythmogenesis. 1D simulaton study. PLoS One Accompanying paper under review:
13. Gomez JF, Cardona K, Romero L, Saiz J, Trenor B (2013) Heterogeneous electrical remodeling of the failing heart modulates the arrhythmogenic substrate. Computing in Cardiology Proceedings 40: 49–52
14. Wiegerinck RF, van Veen TA, Belterman CN, Schumacher CA, Noorman M, et al. (2008) Transmural dispersion of refractoriness and conduction velocity is associated with heterogeneously reduced connexin43 in a rabbit model of heart failure. Heart Rhythm 5: 1178–1185.
15. Wilson LD, Jeyaraj D, Wan X, Hoeker GS, Said TH, et al. (2009) Heart failure enhances susceptibility to arrhythmogenic cardiac alternans. Heart Rhythm 6: 251–259.
16. Moreno JD, Zhu ZI, Yang PC, Bankston JR, Jeng MT, et al. (2011) A computational model to predict the effects of class I anti-arrhythmic drugs on ventricular rhythms. Sci Transl Med 3: 98ra83.
17. Zlochiver S (2010) Subthreshold parameters of cardiac tissue in a bi-layer computer model of heart failure. Cardiovasc Eng 10: 190–200.
18. Turner I, Huang H, Saumarez RC (2005) Numerical simulation of paced electrogram fractionation: relating clinical observations to changes in fibrosis and action potential duration. J Cardiovasc Electrophysiol 16: 151–161.
19. Nayak AR, Shajahan TK, Panfilov AV, Pandit R (2013) Spiral-wave dynamics in a mathematical model of human ventricular tissue with myocytes and fibroblasts. PLoS One 8: e72950.
20. Majumder R, Nayak AR, Pandit R (2012) Nonequilibrium arrhythmic states and transitions in a mathematical model for diffuse fibrosis in human cardiac tissue. PLoS One 7: e45040.
21. McDowell KS, Arevalo HJ, Maleckar MM, Trayanova NA (2011) Susceptibility to arrhythmia in the infarcted heart depends on myofibroblast density. Biophys J 101: 1307–1315.
22. Petrov VS, Osipov GV, Kurths J (2010) Fibroblasts alter spiral wave stability. Chaos 20: 045103.
23. Engelman ZJ, Trew ML, Smaill BH (2010) Structural heterogeneity alone is a sufficient substrate for dynamic instability and altered restitution. Circ Arrhythm Electrophysiol 3: 195–203.
24. Ashihara T, Haraguchi R, Nakazawa K, Namba T, Ikeda T, et al. (2012) The role of fibroblasts in complex fractionated electrograms during persistent/permanent atrial fibrillation: implications for electrogram-based catheter ablation. Circ Res 110: 275–284.
25. Tanaka K, Zlochiver S, Vikstrom KL, Yamazaki M, Moreno J, et al. (2007) Spatial distribution of fibrosis governs fibrillation wave dynamics in the posterior left atrium during heart failure. Circ Res 101: 839–847.
26. Umapathy K, Nair K, Masse S, Krishnan S, Rogers J, et al. (2010) Phase mapping of cardiac fibrillation. Circ Arrhythm Electrophysiol 3: 105–114.
27. Lou Q, Ripplinger CM, Bayly PV, Efimov IR (2008) Quantitative panoramic imaging of epicardial electrical activity. Ann Biomed Eng 36: 1649–1658.
28. Bray MA, Lin SF, Aliev RR, Roth BJ, Wikswo JP Jr (2001) Experimental and theoretical analysis of phase singularity dynamics in cardiac tissue. J Cardiovasc Electrophysiol 12: 716–722.
29. Clayton RH, Taggart P (2005) Regional differences in APD restitution can initiate wavebreak and re-entry in cardiac tissue: a computational study. Biomed Eng Online 4: 54.
30. Grandi E, Pasqualini FS, Bers DM (2010) A novel computational model of the human ventricular action potential and Ca transient. J Mol Cell Cardiol 48: 112–121.
31. Trenor B, Cardona K, Gomez JF, Rajamani S, Ferrero JM Jr, et al. (2012) Simulation and mechanistic investigation of the arrhythmogenic role of the late sodium current in human heart failure. PLoS One 7: e32659.
32. MacCannell KA, Bazzazi H, Chilton L, Shibukawa Y, Clark RB, et al. (2007) A mathematical model of electrotonic interactions between ventricular myocytes and fibroblasts. Biophys J 92: 4121–4132.
33. Taggart P, Sutton PM, Opthof T, Coronel R, Trimlett R, et al. (2000) Inhomogeneous transmural conduction during early ischaemia in patients with coronary artery disease. J Mol Cell Cardiol 32: 621–630.
34. Dupont E, Matsushita T, Kaba RA, Vozzi C, Coppen SR, et al. (2001) Altered connexin expression in human congestive heart failure. J Mol Cell Cardiol 33: 359–371.
35. Rook MB, van Ginneken AC, de JB, el AA, Gros D, et al. (1992) Differences in gap junction channels between cardiac myocytes, fibroblasts, and heterologous pairs. Am J Physiol 263: C959–C977.
36. Vasquez C, Moreno AP, Berbari EJ (2004) Modeling fibroblast-mediated conduction in the ventricle. Computers in Cardiology Proceedings 31: 349–352.
37. Kohl P, Kamkin AG, Kiseleva IS, Noble D (1994) Mechanosensitive fibroblasts in the sino-atrial node region of rat heart: interaction with cardiomyocytes and possible role. Exp Physiol 79: 943–956.
38. Chilton L, Ohya S, Freed D, George E, Drobic V, et al. (2005) K+ currents regulate the resting membrane potential, proliferation, and contractile responses in ventricular fibroblasts and myofibroblasts. Am J Physiol Heart Circ Physiol 288: H2931–H2939.
39. Sachse FB, Moreno AP, Abildskov JA (2008) Electrophysiological modeling of fibroblasts and their interaction with myocytes. Ann Biomed Eng 36: 41–56.
40. Jacquemet V, Henriquez CS (2008) Loading effect of fibroblast-myocyte coupling on resting potential, impulse propagation, and repolarization: insights from a microstructure model. Am J Physiol Heart Circ Physiol 294: H2040–H2052.
41. Kawara T, Derksen R, de Groot JR, Coronel R, Tasseron S, et al. (2001) Activation delay after premature stimulation in chronically diseased human myocardium relates to the architecture of interstitial fibrosis. Circulation 104: 3069–3075.
42. Greisas A, Zlochiver S (2012) Modulation of spiral-wave dynamics and spontaneous activity in a fibroblast/myocyte heterocellular tissue–a computational study. IEEE Trans Biomed Eng 59: 1398–1407.
43. Elshrif MM, Cherry EM (2014) A quantitative comparison of the behavior of human ventricular cardiac electrophysiology models in tissue. PLoS One 9: e84401.
44. Liu YB, Peter A, Lamp ST, Weiss JN, Chen PS, et al. (2003) Spatiotemporal correlation between phase singularities and wavebreaks during ventricular fibrillation. J Cardiovasc Electrophysiol 14: 1103–1109.
45. Rogers JM (2004) Combined phase singularity and wavefront analysis for optical maps of ventricular fibrillation. IEEE Trans Biomed Eng 51: 56–65.
46. Heidenreich EA, Ferrero JM, Doblare M, Rodriguez JF (2010) Adaptive macro finite elements for the numerical solution of monodomain equations in cardiac electrophysiology. Ann Biomed Eng 38: 2331–2345.
47. Clayton RH, Zhuchkova EA, Panfilov AV (2006) Phase singularities and filaments: simplifying complexity in computational models of ventricular fibrillation. Prog Biophys Mol Biol 90: 378–398.
48. Pogwizd SM, Schlotthauer K, Li L, Yuan W, Bers DM (2001) Arrhythmogenesis and contractile dysfunction in heart failure: Roles of sodium-calcium exchange, inward rectifier potassium current, and residual beta-adrenergic responsiveness. Circ Res 88: 1159–1167.
49. Moreno JD, Yang PC, Bankston JR, Grandi E, Bers DM, et al. (2013) Ranolazine for Congenital and Acquired Late INa-Linked Arrhythmias: In Silico Pharmacological Screening. Circ Res 113: e50–e61.
50. Janicki JS, Brower GL (2002) The role of myocardial fibrillar collagen in ventricular remodeling and function. J Card Fail 8: S319–S325.
51. Gonzalez A, Ravassa S, Beaumont J, Lopez B, Diez J (2011) New targets to treat the structural remodeling of the myocardium. J Am Coll Cardiol 58: 1833–1843.
52. Miragoli M, Salvarani N, Rohr S (2007) Myofibroblasts induce ectopic activity in cardiac tissue. Circ Res 101: 755–758.
53. Rohr S (2012) Arrhythmogenic implications of fibroblast-myocyte interactions. Circ Arrhythm Electrophysiol 5: 442–452.
54. Samie FH, Jalife J (2001) Mechanisms underlying ventricular tachycardia and its transition to ventricular fibrillation in the structurally normal heart. Cardiovasc Res 50: 242–250.
55. Davidenko JM, Pertsov AV, Salomonsz R, Baxter W, Jalife J (1992) Stationary and drifting spiral waves of excitation in isolated cardiac muscle. Nature 355: 349–351.
56. Gray RA, Pertsov AM, Jalife J (1998) Spatial and temporal organization during cardiac fibrillation. Nature 392: 75–78.

57. Pandit SV, Jalife J (2013) Rotors and the dynamics of cardiac fibrillation. Circ Res 112: 849–862.
58. Zlochiver S, Munoz V, Vikstrom KL, Taffet SM, Berenfeld O, et al. (2008) Electrotonic myofibroblast-to-myocyte coupling increases propensity to reentrant arrhythmias in two-dimensional cardiac monolayers. Biophys J 95: 4469–4480.
59. Jacquemet V, Henriquez CS (2007) Modelling cardiac fibroblasts: interactions with myocytes and their impact on impulse propagation. Europace 9 Suppl 6: vi29–vi37.
60. Chilton L, Giles WR, Smith GL (2007) Evidence of intercellular coupling between co-cultured adult rabbit ventricular myocytes and myofibroblasts. J Physiol 583: 225–236.
61. Kohl P, Camelliti P, Burton FL, Smith GL (2005) Electrical coupling of fibroblasts and myocytes: relevance for cardiac propagation. J Electrocardiol 38: 45–50.
62. Ashikaga H, Arevalo H, Vadakkumpadan F, Blake RC, III, Bayer JD, et al. (2013) Feasibility of Image-Based Simulation to Estimate Ablation Target in Human Ventricular Arrhythmia. Heart Rhythm.
63. Jacquemet V, Henriquez CS (2009) Genesis of complex fractionated atrial electrograms in zones of slow conduction: a computer model of microfibrosis. Heart Rhythm 6: 803–810.
64. Yun Y, Hwang M, Park JH, Shin H, Shim EB, et al. (2014) The relationship among complex fractionated electrograms, wavebreak, phase singularity, and local dominant frequency in fibrillation wave-dynamics: a modeling comparison study. J Korean Med Sci 29: 370–377.

Identification of a New Target of miR-16, Vacuolar Protein Sorting 4a

Neeta Adhikari[1]⁹, Weihua Guan[2]⁹, Brian Capaldo[6], Aaron J. Mackey[6], Marjorie Carlson[1], Sundaram Ramakrishnan[5], Dinesha Walek[4], Manu Gupta[7], Adam Mitchell[1], Peter Eckman[1], Ranjit John[3], Euan Ashley[8], Paul J. Barton[9], Jennifer L. Hall[1]*

1 Lillehei Heart Institute, Department of Medicine, University of Minnesota, Minneapolis, Minnesota, United States of America, **2** Division of Biostatistics, University of Minnesota, Minneapolis, Minnesota, United States of America, **3** Department of Surgery, Cardiothoracic Surgery Division, University of Minnesota, Minneapolis, Minnesota, United States of America, **4** University of Minnesota Genomics Center, University of Minnesota, Minneapolis, Minnesota, United States of America, **5** Department of Pharmacology, University of Minnesota, Minneapolis, Minnesota, United States of America, **6** Center for Public Health Genomics, University of Virginia, Charlottesville, Virginia, United States of America, **7** National Institute of Heart Research, Cardiovascular Biomedical Research Unit, Royal Brompton and Harefield Trust, London, United Kingdom, **8** Center for Inherited Cardiovascular Disease, Department of Medicine, Stanford University, Stanford, California, United States of America, **9** Heart Science Centre, National Heart and Lung Institute, Imperial College, London, United Kingdom

Abstract

Rationale: The rationale was to utilize a bioinformatics approach to identify miRNA binding sites in genes with single nucleotide mutations (SNPs) to discover pathways in heart failure (HF).

Objective: The objective was to focus on the genes containing miRNA binding sites with miRNAs that were significantly altered in end-stage HF and in response to a left ventricular assist device (LVAD).

Methods and Results: BEDTools v2.14.3 was used to discriminate SNPs within predicted 3′UTR miRNA binding sites. A member of the miR-15/107 family, miR-16, was decreased in the circulation of end-stage HF patients and increased in response to a LVAD ($p<0.001$). MiR-16 decreased Vacuolar Protein Sorting 4a (VPS4a) expression in HEK 293T cells ($p<0.01$). The SNP rs16958754 was identified in the miR-15/107 family binding site of VPS4a which abolished direct binding of miR-16 to the 3′UTR of VPS4a ($p<0.05$). VPS4a was increased in the circulation of end-stage HF patients ($p<0.001$), and led to a decrease in the number of HEK 293T cells *in vitro* ($p<0.001$).

Conclusions: We provide evidence that miR-16 decreases in the circulation of end-stage HF patients and increases with a LVAD. Modeling studies suggest that miR-16 binds to and decreases expression of VPS4a. Overexpression of VPS4a decreases cell number. Together, these experiments suggest that miR-16 and VPS4a expression are altered in end-stage HF and in response to unloading with a LVAD. This signaling pathway may lead to reduced circulating cell number in HF.

Editor: Sudhiranjan Gupta, Texas A & M, Division of Cardiology, United States of America

Funding: This work was supported by NIHR Cardiovascular Biomedical Research Unit of Royal Brompton and Harefield NHS Foundation Trust, Imperial College London (PJB) and the National Institutes of Health (NIH-1 R21 HL104596-01) (JLH). The funders had no role in study design, data collection and analysis, decision to publish, or preparation of the manuscript.

Competing Interests: The authors have declared that no competing interests exist.

* Email: jlhall@umn.edu

⁹ These authors contributed equally to this work.

Introduction

MiRNAs regulate gene function in heart development, physiology and pathology. The miRNA–mRNA interaction is affected by the presence of single nucleotide polymorphisms (SNPs). A SNP within or near the miRNA binding sites of targets has been shown to influence the susceptibility to disease [1,2]. In this study we identified new miRNA/RNA targets using a novel approach of utilizing conserved SNPs in miRNA binding regions as a roadmap. Determining how short RNAs (miRNA and siRNA) impact mRNA target expression within single cells and how this process influences disease initiation and progression is still not known. Recent work has suggested that within each cell, 85% of genes contain fewer than 100 copies [3]. Mullokandov et al provide evidence that only the most abundant miRNA regulate target gene expression [4]. The turnover rate of miRNA has been shown to alter gene expression [5], as well as the secondary structure of the target gene [6].

Several publications have cited circulating expression of miRNA in end-stage HF; however it is challenging to find how the levels of these miRNA compare to others in the circulation [7–11]. These studies identified increases in miR-423-5p and miR-499, and a decrease in miR-126 [7–11]. MiR-16 is one of the highest expressed mRNAs in the circulation. Expression of miR-16 is widely known to be high in all circulating cells [12]. Reticulocytes (immature red blood cells) and platelets exhibit the highest expression of miR-16 [12]. The role of miR-15/107 family members, including miR-16 in peripheral blood in the context of HF has not been defined. MiR-15 -16, -195, -497, -103, -107, -503, share a common sequence "AGCAGC" starting at the first or second nucleotide from the 5′ mature end of the miRNA [13]. This evolutionary conserved family of miRNAs targets a disproportionately high number of cell cycle regulatory genes [14–18]. A predicted target, Vacuolar Protein Sorting 4a, VPS4a, was identified with a SNP rs16958754 in the miR-15/107 family binding site. VPS4a is an ATPase and is one of many vacuolar protein sorting associated proteins involved in diverse cellular processes including multivesicular body formation, cytokinesis, and endosomal trafficking [19].

In this study, we identify miR-16 as the specific member of the miR-15/107 family that decreases in peripheral blood of patients with end stage HF and increases significantly one week post ventricular assist device (LVAD) therapy. The novel target of miR-16, VPS4a that we identified and validated *in vitro*, increases in peripheral blood of end stage HF patients and decreases one week following LVAD therapy. MiR-16 has been identified in CD45 and CD14 positive cells [12]. Overexpression of VPS4a significantly inhibited total cell number, suggesting that the miR-16-VPS4a pathway inhibits proliferation of CD45 and CD14 positive cells in end stage HF.

Methods

An expanded methods section (Text S1) is available as Supporting Information.

Ethics statements

All procedures followed were in accordance with the ethical standards of the responsible committees on human experimentation. Written consents were obtained from eligible patients for being included in this study. Samples were collected from consenting participants and the study was conducted under the Institutional Review Board approval from the University of Minnesota, USA the Royal Brompton and Harefield Cardiovascular Biomedical Research Unit, UK and Stanford University. All samples used in the study and the original repository are listed in Table S5.

Heart samples

Heart samples from patients with end-stage HF were collected at the time of LVAD implant (HF, n = 10) at the University of Minnesota. Non-failing control heart samples (Control, n = 9, 45±5, 57% male) were obtained from Dr. Euan Ashley, Stanford University.

Peripheral blood samples

Blood samples from patients with end-stage HF (n = 9) were collected prior to LVAD implant and 7 days post-implant (n = 9) as described [20] (Table 1). Blood samples from healthy gender and age matched subjects were labeled as controls (n = 6, average age 54±4, 60% male, 83% Caucasian).

DNA samples, genotyping and analysis

DNA samples were obtained from individuals (n = 855) from the Royal Brompton and Harefield NHS Trust Tissue Typing Service, UK, referred for cardiac transplantation due to dilated cardiomyopathy (DCM, n = 234) or ischemic cardiomyopathy (ICM, n = 621), and from individuals at the University of Minnesota (n = 152) referred for heart transplant or placement of a LVAD (DCM, n = 67 and ICM, n = 76) all according to institutional approved protocols. Primers as listed in the Table S4 were used to genotype samples for SNPs in miRNA binding sites on the commercially available high-throughput genotyping Sequenom MassARRAY platform (San Diego, CA, USA) as previously described [21]. SNPs were compared to that in a general population (Caucasian samples from 1000 Genome project, Phase 1 data, (http://www.1000genomes.org/). We identified 853 unique SNPs in 914 unique target sites in 763 unique 3′UTRs in dbSNP. From ESP5500 we identified 343 unique SNPs that were found in 348 unique target sites in 311 unique 3′UTRs (starting from an initial size of 14,024,295 SNPs, and 1,837,369 SNPs in the ESP5500 database). For details see Text S1 and Table S4.

Cell culture and transfection

HEK 293T cells were purchased and maintained according to the manufacturer's guidelines (ATCC). Transient expression of miR-16, -103, -107 or a scrambled control was achieved by using miRVana mimics according to the manufacturer's instruction (Life Technologies). Lipofectamine 2000 was used according to the manufacturer's protocol for transient transfection of HEK 293T cells (Invitrogen). Endpoints were analyzed 48 h post transfection.

RNA isolation and Real Time Quantitative PCR (RTQPCR)

Total RNA was extracted with Trizol according to the manufacturer's directions (Invitrogen). For miRNA, cDNA were synthesized by using the Taqman MicroRNA Reverse Transcription Kit (Applied Biosystems). For mRNA expression cDNA was synthesized by utilizing the SuperScript III kit (Invitrogen) [22]. Data is expressed relative to control and was calculated by the 2^-deltadeltaCT method as described [22]. Taqman primers used in this study are listed in the Table S4.

Dual Luciferase Reporter Assay

HEK 293T cells were co-transfected with either WT or mutated (harboring rs16958754) VPS4a 3′UTR reporter clones for miRNA target validation (Origene) and Renilla luciferase construct (Promega) with miR-16, -103, -107 or a scrambled control mimic according to the manufacturer's protocol (Life Technologies). The 3′UTR of VPS4a was cloned downstream of the luciferase gene. An Internal ribosome entry site (IRES) is located upstream of luciferase. As the miR/RISC complex binds to the target, luciferase activity is reduced. If there is no interaction between the miR and the target, luciferase activity remains high. Luciferase activity was assessed using the Dual Luciferase Reporter Assay System (Promega) [23].

Western Analysis

For details see Text S1.

Cell number and Apoptosis

HEK 293T cells were plated and transfected with VPS4a cDNA plasmid (Origene) or an empty vector (Origene) using Lipofectamine 2000 according to the manufacturer's instruction (Life Technologies). Increase in cells number was assessed every 24 h using a Hemocytometer. Apoptosis was assessed 48 h post transfection by staining with Hoechst 33342 for nuclear morphology, and the percentage of apoptotic nuclei was quantified as previously described [24].

Statistics

A Student's T-test was used for comparison of two groups and a One Way ANOVA with a post-hoc Tukey analysis was used for

Table 1. Characteristics of patients with end-stage HF. Blood samples were obtained prior to LVAD implantation (n = 9) and 7 days post implant (n = 9).

Patient ID	1	2	3	4	5	6	7	8	9
Age	62	65	54	46	63	76	54	70	51
Gender	M	M	M	M	M	M	M	M	F
Ethnicity	C	C	C	C	C	C	C	C	AA
BP	85	87	71	97	111	172	92	88	98
HF etiology	NI	I	I	NI	I	I	NI	I	NI
EF (%)	15–20%	10–15%	15–20%	10–15%	5–10%	5–10%	20–25%	10–15%	22–25%
Diabetes	–	+	–	–	+	–	–	+	–
BNP (pg/mL)	2810	2460	599	6260	7110	9960	991	1507	2550
Creatinine (mg/dL	1.51	1.56	2.07	1.29	1.81	1.55	0.96	1.58	1.03
Beta blocker	+	+	+	+	+	+	+	+	+
ACE/ARB	+		+	+		+	+	+	+
Aldosterone antagonist		+	+	+		+	+		+
Diuretic	+	+	+	+	+	+	+	+	+
Statin		+	+		+	+		+	
Aspirin	+	+	+	+	+	+	+	+	+
Warfarin		+			+	+	+		

M-male, F-female, C-Caucasian, AA-African-American, BP-Blood Pressure, HF-Heart Failure, NI-non Ischemic, I- Ischemic, EF- Ejection fraction, BNP- β-Natriuretic Peptide.

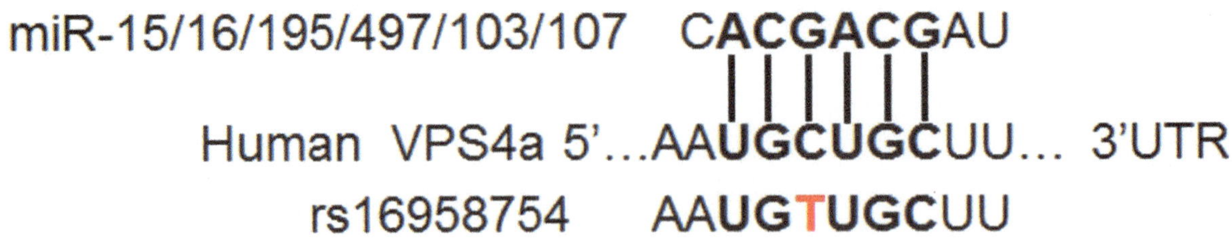

Figure 1. Predicted binding site of miR15/16/195/497/103/107 in 3'UTR of VPS4a. Binding site of miR15/16/195/497/103/107 and the SNP, rs16958754[C/T] in the 3'UTR of human VPS4a.

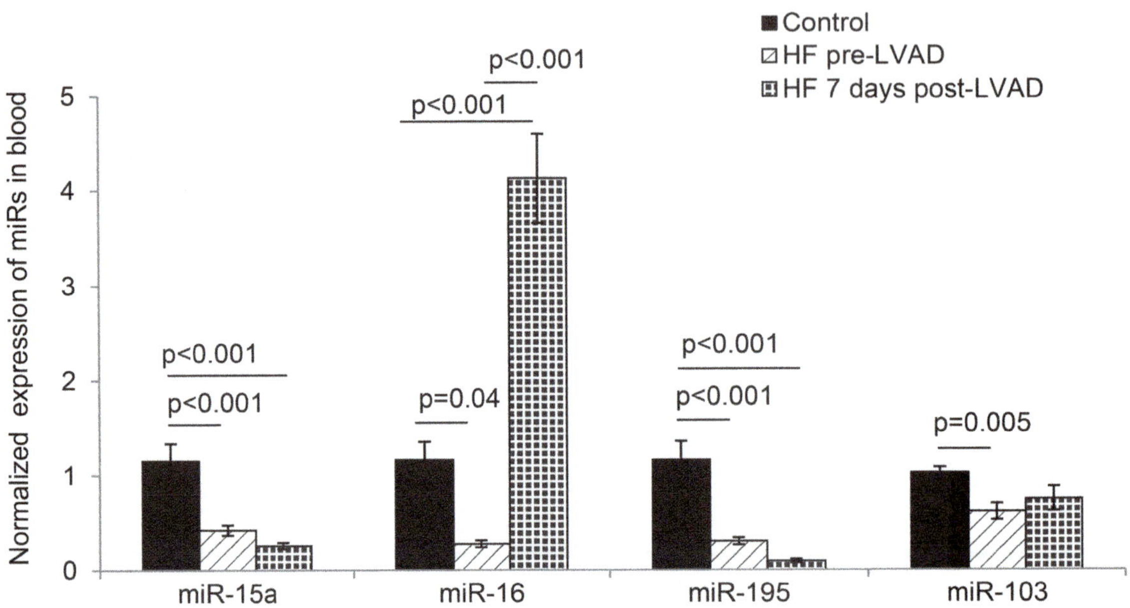

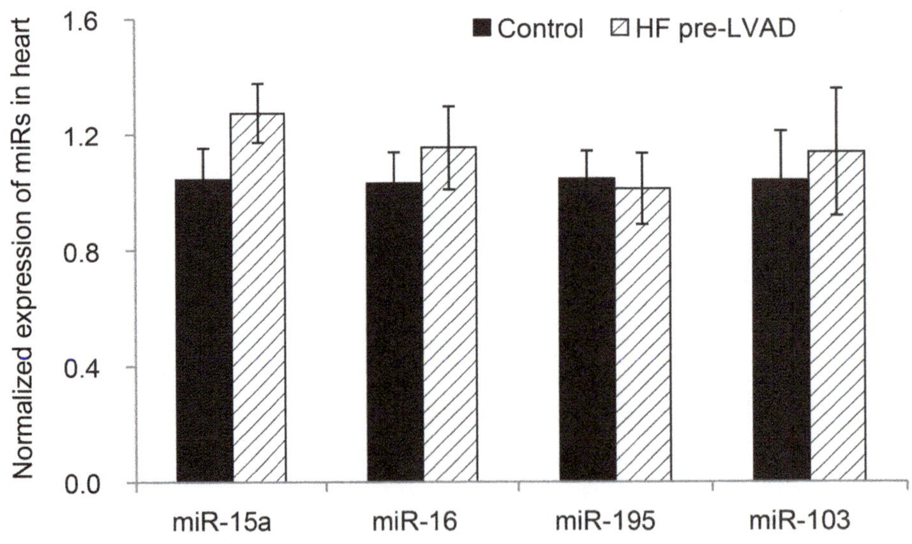

Figure 2. MiR-15a, -16, -195, and -103 expression in peripheral blood and heart tissue in patients with end-stage HF. (**A**) miR-15a, -16, -195, and -103 in peripheral blood were decreased in patients with end-stage HF prior to LVAD implant (pre-LVAD) (n = 9) compared to age, gender, and ethnicity matched healthy controls (n = 6). MiR-16 expression increased from end-stage HF prior to LVAD (HF pre-LVAD, n = 9) compared to patients with end-stage HF 7 days post LVAD (HF 7 days post-LVAD) (n = 9). MiR-15a, -16, -195, and -103 were decreased in patients with HF compared to controls. (**B**) Expression of miR-15/107 family in heart samples was not significantly different between non-failing controls (Controls) (n = 9) and end-stage HF samples (HF pre-LVAD) (n = 10). Samples were in duplicate and target expression normalized to SnU6 for A and B (mean ±SE).

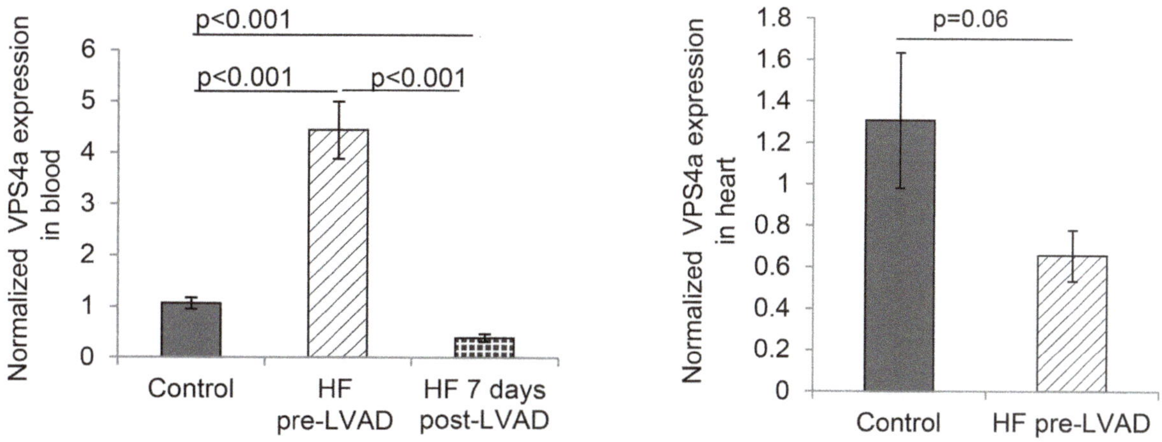

Figure 3. VPS4a expression in peripheral blood and heart tissue in patients with end-stage HF. (**A**) VPS4a transcript is higher in patients with end stage HF pre-LVAD (HF pre-LVAD) (n = 9) and is decreased 7 days post implant (HF 7 days post-LVAD) (n = 9) compared to age and gender matched controls (Control) (n = 6). (**B**) VPS4a transcript in heart was not different in patients with end stage HF (HF pre-LVAD, n = 10) compared to non-failing controls (n = 9). Samples were run in duplicate and target expression was normalized to 18S (mean ± SE).

comparison of multiples groups. P<0.05 was considered significant. All values are presented as mean ± SE.

Results

We identified 1175 SNPs in miRNA binding sites within the 3′ UTR of genes (Table S1). This supplemental table includes targets harboring the same SNP within the binding sites of multiple miRNA families. 137 genes contained a SNP in the 3′ UTR that was within the binding site of more than one miRNA family (Table S1).

24 SNPs were identified in binding sites specific for the miR-15 family. 11 SNPs were identified in binding sites specific for the miR-107 family. One SNP was shared between the miR-15 and the miR-107 family, rs16958754 [C/T] in VPS4a (Fig. 1). miR-15a, -16, -195 and -103 were decreased in peripheral blood samples of individuals with end-stage HF compared to controls (gender, age, and ethnicity matched) ($p<0.02$, Fig. 2A) (Table 1).

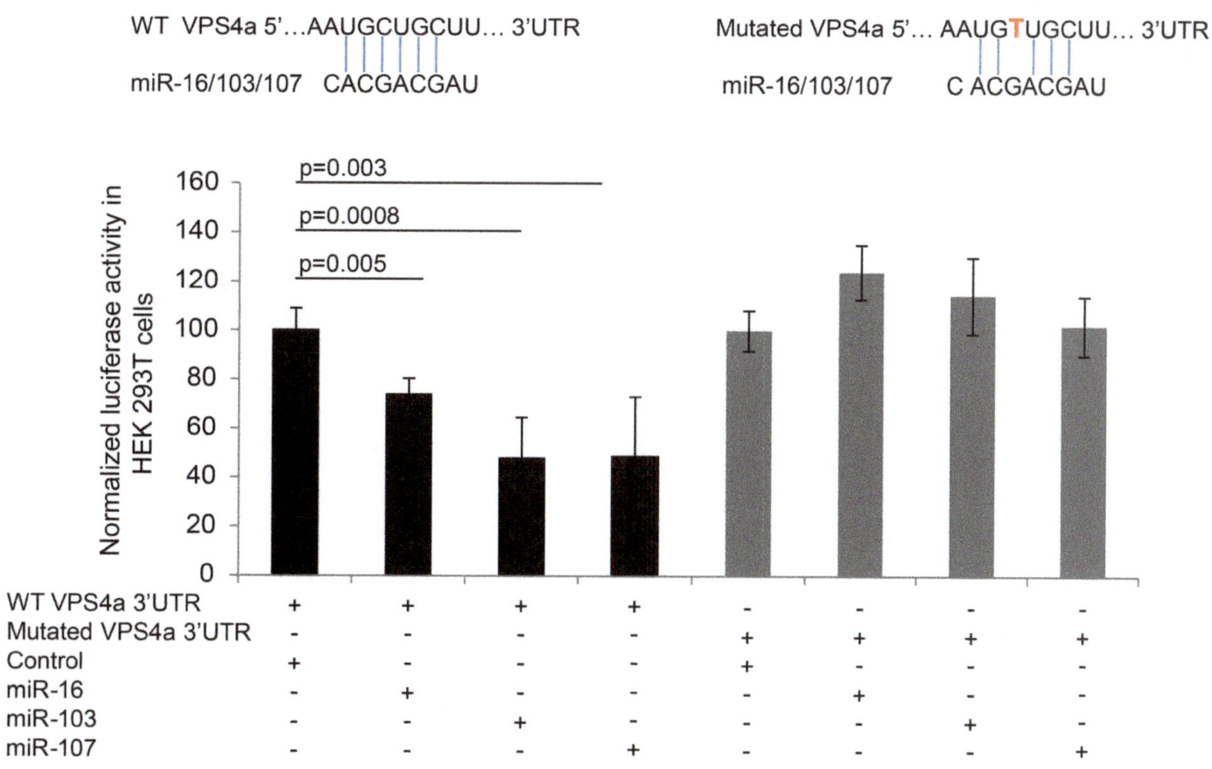

Figure 4. MiR-16, -103 and -107 interact with the 3′UTR of VPS4a. Binding of miR-16, -103 or -107 to WT 3′UTR of VPS4a decreases luciferase activity (n = 10) in HEK 293T cells. The SNP rs16958754[C/T] abolishes the interaction of miR-16, -103 or -107 to the mutated 3′UTR of VPS4a resulting in no change in luciferase activity (n = 10) (mean ± SE).

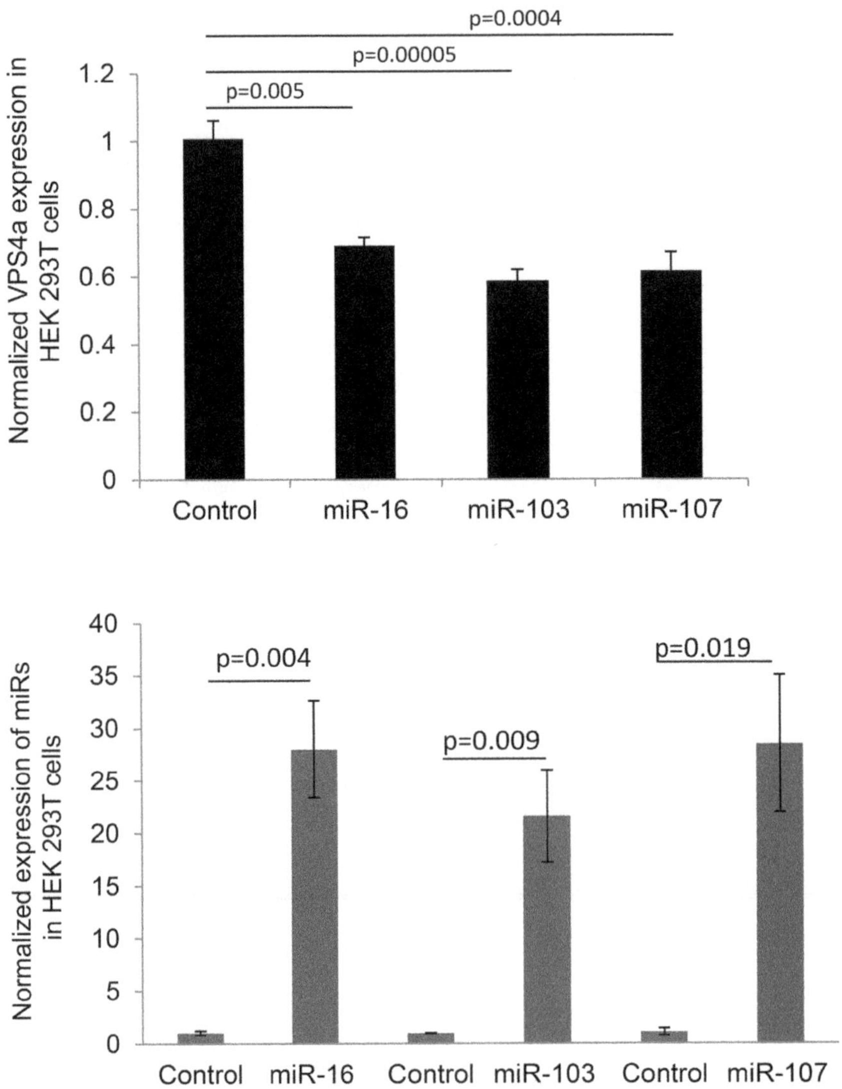

Figure 5. MiR-16, -103 and -107 decrease VPS4a mRNA expression. (**A**) Expression of VPS4a mRNA in HEK 293T cells decreases following overexpression of miR-16, or -103, or -107 (n = 3). Overexpression of a scrambled control mimic (control) had no effect (n = 3). Samples were run in duplicate and VPS4a expression normalized to 18S. (**B**) Overexpression of miR-16, -103 and -107 transcript *vs.* a scrambled control mimic (control) 48 h post transfection in HEK 293T cells (n = 3). Samples were run in duplicate and expression normalized to RNU38B (mean ± SE).

MiR-16 in the peripheral blood was the only miRNA to increase 7 days post LVAD implantation ($p<0.001$, Fig. 2A). Heart tissue from end-stage HF patients (n = 10) showed no change in expression of miR-15a, -16, -195 and -103 compared to controls (n = 9, Fig. 2B).

VPS4a (the gene containing rs16958754 in the miR-15/107 binding site) was increased in peripheral blood from end-stage HF patients and decreased 7 days post-surgery as compared to controls ($p = 0.0001$) (Fig. 3A). VPS4a expression in heart tissue from HF patients was not different from non-failing controls (Fig. 3B).

Studies in vitro showed that miR-16, miR-103 and miR107 inhibited luciferase activity of a 3′ UTR VPS4a reporter construct for mRNA target validation in HEK 293T cells (Fig. 4). Interaction between the 3′UTR VPS4a reporter construct and miR-16 was inhibited by the SNP, rs16958754 (Fig. 4). The endogenous levels of these miRs in HEK 293T cells exhibited crossing thresholds ranging from 23 (miR-16) to 27 (miR-107).

VPS4a mRNA was decreased following overexpression of miR-16, -103 and -107 (Fig. 5A) in HEK 293T cells. Figure 5B shows the overexpression levels of miR-16, -13, -107 transcripts compared to RNU38B, an internal control, 48 h post transfection. Only miR-16 decreased VPS4a protein abundance (Fig. 6). Cell number (HEK 293T) was decreased in response to up-regulation of VPS4a (Fig. 7A). No differences were noted in apoptosis in VPS4a overexpressing cells as compared to cells transfected with an empty vector (0.3±0.2% vs 0.3±0.4%, respectively). The level of VPS4a expression post transfection in HEK 293T cells is shown by Western blotting (Fig. 7B).

The two separate cohorts of end-stage HF samples were genotyped for a subset of the SNPs. The minor allele frequency (MAF) of these SNPs in the two HF populations did not differ significantly from the MAF published in dbSNP or 1000 genomes (Table S2). No SNP showed significant frequency difference between ethnic groups. Using data from the 1000 genomes project (http://www.1000genomes.org/), we were able to map 63

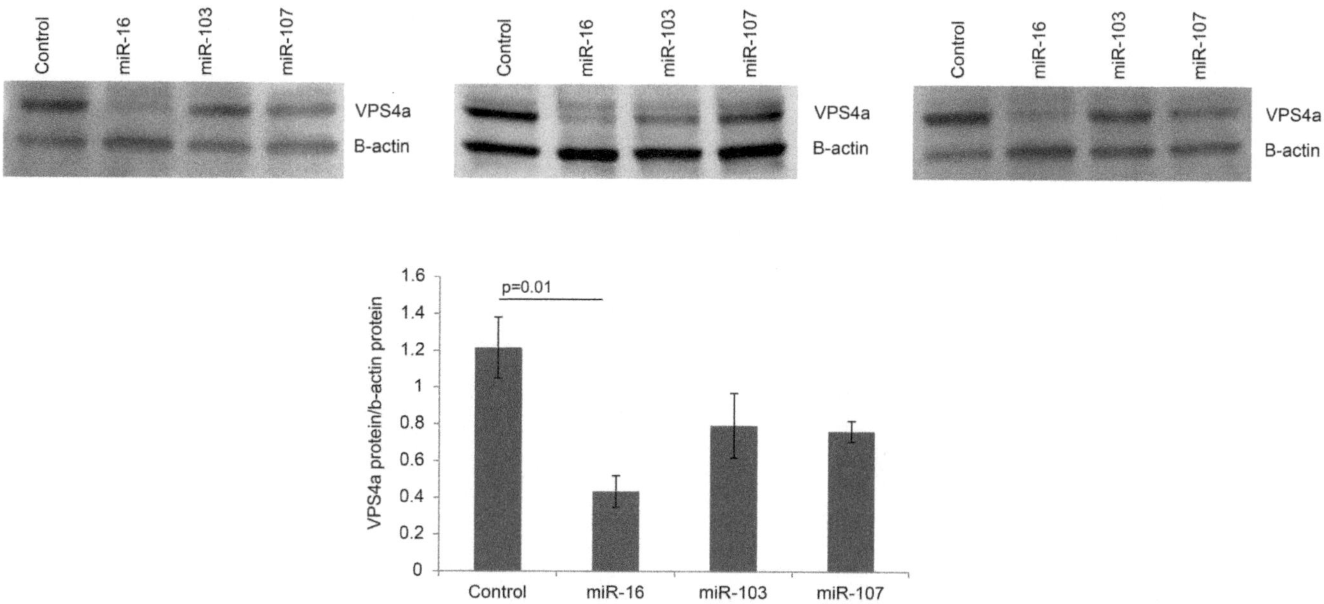

Figure 6. MiR-16 decreases protein expression of VPS4a. VPS4a protein is decreased following overexpression of miR-16. All 3 Western blots are shown along with densitometry. Overexpression of miR-103 and miR-107 or scrambled control had no significant effect. Bands were normalized to β-actin. Densitometry values are mean ± SE, n = 3.

miRNA SNPs by their physical position on the genome. MAFs of these SNPs in Caucasians were compared between our samples and the 1000 genomes samples, and no significant difference was observed. Of interest, we observed several individuals carrying multiple alleles at multiple loci at low frequencies. Specifically, four individuals carry 4 rare alleles (at 4 loci) with frequency <1%, and nine individuals carry 3 rare alleles with frequency <1%. Assuming independence among the miRNA loci, we randomly permuted the rare alleles in our samples to estimate the expected number of individuals carrying multiple rare alleles (Table 2). The excess number of individuals than expected may suggest correlation or interaction between the miRNA loci surveyed in our study.

Discussion

A major finding of this study is that 2–3 miRNA families may bind to a site in the 3′ UTR that contains a single SNP. One of these SNPs, rs16958754, in the gene, VPS4a, was identified in the binding region of both miR-15 and miR-107 families. These families share a common sequence, "AGCAGC". miR-16, a member of the miR-15 family, is one of the top 10 highest expressed mi-RNAs in peripheral blood cells [12]. Expression of miR-16 in the blood was down-regulated in end-stage HF and up-regulated 7 days post unloading with a LVAD. In contrast, the target of miR-16, VPS4a, was up-regulated with HF, and down-regulated post LVAD in the blood (Fig. 3A). Studies *in vitro* validated that miR-16 decreased mRNA level of VPS4a. The presence of the SNP, rs26958754 abolished this effect. Although the presence of the SNP, rs16958754, interfered with miR-16 interaction with VPS4a, the MAF of this SNP in our two heart failure cohorts was rare (0.7 and 2.2%). The MAF of this SNP in normal controls in the 1000 genome project was 0. Taken together, these experiments suggest that miR-16 interacts with VPS4a and that circulating expression of miR-16 is down-regulated with HF while expression of its target, VPS4a, is increased. In response to LVAD therapy, circulating miR-16 is increased along with a concomitant decrease in VPS4a. In the rare case when a subject carries the SNP, rs16958754, it is possible that VPS4a levels have been high prior to HF given that miR-16 was elevated and not binding to the 3′UTR of VPS4a. It is speculated that VPS4a regulation through miR-16 would remain high during HF, given miR-16 is decreased and that miR-16 does not bind efficiently to VPS4a in patients with the SNP. Finally, it is possible that LVAD therapy would not decrease VPS4a through a miR-16 mediated mechanism in these subjects, given that miR-16 would increase with the LVAD yet not interact with its target VPS4a due to the SNP, rs16958754.

To define the cellular role of increased VPS4a in heart failure, we overexpressed VPS4a in HEK 293T cells and showed a significant decrease in cell number. This data agrees with the majority of studies showing that a decrease in miR-16 decreases cell number [25–27]. However not all studies show that miR-16 decreases cell number, which one might expect given miR-16 has multiple downstream targets [28]. VPS4a is thought to be part of an evolutionary ancient membrane remodeling system [19]. VPS4a is regulated by miRNAs 34a, 34c-5p, 449a, 449b, 574-3p, and -515-3p. To our knowledge, these miRNAs have not been reported to be altered in response to HF or LVAD therapy in humans. Furthermore, unlike miR-16, these miRNAs are not expressed at a high level in peripheral blood cells [12]. Expressions of many of the top miRNAs in peripheral blood are increased by 3–4 folds in platelets and reticulocytes including miR-16.

SNPs within miRNA binding sites are currently being used as prognostic and predictive cancer biomarkers [29]. The list of SNPs provided in this study may lead to future work in this direction in the area of cardiovascular disease as well as other diseases outside the realm of cardiovascular disease. The potential to utilize these SNPs and their targets as biomarkers for response to treatment are also future possibilities. We identified many targets with SNPs within a binding site that was recognized by multiple miRNAs. The potential for these SNPs and gene targets to be prognostic markers for blood diseases or immune related diseases in which T and B cells are critical looks to be very promising. This is particularly interesting given that many of the patients have 2

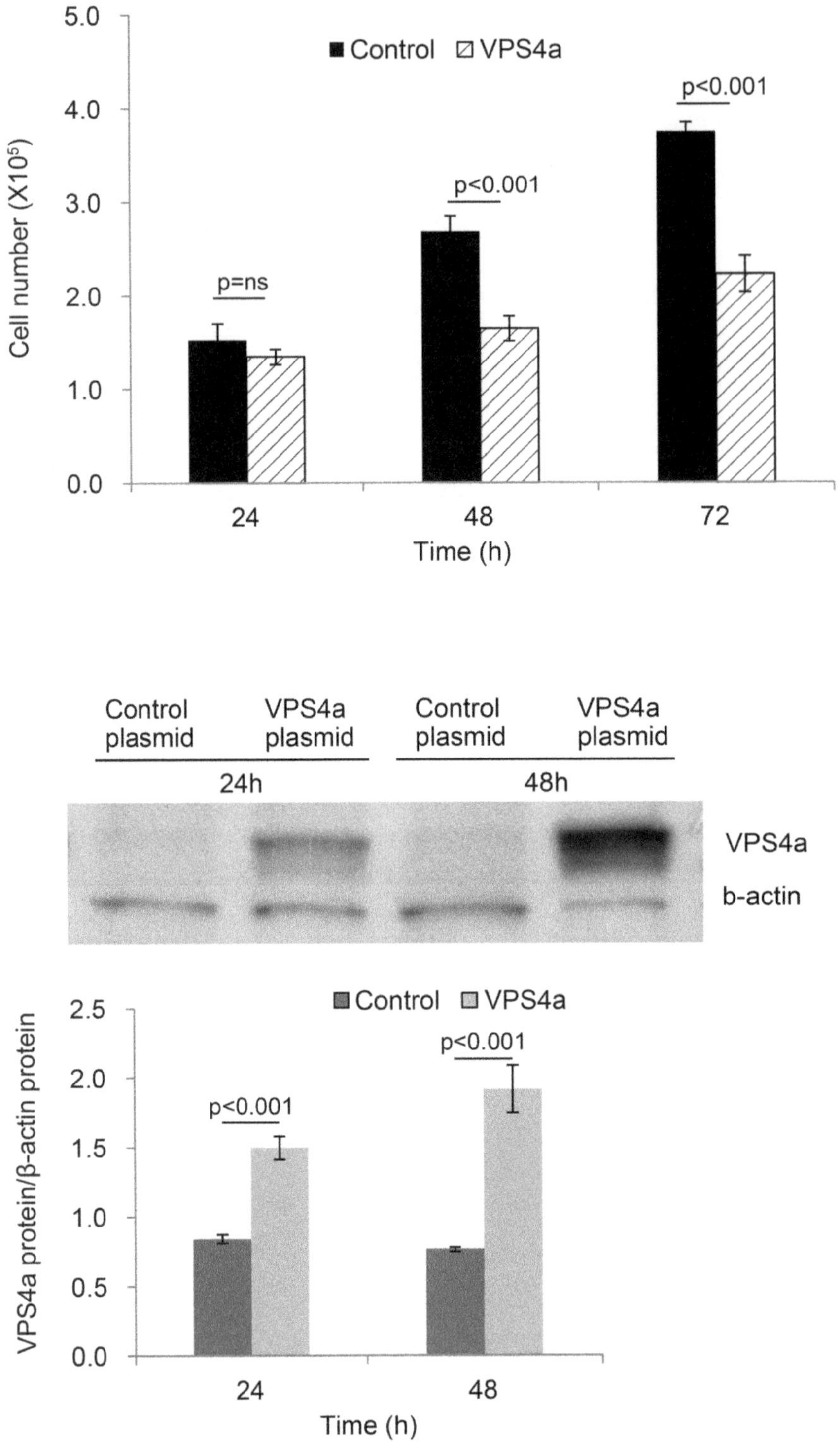

Figure 7. Overexpression of VPS4a decreases cell number. (**A**) Number of HEK 293T cells decreased following transfection with WT VPS4a compared to cells transfected with a control plasmid (Control). Values are mean ± SE, n = 4. (**B**) Western blot showing increased VPS4a protein following VPS4a transfection in HEK 293T cells *vs.* cells transfected with a control plasmid at 24 and 48 hours. Bands were normalized to β-actin. Densitometry values are mean ± SE, n = 3.

SNPs that share a common miRNA that is regulated in the context of cardiovascular disease including miR-129. The complete list of the sample reference numbers and SNPs, miRNAs, and gene targets with more than one SNP is given in the Table S3. In sum, this study shows that SNPs in miRNA binding sites, and/or levels of miRNA expression may impact the progression of heart failure and/or the response to treatment such as a LVAD.

The potential limitations of this study are that the HF cohorts we used to genotype were relatively small. We did genotype two cohorts (one from Minnesota and the other from London), both

Table 2. Number of samples with multiple alleles from the two HF cohorts.

Number of Alleles	Number of samples	
	Observed	Expected*
2	15	9.3
3	9	0.4
4	4	0.1

The complete list of sample ID, SNPs, miRNAs, and gene targets with more than one SNP is given in the Table S3. *The expected numbers were calculated using 1000 permutations.

with end-stage HF. We have provided all of the SNPs identified in the miRNA binding sites for others to utilize. Secondly, the cell type we utilized for the modeling experiments were HEK 293T cells, an epithelial cell line derived from human embryonic kidney. Although experiments in primary cells may have been insightful, the goal was to test if VPS4a was indeed a downstream target of miR-16 and if the SNP interfered with the binding. For these experiments the HEK 293T cells provided clean, interpretable data.

In conclusion, the present study identified and validated VPS4a as a novel target of miR-16. The SNP rs16958754 [C/T] interfered with the binding of miR-16 to VPS4a. Loss of miR-16 in patients with end stage HF and the concomitant rise in VPS4a may lead to a significant decrease in circulating platelets and/or reticulocytes with end stage disease. In response to treatment with a LVAD, miR-16 increases and VPS4a decreases. This suggests a potential role for the miR-16-VPS4a signaling pathway in erythropoiesis.

Supporting Information

Table S1 List of identified chromosomes, miRNA and SNPs with start and stop site.

Table S2 List of SNPs genotyped in this study.

Table S3 Multiple rare alleles identified in individual with end-stage HF.

Table S4 PCR and Extend Primer Sequences of 5 plexes and list of Taqman primers used for miRNA and mRNA expression by RTQPCR.

Table S5 Samples utilized in the study.

Text S1 Expanded Methods.

Acknowledgments

The authors wish to thank John Smith of the Tissue Typing Service Harefield Hospital, Laura Dillon for her help with the clinical data, and Cynthia DeKay for graphics.

Author Contributions

Conceived and designed the experiments: NA JLH PJB PE. Performed the experiments: NA MC DW. Analyzed the data: NA BC AJM WG JLH. Contributed reagents/materials/analysis tools: BC AJM PE AM WG PJB MG RJ EA. Wrote the paper: NA JLH SR. Edited the manuscript: RJ.

References

1. Haas U, Sczakiel G, Laufer SD (2012) MicroRNA-mediated regulation of gene expression is affected by disease-associated SNPs within the 3′-UTR via altered RNA structure. RNA Biol 9: 924–937.
2. Clop A, Marcq F, Takeda H, Pirottin D, Tordoir X, et al. (2006) A mutation creating a potential illegitimate microRNA target site in the myostatin gene affects muscularity in sheep. Nat Genet 38: 813–818.
3. Subkhankulova T, Gilchrist MJ, Livesey FJ (2008) Modelling and measuring single cell RNA expression levels find considerable transcriptional differences among phenotypically identical cells. BMC Genomics 9: 268.
4. Mullokandov G, Baccarini A, Ruzo A, Jayaprakash AD, Tung N, et al. (2012) High-throughput assessment of microRNA activity and function using micro-RNA sensor and decoy libraries. Nat Methods 9: 840–846.
5. Larsson E, Sander C, Marks D (2010) mRNA turnover rate limits siRNA and microRNA efficacy; Larsson E, Sander C, Marks D, editors.
6. Day L, Abdelhadi Ep Souki O, Albrecht AA, Steinhöfel K (2013) Accessibility of microRNA binding sites in metastable RNA secondary structures in the presence of SNPs. Bioinformatics.
7. Corsten MF, Dennert R, Jochems S, Kuznetsova T, Devaux Y, et al. (2010) Circulating MicroRNA-208b and MicroRNA-499 Reflect Myocardial Damage in Cardiovascular Disease. Circulation: Cardiovascular Genetics 3: 499–506.
8. Devaux Y, Vausort M, McCann GP, Kelly D, Collignon O, et al. (2013) A Panel of 4 microRNAs Facilitates the Prediction of Left Ventricular Contractility after Acute Myocardial Infarction. PLoS ONE 8: e70644.
9. Fichtlscherer S, Zeiher AM, Dimmeler S (2011) Circulating MicroRNAs: Biomarkers or Mediators of Cardiovascular Diseases? Arteriosclerosis, Thrombosis, and Vascular Biology 31: 2383–2390.
10. Fukushima Y, Nakanishi M, Nonogi H, Goto Y, Iwai N (2011) Assessment of Plasma miRNAs in Congestive Heart Failure. Circulation Journal 75: 336–340.
11. Tijsen AJ, Creemers EE, Moerland PD, de Windt LJ, van der Wal AC, et al. (2010) MiR423-5p As a Circulating Biomarker for Heart Failure. Circulation Research 106: 1035–1039.
12. Merkerova M, Belickova M, Bruchova H (2008) Differential expression of microRNAs in hematopoietic cell lineages. European Journal of Haematology 81: 304–310.
13. Finnerty JR, Wang W-X, Hébert SS, Wilfred BR, Mao G, et al. (2010) The miR-15/107 Group of MicroRNA Genes: Evolutionary Biology, Cellular Functions, and Roles in Human Diseases. Journal of Molecular Biology 402: 491–509.
14. Bandi N, Zbinden S, Gugger M, Arnold M, Kocher V, et al. (2009) miR-15a and miR-16 are implicated in cell cycle regulation in a Rb-dependent manner and are frequently deleted or down-regulated in non-small cell lung cancer. Cancer Res 69: 5553–5559.
15. Cai CK, Zhao GY, Tian LY, Liu L, Yan K, et al. (2012) miR-15a and miR-16-1 downregulate CCND1 and induce apoptosis and cell cycle arrest in osteosarcoma. Oncol Rep 28: 1764–1770.
16. Rissland Olivia S, Hong S-J, Bartel DP (2011) MicroRNA Destabilization Enables Dynamic Regulation of the miR-16 Family in Response to Cell-Cycle Changes. Molecular Cell 43: 993–1004.
17. Linsley PS, Schelter J, Burchard J, Kibukawa M, Martin MM, et al. (2007) Transcripts Targeted by the MicroRNA-16 Family Cooperatively Regulate Cell Cycle Progression. Molecular and Cellular Biology 27: 2240–2252.
18. Goretti E, Rolland-Turner M, Léonard F, Zhang L, Wagner DR, et al. (2013) MicroRNA-16 affects key functions of human endothelial progenitor cells. Journal of Leukocyte Biology 93: 645–655.
19. Hill CP, Babst M (2012) Structure and function of the membrane deformation AAA ATPase Vps4. Biochimica et Biophysica Acta (BBA) - Molecular Cell Research 1823: 172–181.
20. Mitchell A, Guan W, Staggs R, Hamel A, Hozayen S, et al. (2013) Identification of Differentially Expressed Transcripts and Pathways in Blood One Week and Six Months Following Implant of Left Ventricular Assist Devices. PLoS One 8: e77951.
21. Cotsapas C, Prokunina-Olsson L, Welch C, Saxena R, Weaver C, et al. (2010) Expression analysis of loci associated with type 2 diabetes in human tissues. Diabetologia 53: 2334–2339.
22. Adhikari N, Basi DL, Townsend D, Rusch M, Mariash A, et al. (2010) Heparan sulfate Ndst1 regulates vascular smooth muscle cell proliferation, vessel size and vascular remodeling. Journal of Molecular and Cellular Cardiology 49: 287–293.
23. Wang X, Adhikari N, Li Q, Guan Z, Hall JL (2004) The Role of β-Transducin Repeat-Containing Protein (β-TrCP) in the Regulation of NF-κB in Vascular Smooth Muscle Cells. Arteriosclerosis, Thrombosis, and Vascular Biology 24: 85–90.

24. Basi DL, Adhikari N, Mariash A, Li Q, Kao E, et al. (2007) Femoral artery neointimal hyperplasia is reduced after wire injury in Ref-1+/− mice. Am J Physiol Heart Circ Physiol 292: H516–521.
25. Balakrishnan A, Stearns AT, Park PJ, Dreyfuss JM, Ashley SW, et al. (2010) MicroRNA mir-16 is anti-proliferative in enterocytes and exhibits diurnal rhythmicity in intestinal crypts. Experimental Cell Research 316: 3512–3521.
26. Chamorro-Jorganes A, Araldi E, Penalva LOF, Sandhu D, Fernández-Hernando C, et al. (2011) MicroRNA-16 and MicroRNA-424 Regulate Cell-Autonomous Angiogenic Functions in Endothelial Cells via Targeting Vascular Endothelial Growth Factor Receptor-2 and Fibroblast Growth Factor Receptor-1. Arteriosclerosis, Thrombosis, and Vascular Biology 31: 2595–2606.
27. Chen L, Wang Q, Wang G-D, Wang H-S, Huang Y, et al. (2013) miR-16 inhibits cell proliferation by targeting IGF1R and the Raf1–MEK1/2–ERK1/2 pathway in osteosarcoma. FEBS letters 587: 1366–1372.
28. Lezina L, Purmessur N, Antonov AV, Ivanova T, Karpova E, et al. (2013) miR-16 and miR-26a target checkpoint kinases Wee1 and Chk1 in response to p53 activation by genotoxic stress. Cell Death Dis 4: e953.
29. Preskill C, Weidhaas JB (2013) SNPs in MicroRNA Binding Sites as Prognostic and Predictive Cancer Biomarkers. 18: 327–340.

17

Morning Surge of Ventricular Arrhythmias in a New Arrhythmogenic Canine Model of Chronic Heart Failure Is Associated with Attenuation of Time-Of-Day Dependence of Heart Rate and Autonomic Adaptation, and Reduced Cardiac Chaos

Yujie Zhu, Mohamed A. Hanafy, Cheryl R. Killingsworth, Gregory P. Walcott, Martin E. Young, Steven M. Pogwizd*

Department of Medicine, University of Alabama at Birmingham, Birmingham, Alabama, United States of America

Abstract

Patients with chronic heart failure (CHF) exhibit a morning surge in ventricular arrhythmias, but the underlying cause remains unknown. The aim of this study was to determine if heart rate dynamics, autonomic input (assessed by heart rate variability (HRV)) and nonlinear dynamics as well as their abnormal time-of-day-dependent oscillations in a newly developed arrhythmogenic canine heart failure model are associated with a morning surge in ventricular arrhythmias. CHF was induced in dogs by aortic insufficiency & aortic constriction, and assessed by echocardiography. Holter monitoring was performed to study time-of-day-dependent variation in ventricular arrhythmias (PVCs, VT), traditional HRV measures, and nonlinear dynamics (including detrended fluctuations analysis $\alpha 1$ and $\alpha 2$ (DFA$\alpha 1$ & DFA$\alpha 2$), correlation dimension (CD), and Shannon entropy (SE)) at baseline, as well as 240 days (240d) and 720 days (720d) following CHF induction. LV fractional shortening was decreased at both 240d and 720d. Both PVCs and VT increased with CHF duration and showed a morning rise (2.5-fold & 1.8-fold increase at 6 AM-noon vs midnight-6 AM) during CHF. The morning rise in HR at baseline was significantly attenuated by 52% with development of CHF (at both 240d & 720d). Morning rise in the ratio of low frequency to high frequency (LF/HF) HRV at baseline was markedly attenuated with CHF. DFA$\alpha 1$, DFA$\alpha 2$, CD and SE all decreased with CHF by 31, 17, 34 and 7%, respectively. Time-of-day-dependent variations in LF/HF, CD, DFA $\alpha 1$ and SE, observed at baseline, were lost during CHF. Thus in this new arrhythmogenic canine CHF model, attenuated morning HR rise, blunted autonomic oscillation, decreased cardiac chaos and complexity of heart rate, as well as aberrant time-of-day-dependent variations in many of these parameters were associated with a morning surge of ventricular arrhythmias.

Editor: Marcello Rota, Brigham & Women's Hospital - Harvard Medical School, United States of America

Funding: This work was supported by National Heart, Lung, and Blood Institute Grant HL-097268, SMP. The funders had no role in study design, data collection and analysis, decision to publish, or preparation of the manuscript.

Competing Interests: The authors have declared that no competing interests exist.

* Email: spogwizd@uab.edu

Introduction

Chronic heart failure (CHF), which affects over 5 million people in the US [1], is associated with increased incidence of sudden death primary from ventricular tachycardia (VT) degenerating to ventricular fibrillation [2]. A morning surge (between 6 AM and noon) in sudden deaths and ventricular arrhythmias have been demonstrated in patients with CHF [3]. The onset of other cardiovascular events such as heart attack, stroke and chest pain is also increased in the morning [4,5,6]. The underlying mechanisms are poorly understood, in part due to a lack of characterization of heart rate dynamics, autonomic oscillation and nonlinear dynamics in time-of-day-dependent adverse cardiac events in large animal CHF models. Moreover most studies to date have been done primarily in HF patients and have been limited and influenced by concurrent medication use.

Time-of-day-dependent variations in heart rate (HR) dynamics, autonomic nervous system and nonlinear dynamics are associated with the morning surge in cardiovascular events [3,7]. Heart rate variability (HRV) can assess the regulation of arrhythmogenic substrate in CHF of the failing heart. Traditional linear HRV is analyzed in the time and frequency domain, and markers include SDNN (standard deviation of RR intervals), CV (coefficient of variation of RR intervals), and rMSSD (root mean square of successive differences), spectral power in different frequency range, etc. HRV has been shown to have important prognostic implications [8,9,10,11,12,13]. Heart rate fluctuations have been recognized as complex dynamical behaviors originating from nonlinear processes [8,10,11,12,13,14,15,16,17]. Nonlinear dynamic approaches to HRV are used to determine if HRV has features typical of chaos (complexity & fractal-like behavior) [18]. Nonlinear measures study complex interactions of hemodynamic, electrophysiological, and humoral variables and their regulation by the autonomic and central nervous systems, and have been shown to have prognostic value in CHF [8,9,10,11,12,13]. Cardiac chaos is decreased in human CHF [17] and greater reduction in parameters of cardiac chaos is associated with poorer prognosis in CHF patients [19]. Altered fractal properties, fractal-like scaling exponents and correlation properties of HRV, have been shown to precede the onset of lethal arrhythmias, changes that traditional (i.e. linear) HRV markers failed to detect [20,21].

Despite knowledge of HRV parameters in patients with CHF which are associated with a morning surge in ventricular arrhythmias, the underlying mechanisms contributing to these important observations have remained elusive. We have recently developed a novel arrhythmogenic large animal model of CHF in the canine heart that exhibits decreased LV function and spontaneous ventricular arrhythmia that are initiated and maintained by a focal nonreentrant mechanism [22]. The purpose of the present study was to assess whether there is a morning surge in premature ventricular complexes (PVCs) and VT in our new irreversible arrhythmogenic canine CHF model, and to determine whether this morning surge is associated with alterations in heart rate dynamics, autonomic nervous system and nonlinear dynamics of HRV.

Methods

Animals

All experiments were carried out in strict accordance with the recommendations in the Guide for the Care and Use of Laboratory Animals of the National Institutes of Health (NIH Publication No. 85-23, revised 1996) [23]. The protocols were approved by the Institutional Animal Care and Use Committee of the University of Alabama at Birmingham. Mixed breed dogs of both sexes were housed individually in metal cages with a 12-hr light on (6:00–18:00)/12-hr light off cycle. Neither control dogs nor CHF dogs were on any medication chronically.

Induction of chronic heart failure in dogs

Heart failure was induced by combined aortic insufficiency (AI) and abdominal aortic constriction (AC). For creation of aortic insufficiency, dogs were given Telazol (6 mg/kg, IV) and atropine (0.04 mg/kg, IM). Cefazolin (25 mg/kg IM) and 0.1–0.2 mg/kg Buprenorphine (IM) were subsequently admininistered. The dogs were intubated and ventilated with isoflurane/O_2 mechanically during the surgery. Under continued fluoroscopic imaging, AI was induced by perforating the right and non-coronary aortic valve leaflets using a 5F catheter and a custom-shaped trochar. A 4F Fogarty balloon catheter was passed through the perforation over a guide wire. The balloon was inflated and pulled through the valve to enlarge the perforation. Based on our well-established CHF rabbit model [24], sufficient AI was achieved when the aortic pulse pressure increased by a minimum of 50%. This was confirmed by color flow echocardiography. Eleven dogs were serially studied long term up to 720 days while 15 dogs were used for other terminal studies or died prior to 720 days after AC.

Aortic constriction (AC) to cause pressure overload was created ~6 weeks later, when M-mode echocardiographic measurements indicated that the LV end-diastolic diameter (LVEDD) had increased by 20% compared to baseline. The same anesthesia protocol was used during the surgery. After midline laparotomy, the aorta was isolated at the level of the left renal artery. A 2–0 silk ligature or a sterile polyethylene band was tightened to reduce the aortic diameter until the systolic blood pressure gradient was increased by ~45–50 mm Hg from the pre-ligation measurement. In two dogs, a ligature was also placed around a branch of the renal artery. The aortic systolic pressure gradient was determined using a 4 F catheter passed through a vascular sheath in the femoral artery.

Echocardiography

Prior to any surgical intervention and at approximately 240 days and 720 days following AC, dogs underwent M-mode, 2-D, and color flow echocardiography (sedated with 0.1 mL butorphenol i.v.) using a Philips SONOS 5500 ultrasound system. LV end-systolic (LVESD) and end-diastolic diameter (LVEDD) were measured and the LV fractional shortening (FS = [LVEDD–LVESD]/LVEDD × 100]) was calculated.

Holter monitoring

Prior to surgical intervention and at 240 days and 720 days post AC, digital Holter monitoring (GE SEER Light, GE Healthcare) was obtained from dogs in the conscious state. The chest and back were shaved and five ECG electrodes were applied to the chest secured by a specially-designed nylon jacket. 24-hour period Holter recording were made with the dogs' movements being unrestricted. Holter data were analyzed to quantitate VT & PVCs and their time-of-day occurrence. VT episodes (3 or more consecutive beats), VT beats and PVCs were confirmed by an experienced cardiologist.

HRV analysis

ECG data from Holter recordings were digitized with a sampling rate at 125 Hz. The RR intervals and annotation of heart-beats were exported from the GE MARS Holter system for further analyses using a specially-designed Matlab-based program, as well as Matlab-based Kubios program [25]. Ectopic beats were excluded from HRV analysis.

Power spectral density was assessed using parametric auto-regressive (AR) modeling-based methods. Low frequency power (LF, 0.04–0.15 Hz) mainly reflects sympathetic nerve activity (SNS). High frequency power (HF, 0.15–0.40 Hz) primarily reflects parasympathetic (PNS) modulation of HR. While LF/HF (ratio of LF to HF) have been used as a direct reflection of the ratio of sympathetic to parasympathetic input, it appears to be more of an indicator of overall balance between SNS and PNS [25,26,27]. For example, LF/HF ratio is higher when SNS is predominant, whereas a small LF/HF ratio suggests predominantly PNS control.

Correlation dimension is a measure of dimensionality of the space occupied by a set of points that can be used to measure complexity of the RR interval time series [25,28,29]. Reconstruction of the attractor (vectors with a set of length embedded in m-dimensional space) was performed. Then the correlation integral was calculated with the number of points in the phase space that are closer than a certain threshold r, repeating the process for a certain range of thresholds. Correlation dimension was computed as the slope of the line fitting the log-log plot of the correlation integral as a function of threshold if the number of points was sufficiently large and r was small.

Detrended fluctuation analysis (DFA) quantifies fractal-like scaling exponents and correlation properties of RR intervals [8,25,30]. The RR interval time series was integrated, and detrended within each segment. The root mean square fluctuation of the integrated and detrended data was repeatedly measured over different segment lengths and plotted against different segment lengths on a log-log scale. The scaling exponent DFA α indicates the slope of this regression line. The short-term fluctuation DFA α1 was calculated within range 4≤n≤16 and long-term fluctuation DFA α2 was calculated within range 16≤ n≤64.

Shannon entropy (SE) is a measure of signal complexity of the time series dynamics, and is the information entropy of line segment density distributions from the RR intervals [25,31]. It is measured by the negative sum of the multiplication of the probabilities and base 2 logarithms of probabilities for given line lengths. The probability is the number of length lines divided by the total number of lines.

Statistical analysis

Data are reported as means ± SEM. One-way analysis of variance (ANOVA) was used for measurements obtained from multiple groups. Comparisons between values on two individual groups were done using the two-group (unpaired) t test. Cosinor method for computing rhythm analysis was performed using the nonlinear regression function by SPSS. Rhythmicity was evaluated by fitting the nonlinear cosine function, and a HRV parameter was considered to have a significant time-of-day-dependent oscillation if it fit a cosine wave function for $p<0.05$, with a periodicity of approx. 24 hours. X^2 goodness-of-fit testing was used to determine non-uniform distribution of timing in the 24-hour period.

Results

CHF dogs developed progressive cardiac enlargement & LV dysfunction

Compared with baseline, CHF dogs developed progressive cardiac enlargement and decreased left ventricular (LV) systolic function following AI/AC, as assessed by echocardiography. LV end-diastolic dimension (LVEDD) progressively increased by 59 and 66% after 240 and 720 days post-AC, respectively. Likewise, LV end-systolic dimension (LVESD) increased by 91 and 114% after 240 and 720 days post-AC, respectively. LV fractional shortening progressively decreased from 43.5±0.9% at baseline to 32.0±1.1% at 240 days and 27.5±1.8% at 720 days after AC in CHF dogs (Figures 1 A&B).

Number of VT episodes, VT beats and PVCs show morning rise in CHF dogs

At baseline, there were no episodes of VT and only a total of 3 PVCs in 26 dogs. The incidence of VT episodes, VT beats and PVCs assessed by 24-hr Holter monitoring progressively increased at 240 and 720 days (Figure 2A). Moreover, ventricular arrhythmias exhibited a marked diurnal variation with a rise during the morning in CHF dogs. The number of VT episodes, VT beats and PVCs during 6:00 AM to 12:00 PM was elevated compared with the other time of day (Figure 2B). VT episodes, VT beats and PVCs occurred 1.7, 1.8 and 2.5 times more frequently during 6:00 AM to 12:00 PM than the preceding quartile (between 12:00 AM and 6:00 AM), and all showed a morning rise during 6:00 AM to 12:00 PM at 0.05 significance level by χ^2 goodness-of-fit test. Figure 2C showed representative spontaneously-occurring VT and PVCs in CHF dogs.

Morning (6 AM-noon) HR rise is attenuated in CHF

The average heart rates (HR) for every 3 hours intervals of the day at baseline (N = 26 dogs), and at 240 days (N = 18) and 720 days (N = 11) after AC, are shown in Figure 3A. At baseline, it appears that HR rises rapidly in the morning (with a 13% increase in HR from 6 AM-noon vs midnight-6 AM), which is not observed in the CHF groups at 240 and 720 days. With CHF, the morning HR rise was not as great (ΔHR for 6 AM-noon vs midnight-6 AM of 5.97±1.63 and 6.02±1.62 bpm for 240 & 720 days post-AC, respectively, vs 12.47±1.48 bpm at baseline, $p<0.05$ & 0.05, N = 18, 11, 26; Figure 3C). With development of CHF, mean HR (over 24 hrs) remained unchanged at 240 days but was decreased at 720 days vs baseline (87±2 vs 104±2 bpm, $p<0.01$, N = 11, 26), likely reflecting sinus node dysfunction that is well-described in CHF [32,33].

Morning ANS adaptation is attenuated with CHF

From spectral analyses, the ratio of the low frequency to high frequency (LF/HF) components, a measure of autonomic balance between sympathetic and parasympathetic nervous systems, appears to rise rapidly during the morning at baseline (6 AM-noon vs midnight-6 AM; $p<0.01$ by ANOVA; N = 26, Figure 4A). There was attenuation of the morning rise in LF/HF (from 6 AM-noon vs midnight-6 AM) (Figure 4C) at 240 & 720

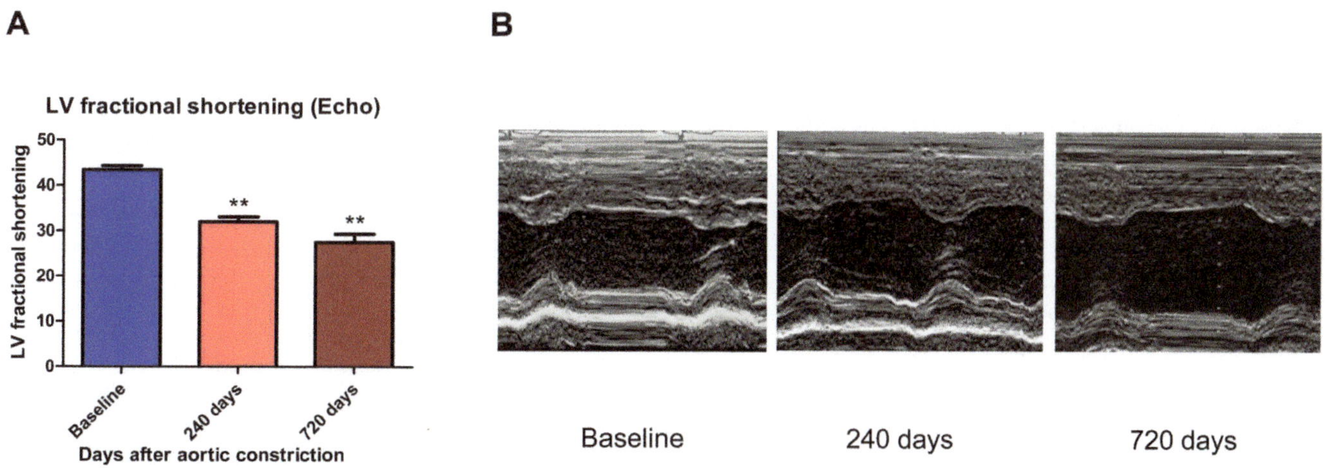

Figure 1. CHF dogs developed LV dysfunction. (A) Histogram of LV fractional shortening (FS) at baseline, 240 days and 720 days after AC (* *, $p<0.01$ vs baseline). (B) 2D echocardiography demonstrates increased LV end-diastolic dimension (LVEDD) and LV end-systolic dimension (LVESD) in CHF dogs.

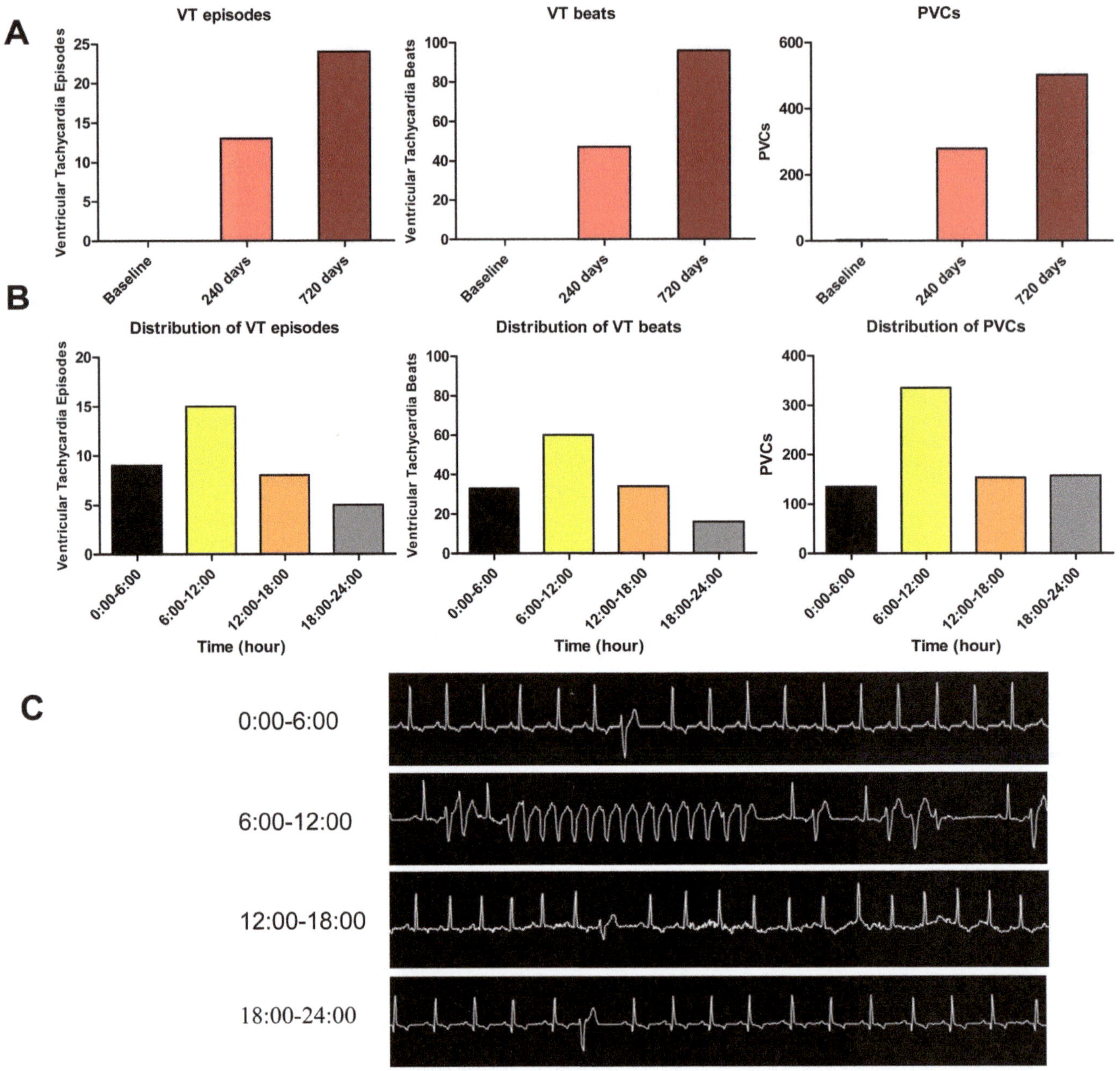

Figure 2. VT episodes, VT beats and PVCs show morning rise in CHF dogs. (A) There is progressive increase in ventricular arrhythmias (VT episodes, VT beats and PVCs) with the duration of CHF. (B) Both VT episodes and VT beats showed a morning rise (1.7-fold & 1.8-fold increase at 6 AM-noon vs midnight-6 AM), and PVCs showed a morning rise (2.5-fold increase at 6 AM-noon vs midnight-6 AM). (C) Representative spontaneously-occurring VT and PVCs in a CHF dog.

days in CHF dogs. With CHF there was a progressive decline in LF/HF such that by 720 days post-AC LF/HF had decreased by 43% ($p<0.01$ by ANOVA; N = 26, 11, Figure 4B).

Correlation dimension progressively decreases with CHF with attenuation of morning rise

CD is one of the nonlinear parameters reflecting cardiac chaos, a decrease of which can be detrimental [34]. Figure 5A shows that CHF provoked consistent progressive reductions in CD. Average 24-hour CD decreased with HF such that by 720 days, CD was reduced by 34% (1.22 ± 0.24 at 720 days vs 1.86 ± 0.13 at baseline, $p<0.05$, N = 11, 26, Figure 5B). At the time of enhanced arrhythmia occurrence (6 AM-noon), CD was reduced by 39% (1.33 ± 0.19 at 720 days vs 2.18 ± 0.17 at baseline, $p<0.01$, N = 11, 26), and there was attenuation of the morning rise in CD both at 240 and 720 days (Figure 5C). Moreover, cosinor analysis revealed that CD significantly oscillated with a periodicity of approx. 24 hours at baseline ($p<0.01$), which was lost at 240 & 720 days ($p>0.05$, $p>0.05$).

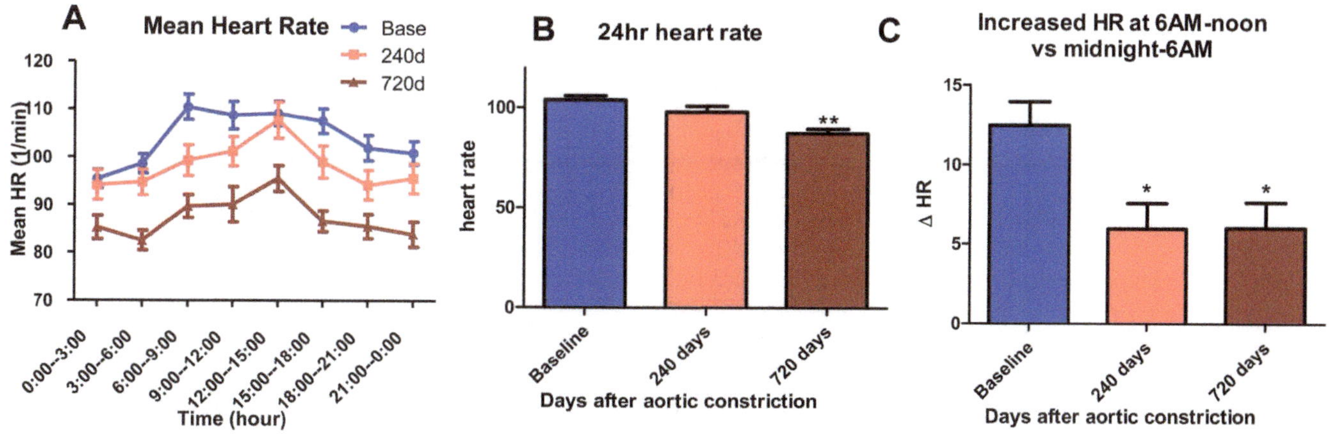

Figure 3. Heart rate at baseline and CHF. (A) Summarized data for mean heart rate at baseline, 240 days and 720 days after AC. Mean heart rate is the average of every 3 hours. (B) Histogram of average 24-hour HR at baseline, 240 days and 720 days after AC (**, $p<0.01$ vs baseline). (C) Histogram of ΔHR at baseline, 240 days and 720 days after AC (*, $p<0.05$ vs baseline). ΔHR represents the increased average heart rate at 6 AM-noon vs midnight-6 AM.

Detrended fluctuations analysis (DFA) α1 and α2 shows progressively decreased fractal properties with CHF with attenuation of morning rise

DFA α1 and α2 reflect the fractal properties of heart rate. Reduced DFA α1 was reported to be a very powerful measure as a predictor of all-cause mortality [8]. Figures 6A and 6D show that at baseline there was a morning rise in DFAα1 and DFAα2 (Figures 6A&D). With CHF the average 24-hour DFA α1 was significantly decreased at 240 and 720 days (0.523±0.039 and 0.456±0.027 at 240 & 720 days, $p<0.05$ & $p<0.01$, N = 18, 11) vs 0.660±0.025 (N = 26) at baseline (Figure 6B). Average 24-hour DFA α2 was significantly decreased only at 720 days vs baseline (0.575±0.029 vs 0.692±0.019 at baseline, $p<0.01$, N = 11, 26; Figure 6E). The potential protective effect of enhanced DFA α1 at the time of increased arrhythmia occurrence was greatly attenuated with CHF (Figure 6C). Rhythm analysis by cosinor method showed that DFAα1 is rhythmic at baseline ($p<0.05$), and loses time-of-day-dependent oscillation at 240d and 720d after AC in CHF dogs ($p>0.05$, $p>0.05$). In contrast there was no significant difference in the morning rise of DFAα2 between baseline and CHF (Figure 6F).

Shannon entropy shows progressive decrease with CHF and lack of morning surge

SE is another analytical approach for complexity of time series, and reduced SE has been reported in heart disease [35]. Figure 7A illustrates that at baseline there was a small morning rise in SE (Figure 7A). With CHF, average 24-hour SE decreased by 7% at 720 days post-AC (2.828±0.051 vs 3.037±0.022 at baseline; $p<0.05$; N = 11, 26; Figure 7B). However the morning rise in SE was practically abolished with CHF (Figure 7C). Cosine curve fitting in SE showed time-of-day-dependence at baseline ($p<0.05$), but loss of time-of-day-dependent variations at 240 and 720 days ($p>0.05$, $p>0.05$).

Discussion

Morning is a time of increased workload, physical activity and heart rate and sympathetic activity [36], associated with increased incidence of adverse cardiac events. In this study we explored

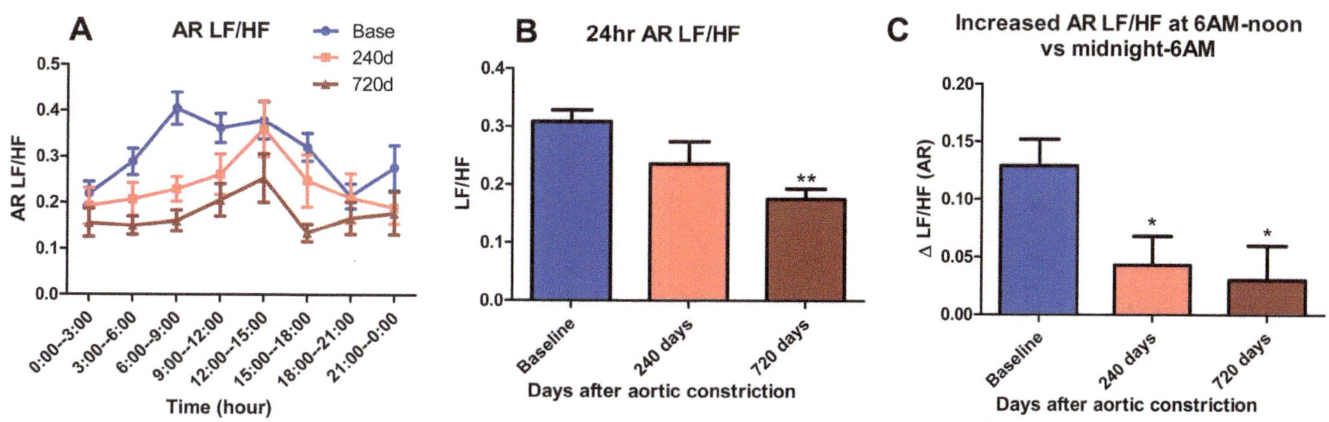

Figure 4. LF/HF at baseline and CHF. (A) Summarized data for mean LF/HF at baseline, 240 days and 720 days after AC. Mean LF/HF is average of every 3 hours. (B) Histogram of average 24-hour LF/HF at baseline, 240 days and 720 days after AC (**, $p<0.01$ vs baseline). (C) Histogram of Δ LF/HF at baseline, 240 days and 720 days after AC (*, $p<0.05$ vs baseline). Δ LF/HF represents the increased average LF/HF at 6 AM-noon vs midnight-6 AM.

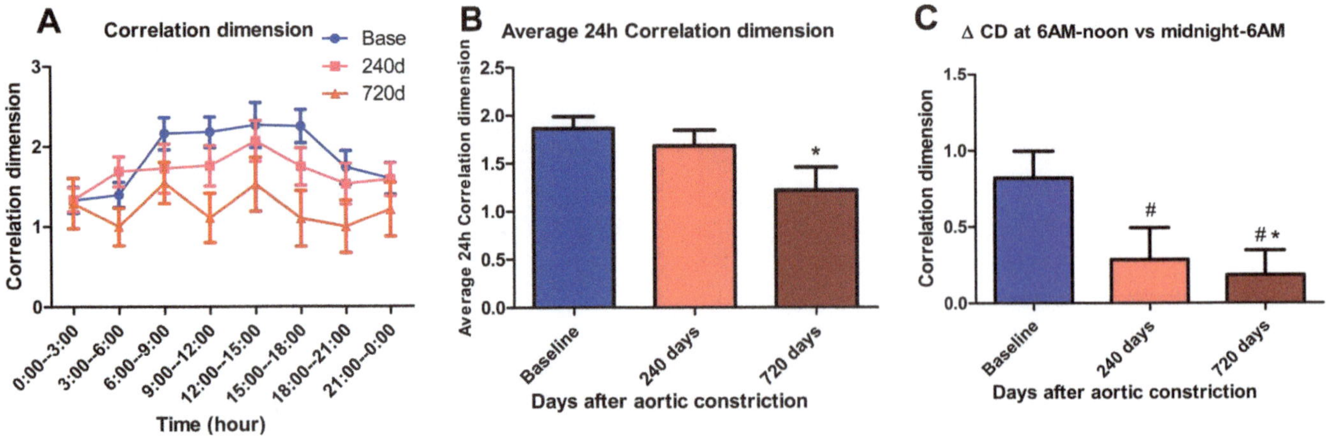

Figure 5. Correlation dimension (CD) decreases with CHF. (A) Summarized data for mean CD at baseline, 240 days and 720 days after AC. Mean CD is average of every 3 hours from 24-hour recordings. (B) Histogram of average 24-hour CD at baseline, 240 days and 720 days after AC (*, $p<0.05$ vs baseline). (C) Histogram of Δ CD at baseline, 240 days and 720 days after AC (*, $p<0.05$ vs baseline; # denotes that CD is arrhythmic at 240d and 720d by rhythm analysis, i.e. exhibits loss of time-of-day dependence). Δ CD represents the change in CD at 6 AM-noon vs midnight-6 AM, and was decreased with CHF.

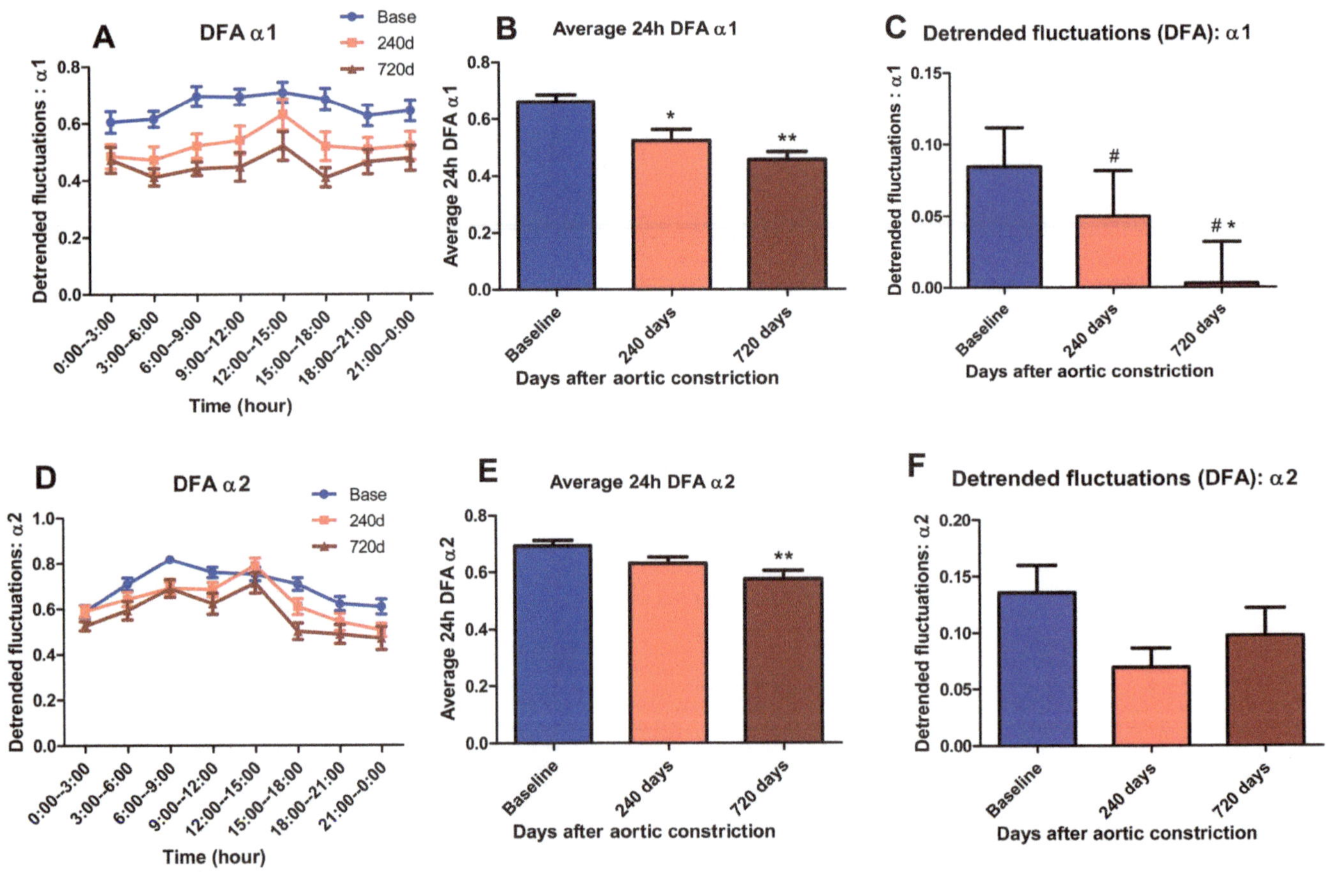

Figure 6. Detrended fluctuations analysis (DFA) α1 and α2. (A) Summarized data of average DFA α1 at baseline, 240 days and 720 days after AC. Mean DFA α1 was the average of every 3 hours. (B) Histogram of average 24-hour DFA α1 at baseline, 240 days and 720 days after AC (*, $p<0.05$ vs baseline; **, $p<0.01$ vs baseline). (C) Histogram of ΔDFA α1 at baseline, 240 days and 720 days after AC (*, $p<0.05$ vs baseline; # denote that DFA α1 is arrhythmic at 240d and 720d by rhythm analysis, i.e. exhibits loss of time-of-day dependence). ΔDFA α1 represents the increased average heart rate at 6 AM-noon vs midnight-6 AM, and was decreased with CHF. (D) Summarized data of average DFA α2 at baseline, 240 days and 720 days after AC. Mean DFA α2 is average of every 3 hours. (E) Histogram of average 24-hour DFA α2 at baseline, 240 days and 720 days after AC (* *, $p<0.01$ vs baseline). (F) Histogram of ΔDFA α2 at baseline, 240 days and 720 days after AC. ΔDFA α2 was decreased in CHF. ΔDFA α2 represents the change in DFA α2 at 6 AM-noon vs midnight-6 AM.

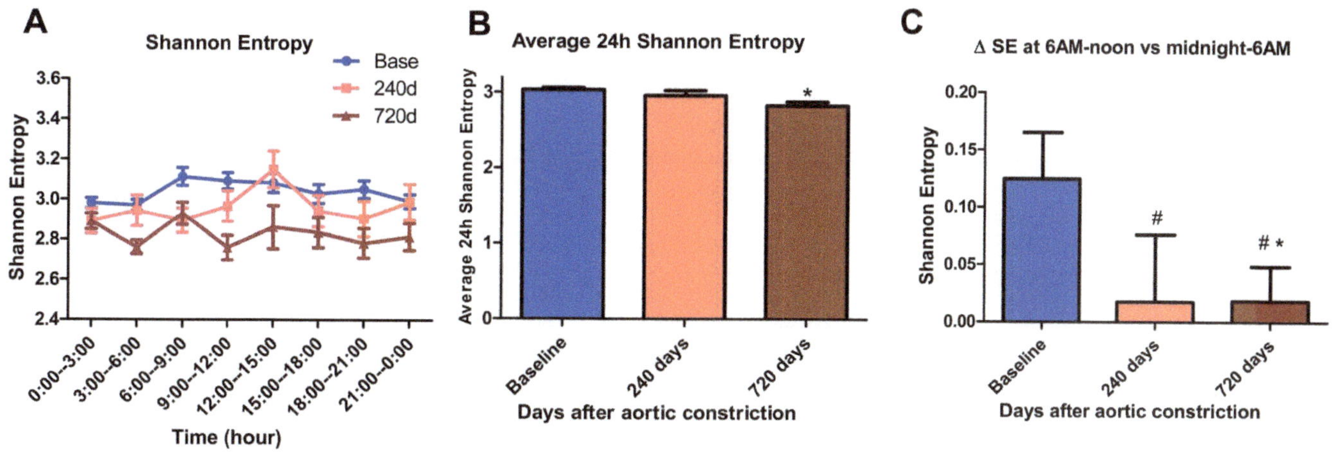

Figure 7. Shannon entropy (SE) decreases with CHF. (A) Summarized data for mean SE at baseline, 240 days and 720 days after AC. Mean SE is the average of every 3 hours. (B) Histogram of average 24-hour SE at baseline, 240 days and 720 days after AC (*, $p<0.05$ vs baseline). (C) Histogram of Δ SE at baseline, 240 days and 720 days after AC (*, $p<0.05$ vs baseline; # denotes that SE is arrhythmic at 240d and 720d by rhythm analysis, i.e. exhibits loss of time-of-day dependence). Δ SE, which represents the change in SE at 6 AM-noon vs midnight-6 AM, was decreased in CHF.

linear and nonlinear dynamics of HRV and their time-of-day-dependent variation in a novel irreversible large animal model of nonischemic CHF in dog. We show, in a large animal model of CHF: a morning surge in ventricular arrhythmias with CHF; a morning rise in HR at baseline that was attenuated in CHF; a morning rise in LF/HF (balance between sympathetic vs parasympathetic system) that was blunted in CHF; reduced chaos in CD, DFA α1 & α2 and SE in CHF; a loss of time-of-day dependence was found in LF/HF, CD, DFA α1 and SE in CHF; and a lack of enhanced chaos at the time of enhanced arrhythmia occurrence. Several unique features of this study include this being the first demonstration of time-of-day-dependent pattern of VT and PVCs in a large animal model of CHF, and this being the first study to characterize chaotic behavior of HRV and its changes with CHF in the canine heart and demonstrating findings similar to those shown in human CHF [30,34,35,37,38,39,40,41].

Normal time-of-day rhythm

At baseline, dogs show normal left ventricular (LV) systolic function and exhibit lack of cardiac arrhythmia. At baseline state, morning HR significantly increased during 6:00 AM to 12:00 PM compared to midnight-6:00 AM. Dogs at baseline also had a significantly higher LF/HF rise in morning (vs 12:00 AM–6:00 AM) compared to CHF dogs. These findings are similar to reports in healthy human subjects [42]. The values of nonlinear dynamics such as CD, DFA α1 and SE are higher at baseline compared to CHF dogs. Cosinor analysis revealed that CD, DFA α1 and SE showed significant time-of-day-dependent oscillation at baseline with a periodicity of approximately 24 hours.

HF model in absence of drug effects

Studies from HF patients have provided important insights into the alterations in autonomic influences that contribute to the arrhythmogenic substrate of the failing heart [8,10,11,12,14], but these studies are typically limited by concurrent medication use such as beta blockers, ACE inhibitors and Ca^{2+} channel blocker. Holter monitoring of HF patients with assessment of HRV to study autonomic imbalance as well as nonlinear dynamics will be influenced by these medication and their drug effects. It is important and essential to study electrophysiological and autonomic regulation in chronic heart failure in the absence of drug effects. This is feasible with studies of HRV (in absence of drug effects) by using a large animal model of CHF that is similar to human nonischemic CHF and which can be used for development of new therapies and for translating basic scientific discoveries from bench to bedside. While there are a number of large animal models of nonischemic HF, the canine rapid pacing HF model is one of the most commonly used. It has provided insights into the complex pathophysiology of HF. However, limitations of the canine pacing HF model include the reversibility of HF with cessation of pacing (making long-term studies of interventions on the failing heart difficult), remodeling different from human CHF, and the lack of hypertrophy [43]. We developed a novel canine model of nonischemic CHF that is both irreversible and arrhythmogenic by induction of combined aortic insufficiency (AI) and abdominal aortic constriction (AC). The hemodynamic burden of combined volume and pressure overload in this canine heart leads to irreversible contractile dysfunction and arrhythmogenesis. We have found that our CHF dogs exhibit a 63% increase in HW/BW [44] and a 66% increase in LVEDD. Moreover this canine model of CHF demonstrates a morning surge in ventricular arrhythmias as well as reduced chaos that will enable us to further define underlying mechanisms in the absence of drug effects so commonly an issue in CHF patients.

Morning surge in adverse cardiovascular event

Prior studies have highlighted the excess risk of adverse cardiovascular events during morning. For example, sudden cardiac death exhibits an increased frequency in the morning [45]. The majority of VT episodes in patients with dilated cardiomyopathy occurred during morning [46], with an increase in the onset of sustained VT at that time [47]. PVCs also increase in the morning [48,49]. In addition to the morning surges in sudden death, VT and PVCs, numerous studies have shown similar morning rise in other cardiovascular events such as chest pain [6], myocardial infarctions [4,6], and stroke [5]. This time-of-day-dependent pattern of excess cardiovascular risk during the morning associated with awakening is an appealing target for therapeutics. However, the lack of a suitable animal model of this phenomenon has hindered our understanding of the mechanisms contributing to the morning rise in these adverse events. Demonstration of time-of-day-dependent oscillations of VT and

PVCs in a large animal model of CHF in the current study provides a unique opportunity to explore underlying mechanisms in the future.

Factors that may be associated with morning surge and time-of-day-dependent variations

Morning rise in heart rate was attenuated in CHF dogs, similar to that in patients with stable coronary artery disease [41,50] and CHF [39], and may be related to altered contribution of autonomic system in the morning or sinus node dysfunction in CHF [32,33]. We found that the morning rise in LF/HF was attenuated in CHF, similar to that shown in patients with coronary artery disease [38] and in patients with morning peak of tachyarrhythmic events [51,52]. Reduced LF power was associated with increased risk of ventricular arrhythmias and cardiac death in patients with CHF in several studies [9,53,54,55,56,57,58]. We also found reduced chaos in CHF, a lack of enhanced chaos at the time of enhanced arrhythmia occurrence, and a loss of time-of-day-dependent variations for LF/HF, CD, DFA $\alpha 1$ and SE in CHF. Non-linear dynamics and chaotic indices in HRV were significantly reduced in patients with a propensity for adverse arrhythmic events which exhibit morning surge [20,59,60,61,62,63]. Reduced chaos was associated with increased arrhythmias [63,64,65]. Thus the changes in linear and nonlinear dynamics in our CHF dogs are similar to that in CHF patients, thereby validating this new arrhythmogenic canine preparation as a valuable model in which to further study molecular, cellular, physiologic and neurohumoral mechanisms in ways not possible in humans.

There are numerous factors that may contribute to this time-of-day elevated incidence in ventricular arrhythmias in dogs as well as in humans. Catecholamines, angiotensin, renin, aldosterone and growth hormone [6] have higher plasma concentrations in morning during maximal sympathetic activity in humans [6]. Protective regulators such as bradykinin, magnesium, potassium, vitamin E and C and melatonin are all low in the morning [6], and may be associated with greater vascular resistance, blood pressure, contractility, coronary artery tone, stroke volume and cardiac output [6]. Additional factors such as acetylcholine, histamine, serotonin, and myocardial oxygen demand [6,41,66] exhibit circadian variation and may contribute to increased risk of adverse cardiovascular events in the morning. All these corresponding biochemical changes in the morning in CHF dogs are reflected by attenuated morning HR rise, blunted autonomic oscillation, decreased cardiac chaos, a loss of time-of-day-dependent rhythm, and a lack of enhanced chaos at the time of enhanced arrhythmia occurrence. Diurnal variation of HRV was reported in healthy human subjects [37,67,68]. We found loss of diurnal variation of HRV in CHF dogs as has been described in human HF [37]. Likewise we found a consistent and progressive decrease in correlation dimension, DFA scaling factor α and SE in CHF dogs as has been shown in human HF [30,34,35,40].

Heart failure and autonomic system

In the current study, the morning rise in LF/HF was attenuated with development of CHF at 240 days and 720 days. Reduction in LF/HF was found in CHF dogs. These may reflect sinus node dysfunction, decreased responsiveness of the sinus node to autonomic input [69] or a CHF-induced reduction in baroreceptor sensitivity in the setting of increased sympathetic tone that has been consistently found in HF [69,70]. Several studies demonstrate that LF power is greatly attenuated [71] and the LF variability of sympathetic nerve activity is absent in patients with heart failure [72,73]. Reduced LF is a powerful predictor of sudden death in CHF patients [9]. In CHF dogs, there was attenuation of the morning rise in LF/HF. On the other hand, ventricular arrhythmias were preceded by elevated sympathetic activation [74,75]. Increased PVCs and VT may correspond to higher sympathetic nerve activation in morning hours [74].

Reduced chaos in heart failure

Several studies have demonstrated reduced complexity and fractal properties in CHF patients. Poon et al found a decrease in complexity of the heartbeat nonlinear dynamics in CHF patients [17]. Ivanov demonstrated that patients with severe heart failure have a reduced HRV complex. CHF patients show a loss of multifractality [16]. DFA $\alpha 1$ remained as a useful prognostic index in multivariate analysis and was a powerful predictor of mortality among class II CHF patients [11]. Patients with cardiovascular disease showed reduced scaling exponents, suggesting a loss of fractal-like HR dynamics ($\alpha 1 < 0.85$, [10]; $\alpha 1 < 0.75$, [8]), and reduced scaling exponent α was a strong predictor of mortality [10]. Costa et al indicated a loss of complexity with CHF [15]. A reduction in HR complexity and fractal scaling properties were reported in CHF patients [30]. Alterations in nonlinear HRV have important prognostic implications. Reduced DFA $\alpha 1$ was a good univariate predictor of mortality in patients with severe left ventricular dysfunction after acute myocardial infarction [8]. The exponent predicted both arrhythmic and non-arrhythmic cardiac death. The reduced chaos in heart failure is likely due to contributors and factors that influence heart rate dynamics to lose partial or full stochastic kinetics of ion channel gating and biochemical processes, thereby making HRV less complex and less fractal. Abnormalities in left ventricular contractility and cardiac autonomic function may both contribute to a decrease in nonlinear dynamic complexity in patients with CHF [17]. The quantification of nonlinear properties of HRV provides important information in risk stratification of CHF. Furthermore, alterations in nonlinear HRV parameters have important predictive implications in arrhythmias. While linear HRV parameters showed no differences prior to VT (in ICD patients), compression entropy before the onset of VT in those HF patients suggest that altered HR dynamics may contribute to VT onset, and nonlinear measures of HRV could have value in improving VT sensing and/or providing a warning to ICD patient of forthcoming shocks [14]. Approximate entropy, a nonlinear index of HR dynamics describing the complexity of the behavior of the RR interval, has provided information on vulnerability to develop atrial fibrillation [13]. DFA fractal scaling exponent has predicted fatal cardiovascular events in various populations [12].

Mechanisms of chaotic properties in beating variability and its effects on arrhythmogenesis

HRV in healthy subjects has important chaotic properties with complexity and fractal properties in RR intervals. HR regulation is one of the most complex systems. RR intervals are influenced by many factors, such as patterns of autonomic nervous system firing, reduced responsiveness to catecholamine and acetylcholine, all of which change during CHF. At the cellular level, the chaotic properties in beating variability are associated with stochastic channel gating, as well as biochemical and molecular processes. Studies support the notion that the stochastic behavior of ion channels could contribute to chaotic beating [76]. Opening of funny channels (I_f) and L-type calcium channels ($I_{Ca,\,L}$) depolarizes cells and increases heart rate, whereas opening of acetylcholine-activated potassium channels (I_{KAch}) hyperpolarizes cells and reduces heart rate. Stochastic open-close kinetics of these and other ionic channels contribute the chaotic heart rate. Stochastic

Ca^{2+} release from sarcoplasmic reticulum, as well as stochastic RyR gating, are also involved in the modulation of chaotic beating rate [77]. Wilders et al. demonstrate the chaotic fluctuations in beat-to-beat interval of pacemaker cells are due to the stochastic open-close kinetics of the gating of membrane ionic channels [78]. Ionic channel turnover represent a stochastic mechanism contributing to such chaotic variations of cellular characteristics. Furthermore, more chaotic variability probably comes from variations in biochemical and molecular processes involving the concentrations of enzymes, metabolites, and second messengers (such as cAMP protein kinase A, phospholamban phosphorylation, and $I_{Ca,\ L}$ phosphorylation) [77]. Additional biochemical factors involved in the control and modulation of chaotic beating are melatonin, plasma cortisol, growth hormone, catecholamines, angiotensin, renin, aldosterone etc. These factors associated with stochastic channel gating and biochemical processes make HRV more complex and fractal. In CHF dogs, the function of some of these factors that influence RR intervals are turned off or show decreased function, so CHF dogs show decreased complexity and loss of fractal property, which may relate to pathological properties of channels and factors in CHF dogs.

Chaos in HRV decreases with progression of CHF patients [17] and in patients with a propensity for adverse arrhythmic events [20,59,60,61,62,63]. Moreover the degree of chaos decreases immediately prior to the onset of ventricular arrhythmias [61,63,65]. However, little is known about the mechanisms by which decreased chaos in HRV is arrhythmogenic in the failing heart. Dvir et al [64] demonstrated low chaotic HRV is a predictor for cardiac arrhythmogenic events and that pacing of ventricular tissue in a stochastic rather than in a deterministic rhythm (to enhance chaos) exerted a protective antiarrhythmic effect due to a consequence of inherent chaotic HRV. Stochastic ventricular pacing reduced spatial action potential duration (APD) heterogeneity, discordant APD alternans and wavebreak initiation [64]. These results suggest that the chaos in HRV provides the heart with a protective mechanism against arrhythmogenesis [64].

Implications

Morning is a time associated with increased workload and physical activity, concomitant with increased sympathetic activity and nonlinear dynamics. Alterations in these parameters with CHF could contribute to increased cardiovascular risk in the morning. The current study characterized heart rate dynamics, autonomic oscillation, and nonlinear dynamics in CHF dogs when there is increased risk of cardiovascular events during morning. Healthy HR fluctuations exhibit fractal-like self-similarity (on time scales ranging from seconds to hours) and complexity, both of which allow for a broad range of adaptive responses. A reduction in HR fractal properties and complexity, lack of morning enhancement of chaotic activity, loss of time-of-day rhythm in autonomic oscillations and nonlinear dynamics, and blunting of the normal morning transition to high heart rate and sympathetic activity could all contribute to altered regulation of the drug-free arrhythmogenic substrate of this new canine CHF model and its morning surge in ventricular arrhythmias. Development of this large animal arrhythmogenic model of CHF that demonstrates a morning surge in ventricular arrhythmias as well as reduced chaos enable us to further define the underlying mechanisms of VT in the failing heart in ways not possible to achieve in humans (i.e. ability to compare CHF to baseline in same animal, absence of drug effects, and later access to tissue & cells for molecular and physiologic studies).

Conclusion

In this new arrhythmogenic canine CHF model, a morning surge in ventricular arrhythmias was associated with attenuated morning HR rise, blunted autonomic adaptation, reduced cardiac chaos and complexity of heart rate, as well as aberrant time-of-day-dependent variations. This novel large animal model will provide an opportunity for further mechanistic studies not easily done in humans that can directly translate to novel therapeutic approaches in patients.

Author Contributions

Conceived and designed the experiments: YZ SMP. Performed the experiments: YZ. Analyzed the data: YZ MAH MEY SMP. Contributed reagents/materials/analysis tools: YZ CRK GPW MEY SMP. Contributed to the writing of the manuscript: YZ MEY SMP.

References

1. Go AS, Mozaffarian D, Roger VL, Benjamin EJ, Berry JD, et al. (2014) Heart Disease and Stroke Statistics–2014 Update: A Report From the American Heart Association. Circulation 129: e28–e292.
2. Packer M (1985) Sudden unexpected death in patients with congestive heart failure: a second frontier. Circulation 72: 681–685.
3. Muller JE, Ludmer PL, Willich SN, Tofler GH, Aylmer G, et al. (1987) Circadian variation in the frequency of sudden cardiac death. Circulation 75: 131–138.
4. Cohen MC, Rohtla KM, Lavery CE, Muller JE, Mittleman MA (1997) Meta-analysis of the morning excess of acute myocardial infarction and sudden cardiac death. Am J Cardiol 79: 1512–1516.
5. Elliott WJ (1998) Circadian variation in the timing of stroke onset: a meta-analysis. Stroke 29: 992–996.
6. Singh RB, Cornelissen G, Weydahl A, Schwartzkopff O, Katinas G, et al. (2003) Circadian heart rate and blood pressure variability considered for research and patient care. Int J Cardiol 87: 9–28; discussion 29–30.
7. Englund A, Behrens S, Wegscheider K, Rowland E (1999) Circadian variation of malignant ventricular arrhythmias in patients with ischemic and nonischemic heart disease after cardioverter defibrillator implantation. European 7219 Jewel Investigators. J Am Coll Cardiol 34: 1560–1568.
8. Huikuri HV, Makikallio TH, Peng CK, Goldberger AL, Hintze U, et al. (2000) Fractal correlation properties of R-R interval dynamics and mortality in patients with depressed left ventricular function after an acute myocardial infarction. Circulation 101: 47–53.
9. La Rovere MT, Pinna GD, Maestri R, Mortara A, Capomolla S, et al. (2003) Short-term heart rate variability strongly predicts sudden cardiac death in chronic heart failure patients. Circulation 107: 565–570.
10. Makikallio TH, Hoiber S, Kober L, Torp-Pedersen C, Peng CK, et al. (1999) Fractal analysis of heart rate dynamics as a predictor of mortality in patients with depressed left ventricular function after acute myocardial infarction. TRACE Investigators. TRAndolapril Cardiac Evaluation. Am J Cardiol 83: 836–839.
11. Makikallio TH, Huikuri HV, Hintze U, Videbaek J, Mitrani RD, et al. (2001) Fractal analysis and time- and frequency-domain measures of heart rate variability as predictors of mortality in patients with heart failure. Am J Cardiol 87: 178–182.
12. Perkiomaki JS, Makikallio TH, Huikuri HV (2005) Fractal and complexity measures of heart rate variability. Clin Exp Hypertens 27: 149–158.
13. Vikman S, Makikallio TH, Yli-Mayry S, Pikkujamsa S, Koivisto AM, et al. (1999) Altered complexity and correlation properties of R-R interval dynamics before the spontaneous onset of paroxysmal atrial fibrillation. Circulation 100: 2079–2084.
14. Baumert M, Baier V, Haueisen J, Wessel N, Meyerfeldt U, et al. (2004) Forecasting of life threatening arrhythmias using the compression entropy of heart rate. Methods Inf Med 43: 202–206.
15. Costa M, Goldberger AL, Peng CK (2005) Multiscale entropy analysis of biological signals. Phys Rev E Stat Nonlin Soft Matter Phys 71: 021906-1-18.
16. Ivanov PC, Amaral LA, Goldberger AL, Havlin S, Rosenblum MG, et al. (1999) Multifractality in human heartbeat dynamics. Nature 399: 461–465.
17. Poon CS, Merrill CK (1997) Decrease of cardiac chaos in congestive heart failure. Nature 389: 492–495.
18. Goldberger AL (1990) Fractal electrodynamics of the heartbeat. Ann N Y Acad Sci 591: 402–409.
19. Arzeno NM, Kearney MT, Eckberg DL, Nolan J, Poon CS (2007) Heart rate chaos as a mortality predictor in mild to moderate heart failure. Conf Proc IEEE Eng Med Biol Soc 2007: 5051–5054.

20. Makikallio TH, Koistinen J, Jordaens L, Tulppo MP, Wood N, et al. (1999) Heart rate dynamics before spontaneous onset of ventricular fibrillation in patients with healed myocardial infarcts. Am J Cardiol 83: 880–884.
21. Wessel N, Ziehmann C, Kurths J, Meyerfeldt U, Schirdewan A, et al. (2000) Short-term forecasting of life-threatening cardiac arrhythmias based on symbolic dynamics and finite-time growth rates. Phys Rev E Stat Phys Plasmas Fluids Relat Interdiscip Topics 61: 733–739.
22. Liu C, Pogwizd SM (2012) Focal Mechanism Underlying Spontaneous And Norepinephrine-Induced Ventricular Tachycardia In A New Arrhythmogenic Canine Model Of Nonischemic Heart Failure. Heart Rhythm 9: S407.
23. Garber JC, Barbee RW, Bielitzki JT, Clayton LA, Donovan JC, et al. (2011) Guide for the care and use of laboratory animals. Washington, D.C.: The National Academies Press. 220 p.
24. Pogwizd SM (1995) Nonreentrant mechanisms underlying spontaneous ventricular arrhythmias in a model of nonischemic heart failure in rabbits. Circulation 92: 1034–1048.
25. Tarvainen MP, Niskanen JP, Lipponen JA, Ranta-Aho PO, Karjalainen PA (2014) Kubios HRV–heart rate variability analysis software. Comput Methods Programs Biomed 113: 210–220.
26. Akselrod S, Gordon D, Ubel FA, Shannon DC, Berger AC, et al. (1981) Power spectrum analysis of heart rate fluctuation: a quantitative probe of beat-to-beat cardiovascular control. Science 213: 220–222.
27. Billman GE (2011) Heart rate variability - a historical perspective. Front Physiol 2: 86.
28. Grassberger P, Procaccia I (1983) Characterization of strange attractors. Phys Rev Lett 50: 346–349.
29. Guzzetti S, Signorini MG, Cogliati C, Mezzetti S, Porta A, et al. (1996) Non-linear dynamics and chaotic indices in heart rate variability of normal subjects and heart-transplanted patients. Cardiovasc Res 31: 441–446.
30. Peng CK, Havlin S, Stanley HE, Goldberger AL (1995) Quantification of scaling exponents and crossover phenomena in nonstationary heartbeat time series. Chaos 5: 82–87.
31. Webber CL Jr, Zbilut JP (1994) Dynamical assessment of physiological systems and states using recurrence plot strategies. J Appl Physiol 76: 965–973.
32. Opthof T, Coronel R, Rademaker HM, Vermeulen JT, Wilms-Schopman FJ, et al. (2000) Changes in sinus node function in a rabbit model of heart failure with ventricular arrhythmias and sudden death. Circulation 101: 2975–2980.
33. Verkerk AO, Wilders R, Coronel R, Ravesloot JH, Verheijck EE (2003) Ionic remodeling of sinoatrial node cells by heart failure. Circulation 108: 760–766.
34. Almoznino-Sarafian D, Sarafian G, Zyssman I, Shteinshnaider M, Tzur I, et al. (2009) Application of HRV-CD for estimation of life expectancy in various clinical disorders. Eur J Intern Med 20: 779–783.
35. Segerson NM, Smith ML, Wasmund SL, Lux RL, Daccarett M, et al. (2008) Heart rate variability measures during sinus rhythm predict cycle length entropy during atrial fibrillation. J Cardiovasc Electrophysiol 19: 1031–1036.
36. Muller JE (1999) Circadian variation and triggering of acute coronary events. Am Heart J 137: S1–S8.
37. Beckers F, Verheyden B, Couckuyt K, Aubert AE (2006) Fractal dimension in health and heart failure. Biomed Tech (Berl) 51: 194–197.
38. Huikuri HV, Niemela MJ, Ojala S, Rantala A, Ikaheimo MJ, et al. (1994) Circadian rhythms of frequency domain measures of heart rate variability in healthy subjects and patients with coronary artery disease. Effects of arousal and upright posture. Circulation 90: 121–126.
39. Panina G, Khot UN, Nunziata E, Cody RJ, Binkley PF (1995) Assessment of autonomic tone over a 24-hour period in patients with congestive heart failure: relation between mean heart rate and measures of heart rate variability. Am Heart J 129: 748–753.
40. Platisa MM, Gal V (2008) Correlation properties of heartbeat dynamics. Eur Biophys J 37: 1247–1252.
41. Quyyumi AA, Panza JA, Diodati JG, Lakatos E, Epstein SE (1992) Circadian variation in ischemic threshold. A mechanism underlying the circadian variation in ischemic events. Circulation 86: 22–28.
42. Boudreau P, Dumont G, Kin NM, Walker CD, Boivin DB (2011) Correlation of heart rate variability and circadian markers in humans. Conf Proc IEEE Eng Med Biol Soc 2011: 681–682.
43. Moe GW, Armstrong P (1999) Pacing-induced heart failure: a model to study the mechanism of disease progression and novel therapy in heart failure. Cardiovasc Res 42: 591–599.
44. Yan J, Killingsworth CR, Walcott GP, Ai X, Pogwizd SM (2013) Connexin43 Downregulation and Dephosphorylation Contribute to Slow Conduction In A New Arrhythmogenic Canine Model of Non-Ischemic Heart Failure. Heart Rhythm 10: S416.
45. Arntz HR, Willich SN, Oeff M, Bruggemann T, Stern R, et al. (1993) Circadian variation of sudden cardiac death reflects age-related variability in ventricular fibrillation. Circulation 88: 2284–2289.
46. Manolis AG, Katsivas A, Lazaris E, Koutsogeogis D, Louvros N (1997) Circadian modulation of ventricular tachycardia cycle length variability in ICD patients with dilated cardiomyopathy. Pacing Clin Electrophysiol 20: 203–207.
47. Twidale N, Taylor S, Heddle WF, Ayres BF, Tonkin AM (1989) Morning increase in the time of onset of sustained ventricular tachycardia. Am J Cardiol 64: 1204–1206.
48. Raeder EA, Hohnloser SH, Graboys TB, Podrid PJ, Lampert S, et al. (1988) Spontaneous variability and circadian distribution of ectopic activity in patients with malignant ventricular arrhythmia. J Am Coll Cardiol 12: 656–661.
49. Siegel D, Black DM, Seeley DG, Hulley SB (1992) Circadian variation in ventricular arrhythmias in hypertensive men. Am J Cardiol 69: 344–347.
50. Ceyhan M, Gunaydin S, Yorgancioglu C, Zorlutuna Y, Uluoglu C, et al. (2003) Comparison of circadian rhythm characteristics of blood pressure and heart rate in patients before and after elective coronary artery bypass surgery. Chronobiol Int 20: 337–349.
51. Fries R, Hein S, J Kn (2002) Reversed circadian rhythms of heart rate variability and morning peak occurrence of sustained ventricular tachyarrhythmias in patients with implanted cardioverter defibrillator. Med Sci Monit 8: CR751–756.
52. Matveev M, Prokopova R, Nachev C (2006) Normal and Abnormal Circadian Characterisitics in Autonomic Cardiac Control: New Opportunities for Cardiac Risk Prevention: Nova Science Publishers.
53. Brunner-La Rocca HP, Esler MD, Jennings GL, Kaye DM (2001) Effect of cardiac sympathetic nervous activity on mode of death in congestive heart failure. Eur Heart J 22: 1136–1143.
54. Chattipakorn N, Incharoen T, Kanlop N, Chattipakorn S (2007) Heart rate variability in myocardial infarction and heart failure. Int J Cardiol 120: 289–296.
55. Frenneaux MP (2004) Autonomic changes in patients with heart failure and in post-myocardial infarction patients. Heart 90: 1248–1255.
56. Galinier M, Pathak A, Fourcade J, Androdias C, Curnier D, et al. (2000) Depressed low frequency power of heart rate variability as an independent predictor of sudden death in chronic heart failure. Eur Heart J 21: 475–482.
57. Guzzetti S, La Rovere MT, Pinna GD, Maestri R, Borroni E, et al. (2005) Different spectral components of 24 h heart rate variability are related to different modes of death in chronic heart failure. Eur Heart J 26: 357–362.
58. Ponikowski P, Anker SD, Chua TP, Szelemej R, Piepoli M, et al. (1997) Depressed heart rate variability as an independent predictor of death in chronic congestive heart failure secondary to ischemic or idiopathic dilated cardiomyopathy. Am J Cardiol 79: 1645–1650.
59. Huikuri HV, Seppanen T, Koistinen MJ, Airaksinen J, Ikaheimo MJ, et al. (1996) Abnormalities in beat-to-beat dynamics of heart rate before the spontaneous onset of life-threatening ventricular tachyarrhythmias in patients with prior myocardial infarction. Circulation 93: 1836–1844.
60. Makikallio TH, Seppanen T, Airaksinen KE, Koistinen J, Tulppo MP, et al. (1997) Dynamic analysis of heart rate may predict subsequent ventricular tachycardia after myocardial infarction. Am J Cardiol 80: 779–783.
61. Skinner JE, Pratt CM, Vybiral T (1993) A reduction in the correlation dimension of heartbeat intervals precedes imminent ventricular fibrillation in human subjects. Am Heart J 125: 731–743.
62. Vybiral T, Glaeser DH, Goldberger AL, Rigney DR, Hess KR, et al. (1993) Conventional heart rate variability analysis of ambulatory electrocardiographic recordings fails to predict imminent ventricular fibrillation. J Am Coll Cardiol 22: 557–565.
63. Wagner CD, Persson PB (1998) Chaos in the cardiovascular system: an update. Cardiovasc Res 40: 257–264.
64. Dvir H, Zlochiver S (2013) Stochastic cardiac pacing increases ventricular electrical stability–a computational study. Biophys J 105: 533–542.
65. Skinner JE, Carpeggiani C, Landisman CE, Fulton KW (1991) Correlation dimension of heartbeat intervals is reduced in conscious pigs by myocardial ischemia. Circ Res 68: 966–976.
66. Muller JE, Tofler GH, Stone PH (1989) Circadian variation and triggers of onset of acute cardiovascular disease. Circulation 79: 733–743.
67. Hu K, Ivanov P, Hilton MF, Chen Z, Ayers RT, et al. (2004) Endogenous circadian rhythm in an index of cardiac vulnerability independent of changes in behavior. Proc Natl Acad Sci U S A 101: 18223–18227.
68. Penzel T, Kantelhardt JW, Grote L, Peter JH, Bunde A (2003) Comparison of detrended fluctuation analysis and spectral analysis for heart rate variability in sleep and sleep apnea. IEEE Trans Biomed Eng 50: 1143–1151.
69. Piccirillo G, Ogawa M, Song J, Chong VJ, Joung B, et al. (2009) Power spectral analysis of heart rate variability and autonomic nervous system activity measured directly in healthy dogs and dogs with tachycardia-induced heart failure. Heart Rhythm 6: 546–552.
70. Moak JP, Goldstein DS, Eldadah BA, Saleem A, Holmes C, et al. (2007) Supine low-frequency power of heart rate variability reflects baroreflex function, not cardiac sympathetic innervation. Heart Rhythm 4: 1523–1529.
71. Sandercock GR, Brodie DA (2006) The role of heart rate variability in prognosis for different modes of death in chronic heart failure. Pacing Clin Electrophysiol 29: 892–904.
72. Notarius CF, Butler GC, Ando S, Pollard MJ, Senn BL, et al. (1999) Dissociation between microneurographic and heart rate variability estimates of sympathetic tone in normal subjects and patients with heart failure. Clin Sci (Lond) 96: 557–565.
73. van de Borne P, Montano N, Pagani M, Oren R, Somers VK (1997) Absence of low-frequency variability of sympathetic nerve activity in severe heart failure. Circulation 95: 1449–1454.
74. Ogawa M, Zhou S, Tan AY, Song J, Gholmieh G, et al. (2007) Left stellate ganglion and vagal nerve activity and cardiac arrhythmias in ambulatory dogs with pacing-induced congestive heart failure. J Am Coll Cardiol 50: 335–343.
75. Zhou S, Jung BC, Tan AY, Trang VQ, Gholmieh G, et al. (2008) Spontaneous stellate ganglion nerve activity and ventricular arrhythmia in a canine model of sudden death. Heart Rhythm 5: 131–139.

76. Guevara MR, Lewis TJ (1995) A minimal single-channel model for the regularity of beating in the sinoatrial node. Chaos 5: 174–183.
77. Ponard JG, Kondratyev AA, Kucera JP (2007) Mechanisms of intrinsic beating variability in cardiac cell cultures and model pacemaker networks. Biophys J 92: 3734–3752.
78. Wilders R, Jongsma HJ (1993) Beating irregularity of single pacemaker cells isolated from the rabbit sinoatrial node. Biophys J 65: 2601–2613.

18

The Plasma B-Type Natriuretic Peptide Levels Are Low in Males with Stable Ischemic Heart Disease (IHD) Compared to Those Observed in Patients with Non-IHD

Kosuke Minai*, Takayuki Ogawa, Makoto Kawai, Kimiaki Komukai, Toshikazu Tanaka, Kazuo Ogawa, Tomohisa Nagoshi, Satoshi Arase, Satoshi Morimoto, Yasunori Inoue, Hiroshi Sekiyama, Akihiro Urabe, Seiichiro Matsuo, Kenichi Hongo, Michihiro Yoshimura

Division of Cardiology, Department of Internal Medicine, The Jikei University School of Medicine, Tokyo, Japan

Abstract

Objective: Although the plasma B-type natriuretic peptide (BNP) level is a marker of heart failure, it is unclear whether BNP *per se* plays a pivotal role for pathogenic mechanisms underlying the development of ischemic heart disease (IHD). In this study, we retrospectively examined the plasma BNP levels in stable patients with IHD and compared to stable patients with cardiovascular diseases other than IHD.

Methods: The study population was 2088 patients (1698 males and 390 females) who were admitted to our hospital due to IHD (n = 1,661) and non-IHD (n = 427) and underwent cardiac catheterization. Measurements of the hemodynamic parameters and blood sampling were performed.

Results: The plasma BNP levels were significantly lower in the IHD group than in the non-IHD group ($p<0.001$). The multiple regression analysis examining the logBNP values showed that age, a male gender, low left ventricular ejection fraction, low body mass index, serum creatinine, atrial fibrillation and IHD *per se* were significant explanatory variables. When the total study population was divided according to gender, the plasma BNP levels were found to be significantly lower in the IHD group than in the non-IHD group among males ($p<0.001$), but not females (p = NS). Furthermore, a multiple logistic regression analysis of IHD showed the logBNP value to be a significant explanatory variable in males (regression coefficient: −0.669, $p<0.001$), but not females (p = NS).

Conclusions: The plasma BNP levels were relatively low in stable patients with IHD compared with those observed in stable patients with non-IHD; this tendency was evident in males. Perhaps, the low reactivity of BNP is causally associated with IHD in males. We hope that this study will serve as a test of future prospective studies.

Editor: Yasuhiro Ikeda, Mayo Clinic, United States of America

Funding: The authors received no specific funding for this work.

Competing Interests: The authors have declared that no competing interests exist.

* Email: heart@jikei.ac.jp

Introduction

A-type natriuretic peptide and B-type natriuretic peptide (BNP), also known as atrial and brain natriuretic peptides, respectively, are cardiac hormones with a wide range of potent biological effects, including vasodilation, natriuresis and inhibition of the renin-angiotensin-aldosterone and sympathetic nervous systems [1–8]. BNP is selectively secreted from the ventricles, and the magnitude of secretion also varies as a function of the severity of heart failure. The BNP value is thus used as a biochemical marker of heart failure.

In addition, we previously reported that, in patients with acute myocardial infarction (AMI), the time course of the changes in the plasma BNP levels just after the onset of AMI exhibited a biphasic pattern, with the first peak occurring approximately 24 hours after the onset and the second peak 3–5 days after the onset. The second peak of plasma BNP was more marked in severe cases of AMI with heart failure [9].

The plasma immunoreactive BNP level is a sensitive biochemical marker of heart failure; although the precise molecular forms of BNP and its precursors have been discussed from different angles [10,11]. BNP increases the cyclic guanosine monophosphate (cGMP) levels [1]. cGMP activated by BNP is protective against cellular injury as it increase particulate guanylate cyclases [12]. BNP may also be beneficial for suppressing the progression of heart failure and atherosclerosis [13,14]. If the plasma BNP level is insufficiently increased for any reason, heart failure and atherosclerosis are likely

Table 1. Baseline characteristics and the past medical history and medication regimen of the study subjects.

	Total			Female			Male		
	Non-IHD (n = 427)	IHD (n = 1,661)	P Value	Non-IHD (n = 144)	IHD (n = 246)	P-Value	Non-IHD (n = 283)	IHD (n = 1,415)	P-Value
Age (yrs ± SD)	63.1±13.1	65.2±10.5	P<0.01	67.5±13.5	70.4±10.2	P<0.05	60.9±12.3	64.4±10.3	P<0.001
Male (%)	66.3	85.1	P<0.001						
Body mass index (kg/m2 ± SD)	23.2±3.6	24.3±3.4	P<0.001	21.9±3.2	23.0±3.5	P<0.01	23.7±3.6	24.5±3.4	P<0.001
Current smoker (%)	21.8	23.2	NS	8.3	12.6	NS	28.6	25.1	NS
Current+past smoker (%)	53.4	69.8	P<0.001	19.4	28.5	P<0.05	70.7	77.0	P<0.05
Hypertension (%)	64.6	76.5	P<0.001	66.0	77.6	P<0.05	64.0	76.3	P<0.001
Diabetes Mellitus (%)	28.8	45.1	P<0.001	27.1	42.7	P<0.01	29.7	45.5	P<0.001
Dyslipidemia (%)	45.7	75.9	P<0.001	43.1	74.0	P<0.001	47.0	76.3	P<0.001
s-Cr (mg/dl ± SD)	1.6±2.4	1.6±2.3	P = 0.001	1.6±2.5	1.5±2.3	NS	1.6±2.3	1.6±2.3	NS
HbA1c (% ± SD)	5.8±1.1	6.0±1.1	P<0.001	5.7±1.1	5.9±0.8	NS	5.8±1.1	6.1±1.1	P<0.001
BNP (pg/ml ± SD)	310.2±650.0	157.6±401.1	P<0.001	319.5±650.4	303.2±668.2	NS	305.5±650.9	132.3±327.4	P<0.001
HD & CAPD (%)	10.8	9.3	NS	13.2	13.0	NS	9.5	8.7	NS
LVEF (% ± SD)	56.0±14.4	57.7±10.8	P<0.05	59.3±12.3	59.5±11.6	NS	54.4±15.1	57.4±10.7	P = 0.001
Heart rate (beat/min ± SD) (At LVG)	74.0±16.4	70.6±13.5	P<0.001	73.3±14.0	72.5±14.3	NS	74.4±17.6	70.3±13.4	P<0.001
LVEDP (mmHg ± SD) (At PreLVG)	16.5±7.2	15.5±6.3	P<0.05	16.4±7.0	16.1±6.9	NS	16.6±7.3	15.5±6.1	P<0.05
LVESVI (ml/m^2 ± SD)	36.5±25.1	28.9±16.3	P<0.001	31.7±19.8	27.3±17.0	P<0.05	39.0±27.2	29.1±16.2	P<0.001
Prior MI (%)	0	38.5	P<0.001	0	35.8	P<0.001	0	38.9	P<0.001
Prior PCI (%)	0	44.6	P<0.001	0	35.8	P<0.001	0	46.1	P<0.001
Prior CABG (%)	0	12.5	P<0.001	0	15.9	P<0.001	0	12.0	P<0.001
Coronary spastic angina	0	8.5	P<0.001	0	12.6	P<0.001	0	7.8	P<0.001
Prior valve repair (%)	4.9	0.7	P<0.001	7.6	1.6	P<0.01	3.5	0.5	P<0.001
Valvular heart disease (%)	30.2	3.4	P<0.001	38.2	6.9	P<0.001	26.1	2.8	P<0.001
Congenital heart disease (%)	5.2	0.36	P<0.001	8.3	0.4	P<0.001	3.5	0.4	P<0.001
Cardiomyopathy (%)	22.7	2.0	P<0.001	20.8	3.3	P<0.001	23.7	1.8	P<0.001
AF (%)	20.6	5.5	P<0.001	19.4	4.9	P<0.001	21.2	5.7	P<0.001
Calcium-channel blockers (%)	39.1	60.6	P<0.001	43.1	59.8	P = 0.001	37.1	60.8	P<0.001
ACE-inhibitors (%)	15.0	21.3	P<0.01	14.6	18.3	NS	15.2	21.8	P<0.05
Angiotensin Receptor Blockers (%)	37.9	41.0	NS	44.4	42.7	NS	34.6	40.7	NS (P = 0.056)
Nitrates (%)	9.1	26.6	P<0.001	8.3	28.5	P<0.001	9.5	26.2	P<0.001
Nicorandil (%)	4.2	20.4	P<0.001	4.2	23.2	P<0.001	4.2	19.9	P<0.001

Table 1. Cont.

	Total			Female			Male		
	Non-IHD (n = 427)	IHD (n = 1,661)	P Value	Non-IHD (n = 144)	IHD (n = 246)	P-Value	Non-IHD (n = 283)	IHD (n = 1,415)	P-Value
Beta-blockers (%)	18.7	34.4	P<0.001	20.8	28.9	NS (P = 0.081)	17.7	35.3	P<0.001
Statins (%)	23.0	59.3	P<0.001	29.9	57.7	P<0.001	19.4	59.6	P<0.001
Fibrates (%)	3.3	3.4	NS	1.4	1.2	NS	4.2	3.8	NS
Diuretics (%)	32.1	19.1	P<0.001	38.2	28.5	P<0.05	29.0	17.5	P<0.001
Oral Hypoglycemic Agents (%)	11.5	23.5	P<0.001	9.7	18.3	P<0.05	12.4	24.5	P<0.001
insulin (%)	5.2	9.9	P<0.01	6.9	10.6	NS	4.2	9.8	P<0.01
Number of vessels disease (0–3)	0	0.95±0.97		0	0.96±0.96		0	0.95±097	

s-Cr, Serum creatinine; BNP, B-type natriuretic peptide; HD & CAPD, Hemodialysis & continuous ambulatory peritoneal dialysis; LVEF, Left ventricular ejection fraction; LVEDP, Left ventricular end-diastolic pressure; LVESVI, Left ventricular end-systolic volume Index; MI, Myocardial Infarction; PCI, Percutaneous coronary intervention; CABG, Coronary artery bypass graft; AF, Atrial Fibrillation.

to advance; therefore, low plasma BNP level, even in patients with high risk factors, may play a causative role in the pathogenetic mechanisms underlying the development of IHD and heart failure. However, the discussion regarding this issue has been insufficient to date, although genetic variations of BNP and related molecules have previously been reported [15–21]. It is also unclear whether the plasma BNP level actually varies according to the individual and whether individual changes in this parameter are associated with disease. Nevertheless, there were a few early reports showing dysregulation of ANP and BNP in patients prone to developing hypertension and other cardiovascular disease [22–24].

Here, we hypothesized that BNP contributes to a pathogenetic mechanism of IHD, and retrospectively examined a possible contribution by comparing the BNP levels between stable patients with IHD and stable patients with cardiovascular diseases other than IHD.

Methods

Study design

The study population was 2088 consecutive patients admitted to the Jikei University Hospital from January 2008 through January 2012 in whom cardiac catheterization, including left ventriculography, and blood sampling for the plasma BNP levels were performed and reviewed. The baseline patient characteristics, including the clinical parameters and the biochemical data, were collected retrospectively from the medical records. The study protocol was approved by the ethics committee of the Jikei University School of Medicine (24–355; 7121).

Recruitment of stable IHD patients and non-IHD patients in this study

The stable IHD patients consisted of 1,661 patients who had coronary stenosis newly diagnosed by angiography, or who had a medical history of coronary artery disease, such as previous myocardial infarction, post-percutaneous coronary intervention and coronary artery bypass graft. A total of 762 patients underwent only one cardiac catheterization, while 359 patients underwent catheterization twice, 50 patients three times, five patients four times, one patient five times and one patient underwent catheterization six times. In order to avoid a selection bias by choosing among the plural data in one patient, we used all consecutive data in this analysis (n = 1661). Patients with coronary spastic angina were included in the stable IHD group if the disease activity of coronary spasm was not clinically high. Coronary spasm was diagnosed by the acetylcholine provocation test. Patients with previously diagnosed coronary spastic angina were also included in the stable IHD group. In contrast, patients requiring urgent catheter intervention for AMI were excluded from this study because the plasma BNP levels are rapidly and extensively changes during the acute phase of AMI [9]. Similarly, patients with acute coronary syndrome were excluded from the stable IHD group in this study. In addition, Also, patients with chest pain syndrome of unknown origin and those with suspected microvascular angina were excluded from the stable IHD group because we were unable to appropriately define cardiac ischemia in such patients. Detailed information of the patients in the stable IHD group were summarized in Table 1.

The non-IHD group consisted of 427 patients; all of those had organic heart diseases such as valvular heart diseases, cardiomyopaty, congenital heart disease and others. All non-IHD patients were clinically stable and admitted to the hospital for evaluation of their underlying cardiac disease. A total of 406 patients underwent cardiac catheterization one time, while nine patients were

Table 2. Comparisons between female and male with and without IHD.

	Non-IHD			IHD		
	Female (n = 144)	Male (n = 283)	P-Value	Female (n = 246)	Male (n = 1,415)	P-Value
Age (yrs ± SD)	67.5±13.5	60.9±12.3	P<0.001	70.4±10.2	64.4±10.3	P<0.001
Body mass index (kg/m2 ± SD)	21.9±3.2	23.7±3.6	P<0.001	23.0±3.5	24.5±3.4	P<0.001
Current smoker (%)	8.3	28.6	P<0.001	12.6	25.1	P<0.001
Current+past smoker (%)	19.4	70.7	P<0.001	28.5	77.0	P<0.001
Hypertension (%)	66.0	64.0	NS	77.6	76.3	NS
Diabetes Mellitus (%)	27.1	29.7	NS	42.7	45.5	NS
Dyslipidemia (%)	43.1	47.0	NS	74.0	76.3	NS
s-Cr (mg/dl ± SD)	1.6±2.5	1.6±2.3	P<0.001	1.5±2.3	1.6±2.3	P<0.001
HbA1c (% ± SD)	5.7±1.1	5.8±1.1	NS	5.9±0.8	6.1±1.1	P<0.05
BNP (pg/ml ± SD)	319.5±650.4	305.5±650.9	P<0.05	303.2±668.2	132.3±327.4	P<0.001
HD & CAPD (%)	13.2	9.5	NS	13.0	8.7	P<0.05
LVEF (% ± SD)	59.3±12.3	54.4±15.1	P<0.001	59.5±11.6	57.4±10.7	P<0.01
Heart rate (beat/min ± SD) (At LVG)	73.3±14.0	74.4±17.6	NS	72.5±14.3	70.3±13.4	P<0.05
LVEDP (mmHg ± SD) (At Pre LVG)	16.4±7.0	16.6±7.3	NS	16.1±6.9	15.5±6.1	NS
LVESVI (ml/m² ± SD)	31.7±19.8	39.0±27.2	P<0.01	27.3±17.0	29.1±16.2	NS
Prior myocardial infarction (%)	0	0		35.8	38.9	NS
Prior PCI (%)	0	0		35.8	46.1	P<0.01
Prior CABG	0	0		15.9	12.0	NS
Coronary spastic angina	0	0		12.6	7.8	P<0.05
Prior valve repair (%)	7.6	3.5	NS	1.6	0.5	P<0.05
Valvular heart disease (%)	38.2	26.1	P = 0.01	6.9	2.8	P = 0.001
Congenital heart disease (%)	8.3	3.5	P<0.05	0.4	0.4	NS
Cardiomyopathy (%)	20.8	23.7	NS	3.3	1.8	NS
AF (%)	19.4	21.2	NS	4.9	5.7	NS
Calcium-channel blockers (%)	43.1	37.1	NS	59.8	60.8	NS
ACE-inhibitors (%)	14.6	15.2	NS	18.3	21.8	NS
Angiotensin Receptor Blockers (%)	44.4	34.6	P<0.05	42.7	40.7	NS
Nitrates (%)	8.3	9.5	NS	28.5	26.2	NS
Nicorandil (%)	4.2	4.2	NS	23.2	19.9	NS
Beta-blockers (%)	20.8	17.7	NS	28.9	35.3	P<0.05
Statins (%)	29.9	19.4	P<0.05	57.7	59.6	NS
Fibrates (%)	1.4	4.2	NS	1.2	3.8	P<0.05
Diuretics (%)	38.2	29.0	NS	28.5	17.5	P<0.001
Oral Hypoglycemic Agents (%)	9.7	12.4	NS	18.3	24.5	P<0.05
insulin (%)	6.9	4.2	NS	10.6	9.8	NS
Number of vessels disease (0–3)	0	0		0.96±0.96	0.95±097	NS

s-Cr, Serum creatinine; BNP, B-type natriuretic peptide; HD & CAPD, Hemodialysis & continuous ambulatory peritoneal dialysis; LVEF, Left ventricular ejection fraction; LVEDP, Left ventricular end-diastolic pressure; LVESVI, Left ventricular end-systolic volume Index; PCI, Percutaneous coronary intervention; CABG, Coronary artery bypass graft;AF, Atrial Fibrillation.

catheterized twice and one patient was catheterized three times. We used all consecutive data in this analysis just as we did in the IHD group (n = 427). We excluded patients suffering from acute heart failure at the time of cardiac cathetherization and blood sampling. Precise information including underlying cardiac disorders was also summarized in Table 1.

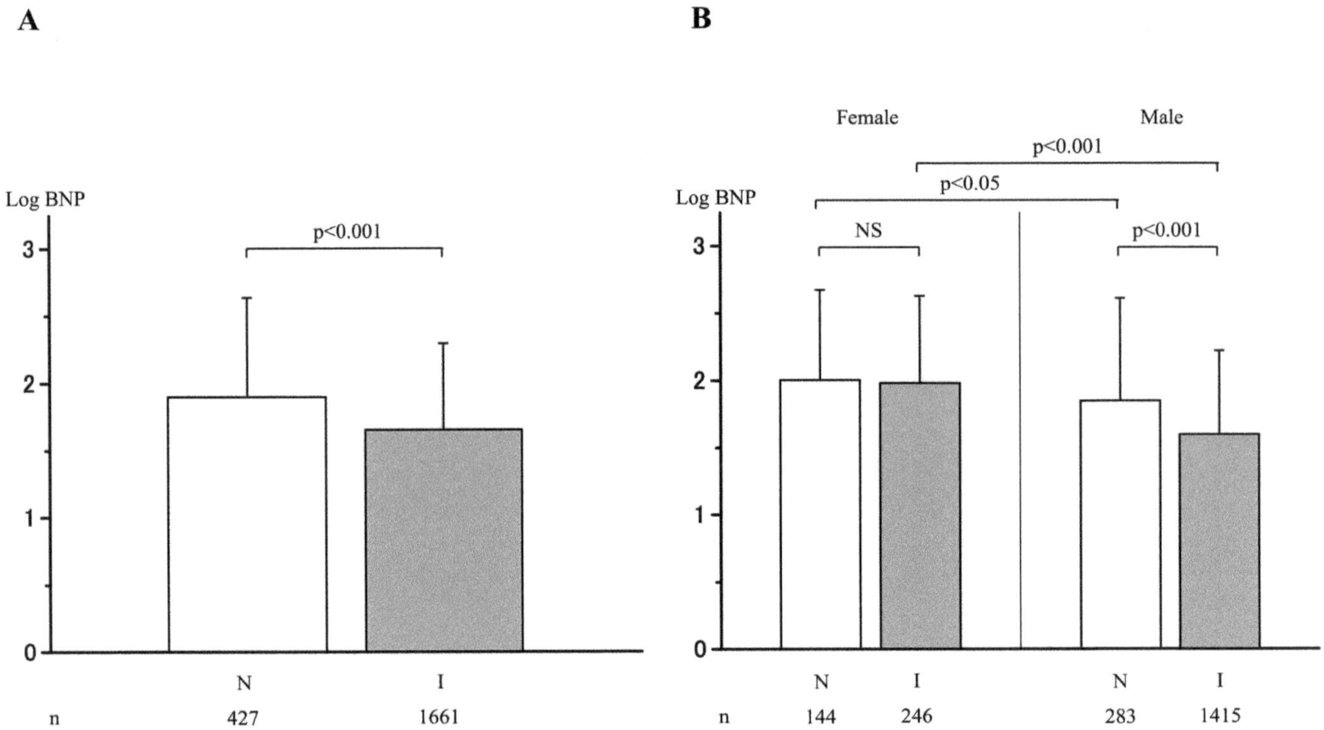

Figure 1. Comparison of the logBNP levels between the non-IHD and IHD groups. A: In the overall population. B: In males and females. N: non-ischemic heart disease group (non-IHD); I: ischemic heart disease group (IHD). BNP: B-type natriuretic peptide.

Measurement of the plasma BNP levels and other parameters

Whole blood (5 ml) was collected in tubes containing potassium EDTA (1 mg/ml blood). The plasma BNP level was determined by an enzyme-linked immunosorbent assay (non-extracted) using an antibody against human BNP (Shionogi Co. Ltd., Tokyo, Japan). Blood sampling was performed immediately before and after the cardiac catheterization whenever possible. The average interval between catheterization and blood sampling was 5.21±8.94 days; 1384 (66.3%) of patients had blood collected for BNP within 72 hours post catheterization. Of these patients, 830 underwent blood collection at the time of the procedure (during, immediately before or just after cardiac catheterization), 1185 underwent blood collection within 24 hours, and 1342 underwent blood collection within 48 hours.

The BMI was calculated as the body weight (kg) divided by the square of the height (m). Hypertension, diabetes mellitus and dyslipidemia were defined as described previously [25].

Statistical analysis

Continuous variables were expressed as the means ± SD. Categorical variables were expressed as percentages. Comparisons between groups were performed using Pearson's chi-square test for categorical variables and the Mann-Whitney U test or Student's t-test for continuous variables, where appropriate. To achieve a normal distribution, the BNP value was log-transformed before the analysis. To assess the dependent determinants of the log BNP, a multiple regression analysis was performed after the simple regression analysis. Age, gender (0 for females and 1 for males), IHD (0 for non-IHD and 1 for IHD), atrial fibrillation (0 for non-AF and 1 for AF), the LVEF, age, BMI, and s-Cr were included as

Table 3. The results of the simple regression analyses for the log BNP in all patients (n = 2088).

Explanatory variable	Regression coefficient	Standard regression coefficient	P	95%CI
Age	0.016	0.270	<0.001	0.014~0.019
Gender	−0.348	−0.203	<0.001	−0.420~−0.276
BMI	−0.047	−0.247	<0.001	−0.055~−0.039
s-Cr	0.119	0.415	<0.001	0.108~0.130
LVEF	−0.027	−0.478	<0.001	−0.030~−0.025
AF	0.597	0.251	<0.001	0.499~0.696
IHD	−0.243	−0.147	<0.001	−0.314~−0.173

BMI, Body mass index; s-Cr, Serum creatinine; LVEF, Left ventricular ejection fraction; AF, Atrial fibrillation; IHD, Ischemic heart disease.

Table 4. The results of the multiple regression analyses for the log BNP in all patients (n = 2088).

Explanatory variable	Regression coefficient	Standard regression coefficient	P	95%CI	VIF
Age	0.015	0.249	<0.001	0.013~0.017	1.125
Gender	−0.272	−0.159	<0.001	−0.327~−0.217	1.120
BMI	−0.015	−0.081	<0.001	−0.022~−0.009	1.128
s-Cr	0.095	0.333	<0.001	0.086~0.104	1.061
LVEF	−0.024	−0.414	<0.001	−0.026~−0.022	1.097
AF	0.325	0.137	<0.001	0.249~0.401	1.107
IHD	−0.115	−0.069	<0.001	−0.168~−0.061	1.131

BMI, Body mass index; s-Cr, Serum creatinine; LVEF, Left ventricular ejection fraction; AF, Atrial fibrillation; IHD, Ischemic heart disease.

variables in the multiple regression analysis. In addition, a gender-segregated multiple logistic regression analysis was performed to determine predictive factors for IHD using age, LVEF, BMI, s-Cr, atrial fibrillation (0 for non-AF and 1 for AF), and logBNP. A value of $p<0.05$ was considered to be statistically significant for all data that were statistically analyzed using the SPSS software package, version 21.0 (SPSS Inc., Chicago, IL).

Results

Clinical characteristics of the study subjects

Table 1 shows the clinical characteristic and the past medical history and medication regimen of the total 2088 patients.

High age, male gender, high BMI, smoking, hypertension, diabetes mellitus and dyslipidemia were more frequently seen in the IHD group than in the non-IHD group. The s-Cr was significantly higher in the non-IHD group than in the IHD group. The heart rate, LVESVI and LVEDP were lower in the IHD group than in the non-IHD group. The LVEF was slightly higher in the IHD group than in the non-IHD group. In this study, AF was more frequently detected in the non-IHD group than in the IHD group, which was due to the higher prevalence of valvular heart disease and cardiomyopathy in the non-IHD groups (precise data not shown in the Results).

The clinical characteristics are shown by gender in Table 2. It is important to compare the clinical characteristics between the females and males in the IHD group. For example, the LVEF was lower and the s-Cr was higher in males, whereas the age was lower and BMI values were higher in this group. With regard to the medical treatments, diuretics were used more frequently in females, and beta-blockers were used more frequently in males, while angiotensin-converting enzyme inhibitors/angiotensin II receptor blockers (ARBs) were used equally in females and males. Every patient had been prescribed the classes and doses of drugs based on his or her individual condition; therefore, it is difficult to compare the drugs more precisely. Nevertheless, the frequency in use and the amount used of major drugs such as enalapril, cavedilol or spironolactones was equivalent between females and males with or without IHD, while only the frequency of use and amount used of furosemide was significantly higher in males than in females (precise data not shown).

Comparison of the plasma BNP levels between the non-IHD and IHD groups and statistical analysis of the logBNP values in the total study population

The plasma BNP levels were significantly lower in the IHD group than in the non-IHD group as shown in Figure 1-A. In order to identify factors contributing to the difference in the plasma BNP levels between the IHD and non-IHD groups among the total study population, statistical analyses was performed, as shown in Table 3 and Table 4. Table 3 is the results of the simple regression analysis of the logBNP values using clinical factors as explanatory variables. Table 4 shows the results of the subsequent multiple regression analysis. Consequently, age, gender, BMI, s-Cr, LVEF, AF, and IHD were found to be significant determinants of the logBNP value. Among these factors, it is noteworthy that IHD *per se* was significantly and inversely correlated with the logBNP value.

Comparison of the plasma BNP levels between the non-IHD and IHD groups based on gender

Figure 1B shows that females with and without IHD had higher levels of plasma BNP compared to males with and without IHD.

Table 5. The results of the logistic regression analysis for IHD in females.

Explanatory variable	Regression coefficient	P	Odds ratio	Odds 95% CI
Log BNP	−0.085	NS (p = 0.719)	0.919	0.579~1.457
LVEF	−0.014	NS (p = 0.232)	0.986	0.963~1.009
Age	0.027	<0.01	1.028	1.007~1.048
BMI	0.101	<0.01	1.106	1.034~1.183
AF	−1.703	<0.001	0.182	0.086~0.388
s-Cr	−0.002	NS (p = 0.965)	0.998	0.901~1.105

BNP, B-type natriuretic peptide; LVEF, Left ventricular ejection fraction; BMI, Body mass index; AF, Atrial fibrillation; IHD, Ischemic heart disease; s-Cr, Serum creatinine.

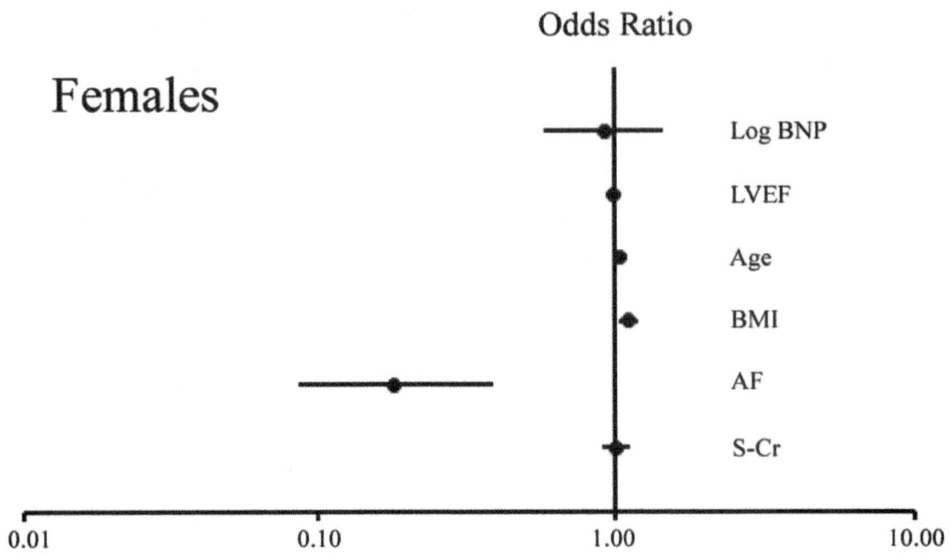

Figure 2. The Forest Plot displaying the odds ratio about risk of IHD in a females. BNP, B-type natriuretic peptide; LVEF, Left ventricular ejection fraction; BMI, Body mass index; AF, Atrial fibrillation; IHD, Ischemic heart disease; s-Cr, Serum creatinine.

The plasma BNP levels were similar in females with and without IHD (p = NS, actually p = 0.725). In contrast, the plasma BNP level was lower in males with IHD compared to males without IHD ($p<0.001$).

The results of the multiple logistic regression analysis for the determination of IHD

We finally examined the factors determining the presence of IHD; a multiple logistic regression analysis was performed for the determination of IHD by using the logBNP, LVEF, age, BMI, AF and s-Cr as explanatory variables in females and males. As shown in Tables 5 and Figure 2 (Females), and Table 6, and Figure 3 (Males), the trend between females and males was similar for age (significant in each gender), BMI (significant in each gender), AF (significant in each gender) and LVEF (not significant in each gender); however, the s-Cr was not significant in females (p = NS) but was significant in males ($p<0.05$). This result may suggest that chronic kidney disease is a more important risk factor for IHD in males than in females. It is noteworthy that the logBNP was not significantly associated with IHD in females (p = NS, actually p = 0.719), but was significantly and inversely associated with IHD in males (Regression coefficient: −0.669, $p<0.001$). Thus, the logBNP may only correlate with IHD in males, and may have a possible causative role, although it is difficult to distinguish between cause and effect based on the present analysis.

Sub-analysis based on the presence or absence of AF

AF was found to be significantly associated with non-IHD in both females and males, as shown in Table 5 and Figure 2 (Females) and Table 6 and Figure 3 (Males). Therefore, an additional analysis would be necessary, and the study population was subsequently divided based on the presence or absence of AF: the AF (+) group and the AF (−) group. There were no significant differences in the plasma BNP levels between the non-IHD and IHD groups among the AF (+) or AF (−) females; however, the plasma BNP levels were significantly lower in the IHD group than in the non-IHD group among AF(+) or AF(−) males. The subgroup analysis of AF therefore suggested that the tendency toward a low plasma BNP level in IHD males was not affected by AF.

Discussion

In the beginning of the study, we found the plasma BNP levels to be specifically lower in the stable patients with IHD than in the stable patients with non-IHD among the total study population. In addition, the multiple regression analysis clearly showed for the

Table 6. The results of the logistic regression analysis for IHD in males.

Explanatory variable	Regression coefficient	P	Odds ratio	Odds 95% CI
Log BNP	−0.669	<0.001	0.512	0.388~0.677
LVEF	−0.007	NS (p = 0.318)	0.993	0.981~1.006
Age	0.049	<0.001	1.050	1.037~1.064
BMI	0.080	<0.001	1.083	1.039~1.128
AF	−1.351	<0.001	0.259	0.172~0.389
s-Cr	0.087	0.01	1.091	1.021~1.167

BNP, B-type natriuretic peptide; LVEF, Left ventricular ejection fraction; BMI, Body mass index; AF, Atrial fibrillation; IHD, Ischemic heart disease; s-Cr, Serum creatinine.

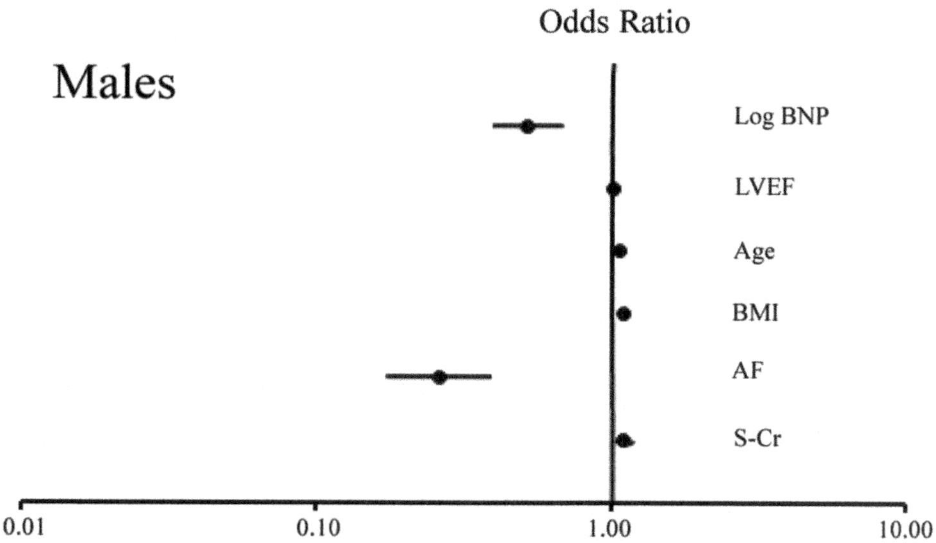

Figure 3. The Forest Plot displaying the odds ratio about risk of IHD in a males. BNP, B-type natriuretic peptide; LVEF, Left ventricular ejection fraction; BMI, Body mass index; AF, Atrial fibrillation; IHD, Ischemic heart disease; s-Cr, Serum creatinine.

first time that IHD *per se* is an independent determinant of the plasma BNP level, in addition to other known factors, such as age, male gender, low BMI, s-Cr, low LVEF and AF [26–31]. Furthermore, when the total study population was divided by gender, significant differences were identified between females and males. For example, it is noteworthy that the plasma BNP levels were significantly lower in the IHD group than in the non-IHD group among males only. In this analysis, the gender-difference observed in the plasma BNP levels in the IHD group was prominent even in consideration of the diverse clinical backgrounds. Therefore, unknown factors likely contributed to the observed gender difference. Next, by a multiple logistic regression analysis conversely performed using IHD as an objective variable and the logBNP as one of the explanatory variables, IHD was inversely determined by the logBNP only in males, but not in females. Hence the statistical analysis clarified that there is a substantial association between IHD *per se* and low plasma BNP level in males only. It is difficult to distinguish between cause and effect based on the present analyses; however, low plasma levels of BNP may be causally associated with IHD in males. In other words, the factor 'low reactivity of the plasma BNP level' may be a new risk factor for IHD in males. This way of thinking is supported by the previous reports showing that a deficiency of ANP and BNP was causatively associated with hypertension and other cardiovascular diseases [22–24].

BNP is biologically active and increases the cGMP levels. BNP is thus beneficial for suppressing the progression of heart failure, and probably atherosclerosis [13,14]. If the BNP level is insufficiently increased, low plasma BNP levels may have a causative role in IHD and heart failure. The reasons for the comparatively low plasma BNP levels or deteriorated response of BNP in IHD are unknown at present. Various factors such as neurohormones or genetic factors associated with gender differences may be linked to the current results. In addition, it is unknown whether a reduction of the synthesis or an augmented clearance of BNP affected the current results. As a next step, we need to examine the precise mechanisms responsible for the low plasma BNP levels seen only in male patients with IHD. The findings of the present and future studies may be able to provide a new strategy to prevent IHD and heart failure by increasing the endogenous natriuretic peptides using agents such as neutral endopeptidase inhibitors.

It is interesting to note a gender difference in the contribution of the plasma BNP level to the pathogenesis of IHD, as a gender difference have generally been reported to be negligible in patients with heart failure to date [27]. The results of this study may therefore help to answer the remaining questions regarding the impact of gender differences in the setting of IHD [32–37]. At present, it remains unknown whether IHD is the only or one of several cardiovascular diseases associated with the gender difference in the plasma BNP levels.

In general, the measurement of the plasma BNP levels is useful for early monitoring of asymptomatic ventricular dysfunction in patients with high risk factors. A value <18.4 pg/ml is considered to be ideal, and less than 40 pg/ml is considered to be within the normal range for patients without cardiac organic disorders visiting the hospital [27]. However, in this study, a considerable number of patients with a low EF (<55%) and low plasma BNP levels (<40 pg/ml) was seen in the IHD group compared with the non-IHD group among males; 153 patients (10.81%) vs. 16 patients (5.65%), $p<0.01$. On the other hand, there were few female patients with the same conditions; only two patients (0.81%) in the IHD group and nine patients (6.25%) in the non-IHD group, $p<0.01$ (precise data not shown in the Results). This indicates that clinicians should take care not to underestimate the degree of heart failure even if the plasma BNP levels are relatively low (less than 40 pg/ml) in male patients with IHD.

It is known that the BNP level increases with inflammation [38]. In this study, we examined the serum C-reactive protein (CRP) levels between 396 patients with IHD and 136 patients with non-IHD via blood samples obtained on the day of the catheterization. The average CRP level was 0.670 ± 1.653 (95%CI: 0.390–0.950) in the non-IHD group and 0.521 ± 1.109 (95%CI: 0.412–0.631) in the IHD group, which was not significantly different ($p=0.239$) (precise data not shown in the Results). Therefore, we thought that the inflammation status would not have influenced the present results.

To avoid a selection bias, the study population was consecutively and non-selectively recruited; therefore, all plural data from one patient were used in this analysis. We essentially performed the analysis by using 1,661 IHD patients and 427 non-IHD patients. However, by way of caution, we performed a similar statistical analysis by using only one dataset from each patient (1178 IHD patients and 416 non-IHD patients) who underwent cardiac catheterization for the first time during this protocol. As a result, the plasma BNP levels were found to be significantly lower in the IHD group than in the non-IHD group ($p<0.001$), the same as in the full dataset. In addition, when the total study population was divided by gender, the plasma BNP levels were significantly lower in the IHD group than in the non-IHD group only in males ($p<0.001$), but not in females ($p = NS$). Thus, the findings of the full dataset and the data from just individual cases were the same.

Finally, this is only a pilot retrospective study of the possible contribution of a low plasma BNP level to the pathogenesis of IHD. Therefore, a prospective study is needed to examine whether male patients with very low levels of plasma BNP, even under conditions of high risk factors, are more likely to develop IHD, for example, by comparing the rates of acute ischemic attack, the progression of IHD and the severity of stenosis in IHD patients grouped by the plasma BNP level.

Study Limitation

First, the number of females was small compared with that of males (1698 males and 390 females); thus, it is difficult to draw any definitive conclusions regarding the gender difference in the contribution of the plasma BNP level to IHD. A larger study including more females is required to arrive at an absolute conclusion. Second, while the plasma BNP level was the primary outcome measurement of the study, the samples were collected on a wide range intervals, and up to 33.7% of the subjects underwent blood collection more than 72 hours after cardiac catheterization. It is ideal to perform simultaneous sampling with hemodynamic measurements during cardiac catheterization; however, this was a retrospective study, and blood sampling for the purpose of measuring the plasma BNP levels was performed in the clinical setting based on the discretion of the attending physician. For this reason, there was a time delay in blood sampling in some patients. However, no statistical differences were noted in the timing of sampling between females and males; the patients who underwent blood sampling after more than 72 hours included 125 females (32.1% of the total 390 females) and 579 males (34.1% of the total 1,698 males) ($P = NS$). Therefore, we do not believe that the time lag in sampling in some cases largely affected the present findings.

Conclusions

The plasma BNP levels were relatively low in stable patients with IHD compared with that observed in the stable patients with non-IHD; this tendency was more evident in males. Perhaps, the low reactivity of BNP is causally associated with IHD in males. We hope this study serves as a test of a prospective study in the future.

Acknowledgments

We thank Mr. Brian Quinn (Japan Medical Communication) for his kind advice regarding the use of the English language.

Author Contributions

Conceived and designed the experiments: KM MY. Performed the experiments: KM TO TT KO TN SA S. Morimoto YI HS AU. Analyzed the data: KM TO MK KK TT S. Matsuo KH MY. Contributed reagents/materials/analysis tools: KM MK MY. Wrote the paper: KM TO KK TT MY.

References

1. Sudoh T, Kangawa K, Minamino N, Matsuo H (1988) A new natriuretic peptide in porcine brain. Nature 332: 78–81.
2. Mukoyama M, Nakao K, Hosoda K, Suga S, Saito Y, et al. (1991) Brain natriuretic peptide as a novel cardiac hormone in humans. Evidence for an exquisite dual natriuretic peptide system, atrial natriuretic peptide and brain natriuretic peptide. J Clin Invest 87: 1402–1412.
3. Yasue H, Yoshimura M, Sumida H, Kikuta K, Kugiyama K, et al. (1994) Localization and mechanism of secretion of B-type natriuretic peptide in comparison with those of A-type natriuretic peptide in normal subjects and patients with heart failure. Circulation 90: 195–203.
4. Omland T, Aakvaag A, Bonarjee VV, Caidahl K, Lie RT, et al. (1996) Plasma brain natriuretic peptide as an indicator of left ventricular systolic function and long-term survival after acute myocardial infarction. Comparison with plasma atrial natriuretic peptide and N-terminal proatrial natriuretic peptide. Circulation 93: 1963–1969.
5. Tsutamoto T, Wada A, Maeda K, Hisanaga T, Maeda Y, et al. (1997) Attenuation of compensation of endogenous cardiac natriuretic peptide system in chronic heart failure: prognostic role of plasma brain natriuretic peptide concentration in patients with chronic symptomatic left ventricular dysfunction. Circulation 96: 509–516.
6. Richards AM, Nicholls MG, Espiner EA, Lainchbury JG, Troughton RW, et al. (2003) B-type natriuretic peptides and ejection fraction for prognosis after myocardial infarction. Circulation 107: 2786–2792.
7. Suzuki S, Yoshimura M, Nakayama M, Mizuno Y, Harada E, et al. (2004) Plasma level of B-type natriuretic peptide as a prognostic marker after acute myocardial infarction: a long-term follow-up analysis. Circulation 110: 1387–1391.
8. Wang TJ, Larson MG, Levy D, Benjamin EJ, Leip EP, et al. (2004) Plasma natriuretic peptide levels and the risk of cardiovascular events and death. N Engl J Med 350: 655–663.
9. Morita E, Yasue H, Yoshimura M, Ogawa H, Jougasaki M, et al. (1993) Increased plasma levels of brain natriuretic peptide in patients with acute myocardial infarction. Circulation 88: 82–91.
10. Hawkridge AM, Heublein DM, Bergen HR III, Cataliotti A, Burnett JC Jr, et al. (2005) Quantitative mass spectral evidence for the absence of circulating brain natriuretic peptide (BNP-32) in severe human heart failure. Proc Natl Acad Sci U S A 102: 17442–17447.
11. Nishikimi T, Okamoto H, Nakamura M, Ogawa N, Horii K, et al. (2013) Direct immunochemiluminescent assay for proBNP and total BNP in human plasma proBNP and total BNP levels in normal and heart failure. PLoS One 8: e53233.
12. Gorbe A, Giricz Z, Szunyog A, Csont T, Burley DS, et al. (2010) Role of cGMP-PKG signaling in the protection of neonatal rat cardiac myocytes subjected to simulated ischemia/reoxygenation. Basic Res Cardiol 105: 643–650.
13. Ogawa Y, Itoh H, Tamura N, Suga S, Yoshimasa T, et al. (1994) Molecular cloning of the complementary DNA and gene that encode mouse brain natriuretic peptide and generation of transgenic mice that overexpress the brain natriuretic peptide gene. J Clin Invest 93: 1911–1921.
14. Nishikimi T, Maeda N, Matsuoka H (2006) The role of natriuretic peptides in cardioprotection. Cardiovasc Res 69: 318–328.
15. Costello-Boerrigter LC, Boerrigter G, Ameenuddin S, Mahoney DW, Slusser JP, et al. (2011) The effect of the brain-type natriuretic peptide single-nucleotide polymorphism rs198389 on test characteristics of common assays. Mayo Clin Proc 86: 210–218.
16. Szabo G, Molvarec A, Stenczer B, Rigo J Jr, Nagy B (2011) Natriuretic peptide precursor B gene (TTTC)(n) microsatellite polymorphism in pre-eclampsia. Clin Chim Acta 412: 1371–1375.
17. Ellis KL, Newton-Cheh C, Wang TJ, Frampton CM, Doughty RN, et al. (2011) Association of genetic variation in the natriuretic peptide system with cardiovascular outcomes. J Mol Cell Cardiol 50: 695–701.
18. Choquet H, Cavalcanti-Proenca C, Lecoeur C, Dina C, Cauchi S, et al. (2009) The T-381C SNP in BNP gene may be modestly associated with type 2 diabetes: an updated meta-analysis in 49 279 subjects. Hum Mol Genet 18: 2495–2501.
19. Poreba R, Poczatek K, Gac P, Poreba M, Gonerska M, et al. (2009) SNP rs198389 (T-381 C) polymorphism in the B-type natriuretic peptide gene promoter in patients with atherosclerotic renovascular hypertension. Pol Arch Med Wewn 119: 219–224.
20. Weber M, Burian M, Dragutinovic I, Moellmann H, Nef H, et al. (2008) Genetic polymorphism of the type A human natriuretic peptide receptor (NPR-A) gene contributes to the interindividual variability in the BNP system. Eur J Heart Fail 10: 482–489.

21. Vassalle C, Andreassi MG, Prontera C, Fontana M, Zyw L, et al. (2007) Influence of ScaI and natriuretic peptide (NP) clearance receptor polymorphisms of the NP System on NP concentration in chronic heart failure. Clin Chem 53: 1886–1890.
22. Ferrari P, Weidmann P, Ferrier C, Dietler R, Hollmann R, et al. (1990) Dysregulation of atrial natriuretic factor in hypertension-prone man. J Clin Endocrinol Metab 71: 944–951.
23. Belluardo P, Cataliotti A, Bonaiuto L, Giuffre E, Maugeri E, et al. (2006) Lack of activation of molecular forms of the BNP system in human grade 1 hypertension and relationship to cardiac hypertrophy. Am J Physiol Heart Circ Physiol 291: H1529–1535.
24. Macheret F, Boerrigter G, McKie P, Costello-Boerrigter L, Lahr B, et al. (2011) Pro-B-type natriuretic peptide(1-108) circulates in the general community: plasma determinants and detection of left ventricular dysfunction. J Am Coll Cardiol 57: 1386–1395.
25. Komukai K, Ogawa T, Yagi H, Date T, Sakamoto H, et al. (2008) Decreased renal function as an independent predictor of re-hospitalization for congestive heart failure. Circ J 72: 1152–1157.
26. Nakane T, Kawai M, Komukai K, Kayama Y, Matsuo S, et al. (2012) Contribution of extracardiac factors to the inconsistency between plasma B-type natriuretic peptide levels and the severity of pulmonary congestion on chest X-rays in the diagnosis of heart failure. Intern Med 51: 239–248.
27. Kawai M, Yoshimura M, Harada M, Mizuno Y, Hiramitsu S, et al. (2013) Determination of the B-type natriuretic peptide level as a criterion for abnormalities in japanese individuals in routine clinical practice: the J-ABS Multi-Center Study (Japan Abnormal BNP Standard). Intern Med 52: 171–177.
28. Cataliotti A, Malatino LS, Jougasaki M, Zoccali C, Castellino P, et al. (2001) Circulating natriuretic peptide concentrations in patients with end-stage renal disease: role of brain natriuretic peptide as a biomarker for ventricular remodeling. Mayo Clin Proc 76: 1111–1119.
29. Redfield MM, Rodeheffer RJ, Jacobsen SJ, Mahoney DW, Bailey KR, et al. (2002) Plasma brain natriuretic peptide concentration: impact of age and gender. J Am Coll Cardiol 40: 976–982.
30. Wang TJ, Larson MG, Levy D, Leip EP, Benjamin EJ, et al. (2002) Impact of age and sex on plasma natriuretic peptide levels in healthy adults. Am J Cardiol 90: 254–258.
31. Knudsen CW, Riis JS, Finsen AV, Eikvar L, Muller C, et al. (2004) Diagnostic value of a rapid test for B-type natriuretic peptide in patients presenting with acute dyspnoe: effect of age and gender. Eur J Heart Fail 6: 55–62.
32. Njolstad I, Arnesen E, Lund-Larsen PG (1996) Smoking, serum lipids, blood pressure, and sex differences in myocardial infarction. A 12-year follow-up of the Finnmark Study. Circulation 93: 450–456.
33. Jousilahti P, Vartiainen E, Tuomilehto J, Puska P (1999) Sex, age, cardiovascular risk factors, and coronary heart disease: a prospective follow-up study of 14 786 middle-aged men and women in Finland. Circulation 99: 1165–1172.
34. Yarnell JW, Beswick AD, Sweetnam PM, Riad-Fahmy D (1993) Endogenous sex hormones and ischemic heart disease in men. The Caerphilly prospective study. Arterioscler Thromb 13: 517–520.
35. Malkin CJ, Pugh PJ, Jones TH, Channer KS (2003) Testosterone for secondary prevention in men with ischaemic heart disease? Qjm 96: 521–529.
36. Schuit SC, Oei HH, Witteman JC, Geurts van Kessel CH, van Meurs JB, et al. (2004) Estrogen receptor alpha gene polymorphisms and risk of myocardial infarction. Jama 291: 2969–2977.
37. Rod NH, Kristensen TS, Diderichsen F, Prescott E, Jensen GB, et al. (2010) Cortisol, estrogens and risk of ischaemic heart disease, cancer and all-cause mortality in postmenopausal women: a prospective cohort study. Int J Epidemiol 39: 530–538.
38. Inoue T, Kawai M, Nakane T, Nojiri A, Minai K, et al. (2010) Influence of low-grade inflammation on plasma B-type natriuretic peptide levels. Intern Med 49: 2659–2668.

19

Estimation of Instantaneous Complex Dynamics through Lyapunov Exponents: A Study on Heartbeat Dynamics

Gaetano Valenza[1,2]*, Luca Citi[1,3], Riccardo Barbieri[1]

1 Neuroscience Statistics Research Laboratory, Department of Anesthesia, Critical Care & Pain Medicine, Harvard Medical School, Massachusetts General Hospital, Boston, Massachusetts, United States of America; and Department of Brain and Cognitive Science, Massachusetts Institute of Technology, Cambridge, Massachusetts, United States of America, **2** Research Center E. Piaggio and Department of Information Engineering, University of Pisa, Pisa, Italy, **3** School of Computer Science and Electronic Engineering, University of Essex, Colchester, United Kingdom

Abstract

Measures of nonlinearity and complexity, and in particular the study of Lyapunov exponents, have been increasingly used to characterize dynamical properties of a wide range of biological nonlinear systems, including cardiovascular control. In this work, we present a novel methodology able to effectively estimate the Lyapunov spectrum of a series of stochastic events in an instantaneous fashion. The paradigm relies on a novel point-process high-order nonlinear model of the event series dynamics. The long-term information is taken into account by expanding the linear, quadratic, and cubic Wiener-Volterra kernels with the orthonormal Laguerre basis functions. Applications to synthetic data such as the Hénon map and Rössler attractor, as well as two experimental heartbeat interval datasets (i.e., healthy subjects undergoing postural changes and patients with severe cardiac heart failure), focus on estimation and tracking of the Instantaneous Dominant Lyapunov Exponent (IDLE). The novel cardiovascular assessment demonstrates that our method is able to effectively and instantaneously track the nonlinear autonomic control dynamics, allowing for complexity variability estimations.

Editor: Ramesh Balasubramaniam, University of California, Merced, United States of America

Funding: The research leading to these results has received partial funding from the Department of Anesthesia, Critical Care & Pain Medicine, Massachusetts General Hospital, and Harvard Medical School, Boston, MA, USA, and European Union Seventh Framework Programme FP7/2007-2013 under Grant No. 601165 of the project "WEARHAP". The funders had no role in study design, data collection and analysis, decision to publish, or preparation of the manuscript.

Competing Interests: The authors have declared that no competing interests exist.

* Email: g.valenza@ieee.org

Introduction

Hearth contractions are regarded by many scientists as the foremost example of a physiological system showing predominantly nonlinear behavior, mainly generated through integration of multiple neural signaling at the level of the sinoatrial node [1]. Accordingly, the fluctuations in the interval between consecutive heartbeats have been widely investigated as output of a nonlinear system revealing and quantifying the complexity of cardiovascular control [2–27].

Among all nonlinearity and complexity measures, Lyapunov exponents (LEs) have been proven to provide an important mathematical tool in characterizing dynamical properties of a nonlinear system [28]. LEs were first defined by Lyapunov [29] in order to study the stability of non-stationary solutions of ordinary differential equations and for more than fifty years they have been extensively studied in many disciplines [30–33]. Specifically, they refer to the average exponential rates of divergence or convergence of neighboring trajectories in the system phase space. In fact, for a system whose characteristic equations are known, there is a straightforward technique for computing the whole Lyapunov spectrum [28]. Several methods for a reliable data-driven LEs estimation, even in short time data records, have been also proposed [34,35]. In a deterministic nonlinear system with no stochastic inputs, a positive LE reflects sensitive dependence to initial conditions and can be taken as a definition of a chaotic system [36]. Nevertheless, a small amount of noise in a limit cycle oscillation could yield a positive LE if the trajectory has regions with large slopes. In chaotic systems [37], stochasticity does not play a crucial role and their dynamics are highly dependent on the initial condition. Although it is straightforward to consider chaotic mathematical systems in which stochastic inputs are suppressed, in actual applications especially related to physiological systems, it is not possible to eliminate such inputs making the chaos assessment simply unreliable [3]. Stationary aperiodic behavior, in fact, can also arise in linear or nonlinear stochastic systems. In light of these considerations, as this work deals with (instantaneous) LEs estimation with applications on heartbeat dynamics, we do not address the issue related to the chaotic behavior of heart rate variability (HRV).

Relying on the approach suggested by Chon et al. [38] and, later, by Armoundas et al. [39], we consider the cardiovascular system both chaotic and stochastic. This concept is in agreement with current physiological knowledge, since healthy HRV dynamics can be considered/modeled as the output of a nonlinear deterministic system (the pacemaker cells of sinus node) being forced by a high-dimensional input (the activity in the nerves innervating the sinus node). Accordingly, we model the heartbeat nonlinear dynamics as a third-order Nonlinear Autoregressive (NAR) model embedded in a point process probabilistic framework. Such statistical approach allows us to estimate the LEs in an instantaneous fashion by fitting the model to the observed data and applying the Fast Orthogonal Search (FOS) algorithm [40]. Point-process theory has been widely recognized as an excellent mathematical tool to characterize the probabilistic generative mechanism of the heartbeat at each moment in time [41]. In the considered model, the intrinsically discrete, unevenly spaced heartbeat intervals are represented by a physiologically-plausible inverse-gaussian (IG) distribution. Defining the first and second-order moments of the IG distribution as function of the past heartbeat intervals (i.e., the RR intervals), it is possible to obtain an effective prediction of the next heartbeat event together with an accurate assessment of instantaneous indices of cardiovascular control. In previous studies [19,41,42], we demonstrated how to estimate heartbeat dynamics even in short recordings under nonlinear and non-stationary conditions using Wiener-Volterra theory for nonlinear systems identification.

Introduction to the Instantaneous Dominant Lyapunov Exponent

In this work, the IG mean is modeled as a third-order nonlinear function of the past RR intervals. In order to perform an effective parameter estimation and retain all the historical information of events, the cubic NAR kernels of the Wiener-Volterra series are expanded using the Laguerre bases [43] leading to the definition of cubic Nonlinear Autoregressive Laguerre (NARL) model. Of note, the NARL definition includes an infinite regression of the past events with a parsimonious use of model parameters. From the NARL point-process model and Fast Orthogonal Search algorithm, we are able to estimate the complete LE spectrum at each moment in time, providing novel information concerning the complexity dynamics and its variability. Of note, to the best of our knowledge, complexity variability measures have never been estimated from instantaneous indices of complexity and could open novel perspectives on the assessment of discrete stochastic physiological systems. We present two applications on synthetic datasets (the Hénon map and Rössler attractor) and two experimental applications portraying the crucial role of the instantaneous Lyapunov Exponents in assessing autonomic changes in humans (ten heathy subjects undergoing postural changes, and fourteen patients with severe heart failure), focusing our attention on the Instantaneous Dominant Lyapunov Exponent (IDLE, λ), which is the first exponent of the Lyapunov spectrum. Preliminary results of these analyses have been presented in [44–46]. We start with a detailed, exhaustive presentation of our methodological framework through the following "Materials and Methods" section.

Materials and Methods

Point-Process Models of Heartbeat Dynamics

A random point process is a stochastic process whose elements are point patterns specified as a locally finite counting measure [47]. Considering the R-waves detected from the Electrocardiogram (ECG) as such events, point process theory can be used to characterize their probability of occurrence [41,42,48]. Mathematically, in the time domain, a simple 1-dimension point process consists of series of timestamps marking the occurrence times $t \in [0,\infty)$ of the random events. Given a set of R-wave events $\{u_j\}_{j=1}^{J}$, let $RR_j = u_j - u_{j-1} > 0$ denote the jth R–R interval, or equivalently, the waiting time until the next R-wave event. Assuming history dependence, the probability distribution of the waiting time $t - u_j$ until the next R-wave event, where u_j denotes the previous R-wave event occurred before time t, follows an inverse Gaussian (IG) model:

$$f(t|\mathcal{H}_t,\xi(t)) = \left[\frac{\xi_0(t)}{2\pi(t-u_j)^3}\right]^{\frac{1}{2}} \exp\left\{-\frac{1}{2}\frac{\xi_0(t)\left[t-u_j-\mu_{RR}(t,\mathcal{H}_t,\xi(t))\right]^2}{\mu_{RR}(t,\mathcal{H}_t,\xi(t))^2(t-u_j)}\right\} \tag{1}$$

where $\mathcal{H}_t = (u_j, RR_j, RR_{j-1},...,RR_{j-M+1})$ is the history of the point process, $\xi(t)$ is the vector of the time-varying parameters, $\mu_{RR}(t,\mathcal{H}_t,\xi(t))$ represents the first-moment statistic (mean) of the distribution, and $\xi_0(t) = \theta > 0$ denotes the shape parameter of the IG distribution (as $\theta/\mu \to \infty$, the IG distribution becomes more like a Gaussian distribution). As $f(t|\mathcal{H}_t,\xi(t))$ indicates the probability of having a beat at time t given that a previous beat has occurred at u_j, $\mu_{RR}(t,\mathcal{H}_t,\xi(t))$ can be interpreted as signifying the average (or expected) waiting time before the next beat. We can also estimate the second-moment statistic (variance) of the IG distribution as $\sigma^2_{RR}(t) = \mu^3_{RR}(t)/\theta$. The use of an IG distribution to characterize the R-R intervals occurrences is motivated by the fact that if the rise of the membrane potential to a threshold initiating the cardiac contraction is modeled as a Wiener process with drift, then the probability density of the times between threshold crossings (the RR intervals) is indeed the inverse Gaussian distribution [41,49]. As a matter of fact, when compared with other distributions, the IG model achieves the overall best fit in terms of smaller KS distance [42]. The instantaneous RR mean, $\mu_{RR}(t,\mathcal{H}_t,\xi(t))$, can be modeled as a generic function of the past RR values $\mu_{RR}(t,\mathcal{H}_t,\xi(t)) = g(RR_{j-1}, RR_{j-2},...,RR_{j-h})$, where RR_{j-k} denotes the previous k^{th} R–R interval occurred prior to the present time t.

Nonlinear Modeling of History Dependence

The general Nonlinear Autoregressive (NAR) formulation can be written as:

$$y(n) = \mathbf{F}(y(n-1), y(n-2),..., y(n-M)) + \epsilon(n) \tag{2}$$

where $\epsilon(n)$ are independent, identically distributed (i.i.d.) Gaussian random variables. The expected value of $y(n)$ can be written as a Taylor expansion under the hypothesis of being infinitely differentiable in a neighborhood of the working point:

$$E[y(n)] = \gamma_0 + \sum_{i=1}^{M}\gamma_1(i)y(n-i) + \sum_{K=2}^{\infty}\sum_{i_1=1}^{M}\cdots\sum_{i_K=1}^{M}\gamma_K(i_1,\ldots,i_K)\prod_{j=1}^{K}y(n-i_j) \tag{3}$$

Due to the autoregressive structure of eq. 3, the system can be identified with only exact knowledge of the output data and with only few assumptions on the input data. In practice, this series will obviously be truncated at some small, finite value. Here, we represent the nonlinear cardiovascular system by taking into account up to the cubic nonlinear terms, i.e. γ_0, $\gamma_1(i)$, $\gamma_2(i,j)$, and $\gamma_3(i,j,k)$. Thus, the model can be written as:

$$E[y(n)] = \gamma_0 + \sum_{i=1}^{M} \gamma_1(i) y(n-i) + \sum_{i=1}^{M}\sum_{j=1}^{M} \gamma_2(i,j) y(n-i) y(n-j) + \sum_{i=1}^{M}\sum_{j=1}^{M}\sum_{k=1}^{M} \gamma_3(i,j,k) y(n-i) y(n-j) y(n-k) \quad (4)$$

where the quadratic and the cubic terms, $\gamma_2(i,j)$ and $\gamma_3(i,j,k)$, are assumed to be permutation invariant. This choice of a third order NAR system further gives robustness against the presence of measurement noise in the data [38].

Laguerre Expansion of the γ_K terms. An important practical limitation in modeling high-order nonlinearities using the model in eq. 4 is the high number of parameters needed to sufficiently fit the observed data. An advocated approach to solve such a limitation has been proposed by using the Laguerre functions [43,50,51]. Let us define the jth-order discrete time orthonormal Laguerre function:

$$\phi_j(n) = \alpha^{\frac{n-j}{2}} (1-\alpha)^{\frac{1}{2}} \sum_{i=0}^{j} (-1)^i \binom{n}{i} \binom{j}{i} \alpha^{j-i} (1-\alpha)^i,$$

where α is the discrete-time Laguerre parameter $(0<\alpha<1)$ which determines the rate of exponential asymptotic decline of these functions, and $n \geq 0$. Given the Laguerre function, $\phi_j(n)$, and the signal, $y(n)$, the jth-order Laguerre filter output is:

$$l_j(n) = \sum_{i=0}^{\infty} \phi_j(i) y(n-i-1) \quad (5)$$

The computation of the Laguerre Filter output can be simplified by using the following recursive relation [43]:

$$l_0(n) = \sqrt{\alpha}\, l_0(n-1) + \sqrt{1-\alpha}\, y(n-1) \quad (6)$$

$$l_j(n) = \sqrt{\alpha}\, l_j(n-1) + \sqrt{\alpha}\, l_{j-1}(n) + \quad (7)$$

$$\sqrt{\alpha}\, l_{j-1}(n-1), j \geq 1 \quad (8)$$

Since the $\{\phi_i(t)\}$ form a complete orthonormal set in functional space $\mathcal{L}_2$, we can write [52]:

$$\gamma_0 = g_0 \quad (9)$$

$$\gamma_1(i) = \sum_{r=0}^{P} g_1(r) \phi_r(i) \quad (10)$$

$$\gamma_2(i,j) = \sum_{r=0}^{Q}\sum_{s=0}^{Q} g_2(r,s) \phi_r(i) \phi_s(j) \text{ if} \quad (11)$$

$i \neq j$ho dimenticato perche avevamo qst

$$\gamma_3(i,j,k) = \sum_{r=0}^{K}\sum_{s=0}^{K}\sum_{t=0}^{K} g_3(r,s,t) \phi_r(i) \phi_s(j) \phi_t(k) \text{ if } i \neq j\,. \quad (12)$$

Here g_0, $g_1(r)$, $g_3(r,s)$ and $g_3(r,s,t)$ are the Laguerre coefficients. Using eq. 5 and eqs. 9–12, the model in eq. 4 for the instantaneous RR mean becomes:

$$\mu_{\text{RR}}(t, \mathcal{H}_t, \xi(t)) = g_0(t) + \sum_{i=0}^{P} g_1(i,t) l_i(t) + \sum_{i=0}^{Q}\sum_{j=0}^{Q} g_2(i,j,t)\, l_i(t)\, l_j(t) + \sum_{i=0}^{K}\sum_{j=0}^{K}\sum_{k=0}^{K} g_3(i,j,k,t)\, l_i(t)\, l_j(t)\, l_k(t)\,. \quad (13)$$

hereinafter called Nonlinear Autoregressive with Laguerre expansion (NARL) model. Here, the Laguerre filter outputs are:

$$l_i(t) = \sum_{n=1}^{\tilde{N}(t)} \phi_i(n) (\text{RR}_{\tilde{N}(t)-n} - \text{RR}_{\tilde{N}(t)-n-1}) \quad (14)$$

with $\tilde{N}(t) = \lim_{\tau \to t^-} N(\tau) = \max\{k : u_k < t\}$ as a left continuous function.

The coefficients g_0,$\{g_1(i)\}$, $\{g_2(i,j)\}$, and $\{g_3(i,j,k)\}$ correspond to the time-varying zero-, first-, second-, and third-order NARL coefficients, respectively. When $\alpha=0$ the filter output becomes $l_j(n) = (-1)^j y(n-j-1)$ and the NARL model corresponds, apart for the sign, to the finite NAR model in eq. 4, whereas for $\alpha \neq 0$ the instantaneous RR mean in terms of NAR equations is theoretically defined as follows:

$$\mu_{\text{RR}}(t, \mathcal{H}_t, \xi(t)) = \text{RR}_{\tilde{N}(t)-1} + \gamma_0 + \sum_{i=1}^{\infty} \gamma_1(i,t)\, \Delta\text{RR}_i + \sum_{i=1}^{\infty}\sum_{j=1}^{\infty} \gamma_2(i,j,t)\, \Delta\text{RR}_i\, \Delta\text{RR}_j + \sum_{i=1}^{\infty}\sum_{j=1}^{\infty}\sum_{k=1}^{\infty} \gamma_3(i,j,k,t)\, \Delta\text{RR}_i\, \Delta\text{RR}_j \Delta\text{RR}_k \quad (15)$$

where $\Delta\text{RR}_h = (\text{RR}_{\tilde{N}(t)-h} - \text{RR}_{\tilde{N}(t)-h-1})$. The autoregressive model is expressed in terms of the derivative RR series, rather than the original RR series, in order to allow the model to cope with highly non-stationary regimes [53].

Moreover, as $\mu_{RR}(t, \mathcal{H}_t, \xi(t))$ is defined in a continuous-time fashion, we can obtain an instantaneous R–R mean estimate at a very fine timescale (with an arbitrarily small bin size Δ), which requires no interpolation between the arrival times of two beats. Given the proposed parametric model, the nonlinear indices of the HR and HRV will be defined as a time-varying function of the parameters $\xi(t) = [\theta(t), g_0(t), g_1(0,t), ..., g_1(P,t), g_2(0,0,t), ..., g_2(Q,Q,t), g_3(0,0,0,t), ..., g_3(K,K,K,t)]$.

Parameter Estimation and Model Goodness-of-fit measures. A local maximum likelihood method [41] is used to estimate the time-varying parameter set $\xi(t)$. Given a local observation interval $(t-l,t]$ of duration l, we consider a subset $U_{m:n}$ of the R-wave events, where $m = \min\{k : u_k > t-l\}$ and $n = \max\{k : u_k \leq t\}$. At each time t, we find the parameter vector $\xi(t)$ that maximizes the local log-likelihood, given the R-wave events recorded in the local observation interval:

$$L(\xi(t) \mid U_{m:n}) = \sum_{k=m+P-1}^{n-1} w(t-u_{k+1}) \log\left[f\left(u_{k+1} \mid \mu_{RR}(u_{k+1}, \mathcal{H}_{u_{k+1}}, \xi(t)), \theta(\xi(t))\right)\right] \quad (16)$$

where $w(\tau) = \exp(\hat{w}\tau)$ with $\hat{w} = 0.02\ s^{-1}$, is an exponential weighting function for the local likelihood. This value has been empirically chosen by considering a range of discrete values ($\hat{w} = \{0.005, 0.01, 0.015, 0.02, 0.025, 0.030\}$), and by choosing the optimum according to KS plots goodness-of-fit analysis, as described in [41]. We use a Newton-Raphson procedure to maximize the local log likelihood in eq. 16 and compute the local maximum-likelihood estimate of $\xi(t)$. Because there is significant overlap between adjacent local likelihood intervals, we start the Newton-Raphson procedure at t with the previous local maximum-likelihood estimate at time $t-\Delta$ in which Δ define how much the local likelihood time interval is shifted to compute the next parameter update. We determined the optimal orders $\{P,Q,K\}$ using the Akaike Information Criterion (AIC) by fitting a subset of the data using local likelihood method [41]) as well as the Kolmogorov-Smirnov (KS) statistic in the *post hoc* analysis. More in detail, we can compare the AIC scores and choose the parameter setup with the minimum AIC value of $AIC = -2L + 2\dim(\xi)$ where L is the maximized value of the likelihood function for the estimated model, and $\dim(\xi)$ is the number of parameters in the statistical model.

It is known from point process theory [41] that the Conditional Intensity Function (CIF) $\beta(t)$ is related to the inter-event probability $p(t)$ with a one-to-one relationship:

$$\beta(t) = \frac{p(t)}{1 - \int_{u_j}^{t} p(\tau) d\tau} \quad (17)$$

The estimated CIF is used to evaluate the goodness-of-fit of the proposed heartbeat interval point process probability model, which is based on the KS test [41].

Instantaneous Lyapunov Exponents Estimation

The Lyapunov Exponent (LE) of a real valued function $f(t)$ defined for $t > 0$ is:

$$\lambda = \lim_{t\to\infty} \sup \frac{1}{t} \log(|f(t)|) \quad (18)$$

More generally, let us consider an n-dimensional linear system in the form $y_i = Y(t)p_i$, where $Y(t)$ is a fundamental solution matrix with $Y(0)$ orthogonal, and $\{p_i\}$ is an orthonormal basis of $\mathbb{R}^n$. Then, the sum of the corresponding n Lyapunov Exponents (λ_i) is minimized, and the orthonormal basis $\{p_i\}$ is called "normal" [54]. One of the key theoretical tools for determining LEs is the continuous QR factorization: $Y(t) = Q(t)R(t)$ [55,56] where $Q(t)$ is orthogonal and $R(t)$ is upper triangular with positive diagonal elements R_{ii}, $i = 1:n$. Therefore we obtain [54–56]:

$$\begin{aligned} \lambda_i &= \lim_{t\to\infty} \frac{1}{t} \log \|Y(t)p_i\| = \lim_{t\to\infty} \frac{1}{t} \log \|R(t)p_i\| \\ &= \lim_{t\to\infty} \frac{1}{t} \log \|R_{ii}(t)\|,\ 1 \leq i \leq n \end{aligned} \quad (19)$$

In our case, the matrix $Y(t)$ corresponds to the Jacobian of the M-dimensional system of the NARL model parameters, where M is the value of the largest model order [39]. Therefore, given the NARL model reported in eq. 13 and using eqs. 9 to 12 bringing back to the NAR framework, it is possible to obtain an M-dimensional state space canonical representation.

Using the Einstein notation, we obtain:

$$\begin{aligned} \mu_{RR}(t, \mathcal{H}_t, \xi(t)) &= \gamma_1(i)\,\Delta RR_i + \gamma_2(i,j)\,\Delta RR_i\,\Delta RR_j \\ &+ \gamma_3(i,j,k)\,\Delta RR_i\,\Delta RR_j \Delta RR_k \end{aligned} \quad (20)$$

Therefore, the elements of the Jacobian can be computed as follows:

$$\begin{aligned} \frac{\partial \mu_{RR}(t,\mathcal{H}_t,\xi(t))}{\partial \Delta RR_p} &= \gamma_1(i)\delta_p + \gamma_2(j,i)\Delta RR_i \delta_{jp} + \\ &\gamma_2(i,j)\Delta RR_i \delta_{ip} + \gamma_3(i,j,k)\delta_{ip}\Delta RR_j \Delta RR_k \\ &+ \gamma_3(i,j,k)\delta_{jp}\Delta RR_i \Delta RR_k \\ &+ \gamma_3(i,j,k)\delta_{kp}\Delta RR_i \Delta RR_j \end{aligned} \quad (21)$$

and considering the symmetry properties of the NAR kernels, we finally obtain:

$$\begin{aligned} \frac{\partial \mu_{RR}(t,\mathcal{H}_t,\xi(t))}{\partial \Delta RR_p} &= \gamma_1(p) + 2\sum_i \gamma_2(i,p)\Delta RR_i \\ &+ 3\sum_i \sum_j \gamma_3(i,j,p)\Delta RR_i \Delta RR_j \end{aligned} \quad (22)$$

Considering N data samples, we evaluate the Jacobian over the time series, and determine the LE by means of the QR decomposition:

$$J(n)Q_{(n-1)} = Q_{(n)}R_{(n)} \quad \text{with } n = 1,2...,N.$$

The matrix $Y(t)$ corresponds to the Jacobian of this system [39]:

$$J(n) = \begin{pmatrix} 0 & 1 & 0 & 0 & \cdots & 0 \\ 0 & 0 & 1 & 0 & \cdots & 0 \\ 0 & 0 & 0 & 1 & \cdots & 0 \\ \vdots & \vdots & \vdots & \vdots & \ddots & \vdots \\ 0 & 0 & 0 & 0 & \cdots & 1 \\ \frac{\partial \mu_{RR}(t,\mathcal{H}_t,\xi(t))}{\partial \Delta RR_1} & \frac{\partial \mu_{RR}(t,\mathcal{H}_t,\xi(t))}{\partial \Delta RR_2} & \frac{\partial \mu_{RR}(t,\mathcal{H}_t,\xi(t))}{\partial \Delta RR_3} & \frac{\partial \mu_{RR}(t,\mathcal{H}_t,\xi(t))}{\partial \Delta RR_4} & \cdots & \frac{\partial \mu_{RR}(t,\mathcal{H}_t,\xi(t))}{\partial \Delta RR_M} \end{pmatrix}.$$

This decomposition is unique except in the case of zero diagonal elements. Then, the LEs λ_i are given by

$$\lambda_i = \frac{1}{\tau N} \sum_{j=0}^{N-1} \ln R_{(j)ii} \tag{23}$$

where τ is the sampling time step. The estimation of the LEs is performed at each time t from the corresponding time-varying vector of parameters, $\xi(t)$. We define the first LE ($\lambda_1(t)$) as the instantaneous dominant Lyapunov exponent (IDLE). In particular, the median IDLE ($\overline{\lambda_{RR}}$) and its median absolute deviation ($\sigma_{\lambda_{RR}}$) were considered as group features.

Standard and Nonlinear Measures of Heartbeat Dynamics

In order to perform a comparison analysis with standard and nonlinear estimates of heartbeat dynamics, we also calculated the standard mean of the RR intervals (Mean RR), the root mean square of successive differences of intervals (RMSSD) and the number of successive differences of intervals which differ by more than 50 ms (pNN50% expressed as a percentage of the total number of heartbeats analyzed) [57]. Referring to morphological patterns of HRV, the triangular index is obtained as the integral of the histogram (i.e. total number of RR intervals) divided by the height of the histogram which depends on the selected bin width [57]. Moreover, we performed the estimation of the dominant Lyapunov exponent according to the algorithm described by Wolf et al. [34] (L_{D_1}) and Rosenstein et al. [58] (L_{D_2}). Both algorithms are suitably applied to experimental noisy data. Finally, other nonlinear measures such as the approximate entropy (ApEn) [59], Sample Entropy [60], and the Detrended Fluctuation Analysis (DFA) [61] were evaluated.

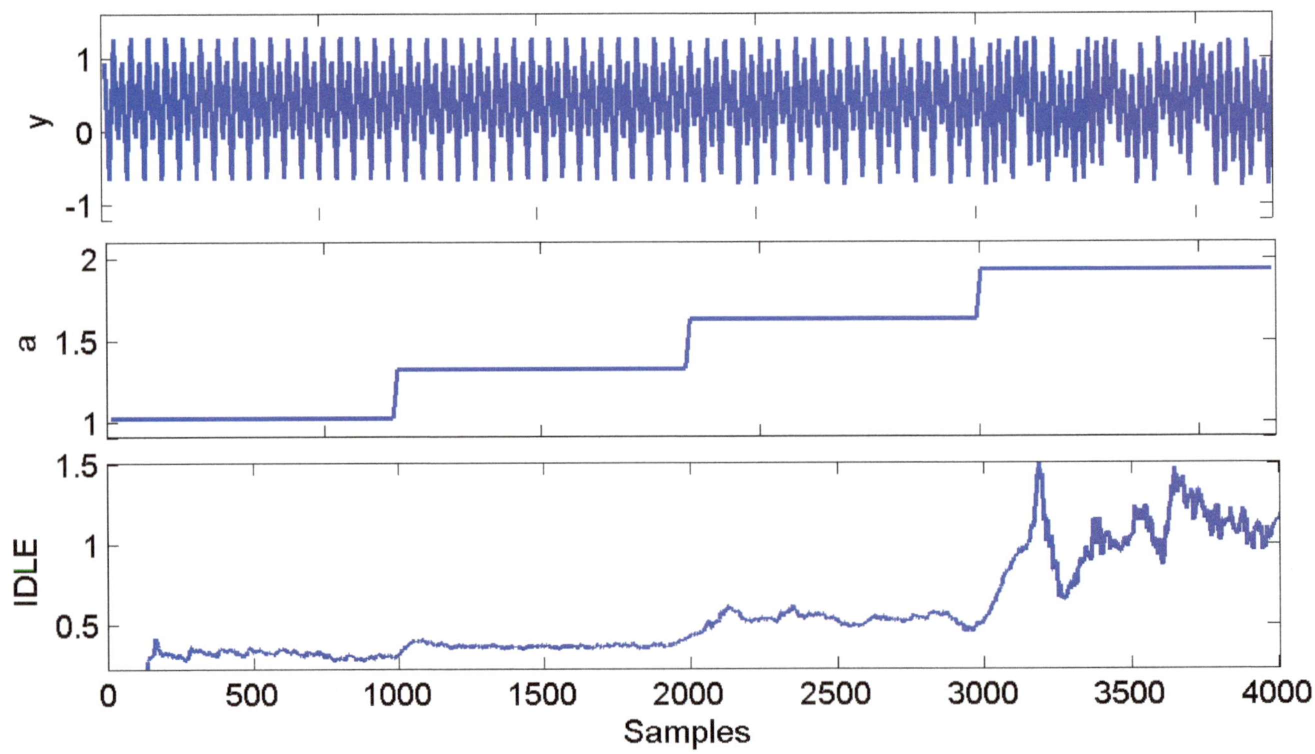

Figure 1. Simulation results using the Hénon equations. (Top) Synthetic interval series from the Hénon map, (Middle) the a stepping, and (Bottom) IDLE averaged estimate from 100 realizations using NARL model with noise level of $k = 0.001$.

Experimental Data

Synthetic Data

Before reporting the implementation of the synthetic datasets, it is important to clarify some important differences from standard definitions that are introduced by our methodology. In fact, standard nonlinear systems such as the Hénon Map and Rössler Attractor are intrinsically defined in the continuos time domain, whereas our methodology deals with stochastic point processes which are a sequence of events. Moreover, additive noise terms have to be considered as well. Therefore, starting from the canonical equations of each nonlinear system, we slightly modify the system equations by adding a noise term. Then, the output of the system is taken as an input of an integrate-and-fire system. The output of such an integrate-and-fire system constitutes the series modeled by the proposed cubic NARL model within the point-process framework.

Hénon Map. In order to test the efficiency of the proposed cubic NARL model in tracking the complexity of a synthetic stochastic series through the IDLE index, we simulated a modified version of the well-known chaotic Hénon Map as suggested in [39]. Such a complex system, in which stochastic terms are also considered, is governed by the following differential equations:

$$\begin{aligned} y_{n+1} &= bx_n + k\epsilon(t); \\ x_{n+1} &= 1 - ax_n^2 + y_n + k\epsilon(t); \end{aligned} \tag{24}$$

The time series y_n were taken into account fixing $b=0.3$. The term $\epsilon(t)$ is an independent identically distributed Gaussian random variable with zero mean and standard deviation of 1, which is modulated by the coefficient k. The coefficient a is taken as a time-varying variable from $a=1$ to $a=1.09$ with step size 0.03. Note that the value $a=1.07$, in a purely deterministic domain, corresponds to the transition between the non-chaotic and chaotic regime. A total of 100 realizations the Hénon Map series were simulated, each of which was comprised of 4000 data

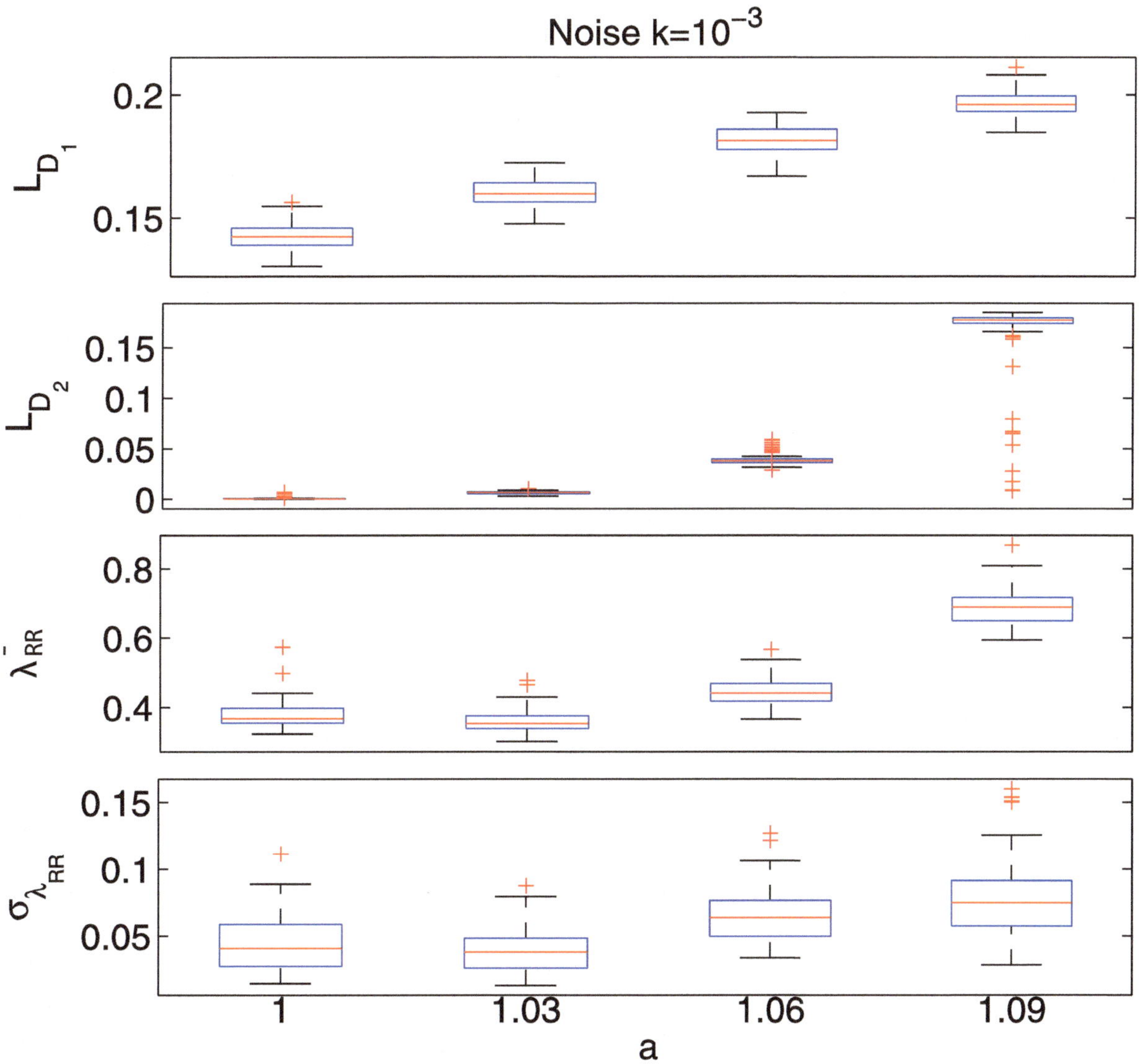

Figure 2. Simulation results using the Rössler equations. (Top) Synthetic interval series from the Rössler system, (Middle) the a stepping, and (Bottom) IDLE estimates using NARL model. The dotted vertical line indicates the transition between the non-chaotic and chaotic regime.

points with 1000 samples for each of the four a-values. A realization of the simulated time series is illustrated in Fig. 1 along with the a-values and the corresponding IDLE results.

Rössler Attractor. As a further validation, we simulated a modified version of the well-known chaotic Rössler time series (see previous work [19]). Such a complex system, in which stochastic terms are also considered, is governed by the following differential equations:

$$\frac{dx}{dt} = -z - y + k\epsilon(t); \quad \frac{dy}{dt} = x + ay + k\epsilon(t); \quad \frac{dz}{dt} = b + z(x-c) + k\epsilon(t); \tag{25}$$

The time series were implemented with sampling time of 0.01 using the Runge-Kutta integration and fixing $b=2$, and $c=4$. The term $\epsilon(t)$ is an independent identically distributed Gaussian random variable with zero mean and standard deviation of 0.01. The coefficient a is taken as a time-varying variable from $a=0.35$ to $a=0.45$ with step size 0.025. Note that the value $a=0.432$, in a purely deterministic domain, corresponds to the transition between the non-chaotic and chaotic regime. A total of 75000 data points were generated with 15000 samples for each of the five a-values. The simulated time series is illustrated in Fig. 2 along with the a-values and the corresponding results on the IDLE. The IDLE transitions to positive values reflect the simulated switch to chaotic behavior.

Experimental Data

In order to validate the proposed algorithms performance as related to actual cardiovascular dynamics, we have considered two experimental datasets. Since the experimental protocols are fully described in [19,41] in this paragraph we provide only briefly descriptions of the two datasets.

Postural Changes. In order to validate the proposed algorithms performance as related to actual cardiovascular dynamics, we studied the complexity of RR interval series recorded from 10 healthy subjects for the study of cardiovascular and autonomic regulation undergoing a tilt-table protocol. This choice is motivated by the high presence of nonlinearity and non-stationarity in such time series. In this study, a subject lying horizontally in a supine position is then actively or passively tilted to the vertical position. The rest (supine) and upright sessions alternated six times with three possible modality of transition: active stand-up, slow and fast passive tilt. A single-lead ECG was

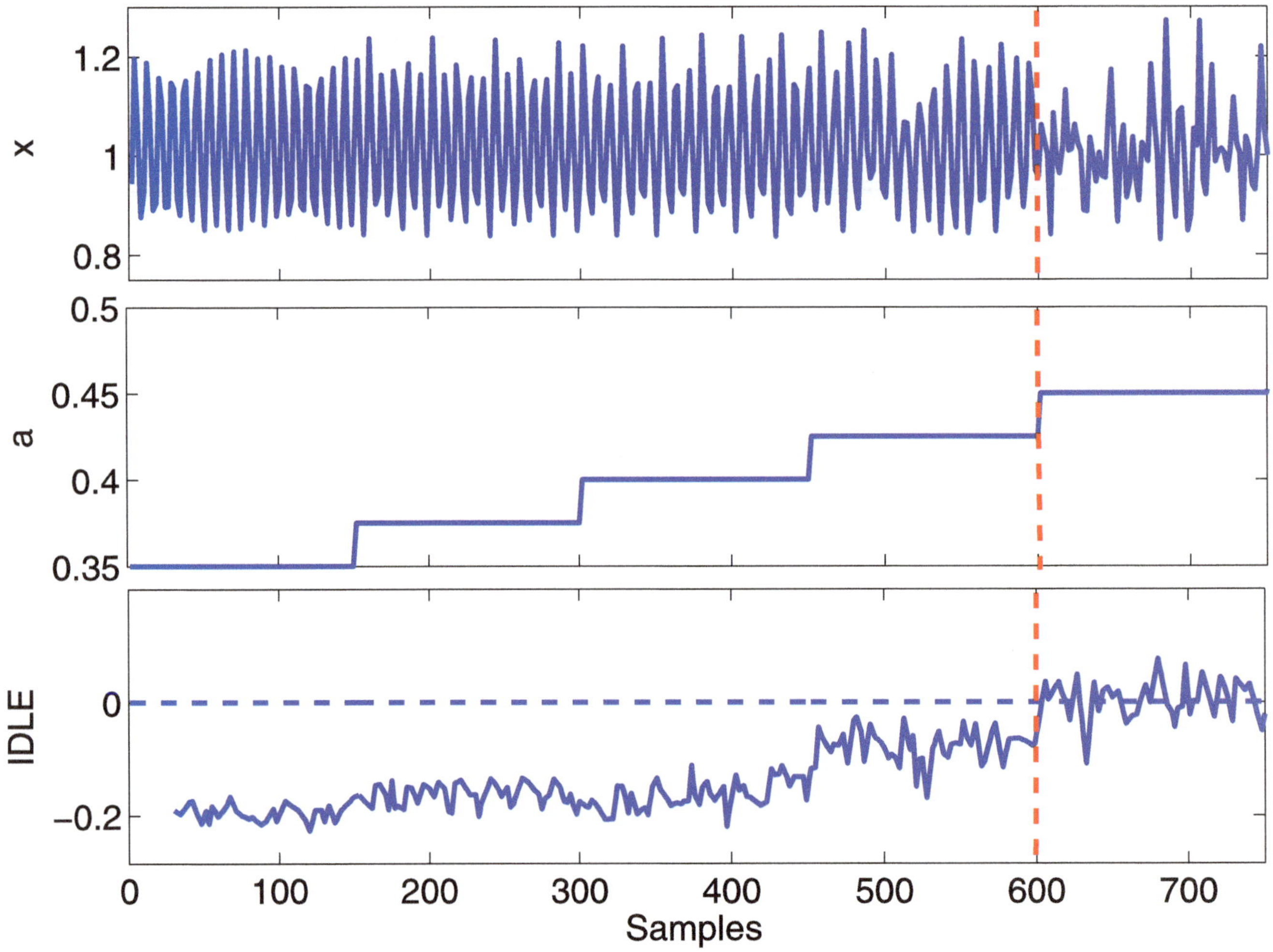

Figure 3. Box plots of standard and proposed Lyapunov estimations performed on the Hénon map among the a−stepping with noise level of $k=0.001$.

Table 1. IDLE Results from the Hénon map Synthetic Dataset.

a-values	1	1.03	1.06	1.09	
Noise k = 0.001					p-value
L_{D_1}	0.1424 ± 0.0035	0.1598 ± 0.0041	0.1814 ± 0.0040	0.1960 ± 0.0030	$<10^{-12}$
L_{D_2}	0.0004 ± 0.0002	0.0064 ± 0.0009	0.0377 ± 0.0019	0.1772 ± 0.0030	$<10^{-12}$
$\overline{\lambda_{RR}}$	0.3679 ± 0.0195	0.3530 ± 0.0179	0.4410 ± 0.0268	0.6885 ± 0.0349	$<10^{-12}$
$\sigma_{\lambda_{RR}}$	0.0407 ± 0.0151	0.0379 ± 0.0112	0.0636 ± 0.0130	0.0747 ± 0.0170	$<10^{-12}$
Noise k = 0.01					p-value
L_{D_1}	2.5488 ± 0.0251	2.5552 ± 0.0387	2.5537 ± 0.0280	2.5573 ± 0.0238	>0.05
L_{D_2}	0.3038 ± 0.0070	0.3049 ± 0.0077	0.3037 ± 0.0085	0.3033 ± 0.0083	>0.05
$\overline{\lambda_{RR}}$	1.2240 ± 0.3232	1.5006 ± 0.4380	1.4822 ± 0.5034	1.4962 ± 0.5237	$<5{*}10^{-4}$
$\sigma_{\lambda_{RR}}$	0.4511 ± 0.1559	0.6884 ± 0.2008	0.5780 ± 0.2476	0.7137 ± 0.2830	$2<10^{-5}$
Noise k = 0.1					p-value
L_{D_1}	2.6704 ± 0.0265	2.6710 ± 0.0283	2.6756 ± 0.0306	2.6719 ± 0.0350	>0.05
L_{D_2}	0.2069 ± 0.0997	0.2161 ± 0.1221	0.2320 ± 0.1334	0.2334 ± 0.1459	>0.05
$\overline{\lambda_{RR}}$	0.1180 ± 0.0517	0.1383 ± 0.0565	0.1319 ± 0.0487	0.1566 ± 0.0468	>0.05
$\sigma_{\lambda_{RR}}$	0.1348 ± 0.0376	0.1398 ± 0.0314	0.1360 ± 0.0378	0.1369 ± 0.0247	>0.05
Noise k = 1					p-value
L_{D_1}	0.2949 ± 0.0033	0.2953 ± 0.0031	0.2949 ± 0.0031	0.2947 ± 0.0023	>0.05
L_{D_2}	0.0023 ± 0.0022	0.0015 ± 0.0015	0.0011 ± 0.0011	0.0017 ± 0.0016	>0.05
$\overline{\lambda_{RR}}$	−0.1032 ± 0.0104	−0.1018 ± 0.0107	−0.0998 ± 0.0098	−0.0993 ± 0.0119	>0.05
$\sigma_{\lambda_{RR}}$	0.0318 ± 0.0056	0.0311 ± 0.0071	0.0337 ± 0.0066	0.0319 ± 0.0071	>0.05

continuously recorded for each subject during the study, and the RR intervals were extracted using a curve length-based QRS detection algorithm [62]. Further details on the experimental protocol can be found in [19,41]. The study was conducted at the Massachusetts Institute of Technology (MIT) General Clinical Research Center (GCRC) and was approved by the MIT Institutional Review Board and the GCRC Scientific Advisory Committee. Patient records/information was anonymized and de-identified prior to analysis.

Congestive Heart Failure. The second heartbeat dataset was constituted from data gathered from Congestive Heart Failure (CHF) and reference healthy subjects on a public source: Physionet (http://www.physionet.org/) [63]. The RR time series were recorded from 14 CHF patients (from $BIDMC-CHF$ Database) as well as 16 healthy subjects (from $MIT-BIH$ Normal Sinus Rhythm Database). Each RR time series was artifact-free (upon human's visual inspection and artifact rejection) and lasted about 50 min (small segments of the original over longer recordings). These recordings have been taken as landmark for studying complex heartbeat interval dynamics [3,8].

Results

Instantaneous Complex Dynamics on Synthetic Data

Hénon Map. We performed the IDLE estimation by fitting the NARL model on y series from the modified stochastic Hénon Map time series (see eq. 24). The series were generated a hundred times for each of the four considered noise levels $k=\{0.001, 0.01, 0.1, 1\}$. For $k>0.001$, a further constrain of $x_n=0.1\epsilon(t)$ was imposed as $x_n<=-0.1$ or $x_n>=-0.5$ in order to prevent the system to become unstable. The model orders were set as $P=3$, $Q=1$, $K=1$, and $\alpha=0.4$ were chosen by preliminary KS plots goodness-of-fit analysis, according to [41]. The simulated time series along with the resulted IDLE series are shown in Fig. 1, whereas the corresponding box plots are shown in Fig. 3 in terms of IDLE median $(\overline{\lambda_{RR}})$ and its median absolute deviation $\sigma_{\lambda_{RR}}$. The proposed IDLE is able to track the complexity variation at each moment in time. As a matter of fact, the IDLE goes increasingly high from the non-chaotic behavior to the chaotic one. Remarkably, the non-chaos–chaos transition is instantaneously detected, although a significant oscillatory dynamics is present in the chaotic region. The related IDLE values are reported in Table 1 along with standard estimates of the dominant Lyapunov exponents. A non-parametric statistical analysis has been performed in order to quantify the differences between the considered a-values for each of the considered noise level.

Considering the noise level $k=0.001$, the Kruskal-Wallis test reveals significant differences ($p<10^{-12}$) for both the standard Lyapunov estimates and the proposed $\overline{\lambda_{RR}}$ and complexity variability index $\sigma_{\lambda_{RR}}$. In this case, the Dunn test for multiple comparison, which considers a Tukey-Kramer correction, shows that each group of standard estimates of L_{D_1} and L_{D_2} having coherent a parameter are different with all the other groups ($p<10^{-3}$), whereas coherent a-values of $\overline{\lambda_{RR}}$ are different with all the other groups ($p<10^{-3}$) except for $a=\{1-1.03\}$ ($p>0.05$).

Considering the noise level $k=0.01$, the Kruskal-Wallis test reveals significant differences ($p<5{*}10^{-4}$) only for the proposed $\overline{\lambda_{RR}}$ and complexity variability index $\sigma_{\lambda_{RR}}$. In this case, the Dunn test for multiple comparison, which considers a Tukey-Kramer correction, shows that coherent $a=1$ values are different with all the other groups ($p<10^{-3}$), with $a=\{1.03, 1.06, 1.09\}$ equal between each other ($p>0.05$). For noise level $k=0.1$ and $k=1$,

Table 2. Median and MAD of IDLE evaluated in the Tilt-Table Experimental Dataset.

Subject	P-Value	KS dist.	Rest	Stend-Up	Rest	Slow Tilt	Rest	Fast Tilt
1	0.0320	0.0458	0.0264 ± 0.0298	0.0108 ± 0.077	0.0304 ± 0.0466	-0.0340 ± 0.0514	0.0518 ± 0.0227	-0.1165 ± 0.0326
2	0.0340	0.0603	0.1469 ± 0.1712	0.0120 ± 0.1794	0.2534 ± 0.1007	0.0050 ± 0.1372	0.2226 ± 0.0988	0.0075 ± 0.0515
3	$< e^{-8}$	0.0355	0.0435 ± 0.0552	0.0207 ± 0.0232	0.0439 ± 0.0745	-0.0200 ± 0.0423	-0.0222 ± 0.0662	-0.0313 ± 0.0574
4	0.0300	0.0227	-0.0551 ± 0.0150	-0.0550 ± 0.0185	0.0557 ± 0.0679	-0.0585 ± 0.0315	0.0649 ± 0.0785	0.0084 ± 0.0365
5	0.0220	0.0451	-0.0719 ± 0.0613	-0.0578 ± 0.0547	-0.0045 ± 0.0441	-0.0403 ± 0.0355	-0.0137 ± 0.0595	-0.0388 ± 0.0226
6	0.0020	0.0409	0.0520 ± 0.0894	-0.0665 ± 0.0368	-0.0032 ± 0.0692	-0.0734 ± 0.0442	-0.0007 ± 0.0786	-0.0362 ± 0.0303
7	0.0020	0.0458	0.0339 ± 0.0448	-0.0346 ± 0.0589	0.0278 ± 0.0343	-0.0665 ± 0.0341	0.0969 ± 0.0406	-0.0258 ± 0.1049
8	0.0760	0.0408	-0.0352 ± 0.0467	-0.0103 ± 0.0668	-0.0159 ± 0.0571	-0.0783 ± 0.0405	0.0093 ± 0.0518	-0.0612 ± 0.0375
9	$< e^{-6}$	0.0571	-0.0079 ± 0.048	-0.0033 ± 0.0703	-0.0217 ± 0.0365	0.0216 ± 0.0391	0.0058 ± 0.0394	-0.0042 ± 0.0145
10	$< e^{-8}$	0.0572	0.6521 ± 0.4771	0.0324 ± 0.0830	0.2316 ± 0.1737	-0.0052 ± 0.0650	0.2662 ± 0.1708	0.0384 ± 0.1653

P-values are obtained from the nonlinearity test.

the difference between the a-values are not revealed by standard and proposed dominant Lyapunov estimates.

Rössler System. We performed the IDLE estimation by fitting the NARL model on the x series from the modified stochastic Rössler time series (see eq. 25). The model orders were set as $P=3$, $Q=1$, $K=1$, and $\alpha=0.2$ were chosen by preliminary KS plots goodness-of-fit analysis, according to [41]. The simulated time series along with the resulted IDLE series are shown in Fig. 2. Clearly, the proposed IDLE is able to track the complexity variation at each moment in time. As a matter of fact, the IDLE goes increasingly high from the non-chaotic behavior to the chaotic one. Remarkably, the non-chaos–chaos transition is instantaneously detected, although a significant oscillatory dynamics is present in the chaotic region. Intervals expressed as median $\pm$ M.A.D. are as follows: -0.0973 ± 0.0044 for $a=0.350$, -0.0813 ± 0.0065 for $a=0.375$, -0.0850 ± 0.0077 for $a=0.400$, -0.0375 ± 0.0075 for $a=0.425$, 0.0033 ± 0.0092 for $a=0.450$. A non-parametric statistical analysis has been performed in order to quantify the differences between the considered a-values. The Kruskal-Wallis test reveals significant differences ($p<10^{-6}$) and the Dunn test for multiple comparison, which considers a Tukey-Kramer correction, shows that each IDLE group having coherent a-values is different with all the other group ($p<10^{-5}$) except for $a=\{0.375-0.4\}$ ($p>0.05$).

Instantaneous Complex Dynamics on Postural Changes

Before estimating the IDLE from the experimental datasets, we first considered a specific time-domain method [64] for testing the presence of nonlinearity in the heartbeat intervals. The null hypothesis of the test states that the given time series is linear. In the considered recordings, we restricted the test to short-term dependence by setting the number of laps $M=8$, and a total of 500 bootstrap replications. Concerning the RR series gathered during postural changes, the nonlinearity test shows that the level of nonlinearity of the considered RR intervals is statistically significant for all the considered subjects but one (see Table 2. As also shown in Table 2, the NARL modeling always gives a good model fit, with KS distance <0.0604 in all cases. Specifically, concerning the three experimental sessions, i.e. stand-up, slow-tilt, and fast-tilt, a decrease of the IDLE with respect to the relative rest condition is shown in 25 out of 30 epochs. In particular, in the fast-tilt condition the decrease happens for all subjects, and is more significant than stand-up and slow-tilt. Group statistics of standard and proposed instantaneous measures are shown in Table 3, whose inter-subject analysis was performed using a non-parametric rank-sum test. Results on the proposed IDLE show a non-significant statistical difference between the stand-up epochs and their relative rest epochs ($p>0.05$) and a significant difference for the slow-tilt epochs ($p<0.05$). The highest significance was found comparing the fast-tilt epochs with their relative rest ($p<0.001$). These trends are confirmed by the standard DLE estimation according to the Rosenstein et al. [58] technique, whereas the one suggested by Wolf et al. [34] did not show such significant differences. IDLE dynamics for one representative subject are shown in Fig. 4, whereas the averaged IDLEs for all 10 subjects are shown in Fig. 5, providing a clear portrayal of how different postural stimuli elicit different changes in the dynamic signatures of complexity. Concerning other standard and instantaneous indices, we report significant differences on three session on μ_{RR}, ApEn, and SampEn, whereas RMSSD and pNN50% showed significant differences during the slow and fast tilt sessions.

Using this dataset, we further evaluate the effect of the Laguerre parameter α on the IDLE estimates. Tracking for values $\alpha=\{0.1,0.2,0.3,...,0.8\}$ from a representative subject undergoing

Table 3. Group Statistics of Standard and Instantaneous Heartbeat Dynamics Measures from the Tilt-Table Experimental Dataset.

Feature	Rest	Stand-up	p-value	Rest	Slow Tilt	p-value	Rest	Fast Tilt p-value	
Standard and Instantaneous Time Domain Measures of HRV									
Mean RR (ms)	910.94 ± 123.08	781.92 ± 55.96	<0.003	871.86 ± 74.27	772.82 ± 46.10	<0.0002	860.50 ± 80.47	774.66 ± 44.34	<0.0004
RMSSD	0.0279 ± 0.0123	0.0202 ± 0.0055	>0.05	0.0325 ± 0.0127	0.0202 ± 0.0048	<0.03	0.0296 ± 0.0127	0.0200 ± 0.0042	<0.03
pNN50%	6.4335 ± 6.4335	2.3472 ± 2.3472	>0.05	10.0744 ± 9.4524	1.6860 ± 1.5708	<0.05	7.6677 ± 7.2816	2.0339 ± 2.0339	<0.05
HRV Triangular Index	4.1644 ± 0.6832	3.9065 ± 0.4754	>0.05	3.3012 ± 0.5142	3.5347 ± 0.3497	>0.05	3.6429 ± 0.9743	4.3333 ± 0.6352	>0.05
μ_{RR}(ms)	915.10 ± 122.16	769.77 ± 78.22	<0.02	879.60 ± 74.80	773.23 ± 62.29	<0.001	890.17 ± 95.18	776.92 ± 57.40	<0.005
σ^2_{RR} (ms^2)	394.15 ± 319.26	233.09 ± 139.09	>0.05	435.36 ± 237.42	208.07 ± 112.84	<0.03	440.76 ± 302.71	220.71 ± 108.79	>0.05
Standard and Instantaneous Nonlinear Measures of HRV									
ApEn	1.122 ± 0.055	0.944 ± 0.079	$<10^{-3}$	1.167 ± 0.091	0.927 ± 0.125	$<10^{-3}$	1.087 ± 0.116	0.964 ± 0.072	<0.004
SampEn	1.501 ± 0.192	1.243 ± 0.245	<0.025	1.495 ± 0.173	0.900 ± 0.247	$<10^{-3}$	1.320 ± 0.247	1.197 ± 0.233	>0.05
DFA-α_1	0.9806 ± 0.1039	0.9968 ± 0.1624	>0.05	0.9892 ± 0.0952	1.2128 ± 0.1126	>0.05	0.9788 ± 0.0990	1.0137 ± 0.1425	>0.05
L_{D_1}	0.0128 ± 0.0014	0.0125 ± 0.0013	>0.05	0.0133 ± 0.0017	0.0135 ± 0.0015	>0.05	0.0137 ± 0.0013	0.0128 ± 0.0008	>0.05
L_{D_2}	0.0029 ± 0.0005	0.0028 ± 0.0005	>0.05	0.0037 ± 0.0006	0.0024 ± 0.0004	<0.005	0.0033 ± 0.0006	0.0020 ± 0.0007	<0.001
$\overline{\lambda_{RR}}$	−0.0128 ± 0.0480	−0.0390 ± 0.0330	>0.05	0.0205 ± 0.0372	−0.0491 ± 0.0236	<0.0005	−0.0022 ± 0.0332	−0.0404 ± 0.0232	<0.001
$\sigma_{\lambda_{RR}}$	0.0585 ± 0.0213	0.0652 ± 0.0178	>0.05	0.0693 ± 0.0098	0.0582 ± 0.0113	>0.05	0.0617 ± 0.0131	0.0500 ± 0.0144	>0.05

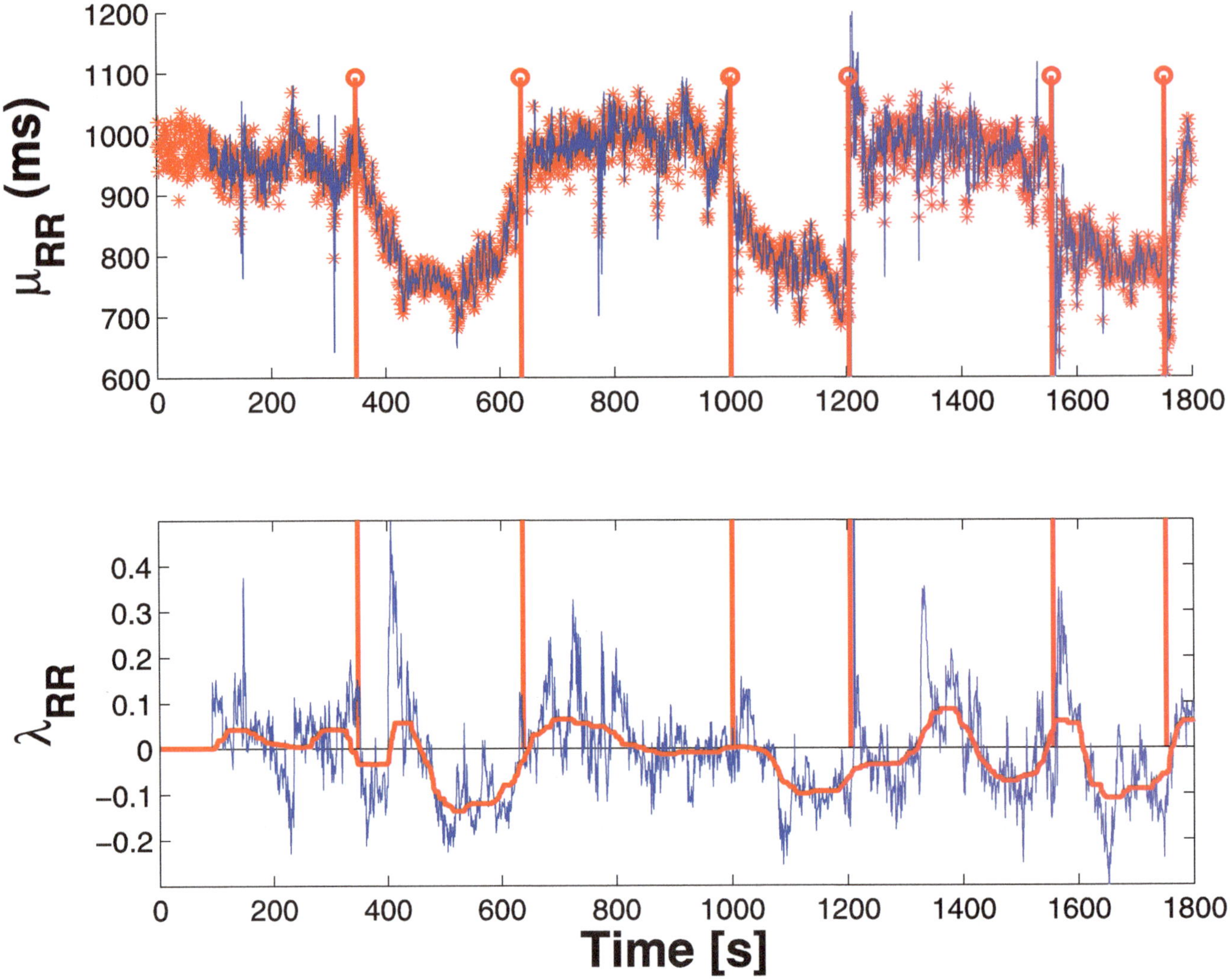

Figure 4. Instantaneous heartbeat statistics computed from a representative subject (subject 1) from the tilt-table protocol. In the top panel, the estimated $\mu_{RR}(t)$ is superimposed on the recorded RR series. In the bottom panel, the instantaneous averaged IDLE is superimposed on the original IDLE.

postural changes are shown in Fig. 6. Indeed, the IDLE estimates are affected by the choice of the Laguerre parameter α. However, such a variability is significantly less than the variability of the IDLE dynamics within session. As a matter of fact, quantitative results reported in Table 4 show that these differences are associated to a p-value less than $2e^{-4}$ for each experimental session.

Finally, we report further results on the nonlinearity test separately performed for each of the experimental session, instead of the whole recordings (see Table 2). As a result, under the null hypothesis of linearity according to the time-domain method described in [64] for testing the presence of nonlinearity in the heartbeat intervals, the 49.12% of the resting state (28/57 sessions) were associated to a significant p-value <0.05, along with the 44.4% of the stand-up (8/18 sessions) protocol, the 20% of the slow-tilt (4/20 sessions) protocol, the 10.53% of the fast-tilt (2/19 sessions) protocol.

Instantaneous Complex Dynamics on CHF patients

The results of the second experimental dataset (on CHF) are shown in Table 5. According to the nonlinearity test, 15 out of 16 RR time series from the healthy subjects showed significant nonlinearity ($p<0.05$), whereas in the CHF group, 6 out of 14 RR time series failed to reach significance ($p>0.05$). The fact that a lower degree of nonlinearity was found in the CHF patients suggests that pathological conditions might reduce the nonlinearity in the heartbeat interval series, which is also consistent with previous finding that a healthy heartbeat presents more pronounced nonlinear dynamics [3,6,8,65]. Table 5 also demonstrates that the NARL model well fit both pathological and healthy heartbeat series with KS distance <0.082 in all cases. Results averaged among groups are reported in Table 6. We report that standard and instantaneous time domain measures are able to discern the two groups with high statistical significance ($p < 5e^{-4}$). On the other hand, comparing the standard and proposed instantaneous complexity measures, only the DFA-α_2 and the complexity variability $\sigma_{\lambda_{RR}}$ are able to provide significant

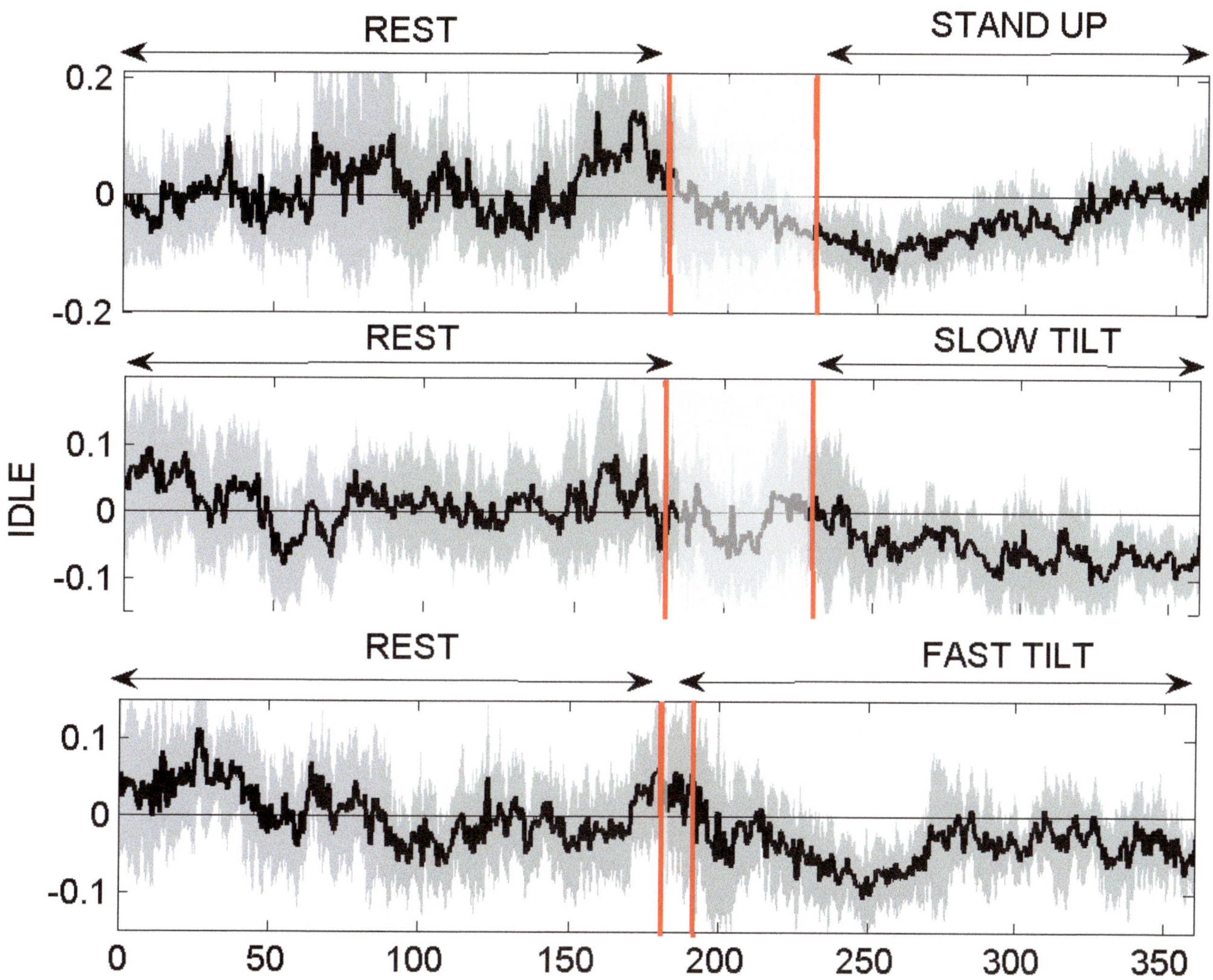

Figure 5. IDLE dynamics averaged for all 10 subjects. The vertical red lines indicate the transition from the supine to the upright position after stand up (top panel), after slow tilt (middle panel), and after fast tilt (bottom panel).

discrimination capability between the two populations with $p < 0.05$.

Discussion and Conclusion

Novelties and Impact of the proposed Methodology

We presented a novel methodology able to instantaneously characterize the complex nonlinear dynamics of a stochastic series of events by using the LEs. The proposed approach relies on the previous literature for the LEs mathematical definition [38,39] and is embedded in a novel IG-based point-process nonlinear framework defined through a third-order Wiener-Volterra representation, thus advancing on the previous models [19]. As a consequence, the novel instantaneous LEs definition is able to provide a reliable complexity measure tool to examine the unevenly spaced events at very high temporal resolutions, without resorting to any interpolation method. Moreover, goodness of fit measures such as KS distance and autocorrelation plots quantitatively allow to verify the model fit as well as to choose the proper model order, which represents another open issue of current parametric approaches.

The effective procedure for the time-varying parameter identification is ensured by the combined use of the discrete-time Laguerre expansions for the Wiener-Volterra terms and local maximum likelihood method. In particular, expanding the Volterra terms with the orthonormal Laguerre bases requires a reduced number of parameters to retain the information of all the past events. The nonlinear regression is further performed on the derivative series to better account for nonstationarity [53]. Importantly, unlike other methods that might require large sample size, our method is potentially useful to perform complexity measures in short recordings of the signals of interest.

Importantly, the proposed measures also allows for the study of the *complexity variability*, i.e., the analysis of complex systems referring to the fluctuations in complexity instead of analysis of central tendency. Within the proposed framework, it is always possible to incorporate physiological covariates (such as respiration or blood pressure measures) and produce further instantaneous indices from their dynamic cross spectrum and cross bispectrum [48]. Unlike other paradigms for estimating nonlinearity indices developed in the literature [7,59,66,67], our method is formulated within a probabilistic framework specifically developed for point-

Table 4. IDLE Variability evaluated through $\alpha=\{0.1,0.2,0.3,...,0.8\}$ and within each session of the postural changes protocol.

Session	Through α-values	Within Session	p-Value
Resting State	0.0117 ± 0.0044	0.0585 ± 0.0213	$<5e^{-6}$
Stand-Up	0.0125 ± 0.0082	0.0652 ± 0.0178	$2e^{-5}$
Resting State	0.0170 ± 0.0240	0.0693 ± 0.0098	$7e^{-5}$
Slow Tilt	0.0119 ± 0.0128	0.0582 ± 0.0113	$<2e^{-6}$
Resting State	0.0167 ± 0.0192	0.0617 ± 0.0131	$2e^{-4}$
Fast Tilt	0.0119 ± 0.0128	0.0500 ± 0.0144	$2e^{-6}$

P-values are obtained from the Mann-Whitney test with null hypothesis of equal medians between the two groups. Values are expressed as $X = \text{Median}(X) \pm \text{MAD}(X)$.

process observations (e.g. RR intervals), which already produced important nonlinear quantifiers for autonomic assessment, based on second- and third-order statistics (instantaneous spectrum and bispectrum) [19]. Most other nonlinearity indices are derived from non-parametric models, whereas our model is purely parametric and the analytically derived indices can be evaluated in a dynamic and instantaneous fashion. We believe these strengths enable our method as a useful tool for assessing nonlinear dynamics of heartbeat intervals in a non-stationary environment.

Study of the Instantaneous Cardiovascular Complex Dynamics

The novel IDLE index was evaluated in both synthetic and experimental heartbeat series. Estimations on the synthetic dataset were performed on a stochastic version of the well-known chaotic Hénon Map and Rössler attractor. The use of such a modified version of the Hénon Map and Rössler system alongside the obtained IDLE results need to be discussed. We are aware that in purely deterministic Rössler equations the first LE should be zero in the non-chaotic region, whereas it should be increasingly positive in the chaotic region. However, the IDLE results show slightly negative values in the non-chaotic region. Such a behavior may be ascribed to the stochastic input and to the additional integrate-and-fire step which affect the estimation of all complexity measures, including LEs. To this extent, in order to further investigate the effect of noise, results from the Hénon Map equations were gathered as a function of the noise level. We demonstrate that, for small amount of noise ($k=0.001$), standard and instantaneous estimates of the dominant Lyapunov exponent achieve similar results. However, considering Hénon Map dynamics with $k=0.01$, the IDLE is exclusively able to discern the different behavior of the nonlinear system. Of note, for $k \geq 0.1$,

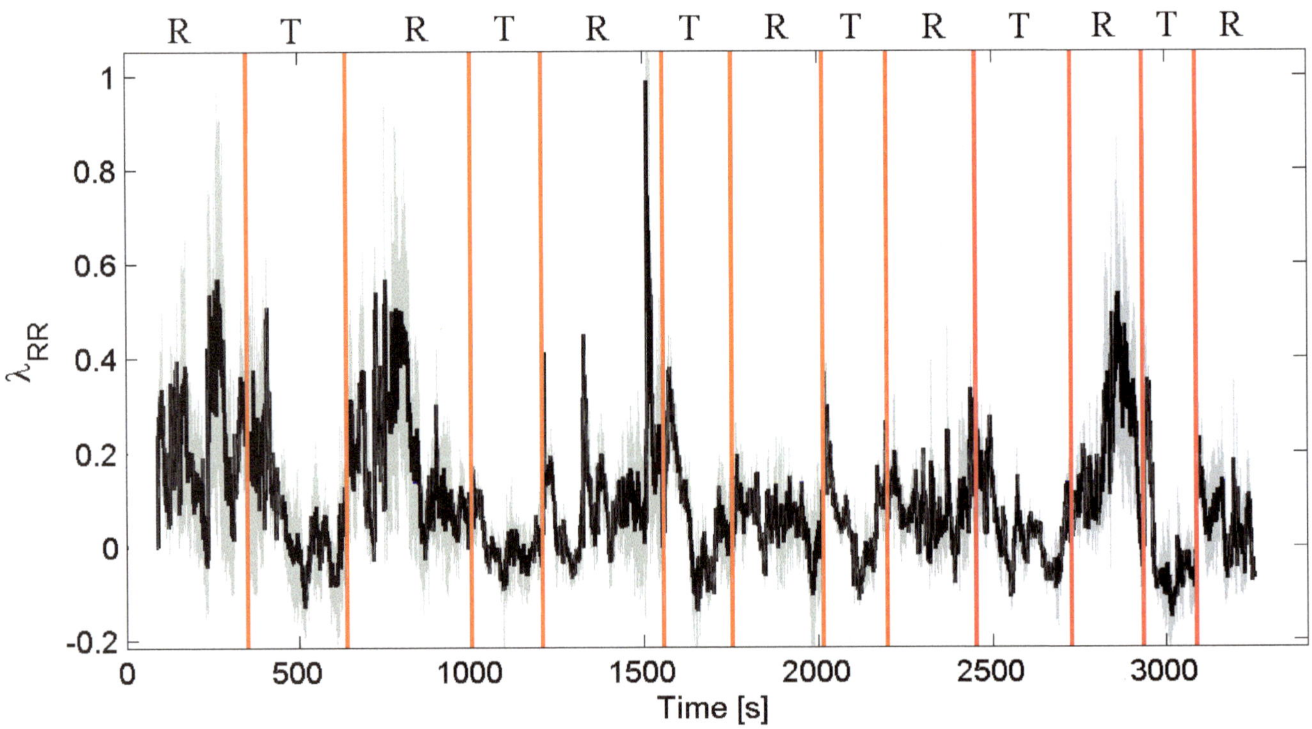

Figure 6. IDLE dynamics averaged for $\alpha=\{0.1,0.2,0.3,...,0.8\}$ from a representative subject undergoing postural changes. Resting state (R) sessions during supine position alternate with upright session after tilt (T). The bold line and gray area indicate the IDLE median and MAD, respectively. Averaged values for all subjects are shown in Table 4.

Table 5. Results from the CHF-Healthy Experimental Dataset.

Subject	Group	μ_{RR}(ms)	p-value	KS dist.	$\overline{\lambda_{RR}}$	$\sigma_{\lambda_{RR}}$
01	CHF	995.4 ± 26.4	>0.05	0.0445	0.2268	0.1123
03	CHF	910.25 ± 28.9	>0.05	0.0552	0.2165	0.1257
04	CHF	603.09 ± 22.7	<0.02	0.0456	0.0676	0.0896
05	CHF	655.6 ± 13.3	>0.05	0.0297	−0.0114	0.0507
06	CHF	637.4 ± 15.9	<0.001	0.0802	0.0757	0.0659
07	CHF	778.0 ± 7.3	>0.05	0.0363	0.0762	0.0793
08	CHF	800.1 ± 14.1	<0.01	0.0357	−0.0965	0.0327
09	CHF	602.5 ± 5.4	>0.05	0.0305	−0.0121	0.0555
10	CHF	486.9 ± 6.9	<0.001	0.0329	−0.0622	0.0444
11	CHF	685.1 ± 16.0	<0.02	0.0354	−0.0014	0.0578
12	CHF	722.8 ± 27.2	<0.001	0.0326	−0.0798	0.0380
13	CHF	619.7 ± 5.1	<0.001	0.0386	0.0550	0.0655
14	CHF	837.7 ± 23.4	>0.05	0.0367	0.0041	0.0613
15	CHF	652.15 ± 20.6	<0.005	0.0265	−0.0322	0.0550
16265	healthy	1023.9 ± 38.9	<0.001	0.0527	0.0162	0.0438
16272	healthy	924.7 ± 30.6	<0.001	0.0539	−0.0304	0.0557
16273	healthy	1046.2 ± 68.7	<0.001	0.0764	0.0998	0.0543
16420	healthy	849.9 ± 39.2	<0.001	0.0394	0.0107	0.0410
16483	healthy	818.5 ± 24.9	<0.001	0.0336	−0.0254	0.0396
16539	healthy	831.5 ± 47.9	<0.001	0.0592	0.0736	0.0485
16773	healthy	1238.9 ± 74.7	<0.001	0.0819	0.0842	0.0613
16786	healthy	945.1 ± 37.0	<0.001	0.0503	0.0226	0.0527
16795	healthy	889.4 ± 61.8	<0.001	0.0442	−0.0214	0.0462
17052	healthy	939.8 ± 33.3	>0.05	0.0487	0.0682	0.0819
17453	healthy	816.6 ± 31.9	<0.001	0.0416	0.0310	0.0466
18177	healthy	639.3 ± 25.7	<0.001	0.0267	0.0058	0.0608
18184	healthy	831.2 ± 31.7	<0.001	0.0392	−0.0373	0.0438
19090	healthy	993.54 ± 41.0	<0.001	0.0565	−0.0101	0.0393
19140	healthy	849.1 ± 49.9	<0.001	0.0353	0.0459	0.0513
19830	healthy	821.2 ± 29.4	<0.001	0.0452	−0.0795	0.0332

P-values are obtained from the nonlinearity test.

the noise has an amplitude comparable with the output of the system, thus destroying the different behaviors among the a-values.

The use of the Laguerre expansion of the Wiener-Volterra kernels was also investigated through experimental analysis. As the zero-order Laguerre basis is an exponential function, the IDLE estimates present a mild dependence on the α value of the Laguerre functions. Nevertheless, we demonstrated that the actual information needed to characterize the experimental sessions, i.e., the variability within each session, is significantly higher than the variability among all the α values. Anyway, using the hereby proposed approach we clearly demonstrate the ability of the IDLE in tracking the system complexity in an instantaneous fashion. The IDLE, in fact, becomes higher when the simulated system switches from non-chaotic to chaotic behavior (see Fig. 2). In all applications, an IG probability model was used as a stochastic version of the widely-applied deterministic integrate-and-fire models used to simulate heartbeats. Regarding the experimental datasets, we demonstrated that our approach is useful in characterizing the inherent nonlinearity of the cardiovascular system. For the first time, tracking complexity by instantaneous Lyapunov Exponents was performed and evaluated during postural changes. During the resting condition the cardiovascular and autonomic nervous system are more sensitive to the initial conditions (positive IDLE), whereas a more regular dynamics (negative IDLE values) appear during the tilt phases (see Fig. 4). These results are in agreement with previous findings that complex vagally-driven dynamics are blunted under sympathetic drive [68] and with more recent reports on loss of complexity during states of arousal [20]). Our instantaneous measures also confirm that the instantaneous complexity reflects instantaneous autonomic nervous system (ANS) control on the cardiovascular dynamics. We have shown that tracking ANS complexity on healthy subjects undergoing postural changes not only confirms previous results [69,70], but further improves sympathovagal assessment as elicited by different dynamic gravitational stimuli.

Our experimental findings on the nonlinearity test performed on each experimental session (resting state, stand-up, slow tilt, and fast tilt) suggest that loss of instantaneous heartbeat complexity as a function of velocity of the postural changes is reasonably due to changes in the nonlinearity of the cardiovascular system (instead

Table 6. Group Statistics of Standard and Instantaneous Heartbeat Dynamics Measures from CHF-Healthy Experimental Dataset.

	CHF (n = 14)	Healthy (n = 16)	p-value
Standard and Instantaneous Time Domain Measures of HRV			
Mean RR (ms)	669.73 ± 68.66	855.74 ± 56.14	<0.002
RMSSD	0.0121 ± 0.0036	0.0432 ± 0.0145	$<4e^{-4}$
pNN50%	0.2357 ± 0.2246	21.5406 ± 15.4908	$<1e^{-4}$
HRV Triangular Index	2.9551 ± 0.5769	2.5628 ± 0.3593	>0.05
μ_{RR}(ms)	671.55 ± 69.6	864.7 ± 53.3	$<4e^{-3}$
σ_{RR}(ms)	8.31 ± 2.2	24.7 ± 7.0	$<5e^{-4}$
Standard and Instantaneous Nonlinear Measures of HRV			
ApEn	1.2130 ± 0.1032	1.2177 ± 0.1066	>0.05
SampEn	1.5670 ± 0.2690	1.4092 ± 0.1522	>0.05
DFA-α_1	0.8498 ± 0.2191	1.0820 ± 0.1467	>0.05
DFA-α_2	1.1552 ± 0.1335	0.9286 ± 0.0544	<0.05
L_{D_1}	0.0167 ± 0.0025	0.0165 ± 0.0012	>0.05
L_{D_2}	0.0029 ± 0.0008	0.0033 ± 0.0005	>0.05
$\overline{\lambda_{RR}}$	0.0014 ± 0.0649	0.0135 ± 0.0368	>0.05
$\sigma_{\lambda_{RR}}$	0.0595 ± 0.0120	0.0476 ± 0.0066	<0.05

P-values are obtained from the Mann-Whitney test with null hypothesis of equal medians between the CHF and healthy subject groups. Values are expressed as $X = \mathrm{Median}(X) \pm \mathrm{MAD}(X)$.

of, for example, changes on the noise properties). Of note, we have previously reported that the standard HRV indices defined in the time and frequency domain are unable to distinguish the three possible modality of transition through different p-values [19].

Moreover, the novel complexity features $\{\overline{\lambda_{RR}};\ \sigma_{\lambda_{RR}}\}$ give important information in the complexity evaluation, also useful in distinguishing heartbeat dynamics coming from patients with CHF and healthy subjects. We found that pathological heartbeat dynamics are associated with increased complexity variability, providing an unique measure of complexity able to discern the CHF and healthy populations. Of note, some of the standard measures defined in the time domain have similar p-value than the point-process measures, as well as DFA-α_2 shows similar performances than the IDLE median absolute deviation. Nevertheless, we point out that we aimed at showing the performances of novel instantaneous measures of complexity based on Lyapunov exponents, providing novel insights on the complexity characterization of stochastic time-varying discrete point-process systems. In other words, although other HRV-based measures are able to discern CHF from healthy subjects, no other measures have been proposed to characterize the time-varying complexity behavior occurring in pathological vs. a healthy cardiovascular system. In particular, while confirming the results reported in the current literature (i.e., several measures of complexity are not able to characterize the CHF and healthy subjects groups), we show a novel key complexity behavior through the proposed complexity variability framework. These findings can be linked to the current literature whereby cardiovascular disorders affect complexity and variability, and may lead to serious pathological events such as heart failure [71].

Concerning other preliminary applications, the proposed IDLE methodology has been revealed as a powerful tool also in tracking the instantaneous complexity during loss of consciousness induced by anesthetic drugs [46]. Looking at the overall results shown using actual heartbeat dynamics data, it seems that the median IDLE is sensitive to changes in ANS regulation induced by orthostatic stress, while IDLE median absolute deviation is sensitive to changes in ANS regulation induced by CHF. However, this conclusion cannot be made without speculation at this time as the data used for the comparison between CHF patients and healthy subjects is related to long-term ECG monitoring during unstructured activity, whereas the data from the tilt-table experimental dataset is structured. Therefore, the observed sensitivity of the IDLE measures could be due to different physiological behavior occurring in CHF subjects or to differences related to the kind of experimental protocol. Future works are related to pursue this direction in further investigating the potential of these high-order nonlinear models in producing new real-time measures for the underlying complexity of physiological systems, and to the investigation of the instantaneous complexity, along with the baroreflex sensitivity and respiratory sinus arrhythmia, during postural changes in CHF subjects, thus allowing some conclusions on the complex physiological behavior of the cardiovascular system in CHF subjects.

Acknowledgments

The authors are grateful to Roger G. Mark and Thomas Heldt (Harvard-MIT Division of Health Sciences and Technology) for kindly providing the tilt-table data analyzed in this study. Early versions of this work have been reported in Proceedings of IEEE-EMBC 2012, San Diego (USA), and IEEE-EMBC 2013, Osaka (Japan).

Author Contributions

Analyzed the data: GV LC RB. Wrote the paper: GV LC RB. Conceived and designed the methodology and experiments: GV LC RB.

References

1. Sunagawa K, Kawada T, Nakahara T (1998) Dynamic nonlinear vago-sympathetic interaction in regulating heart rate. Heart and Vessels 13: 157–174.
2. Atyabi F, Livari M, Kaviani K, Tabar M (2006) Two statistical methods for resolving healthy individuals and those with congestive heart failure based on extended self-similarity and a recursive method. Journal of Biological Physics 32: 489–495.
3. (2009) Special issues on nonlinearity on heart rate. Chaos 19.
4. Valenza G, Citi L, Lanatá A, Scilingo EP, Barbieri R (2014) Revealing real-time emotional responses: a personalized assessment based on heartbeat dynamics. Nature Scientific reports 4.
5. Valenza G, Citi L, Lanata A, Scilingo EP, Barbieri R (2013) A nonlinear heartbeat dynamics model approach for personalized emotion recognition. In: Engineering in Medicine and Biology Society (EMBC), 2013 35th Annual International Conference of the IEEE. IEEE, pp. 2579–2582.
6. Glass L (2001) Synchronization and rhythmic processes in physiology. Nature 410: 277–284.
7. Goldberger A, Peng C, Lipsitz L (2002) What is physiologic complexity and how does it change with aging and disease? Neurobiology of aging 23: 23–26.
8. Poon C, Merrill C (1997) Decrease of cardiac chaos in congestive heart failure. Nature 389: 492–495.
9. Lanata A, Valenza G, Mancuso C, Scilingo EP (2011) Robust multiple cardiac arrhythmia detection through bispectrum analysis. Expert Systems with Applications 38: 6798–6804.
10. Wu G, Arzeno N, Shen L, Tang D, Zheng D, et al. (2009) Chaotic signatures of heart rate variability and its power spectrum in health, aging and heart failure. PloS one 4: e4323.
11. Valenza G, Lanata A, Scilingo EP (2012) Oscillations of heart rate and respiration synchronize during affective visual stimulation. IEEE Transactions on Information Technology in Biomedicine 16: 683–690.
12. Winfree A (1994) Electrical turbulence in three-dimensional heart muscle. Science 266: 1003–1006.
13. Valenza G, Nardelli M, Lanata A, Gentili C, Bertschy G, et al. (2014) Wearable monitoring for mood recognition in bipolar disorder based on history-dependent long-term heart rate variability analysis. IEEE Journal of Biomedical and Health Informatics.
14. Chialvo DR, Gilmour Jr RF, Jalife J (1990) Low dimensional chaos in cardiac tissue. Nature 343: 653–657.
15. Valenza G, Lanatá A, Scilingo EP (2013) Improving emotion recognition systems by embedding cardiorespiratory coupling. Physiological measurement 34: 449.
16. Kanters JK, Højgaard MV, Agner E, Holstein-Rathlou NH (1996) Short-and long-term variations in non-linear dynamics of heart rate variability. Cardiovascular Research 31: 400–409.
17. Schmidt G, Monfill G (1995) Nonlinear methods for heart rate variability assessment. Heart rate variability Armonk: Futura: 87–98.
18. Jelinek HF, Khandoker AH, Quintana D, Imam MH, Kemp A (2011) Complex correlation measure as a sensitive indicator of risk for sudden cardiac death in patients with depression. In: Computing in Cardiology, 2011. IEEE, pp. 809–812.
19. Valenza G, Citi L, Scilingo E, Barbieri R (2013) Point-process nonlinear models with laguerre and volterra expansions: Instantaneous assessment of heartbeat dynamics. IEEE Transactions on Signal Processing 61: 2914–2926.
20. Valenza G, Allegrini P, Lanatà A, Scilingo EP (2012) Dominant lyapunov exponent and approximate entropy in heart rate variability during emotional visual elicitation. Frontiers in neuroengineering 5.
21. Schmitt DT, Stein PK, Ivanov PC (2009) Stratification pattern of static and scale-invariant dynamic measures of heartbeat fluctuations across sleep stages in young and elderly. IEEE Transactions on Biomedical Engineering 56: 1564–1573.
22. Valenza G, Citi L, Gentili C, Lanata A, Scilingo E, et al. (2014) Characterization of depressive states in bipolar patients using wearable textile technology and instantaneous heart rate variability assessment. IEEE Journal of Biomedical and Health Informatics.
23. Bär KJ, Boettger MK, Koschke M, Schulz S, Chokka P, et al. (2007) Non-linear complexity measures of heart rate variability in acute schizophrenia. Clinical neurophysiology 118: 2009–2015.
24. Tarvainen MP, Georgiadis S, Laitio T, Lipponen JA, Karjalainen PA, et al. (2012) Heart rate variability dynamics during low-dose propofol and dexmedetomidine anesthesia. Annals of biomedical engineering 40: 1802–1813.
25. Valenza G, Citi L, Scilingo EP, Barbieri R (2014) Inhomogeneous point-process entropy: An instantaneous measure of complexity in discrete systems. Physical Review E 89: 052803.
26. Orini M, Laguna P, Mainardi L, Bailón R (2012) Assessment of the dynamic interactions between heart rate and arterial pressure by the cross time–frequency analysis. Physiological measurement 33: 315.
27. Valenza G, Nardelli M, Bertschy G, Lanata A, Scilingo E (2014) Mood states modulate complexity in heartbeat dynamics: A multiscale entropy analysis. EPL (Europhysics Letters) 107: 18003.
28. Shimada I, Nagashima T (1979) A numerical approach to ergodic problem of dissipative dynamical systems. Progress of Theoretical Physics 61: 1605–1616.
29. Lyapunov A (1949) Problem general de la stabilite du mouvement. Ann Math Stud 17.
30. Keller J, Hense A, Rhodin A (2010) Estimating uncertainty in atmospheric models-application and new approaches of lyapunov vector estimations. In: AGU Fall Meeting Abstracts. volume 1, p. 1319.
31. Hernández-Carrasco I, López C, Hernández-García E, Turiel A (2011) How reliable are finite-size lyapunov exponents for the assessment of ocean dynamics? Ocean Modelling 36: 208–218.
32. Lindsay DH, Campbell A (2011) A chaos approach to bankruptcy prediction. Journal of Applied Business Research (JABR) 12: 1–9.
33. Hu J, Gao J, Tung Ww (2009) Characterizing heart rate variability by scale-dependent lyapunov exponent. Chaos: An Interdisciplinary Journal of Nonlinear Science 19: 028506–028506.
34. Wolf A, Swift JB, Swinney HL, Vastano JA (1985) Determining lyapunov exponents from a time series. Physica D: Nonlinear Phenomena 16: 285–317.
35. Abarbanel HD, Gollub JP (1996) Analysis of observed chaotic data. Physics Today 49: 86.
36. Ruelle D (1994) Where can one hope to profitably apply the ideas of chaos? Physics Today 47: 24.
37. Gao J, Cao Y, Tung Ww, Hu J (2007) Multiscale analysis of complex time series: integration of chaos and random fractal theory, and beyond. John Wiley & Sons.
38. Chon K, Yip K, Camino B, Marsh D, Holstein-Rathlou NH (2000) Modeling nonlinear determinism in short time series from noise driven discrete and continuous systems. International Journal of Bifurcation and Chaos 10: 2745–2766.
39. Armoundas A, Ju K, Iyengar N, Kanters J, Saul P, et al. (2002) A stochastic nonlinear autoregressive algorithm reflects nonlinear dynamics of heart-rate fluctuations. Annals of biomedical engineering 30: 192–201.
40. Korenberg M (1989) A robust orthogonal algorithm for system identification and time-series analysis. Biological Cybernetics 60: 267–276.
41. Barbieri R, Matten E, Alabi A, Brown E (2005) A point-process model of human heartbeat intervals: new definitions of heart rate and heart rate variability. American Journal of Physiology-Heart and Circulatory Physiology 288: H424.
42. Chen Z, Brown E, Barbieri R (2009) Assessment of autonomic control and respiratory sinus arrhythmia using point process models of human heart beat dynamics. IEEE Transactions on Biomedical Engineering 56: 1791–1802.
43. Marmarelis V (1993) Identification of nonlinear biological system using laguerre expansions of kernels. Ann Biomed Eng 21.
44. Valenza G, Citi L, Barbieri R (2013) Instantaneous nonlinear assessment of complex cardiovascular dynamics by laguerre-volterra point process models. In: Engineering in Medicine and Biology Society (EMBC), 2013 35th Annual International Conference of the IEEE. IEEE, pp. 6131–6134.
45. Citi L, Valenza G, Barbieri R (2012) Instantaneous estimation of high-order nonlinear heartbeat dynamics by lyapunov exponents. In: Proceeding of the IEEE-EMBC. pp. 13–16.
46. Citi L, Valenza G, Purdon PL, Brown EN, Barbieri R (2012) Monitoring heartbeat nonlinear dynamics during general anesthesia by using the instantaneous dominant lyapunov exponent. In: Engineering in Medicine and Biology Society (EMBC), 2012 Annual International Conference of the IEEE. IEEE, pp. 3124–3127.
47. Daley D, Vere-Jones D (2003) An introduction to the theory of point processes, vol. I: Elementary Theory and Methods, volume 2. Springer Verlag.
48. Chen Z, Purdon P, Harrell G, Pierce E, Walsh J, et al. (2011) Dynamic assessment of baroreflex control of heart rate during induction of propofol anesthesia using a point process method. Annals of biomedical engineering: 1–17.
49. Citi L, Brown E, Barbieri R (2012) A real-time automated point process method for detection and correction of erroneous and ectopic heartbeats.
50. Akay M (2000) Nonlinear Biomedical Signal Processing Vol. II: Dynamic Analysis and Modeling. Wiley-IEEE Press.
51. Korenberg M (1991) Parallel cascade identification and kernel estimation for nonlinear systems. Annals of biomedical engineering 19: 429–455.
52. Schetzen M (1980) The volterra and wiener theories of nonlinear systems.
53. Granger C, Joyeux R (1980) An introduction to long-memory time series models and fractional differencing. Journal of time series analysis 1: 15–29.
54. Dieci L, Russell R, Van Vleck E (1997) On the computation of lyapunov exponents for continuous dynamical systems. SIAM journal on numerical analysis: 402–423.
55. Holzfuss J, Parlitz U (1991) Lyapunov exponents from time series. Lyapunov Exponents: 263–270.
56. Geist K, Parlitz U, Lauterborn W (1990) Comparison of different methods for computing lyapunov exponents. Prog Theor Phys 83: 875–893.
57. Rajendra Acharya U, Paul Joseph K, Kannathal N, Lim C, Suri J (2006) Heart rate variability: a review. Medical and Biological Engineering and Computing 44: 1031–1051.
58. Rosenstein MT, Collins JJ, De Luca CJ (1993) A practical method for calculating largest lyapunov exponents from small data sets. Physica D: Nonlinear Phenomena 65: 117–134.
59. Pincus S (1991) Approximate entropy as a measure of system complexity. Proceedings of the National Academy of Sciences 88: 2297.

60. Richman J, Moorman J (2000) Physiological time-series analysis using approximate entropy and sample entropy. American Journal of Physiology-Heart and Circulatory Physiology 278: H2039.
61. Peng C, Buldyrev S, Havlin S, Simons M, Stanley H, et al. (1994) Mosaic organization of dna nucleotides. Physical Review E 49: 1685.
62. Zong W, Moody G (2003) Wqrs-single-channel qrs detector based on length transform. Physionet http://wwwphysionetorg/physiotools/wag/wqrs-1htm.
63. Goldberger A, Amaral L, Glass L, Hausdorff J, Ivanov P, et al. (2000) Physiobank, physiotoolkit, and physionet: Components of a new research resource for complex physiologic signals. Circulation 101: e215.
64. Barnett A, Wolff R (2005) A time-domain test for some types of nonlinearity. IEEE Transactions on Signal Processing. 53: 26–33.
65. Baillie R, Cecen A, Erkal C (2009) Normal heartbeat series are nonchaotic, nonlinear, and multifractal: New evidence from semiparametric and parametric tests. Chaos: An Interdisciplinary Journal of Nonlinear Science 19: 028503.
66. Costa M, Goldberger A, Peng C (2002) Multiscale entropy analysis of complex physiologic time series. Physical Review Letters 89: 68102.
67. Thuraisingham R, Gottwald G (2006) On multiscale entropy analysis for physiological data. Physica A: Statistical Mechanics and its Applications 366: 323–332.
68. Hagerman I, Berglund M, Lorin M, Nowak J, Sylvén C (1996) Chaos-related deterministic regulation of heart rate variability in time-and frequency domains: effects of autonomic blockade and exercise. Cardiovascular research 31: 410–418.
69. Porta A, Gnecchi-Ruscone T, Tobaldini E, Guzzetti S, Furlan R, et al. (2007) Progressive decrease of heart period variability entropy-based complexity during graded head-up tilt. Journal of applied physiology 103: 1143–1149.
70. Tulppo MP, Mäkikallio TH, Seppänen T, Shoemaker K, Tutungi E, et al. (2001) Effects of pharmacological adrenergic and vagal modulation on fractal heart rate dynamics. Clinical Physiology 21: 515–523.
71. Schwartz PJ, De Ferrari GM (2011) Sympathetic–parasympathetic interaction in health and disease: abnormalities and relevance in heart failure. Heart failure reviews 16: 101–107.

Cardiac Overexpression of Constitutively Active Galpha q Causes Angiotensin II Type1 Receptor Activation, Leading to Progressive Heart Failure and Ventricular Arrhythmias in Transgenic Mice

Naoko Matsushita[1,2], Toshihide Kashihara[3], Hisashi Shimojo[4], Satoshi Suzuki[5], Tsutomu Nakada[3], Yasuchika Takeishi[5], Ulrike Mende[6], Eiichi Taira[2], Mitsuhiko Yamada[3], Atsushi Sanbe[7], Masamichi Hirose[1]*

1 Department of Molecular and Cellular Pharmacology, Iwate Medical University School of Pharmaceutical Sciences, Shiwa, Iwate, Japan, **2** Department of Pharmacology, Iwate Medical University School of Medicine, Shiwa, Iwate, Japan, **3** Department of Molecular Pharmacology, Shinshu University School of Medicine, Matsumoto, Nagano, Japan, **4** Department of Pathology, Shinshu University School of Medicine, Matsumoto, Nagano, Japan, **5** Department of Cardiology and Hematology, Fukushima Medical University, Fukushima, Fukushima, Japan, **6** Cardiovascular Research Center, Division of Cardiology, Rhode Island Hospital & The Alpert Medical School of Brown University, Providence, Rhode Island, United States of America, **7** Department of Pharmacotherapeutics, Iwate Medical University School of Pharmaceutical Sciences, Shiwa, Iwate, Japan

Abstract

Background: Transgenic mice with transient cardiac expression of constitutively active Galpha q ($G\alpha_q$-TG) exhibt progressive heart failure and ventricular arrhythmias after the initiating stimulus of transfected constitutively active $G\alpha_q$ becomes undetectable. However, the mechanisms are still unknown. We examined the effects of chronic administration of olmesartan on heart failure and ventricular arrhythmia in $G\alpha_q$-TG mice.

Methodology/Principal Findings: Olmesartan (1 mg/kg/day) or vehicle was chronically administered to $G\alpha_q$-TG from 6 to 32 weeks of age, and all experiments were performed in mice at the age of 32 weeks. Chronic olmesartan administration prevented the severe reduction of left ventricular fractional shortening, and inhibited ventricular interstitial fibrosis and ventricular myocyte hypertrophy in $G\alpha_q$-TG. Electrocardiogram demonstrated that premature ventricular contraction (PVC) was frequently (more than 20 beats/min) observed in 9 of 10 vehicle-treated $G\alpha_q$-TG but in none of 10 olmesartan-treated $G\alpha_q$-TG. The collected QT interval and monophasic action potential duration in the left ventricle were significantly shorter in olmesartan-treated $G\alpha_q$-TG than in vehicle-treated $G\alpha_q$-TG. CTGF, collagen type 1, ANP, BNP, and β-MHC gene expression was increased and olmesartan significantly decreased the expression of these genes in $G\alpha_q$-TG mouse ventricles. The expression of canonical transient receptor potential (TRPC) 3 and 6 channel and angiotensin converting enzyme (ACE) proteins but not angiotensin II type 1 (AT_1) receptor was increased in $G\alpha_q$-TG ventricles compared with NTG mouse ventricles. Olmesartan significantly decreased TRPC6 and tended to decrease ACE expressions in $G\alpha_q$-TG. Moreover, it increased AT_1 receptor in $G\alpha_q$-TG.

Conclusions/Significance: These findings suggest that angiotensin II type 1 receptor activation plays an important role in the development of heart failure and ventricular arrhythmia in $G\alpha_q$-TG mouse model of heart failure.

Editor: Junichi Sadoshima, Rutgers New Jersey Medical School, United States of America

Funding: This study was supported in part by a Grant-in-Aid for Scientific Research from Ministry of Education, Culture, Sports, Science and Technology, Japan (No. 21590276) (M.H.) and the grant from KEIRYOKAI research foundation (M.H.). The funders had no role in study design, data collection and analysis, decision to publish, or preparation of the manuscript.

Competing Interests: The authors have declared that no competing interests exist.

* Email: mhirose@iwate-med.ac.jp

Introduction

Our previous study showed that transient expression of a constitutively active the GTP-binding protein α_q subunit in hearts of transgenic mice ($G\alpha_q$-TG mice) is sufficient to induce cardiac hypertrophy and heart failure (HF) [1]. In fact, although the $G\alpha_q$ protein decreases at 4 weeks and is undetectable until 10 weeks, the mice develop cardiac hypertrophy and dilatation, leading to HF until 16 to 32 weeks of age [1–4]. When the cardiac hypertrophy and dilatation develop, endogenous but not transfected $G\alpha_q$ rises in the heart. Basal and G_q-coupled receptor agonist stimulated activity of phospholipase Cß (PLCß), leading to generatiton of inositol trisphosphate (IP_3) and diacylglycerol (DAG), which is elevated in ventricles at 10 week age in $G\alpha_q$-TG mice, presumably at least in part because of the rise in endogenous $G\alpha_q$ [1,5]. Therefore, the pathological changes initiated by early transient constitutively active $G\alpha_q$ expression may be maintained by multiple and persistent changes in signal transduction pathways [1,5]. Our more recent studies demonstrated that diacylglycerol kinase zeta, which catalyzes DAG, rescues HF [2] and inhibited atrial [3] and ventricular [4] arrhythmias in $G\alpha_q$-TG mice, suggesting that DAG plays a critical role in the development of cardiac hypertrophy and HF in this mouse model. However, it is still unknown what factors act upstream of DAG. It is well known that the renin-angiotensin system, which increases the level of DAG, plays a critical role in the development of cardiac hypertrophy and HF [6–8]. We hypothesized that the renin-angiotensin system plays an important role in the development of cardiac hypertrophy and HF in this transgenic mouse model after the initiating stimulus of transfected constitutively active $G\alpha_q$ becomes undetectable. Olmesartan is an angiotensin II type 1 receptor antagonist, which can inhibit angiotensin II-induced cardiac remodeling and HF [9,10]. In the present study, therefore, we investigated the inhibitory effects of olmesartan on ventricular remodeling, leading to HF and ventricular arrhythmias in $G\alpha_q$-TG mice.

Materials and Methods

Ethics

This study was carried out in strict accordance with the recommendations in the Guide for the Care and Use of Laboratory Animals of the National Institutes of Health. This study was approved by the Animal Care Committee of the Iwate Medical University and Shinshu University. The protocol was approved by the Committee on the Ethics of Animal Experiments of the Iwate Medical University (Permit Number: 22–39) and the Shinshu University (Permit Number: 200044). All surgery was performed under sodium pentobarbital anesthesia, and all efforts were made to minimize suffering.

Experimental Animals

A transgenic mouse ($G\alpha_q$-TG mouse) with transient, modest expression of $HA\alpha^*_q$ was used [1]. The genotypes of the non-transgenic (NTG) and $G\alpha_q$-TG mice were identified by polymerase chain reaction (PCR) with the use of tail genomic DNA as a template, as previously reported [1]. Our previous studies demonstrated that $G\alpha_q$-TG mice developed HF but not ventricular arrhythmias at the age of 16 weeks, whereas they developed ventricular arrhythmias by 32 weeks [4]. We measured the systemic blood pressure and heart rate using the tail-cuff method. (BP-98A Softron, Tokyo, Japan) and demonstrated that olmesartan at a dose of 1 mg/kg/day did not decrease the systemic blood pressure (Table 1). Therefore, to examine the effects of chronic olmesartan administration on HF and ventricular arrhythmias, olmesartan (1 mg/kg/day) was orally administered to $G\alpha_q$-TG

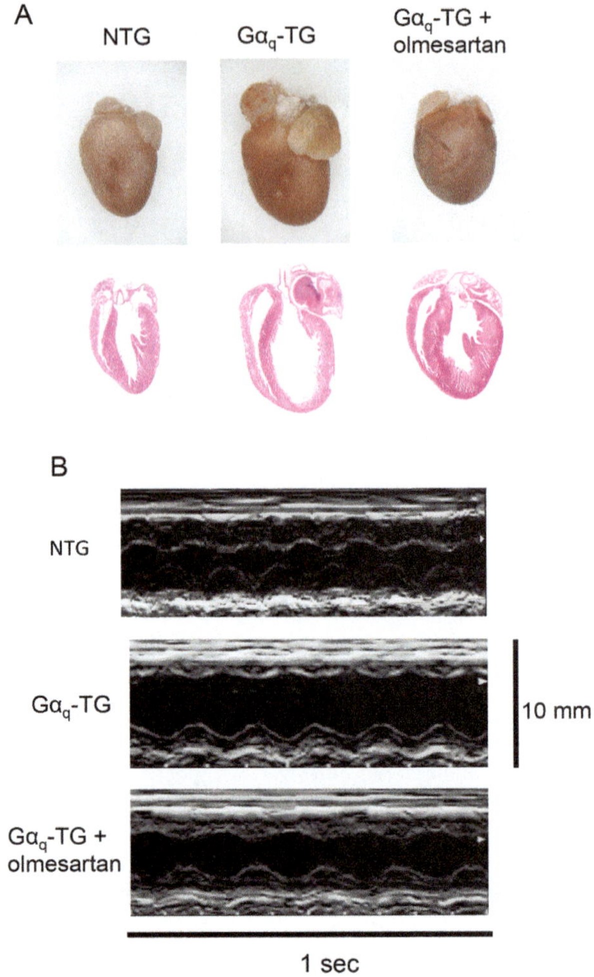

Figure 1. Effects of olmesartan on cardiac morphology and on the left ventricular contractile function. Panel A: Gross examination of a heart and its four-chamber view histology stained with hematoxylin/eosin in NTG, $G\alpha_q$-TG, and $G\alpha_q$-TG+olmesartan mouse hearts. The four-chamber view histology revealed all chambers to be dilated in the vehicle-treated $G\alpha_q$-TG heart compared with those in NTG and olmesartan-treated Gαq-TG hearts. Original magnification: 1.25×. Mice at the age of 32 weeks were used. Panel B: Representative M-mode echocardiograms of NTG, $G\alpha_q$-TG, and $G\alpha_q$-TG+olmesartan mice at the age of 32 weeks.

Table 1. Systemic blood pressure (BP) and heart rates in NTG, $G\alpha_q$-TG, and $G\alpha_q$-TG+olmesartan mice.

Parameters	NTG	$G\alpha_q$-TG	$G\alpha_q$-TG+olmesartan
HR (beats/min)	613±23	566±45	651±20
SBP (mmHg)	102±6	94±3	103±3
DBP (mmHg)	62±3	60±4	64±2
MBP(mmHg)	75±4	72±5	77±1

Data are the mean ± SE obtained from 7 mice for each group. SBP, systolic BP; DBP, diastric BP; MBP, mean BP.

Table 2. General parameters and the incidence of premature ventricular contraction (PVC) in NTG, Gα_q-TG, and Gα_q-TG+ olmesartan mice.

Parameters	NTG	Gα_q-TG	Gα_q-TG+olmesartan
BW (g)	26.5±1.9	27.8±2.0	32.0±1.9
HW (mg)	133±5.5	206±20.4^c	172±8.9^a
HW/BW (mg/g)	5.1±0.4	7.5±0.7^b	5.4±0.5$^+$
LA/TL (mm/mm)	0.14±0.06	0.33±0.03^c	0.19±0.02$^\$$
PVC (>20 beats/min)	0/10	9/10^c	0/10$^+$

Data are the mean ± SE obtained from 10 mice for each group. ^{a}p<0.05, ^{b}p<0.01, ^{c}p<0.001 vs. NTG, $^+$p<0.01, $^\$$p<0.001 vs. values in corresponding parameters of Gα_q-TG.

mice from 6 to 32 weeks of age. All experiments were performed in 32-week-old mice. As described in detail previously [11], all mice were anesthetized with sodium pentobarbital (30 mg/kg) applied intraperitoneally, and the adequacy of anesthesia was monitored by observing heart rate and the frequency and the degree of motion of the sternum as well as movement of the extremities.

Echocardiography

Vehicle-treated NTG, vehicle-treated Gα_q-TG, and olmesartan-treated Gα_q-TG mice (n =7 each) were anesthetized, and cardiac function was assessed by echocardiography (GE Yokogawa Medical System, Tokyo, Japan). As described in detail previously [12], the level of the papillary muscles along the short axis was used to view heart. The average of three consecutive beats in M-mode tracings was used to measure the following parameters: interventricular septum thickness, left ventricular end-diastolic dimension (LVEDd), end-systolic dimension (LVESd), and fractional shortening (LVFS), which was calculated as follows: (LVEDd - LVESd)/LVEDd×100%.

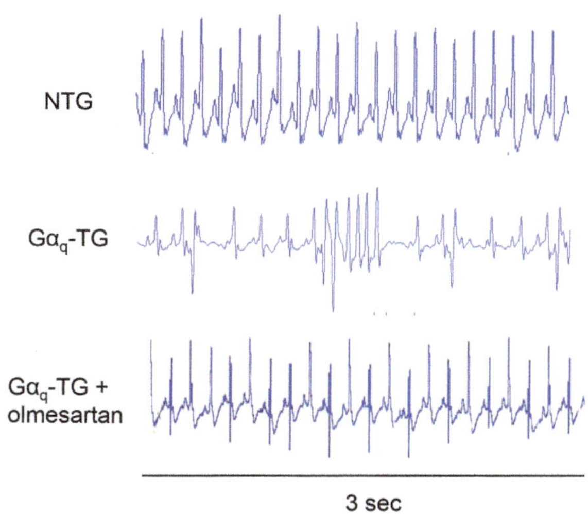

Figure 2. Electrocardiogram (ECG) lead II recordings from NTG, Gα_q-TG, and Gα_q-TG+olmesartan mice. The middle ECG shows ventricular arrhythmias recorded from vehicle-treated Gα_q-TG mice. PVC was frequently observed. In contrast, the upper and lower ECGs recorded from an NTG and olmesartan-treated Gα_q-TG mouse showed P waves and QRS complexes with regular RR intervals without any arrhythmia, indicating a sinus rhythm. Mice at the age of 32 weeks were used.

Electrocardiography (ECG) and Electrophysiological Measurement

Vehicle-treated NTG, vehicle-treated Gα_q-TG, and olmesartan-treated Gα_q-TG mice (n = 7 each) were anesthetized with sodium pentobarbital (30 mg/kg) applied intraperitoneally. Electrocardiography (ECG) lead II was recorded for 10 min in all mice. As described in detail previously [11], surface ECG was recorded and filtered (0.1 to 300 Hz), digitized with 12-bit precision at a sampling rate of 1000 Hz per channel (Microstar Laboratories Inc., Bellevue, WA, USA), transmitted into a microcomputer and saved on a CD-ROM.

In all mice examined, P, PR, QRS complex, QT, and RR intervals were measured from ECG lead II. The number of premature ventricular contractions (PVCs) per minute was calculated from ECG lead II. A high incidence of PVCs (High PVC) was defined as more than 20 beats/min of PVC.

Gross Anatomy and Histology

After vehicle-treated NTG, vehicle-treated Gα_q-TG, and olmesartan-treated Gα_q-TG mice (n = 10 each) were anesthetized, hearts were quickly excised. To examine gross anatomy and histology, the heart preparation was prepared. As described in detail previously [11], the hearts were fixed with a 30% solution of formalin in phosphate-buffered saline at room temperature for more than 24 hours, embedded in paraffin, and then cut serially from the apex to the base. Six sections were stained with hematoxylin/eosin or Masson's trichrome for histopathological analysis. To measure the cross-sectional diameter of cardiomyocytes, the diameter of at least 20 cardiomyocytes in each section was measured using the image analyzing software MacSCOPE (MITANI Corporation, Tokyo) on a Macintosh computer. The measurements were performed on 3 sections in each preparation and averaged. The degree of fibrosis was assessed by digital microscopic images taken from the sections stained with Masson's trichrome stain using light microscopy with a digital camera system. As described in detail previously [3], the measurements were performed on 3 images from different parts of the left ventricle in each preparation. The fibrosis fraction was obtained by calculating the ratio of total connective area to total myocardial area from 3 images in each preparation.

Western Blot Analysis

The ventricular myocardium of anesthetized NTG, vehicle-treated Gα_q-TG, and olmesartan-treated Gα_q-TG mice (n = 6 each) was prepared to extract the total protein using a lysis buffer (Cell Signaling Technology, Inc., Danvers, MA). The protein expression of canonical transient receptor potential (TRPC) and

Table 3. Echocardiographic parameters in NTG, Gα_q-TG, and Gα_q-TG+olmesartan mice.

Parameters	NTG	Gα_q-TG	Gα_q-TG+olmesartan
IVS (mm)	0.73±0.03	0.62±0.05	0.75±0.07
LVEDd (mm)	2.6±0.2	3.5±0.1^c	2.8±0.2$^+$
LVFS (%)	50.9±2.5	25.4±1.7^c	44.2±2.5$^{a,\$}$

Data are the mean ± SE obtained from 7 mice for each group. ^{a}p<0.01, ^{c}p<0.001 vs. NTG, $^+$p<0.01, $^\$$p<0.001 vs. values in corresponding parameters of Gα_q-TG. LVEDd, left ventricular end-diastolic dimension; IVS, intraventricular septum.

angiotensin-converting enzyme (ACE) isoforms was examined. As described in detail previously [11], protein concentrations were assayed, and equal amounts of the proteins were subjected to 10% SDS-PAGE and transferred to PVDF membranes. To ensure equivalent protein loading and to verify efficient protein transfer, membranes were stained with Ponceau S before incubating with primary isoform-specific antibodies against TRPC isoforms (TRPC 3 and 6; SIGMA, St. Louis, MO), ACE isoforms (ACE and ACE2; SIGMA, St. Louis, MO) and actin. [13] Immunoreactive bands were detected with an ECL kit (Amersham Biosciences Corp., Piscataway, NJ). The densitometric intensity of bands representing TRPC and ACE isoforms was normalized to that of actin. The protein expression levels of angiotensin II type 1 (AT_1) receptor in the ventricular myocardium of anesthetized NTG, vehicle-treated Gα_q-TG, and olmesartan-treated Gα_q-TG mice (n = 6 each) were also examined, as described in detail previously [14–15]. Western blot analyses were performed using anti-GAPDH antibody (Chemicon International, Temecula, CA, USA) and anti-AT_1 receptor antibody (Santa Cruz Biotechnology, Dallas, TX, USA).

Quantification of mRNA by Real-Time PCR

Total RNA was prepared from the ventricular myocardium of anesthetized NTG, vehicle-treated Gα_q-TG and olmesartan-treated Gα_q-TG mice (n = 7 each) with NucleoSpin RNA II (TAKARA Co. Ltd., Tokyo, Japan) according to the manufacturer's instructions. The mRNA levels of atrial natriuretic factor (ANF), B-type natriuretic peptide (BNP), β-myosin heavy chain (β-MHC), connective tissue growth factor (CTGF), collagen type 1, and acidic ribosomal protein P0 (ARPP0) were examined. As described in detail previously [11], one microgram of total RNA was used as a template for reverse transcription with the SuperScript III First-Strand synthesis system for qRT-PCR (Invitrogen, Carlsbad, CA). Partial cDNA fragments of ANF, BNP, β-MHC, CTGF, collagen type 1, and ARPP0 were amplified from the heart cDNA by PCR with DNA polymerase Fast SYBR Green Master Mix (Takara Bio, Shiga, Japan) to generate a standard curve for mRNA quantification. Real-time PCR was performed with an ABI Step One Real-Time PCR System (Applied Biosystems, Foster City, CA). The PCR mixture (10 μl) contained Fast SYBR Green Master (Mix) (Roche Diagnostics), standard cDNA (5×10^2 ng per reaction), and 200 nM forward and reverse primers. All primers used are listed in Table S1. The expression of each gene was normalized to that of ARPP0 mRNA because the expression of ARPP0 mRNA was most consistent among the groups. The specificity of the method was confirmed by dissociation analysis according to the instructions supplied by Applied Biosystems.

Monophasic action potential (MAP) measurement

Vehicle-treated NTG, vehicle-treated Gα_q-TG, and olmesartan-treated Gα_q-TG mice (n = 6 each) were anesthetized with sodium pentobarbital (30 mg/kg) applied intraperitoneally, and then treated with sodium heparin (500 USP units/kg i.v.). After the hearts were quickly excised, we connected them to a Langendorff apparatus. We used a polyterafluoroethylene-coated silver bipolar electrode to stimulate the epicardial surface of the left ventricle at the twice diastolic threshold current with a duration of 1 ms. As described in detail previously [11], to measure the monophasic action potential (MAP) duration, we put on MAP electrode on the epicardial surface of the posterior left ventricle. MAPs were recorded for 5 sec at a basic cycle length of 200 ms. Each heart preparation was perfused under constant pressure conditions (65 mmHg) with oxygenated (95% oxygen, 5% CO_2) Tyrode's solution containing, in mM: NaCl, 141.0; KCl, 5.0; $CaCl_2$, 1.8; $NaHCO_3$, 25.0; $MgSO_4$, 1.0; NaH_2PO_4, 1.2; HEPES, 5; and dextrose, 5.0 (pH of 7.4 at 36±1°C). The MAP signals were filtered (0.3 to 300 Hz), amplified (1,000×), and recorded. As described in detail previously [11], the MAP duration was calculated from MAP signals of all Langendorff hearts.

Table 4. Electrocardiographic parameters in NTG, Gα_q-TG, and Gα_q-TG+olmesartan mice.

Parameters	NTG	Gα_q-TG	Gα_q-TG+olmesartan
P (msec)	21±1	29±1^b	22±1$^\$$
RR (msec)	182±12	218±29	229±19
PR (msec)	49±5	87±8^a	50±4$^\&$
QRS (msec)	15±0.6	20±1^a	21±1^a
QT (msec)	33±1	43±2^b	37±1$^{a,+}$

Data are the mean ± SE obtained from 7 mice for each group. ^{a}p<0.05, ^{b}p<0.001 vs. WT, $^+$p<0.05, $^\&$p<0.01, $^\$$p<0.001 vs. values in corresponding parameters of vehicle-treated Gα_q-TG.

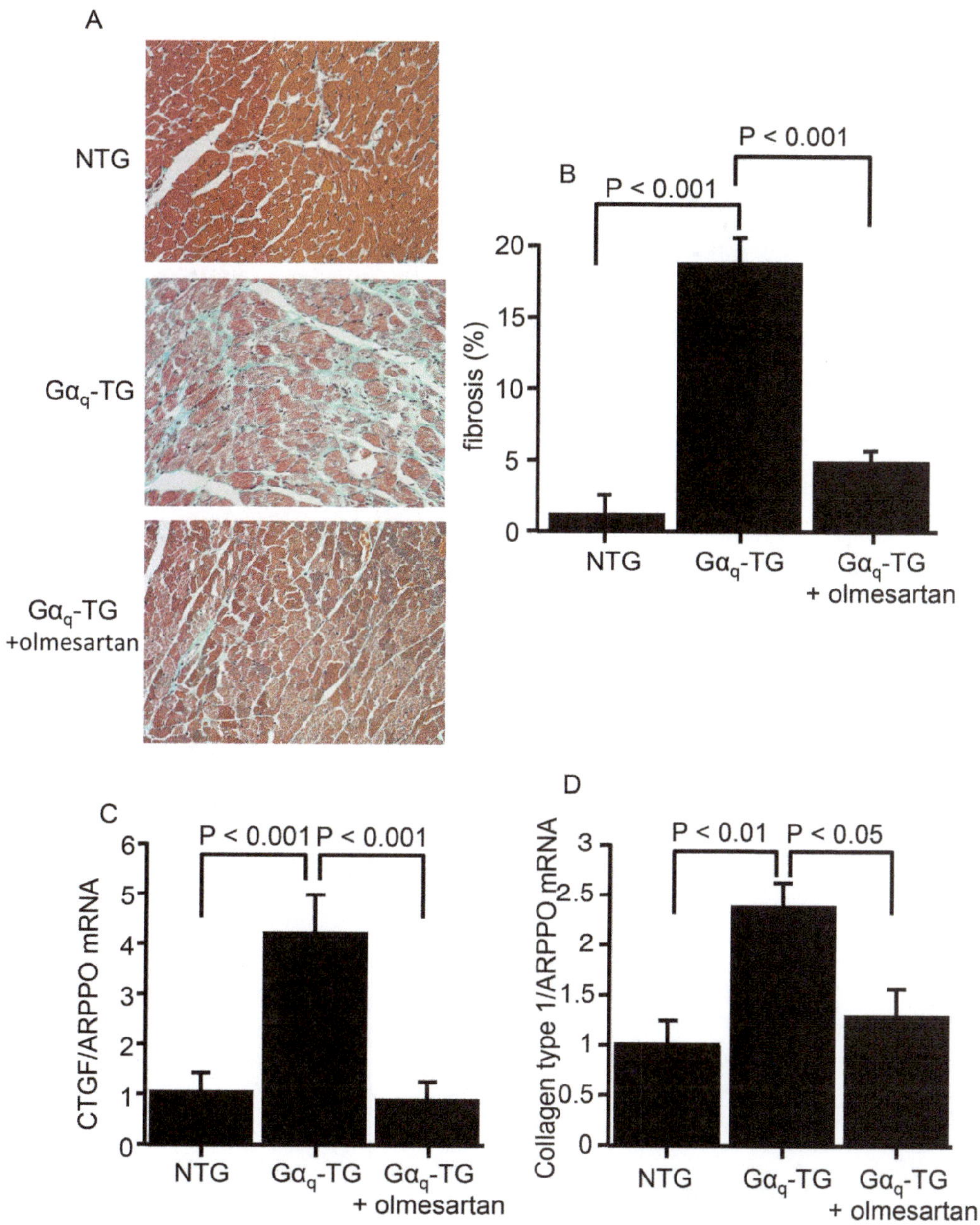

Figure 3. Effects of olmesartan on the left ventricular fibrosis and on connective tissue growth factor (CTGF) and collagen type 1 gene expression. Panel A: Histology of the left ventricle stained with Masson's trichrome in NTG, $G\alpha_q$-TG, and $G\alpha_q$-TG+olmesartan mice. Original magnification: 40×. Panel B: Comparison of the fibrosis fraction in the left ventricle in NTG, $G\alpha_q$-TG, and $G\alpha_q$-TG+olmesartan mice. Panels C and D: Quantitative analyses of CTGF (C) and collagen type 1 (D) gene expression by real-time reverse transcriptase-polymerase chain reaction (RT-PCR) in NTG, $G\alpha_q$-TG, and $G\alpha_q$-TG+olmesartan hearts. Data for CTGF and collagen type 1 were normalized to those for ARPP0. Data are the mean ± SE obtained from 6 mice for each group.

Data Analysis

All data are shown as the mean ± SE. The statistical analysis of multiple comparisons of data was calculated using An analysis of variance with Bonferroni's test. The incidence of High PVC between different conditions was compared using Fisher's exact test. $P<0.05$ was considered statistically significant.

Drug

Olmesartan was kindly provided by Daiichi Sankyo Pharmaceutical Co. (Tokyo, Japan).

Results

Effects of Olmesartan on the Development of Cardiomegaly and Contractile Dysfunction in $G\alpha_q$-TG Mice

Effects of chronic administration of olmesartan on cardiac morphology was examined in NTG, vehicle-treated $G\alpha_q$-TG, and olmesartan-treated $G\alpha_q$-TG mice at the age of 32 weeks. All four-chambers were dilated in the vehicle-treated $G\alpha_q$-TG heart compared with those in NTG and olmesartan-treated Gαq-TG hearts (Fig. 1A). The marked cardiomegaly was observed in the

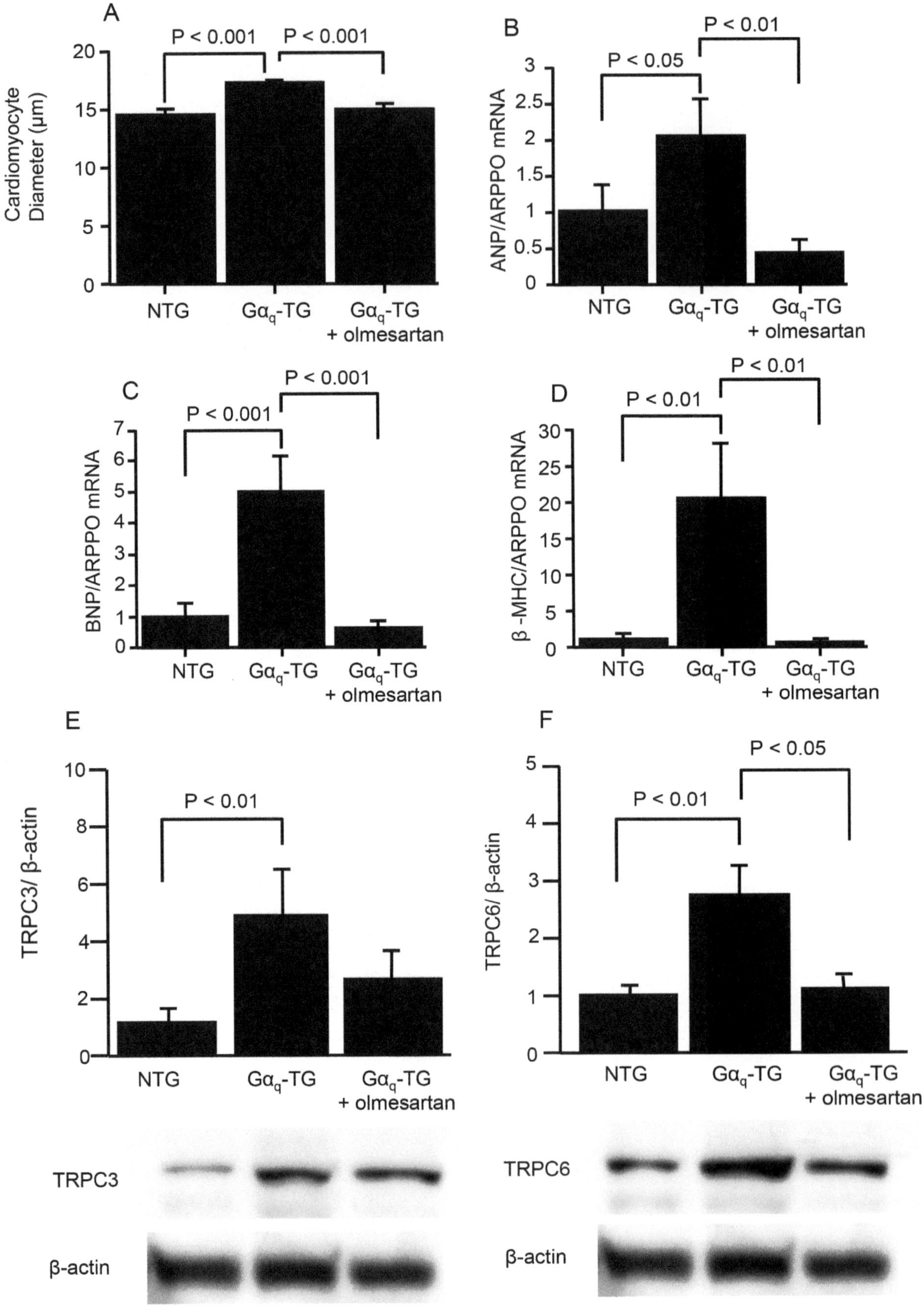
A
P < 0.001
P < 0.001
Cardiomyocyte Diameter (μm)
20
15
10
5
0
NTG
Gαq-TG
Gαq-TG + olmesartan
B
P < 0.01
P < 0.05
ANP/ARPPO mRNA
3
2.5
2
1.5
1
0.5
0
NTG
Gαq-TG
Gαq-TG + olmesartan
C
P < 0.001
P < 0.001
BNP/ARPPO mRNA
7
6
5
4
3
2
1
0
NTG
Gαq-TG
Gαq-TG + olmesartan
D
P < 0.01
P < 0.01
β -MHC/ARPPO mRNA
30
25
20
15
10
5
0
NTG
Gαq-TG
Gαq-TG + olmesartan
E
P < 0.01
TRPC3/ β-actin
10
8
6
4
2
0
NTG
Gαq-TG
Gαq-TG + olmesartan
TRPC3
β-actin
F
P < 0.05
P < 0.01
TRPC6/ β-actin
5
4
3
2
1
0
NTG
Gαq-TG
Gαq-TG + olmesartan
TRPC6
β-actin

Figure 4. Effects of olmesartan on the left ventricular hypertrophy, on ANP, BNP, and β-MHC gene expression, and on protein expression of canonical transient receptor potential (TRPC) channel isoforms. Panel A: Comparison of cardiomyocyte size in the left ventricle in NTG, $G\alpha_q$-TG, and $G\alpha_q$-TG+olmesartan mice. Panels B–D: Quantitative analyses of ANP (B), BNP (C), and β-MHC (D) gene expression by real-time RT-PCR in NTG, $G\alpha_q$-TG, and $G\alpha_q$-TG+olmesartan hearts. Data for ANP, BNP, and β-MHC were normalized to those for ARPP0. Data are the mean ± SE obtained from 6 mice for each group. Panel E: Expression of TRPC channel isoforms in NTG, $G\alpha_q$-TG, and $G\alpha_q$-TG+olmesartan hearts. TRPC isoform expression was normalized to actin expression and is expressed relative to wt (set at 1). Data are the mean ± SE obtained from 6 mice for each group. ANF, atrial natriuretic factor; BNP, B-type natriuretic peptide; β-MHC, β-myosin heavy chain; ARPP0, acidic ribosomal protein P0. Mice at the age of 32 weeks were used.

vehicle-treated $G\alpha_q$-TG mouse. The heart/body weight ratio increased in vehicle-treated $G\alpha_q$-TG mice compared with that in NTG mice. Olmesartan significantly reduced the ratio in $G\alpha_q$-TG mice (Table 2). The left atrial size/tibial length ratio was also increased in vehicle-treated $G\alpha_q$-TG compared with that in NTG hearts. Olmesartan also decreased the ratio in $G\alpha_q$-TG hearts (Table 2). Representative M-mode echocardiograms are shown in Figure 1B. Compared with the NTG mice, vehicle-treated $G\alpha_q$-TG mice showed the markedly reduced LVFS and the increased LVEDd (Fig. 1B and Table 3). Interestingly, olmesartan significantly improved the reduced LVFS and increased LVEDd in $G\alpha_q$-TG mice (Fig. 1B and Table 3).

Olmesartan-induced Reduction of the Number of Premature Ventricular Contractions (PVCs) in $G\alpha_q$-TG Mice

Figure 2 shows representative ECGs recorded form anesthetized NTG, vehicle-treated $G\alpha_q$-TG, and olmesartan-treated $G\alpha_q$-TG mice. The middle ECG shows ventricular arrhythmias recorded from vehicle-treated $G\alpha_q$-TG mice. Premature ventricular contraction (PVC) and non-sustained ventricular tachyarrhythmia (VT) were frequently observed. In contrast, the upper and lower ECGs recorded from an NTG- and olmesartan-treated $G\alpha_q$-TG mouse showed P waves and QRS complexes with regular RR intervals without any arrhythmia, indicating a sinus rhythm. Table 2 shows the overall data for ventricular arrhythmias. NTG mice did not induce ventricular arrhythmias such as a high PVC count (more than 20 beats/min). In contrast, a high number of PVCs was observed in 9 of 10 vehicle-treated $G\alpha_q$-TG mice (Table 2). Moreover, non of olmesartan-treated $G\alpha_q$-TG mice induced a high PVC count, indicating a significant reduction of ventricular arrhythmias in olmesartan-treated $G\alpha_q$-TG mice compared with that in vehicle-treated $G\alpha_q$-TG mice.

Effects of Olmesartan on Changes in Electrocardiogram Parameters in $G\alpha_q$-TG Mice

Overall data for the electrophysiological parameters in NTG, vehicle-treated $G\alpha_q$-TG, and olmesartan-treated $G\alpha_q$-TG mice at 32 weeks of age are shown in Table 4. P, PR, QRS, and QT interval were longer in vehicle-treated $G\alpha_q$-TG mice than in NTG mice. Interestingly, while the prolonged QRS interval was still observed in olmesartan-treated $G\alpha_q$-TG mice compared with NTG mice, the P, PR, and QT intervals were restored to normal levels in olmesartan-treated $G\alpha_q$-TG compared with those in vehicle-treated $G\alpha_q$-TG mice.

Effects of Olmesartan on Myocardial Fibrosis and the mRNA Expression of Profibrotic Genes in $G\alpha_q$-TG Mice

The effects of chronic olmesartan administration on left ventricular myocardial fibrosis and profibrotic gene expressions of $G\alpha_q$-TG mice at the age of 32 weeks are shown in figure 3. Vehicle-treated $G\alpha_q$-TG hearts induced extensive interstitial fibrosis in the left ventricle compared with that in NTG and olmesartan-treated $G\alpha_q$-TG hearts. The degree of myocardial fibrosis in the left ventricle was significantly greater in vehicle-treated $G\alpha_q$-TG mice compared with that in NTG mice (Fig. 3B). Olmesartan-tretated $G\alpha_q$-TG mice showed the reduced interstitial fibrosis compared with vehicle-treated $G\alpha_q$-TG mice (Fig. 3B). Interestingly, compared with NTG mouse hearts CTGF and collagen type 1 mRNA expression levels were significantly upregulated in vehicle-treated $G\alpha_q$-TG mouse hearts (Fig. 3C and D). Olmesartan significantly decreased the increased expression of those profibrotic genes in $G\alpha_q$-TG hearts (Fig. 3C and D).

Effects of Olmesartan on Cardiomyocyte Hypertrophy, Fetal Gene Expression and TRPC 6 Channel Protein Levels in $G\alpha_q$-TG Mice

The effects of olmesartan on the cardiomyocyte hypertrophy and the mRNA expression of fetal type genes such as ANF, β-MHC, and BNP in $G\alpha_q$-TG mice are shown in figure 4. The cross-sectional diameter of cardiomyocytes in vehicle-treated $G\alpha_q$-TG mice was longer than that in NTG mice (Fig. 4A). The increased cross-sectional diameter was significantly decreased in olmesartan-treated $G\alpha_q$-TG mice (Fig. 4A). Moreover, the mRNA expression levels of ANF, BNP, and β-MHC were significantly upregulated in $G\alpha_q$-TG hearts compared with that in NTG mouse hearts (Figs. 4B, C, and D). The increased gene expression of ANF, BNP, and β-MHC was decreased in olmesartan-treated $G\alpha_q$-TG hearts (Figs. 4B, C, and D). Recent studies have suggested that the activation of TRPC channels plays important roles in the generation of cardiac hypertrophy and cardiac arrhythmia induction [4,16]. Moreover, TRPC3 and 6 protein expression levels were increased in $G\alpha_q$-TG mouse hearts [4]. Therefore, we examined the effects of olmesartan on the protein expression of TRPC3 and 6 channels in $G\alpha_q$-TG hearts. Compared with NTG hearts, the vehicle-treated $G\alpha_q$-TG hearts exhibited the increased TRPC 3 and 6 protein levels (Figs. 4E and F). The increased expression of TRPC 6 protein was decreased in olmesartan-treated $G\alpha_q$-TG mouse hearts (Fig. 4F).

Effects of Olmesartan on Angiotensin Converting Enzyme (ACE) and Angiotensin II Type 1 (AT_1) Receptor Protein Expression in $G\alpha_q$-TG Mice

We examined the protein expression levels of ACE, ACE2, and AT_1 receptor in NTG, vehicle-treated $G\alpha_q$-TG, and olmesartan-treated $G\alpha_q$-TG mice at the age of 32 weeks. The level of ACE but not ACE2 was significantly increased in $G\alpha_q$-TG hearts compared with that in NTG hearts (Figs. 5A and B). Olmesartan tended to decrease the increased expression of ACE in $G\alpha_q$-TG mouse hearts (Fig. 5A). The level of AT_1 receptor was not changed in $G\alpha_q$-TG hearts compared with that in NTG hearts (Fig. 5C). Olmesartan significantly increased the expression of AT_1 receptor in $G\alpha_q$-TG mouse hearts (Fig. 5C).

Effects of Olmesartan on Ventricular Monophasic Action Potential (MAP) in $G\alpha_q$-TG Mice

Figure 6A showed examples of left ventricular MAPs in Langendorff-perfused NTG, $G\alpha_q$-TG, and olmesartan-treated

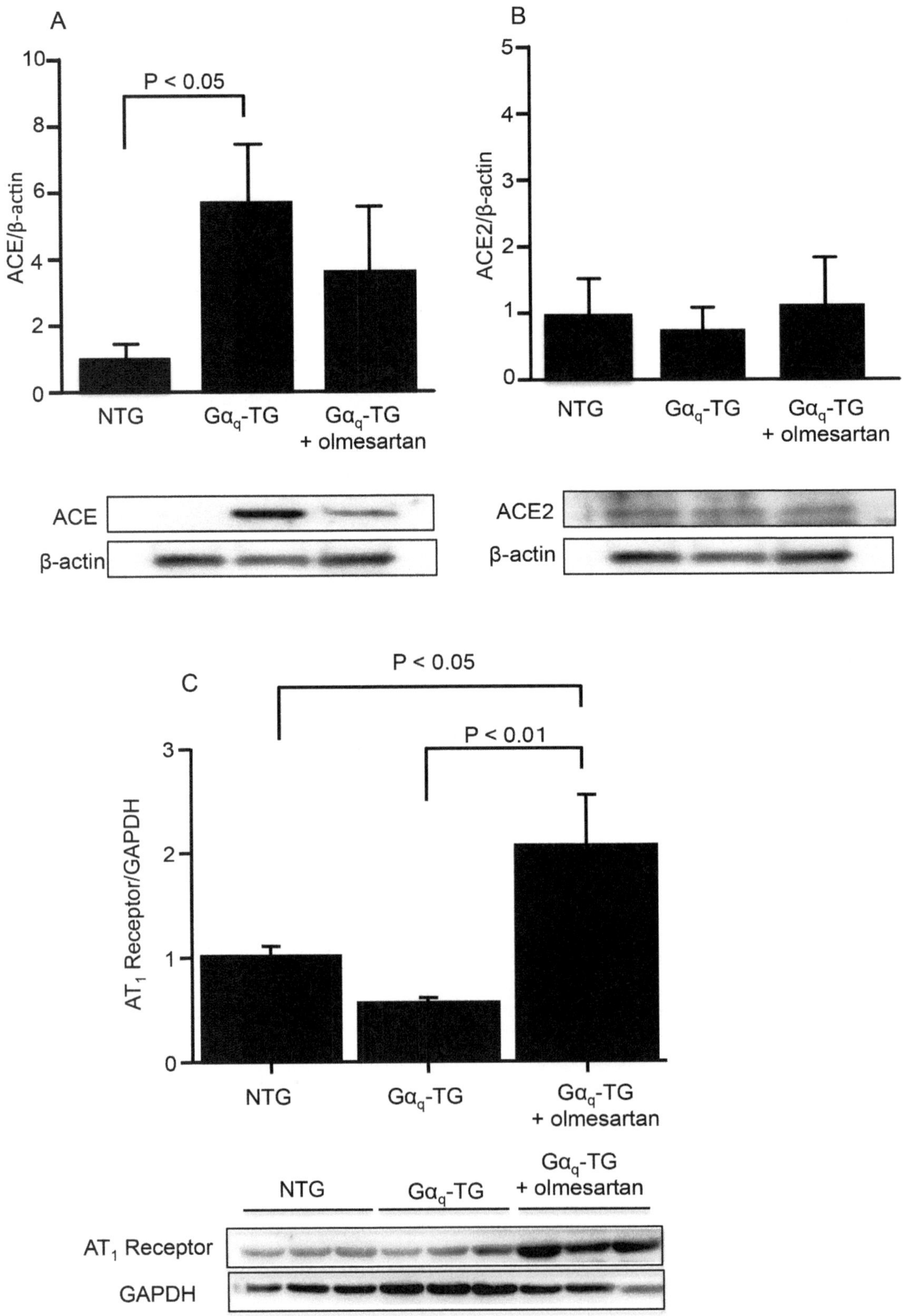

Figure 5. Effects of olmesartan on protein expression of angiotensin converting enzyme (ACE) isoforms and angiotensin II type 1 (AT_1) receptor. Expression of ACE (A), ACE2 (B), and AT_1 receptor (C) in NTG, $G\alpha_q$-TG, and $G\alpha_q$-TG+olmesartan hearts. ACE isoform expression was normalized to actin expression and is expressed relative to NTG (set at 1). AT_1 receptor was normalized to GAPDH and is expressed relative to NTG (set at 1). Data are the mean ± SE obtained from 6 mice for each group. Mice at the age of 32 weeks were used.

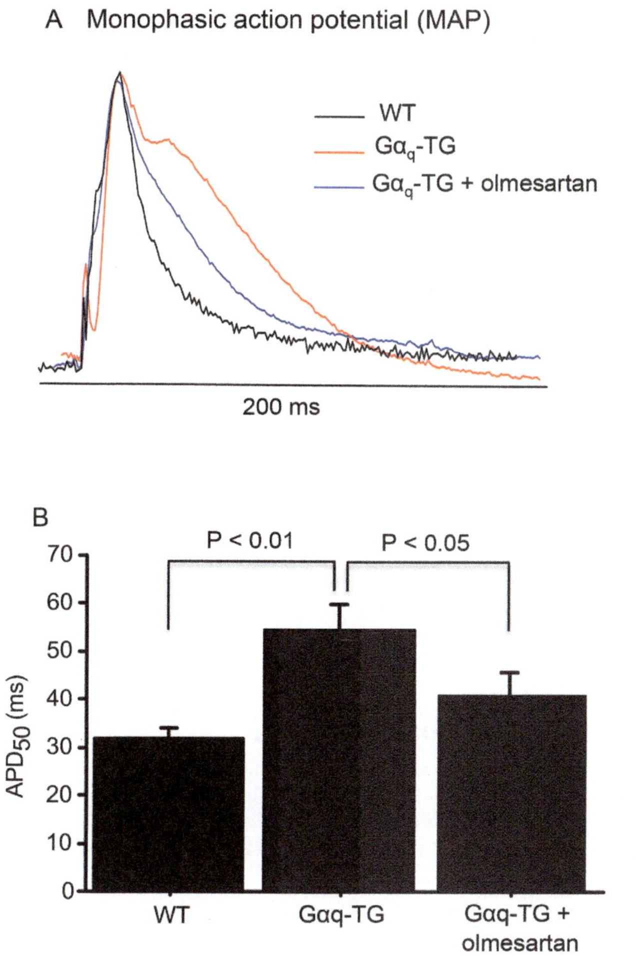

Figure 6. Effects of chronic olmesartan treatment on ventricular monophasic action potential (MAP) duration. Panel A: Representative examples of MAPs recorded from the posterior left ventricle in a Langendorff-perfused in NTG, $G\alpha_q$-TG, and $G\alpha_q$-TG+ olmesartan hearts during steady state pacing at a cycle length of 200 msec. Panel B: Overall data of MAP duration in in NTG, $G\alpha_q$-TG, and $G\alpha_q$-TG+olmesartan hearts.

$G\alpha_q$-TG mouse heart. The MAP duration prolonged in the $G\alpha_q$-TG heart compared with that in the NTG and olmesartan-treated $G\alpha_q$-TG mouse hearts. The overall data demonstrated that the chronic administration of olmesartan significantly shortened the ventricular MAP duration in $G\alpha_q$-TG hearts.

Discussion

In this study, we found that ACE but not ACE2 and AT_1 receptor protein expression was increased in vehicle-treated $G\alpha_q$-TG mouse hearts. Moreover, chronic administration of olmesartan for 26 weeks prevented the progression of heart failure and ventricular arrhythmia in $G\alpha_q$-TG mice. We also found that olmesartan inhibited ventricular interstitial fibrosis and ventricular myocyte hypertrophy in $G\alpha_q$-TG. CTGF, collagen type 1, ANP, BNP, and β-MHC gene expression was increased in vehicle-treated $G\alpha_q$-TG. Olmesartan significantly decreased the expression of these genes in $G\alpha_q$-TG mice. Electrocardiogram demonstrated that premature ventricular contraction (PVC) was frequently observed in 9 of 10 vehicle-treated $G\alpha_q$-TG but in none of 10 olmesartan-treated $G\alpha_q$-TG. These results suggest that angiotensin II type 1receptor activation plays crucial roles in cardiac remodeling and ventricular arrhythmia in $G\alpha_q$-TG mice.

Clinical and experimental studies have demonstrated that the G_q-phosphoinositide signaling pathway plays important roles in the development of cardiac hypertrophy and heart failure [17–21]. It is well known that several bioactive factors such as angiotensin, endothelin, and norepinephrine activate the cardiac G_q-phosphoinositide signaling pathway. Our previous study showed that transient expression of a constitutively active mutant of $G\alpha_q$ in hearts of transgenic mice is sufficient to induce cardiac hypertrophy and dilatation. In fact, after the initiating stimulus of the transgenic constitutively active $G\alpha_q$ was not detected the cardiac hypertrophy and dilatation continued to progress [1]. We showed that the multiple and persistent changes in signal transduction pathways maintained cardiac pathological changes initiated by early transient expression of constitutively active $G\alpha_q$ [1,5]. It is well known that the renin-angiotensin system, which increases the level of DAG, plays a critical role in the development of cardiac hypertrophy and HF [6–8]. In addition, cardiac renin-angiotensin system activation (i.e. local) is important in the development of cardiac hypertrophy [22]. Moreover, increased cardiac tissue ACE is known to play important roles in cardiac remodeling [23]. In this study, the protein expression of ACE was increased significantly in $G\alpha_q$ TG mouse hearts compared with that in NTG mouse hearts. In addition, left ventricular myocyte hypertrophy was observed and olmesartan significantly inhibited it (Fig. 4A), which was associated with the prevention of HF and ventricular arrhythmia induction in $G\alpha_q$-TG mice (Fig. 4A). Moreover, mRNA expression of ANF, β-MHC, and BNP was significantly upregulated in $G\alpha_q$-TG hearts compared with that in NTG mouse hearts and decreased by olmesartan in $G\alpha_q$-TG hearts (Figs. 4B, C, and D). These results suggest that transient $G\alpha_q$ activation causes activation of the local renin-angiotensin system, leading to progressive heart failure and ventricular arrhythmias in $G\alpha_q$-TG mice. These findings suggest that the cardiac renin-angiotensin system plays an important role in the development of cardiac hypertrophy and heart failure, even if the initiating stimulus of cardiac $G\alpha_q$ activation does not result from angiotensin II type I (AT_1) receptor stimulation.

Several studies have demonstrated that cardiac remodeling is associated with increases in AT_1 receptor protein expression [24–26]. Moreover, olmesartan suppressed cardiac AT_1 receptor levels in hypertensive rats [24]. In this study, the protein expression levels of AT_1 receptor were not changed in $G\alpha_q$-TG hearts compared with those in NTG hearts (Fig. 5C). Moreover, olmesartan significantly increased the expression of AT_1 receptor in $G\alpha_q$-TG mouse hearts (Fig. 5C). The reason for the discrepancy between the previous and present results is uncertain. In fact, cardiac dysfunction is severe in this $G\alpha_q$-TG mouse compared with that in animals used in previous studies [24,26]. Moreover, the duration of olmesartan treatment was much longer in this study than in the previous study [24]. Those differences may explain the discrepancy. In any case, our present results suggest that AT_1 receptor activation plays important roles in the development of heart failure and ventricular arrhythmias in this model.

It is known that myocardial ACE is a possible substrate for cardiac fibrosis [23]. In this study, the protein expression of ACE was increased significantly in $G\alpha_q$ TG mouse hearts compared with that in NTG mouse hearts. Moreover, the left ventricular fibrosis and mRNA expression of CTGF and collagen type I were also significantly increased in $G\alpha_q$-TG mouse hearts. Olmesartan decreased the increased left ventricular fibrosis and the mRNA expression of CTGF and collagen type I, suggesting that the renin-angiotensin system participates in the development of cardiac fibrosis in this model. Importantly, together these findings suggest that the cardiac renin-angiotensin system plays an important role in the development of cardiac hypertrophy, fibrosis and heart even if the initiating stimulus of cardiac $G\alpha_q$ activation does not result from AT_1 receptor stimulation.

It has been shown that mechanical stress activates AT_1 receptor independently of angiotensin II, and this activation can be inhibited by an inverse agonist of the AT_1 receptor [27–28]. Our previous study demonstrated that the left ventricular end-diastolic pressure was increased in $G\alpha_q$-TG compared with that in NTG mice [2], suggesting that mechanical stretching of the myocardium was induced in $G\alpha_q$-TG mice, leading to activation of AT_1 receptors. Recent study has demonstrated that olmesartan has strong inverse agonist activities against the constitutively active AT_1 receptor and the stretch-induced activation of AT_1 receptor, respectively [28]. Therefore, olmesartan induced inhibition of ventricular myocyte hypertrophy and interstitial fibrosis in $G\alpha_q$-TG may be caused in part through inverse agonistic action.

In this study, chronic administration of olmesartan prevented the progression of heart failure and ventricular arrhythmia in $G\alpha_q$-TG mice. In fact, electrocardiogram demonstrated that PVC was frequently (more than 20 beats/min) observed in 9 of 10 vehicle-treated $G\alpha_q$-TG mice but in none of 10 olmesartan-treated $G\alpha_q$-TG mice. In addition, the QT interval was significantly shorter in olmesartan-treated $G\alpha_q$-TG than in vehicle-treated $G\alpha_q$-TG mice. Moreover, the MAP duration was also significantly shorter in olmesartan-treated $G\alpha_q$-TG than in vehicle-treated $G\alpha_q$-TG mice. It is well known that ventricular arrhythmias are common in heart failure. However, a recent study demonstrated that chronic angiotensin II stimulation in the heart directly induced QT prolongation through down-regulation of potassium channels, [29] which can induce triggered activity, leading to the production of PVC. Moreover, a recent study clearly demonstrated that AT_1 receptor signaling in the heart directly contributed to the increased arrhythmogenicity in cardiac hypertrophy [30]. In fact, our previous study demonstrated that early-after depolarization by the prolongation of action potential duration caused triggered activity. Therefore, in addition to improvement of heart failure olmesartan might directly inhibit PVC induction because of the shortening of action potential duration. We previously demonstrated that the protein levels of TRPC3 and 6 are increased in $G\alpha_q$-TG hearts [4] and suggested that the activation of TRPC channels participates in the generation of cardiac arrhythmia induction. Interestingly, olmesartan decreased the increased expression of TRPC 6 in $G\alpha_q$-TG mouse hearts (Fig. 4F) in this study, suggesting that AT_1 receptor activation contributes to an increase in TRPC6 expression, leading to ventricular arrhythmia induction.

Supporting Information

Table S1 Primers used in this study.

Acknowledgments

We are grateful to Ms. Reiko Sakai for her secretarial assistance.

Author Contributions

Conceived and designed the experiments: MH NM. Performed the experiments: NM SS TK HS TN MH AS. Analyzed the data: NM SS TK HS TN MH MY AS. Contributed reagents/materials/analysis tools: MY UM YT ET. Contributed to the writing of the manuscript: UM MH MY ET YT.

References

1. Mende U, Kagen A, Cohen A, Aramburu J, Schoen FJ, et al. (1998) Transient cardiac expression of constitutively active Gaq leads to hypertrophy and dilated cardiomyopathy by calcineurin-dependent and independent pathways. Proc Natl Acad Sci USA 95: 13893–13898.
2. Niizeki T, Takeishi Y, Kitahara T, Arimoto T, Koyama Y, et al. (2008) Diacylglycerol kinase zeta rescues G alpha q-induced heart failure in transgenic mice. Circ J 72: 309–317.
3. Hirose M, Takeishi Y, Niizeki T, Shimojo H, Nakada T, et al. (2009) Diacylglycerol kinase ζ inhibits Gαq-induced atrial remodeling in transgenic mice. Heart Rhythm 6: 78–84.
4. Hirose M, Takeishi Y, Niizeki T, Nakada T, Shimojo H, et al. (2011) Diacylglycerol kinase ζ inhibits ventricular tachyarrhythmias in a mouse model of heart failure: Roles of canonical transient receptor potential (TRPC) channels. Circ J 75: 2333–2342.
5. Mende U, Kagen A, Meister M, Neer EJ (1999) Signal transduction in atria and ventricles of mice with transient cardiac expression of activated G protein alpha(q). Circ Res 85: 1085–1091.
6. Granger CB, McMurray JJ, Yusuf S, Held P, Michelson EL, et al. (2003) Effects of candesartan in patients with chronic heart failure and reduced left-ventricular systolic function intolerant to angiotensin converting enzyme inhibitors: the CHARM-Alternative trial. Lancet 362: 772–776.
7. The SOLVD Investigators (1991) Effect of enalapril on survival in patients with reduced left ventricular ejection fractions, and congestive heart failure. N Engl J Med 325: 293–302.
8. Farmer JA, Torre-Amione G (2001) The renin angiotensin system as a risk factor for coronary artery disease. Curr Atheroscler Rep 3: 117–124.
9. Nishio M, Sakata Y, Mano T, Yoshida J, Ohtani T, et al. (2007) Therapeutic effects of angiotensin II type 1 receptor blockerat an advanced stage of hypertensive diastolic heart failure. J Hypertens 25: 455–461.
10. Yoshida K, Kohzuki M (2004) Clinical and experimental aspects of olmesartan medoxomil, a new angiotensin II receptor antagonist. Cardiovasc Drug Rev 22: 285–308.
11. Hirose M, Takeishi Y, Nakada T, Shimojo H, Kashihara T, et al. Nicorandil prevents $G\alpha_q$-induced progressive heart failure and ventricular arrhythmias in transgenic mice. PLoS One 7;e52667, 2012.
12. Kamiyoshi Y, Takahashi M, Yokoseki O, Yazaki Y, Hirose S, et al. (2005) Mycophenolate mofetil prevents the development of experimental autoimmune myocarditis. J Mol Cell Cardiol 39: 467–477.
13. Niizeki T, Takeishi Y, Kitahara T, Arimoto T, Ishino M, et al. (2008) Diacylglycerol kinase-ε restores cardiac dysfunction under chronic pressure overload: a new specific regulator of Gαq signaling cascade. Am J Physiol 295: H245–H255.
14. Sanbe A, Daicho T, Mizutani R, Endo T, Miyauchi N, et al. (2009) Protective effect of geranylgeranylacetone via enhancement of HSPB8 induction in desmin-related cardiomyopathy. PLoS One 4: e5351.
15. Sanbe A, Marunouchi T, Yamauchi J, Tanonaka K, Nishigori H, et al. (2011) Cardioprotective effect of nicorandil, a mitochondrial ATP-sensitive potassium channel opener, prolongs survival in HSPB5 R120G transgenic mice. PLoS ONE 25: e18922.
16. Onohara N, Nishida M, Inoue R, Kobayashi H, Sumimoto H, et al. (2006) TRPC3 and TRPC6 are essential for angiotensin II-induced cardiac hypertrophy. EMBO J 25: 5305–5316.
17. Harada K, Komuro I, Shiojima I, Hayashi D, Kudoh S, et al. (1998) Pressure overload induces cardiac hypertrophy in angiotensin II type 1A receptor knockout mice. Circulation 97: 1952–1959.
18. Schultz Jel J, Witt SA, Glascock BJ, Nieman ML, Reiser PJ, et al. (2002) TGF-1 mediates mediates the hypertrophic cardio-myocyte growth induced by angiotensin II. J Clin Invest 109: 787–796.
19. Izumiya Y, Kim S, Izumi Y, Yoshida K, Yoshiyama M, et al. (2003) Apoptosis signal-regulating kinase 1 plays a pivotal role in angiotensin II–induced cardiac hypertrophy and remodeling. Circ Res 93: 874–883.
20. Takeishi Y, Jalili T, Ball NA, Walsh RA (1999) Responses of cardiac protein kinase C isoforms to distinct pathological stimuli are differentially regulated. Circ Res 85: 264–271.
21. Hunter JJ, Chien KR (1999) Signaling pathways for cardiac hypertrophy and failure. N Engl J Med 341: 1276–1283.
22. Mazzolai L, Nussberger J, Aubert JF, Brunner DB, Gabbiani G, et al. (1998) Blood pressure-independent cardiac hypertrophy induced by locally activated renin-angiotensin system. Hypertension 31: 1324–1330.
23. Sun Y, Weber KT (1994) Fibrosis and myocardial ACE: possible substrate and independence from circulating angiotensin II. J Card Fail 1: 81–89.
24. Fukui S, Fukumoto Y, Suzuki J, Saji K, Nawata J, et al. (2009) Diabetes mellitus accelerates left ventricular diastolic dysfunction through activation of the renin-angiotensin system in hypertensive rats. Hypertens Res 32: 472–480.
25. Wang XH, Wang WF, Cao YX, Ma AQ (2013) Ang II receptor expression and effect of Ang II receptor blockade in thyrotoxic rat myocardium. Eur Rev Med Pharmacol Sci 17: 2619–2627.

26. Lin L, Xu J, Ye Y, Ge J, Zou Y, et al. (2014) Isosorbide dinitrate inhibits mechanical stress-induced cardiac hypertrophy and autophagy through downregulation of angiotensin II type 1 receptor. J Cardiovasc Pharmacol 2014Epub ahead of print.
27. Zou Y, Akazawa H, Qin Y, Sano M, Takano H, et al. (2004) Mechanical stress activates angiotensin II type 1 receptor without the involvement of angiotensin II. Nat Cell Biol 6: 499–506.
28. Qin Y, Yasuda N, Akazawa H, Ito K, Kudo Y, et al. (2009) Multivalent ligand-receptor interactions elicit inverse agonist activity of AT_1 receptor blockers against stretch-induced AT_1 receptor activation. Hypertens Res 32: 875–883.
29. Domenighetti AA, Boixel C, Cefai D, Abriel H, Pedrazzini T (2007) Chronic angiotensin II stimulation in the heart produces an acquired long QT syndrome associated with IK_1 potassium current downregulation. J Mol Cell Cardiol 42: 63–70.
30. Yasuno S, Kuwahara K, Kinoshita H, Yamada C, Nakagawa Y, et al. (2013) Angiotensin II type 1a receptor signalling directly contributes to the increased arrhythmogenicity in cardiac hypertrophy. Br J Pharmacol 170: 1384–1395.

Calcium-Activated Potassium Current Modulates Ventricular Repolarization in Chronic Heart Failure

Ingrid M. Bonilla[1,2], Victor P. Long, III[1,2], Pedro Vargas-Pinto[3¤], Patrick Wright[2], Andriy Belevych[2], Qing Lou[2], Kent Mowrey[4], Jae Yoo[1], Philip F. Binkley[2], Vadim V. Fedorov[2], Sandor Györke[2], Paulus M. L. Janssen[2], Ahmet Kilic[2], Peter J. Mohler[2], Cynthia A. Carnes[1,3]*

1 College of Pharmacy, The Ohio State University, Columbus, Ohio, United States of America, **2** Dorothy M. Davis Heart and Lung Research Institute, The Ohio State University Wexner Medical Center, Columbus, Ohio, United States of America, **3** College of Veterinary Medicine, The Ohio State University, Columbus, Ohio, United States of America, **4** St Jude Medical, Sylmar, California, United States of America

Abstract

The role of I_{KCa} in cardiac repolarization remains controversial and varies across species. The relevance of the current as a therapeutic target is therefore undefined. We examined the cellular electrophysiologic effects of I_{KCa} blockade in controls, chronic heart failure (HF) and HF with sustained atrial fibrillation. We used perforated patch action potential recordings to maintain intrinsic calcium cycling. The I_{KCa} blocker (apamin 100 nM) was used to examine the role of the current in atrial and ventricular myocytes. A canine tachypacing induced model of HF (1 and 4 months, n = 5 per group) was used, and compared to a group of 4 month HF with 6 weeks of superimposed atrial fibrillation (n = 7). A group of age-matched canine controls were used (n = 8). Human atrial and ventricular myocytes were isolated from explanted end-stage failing hearts which were obtained from transplant recipients, and studied in parallel. Atrial myocyte action potentials were unchanged by I_{KCa} blockade in all of the groups studied. I_{KCa} blockade did not affect ventricular myocyte repolarization in controls. HF caused prolongation of ventricular myocyte action potential repolarization. I_{KCa} blockade caused further prolongation of ventricular repolarization in HF and also caused repolarization instability and early afterdepolarizations. SK2 and SK3 expression in the atria and SK3 in the ventricle were increased in canine heart failure. We conclude that during HF, I_{KCa} blockade in ventricular myocytes results in cellular arrhythmias. Furthermore, our data suggest an important role for I_{KCa} in the maintenance of ventricular repolarization stability during chronic heart failure. Our findings suggest that novel antiarrhythmic therapies should have safety and efficacy evaluated in both atria and ventricles.

Editor: Blanca Rodriguez, University of Oxford, United Kingdom

Funding: Pacemakers and leads provided by St. Jude Medical, Sylmar, CA as an in-kind donation (Carnes). Research supported in part by NIH grants (R01-HL115580 to CAC and VVF; R01-HL089836 to CAC; HL074045 to SG; HL084583, HL083422, HL114383 to PJM) and the American Heart Association (PJM). The funders had no role in study design, data collection and analysis, decision to publish or preparation of the manuscript.

Competing Interests: The authors have declared that no competing interests exist.

* Email: carnes.4@osu.edu

¤ Current address: University of LaSalle, Bogota, Columbia

Introduction

Heart failure (HF) is a chronic disease that develops over months to years, and is defined by insufficient cardiac output to meet the physiologic and metabolic needs of the body. Atrial fibrillation (AF) and HF are common coexisting disease states, and HF results in a 4.5 to 5.9 fold increase in the risk of developing AF. [1] Moreover, in patients with HF, the development of AF significantly increases the risk of death. [2] Thus, identifying and elucidating pharmacological targets to treat AF may significantly reduce mortality and morbidity in HF.

Small-conductance Ca^{2+}- activated K^+ (SK) channels are expressed in multiple tissues such as skeletal and smooth muscle, the central and peripheral nervous system and the heart.[3–5] Cardiac myocytes express SK1, SK2 and SK3 gene products. [6] SK- encoded current is voltage-independent and activated by intracellular calcium. [7] All three members of the SK family have similar calcium sensitivity for activation (0.6–0.7 μM) [8]. SK-encoded current is blocked by apamin, a constituent of bee venom, which appears to be highly selective for I_{KCa}. [7,9,10].

I_{KCa}, the potassium current conducted by SK channels, contributes to repolarization, [3,11] but the importance of I_{KCa} in repolarization remains poorly elucidated. For example, ventricular I_{KCa} shortens repolarization and promotes peri-infarct arrhythmias in rats. [12] Conversely, blockade of I_{KCa} promotes ventricular arrhythmias in human HF and a non-ischemic rabbit HF model, suggesting a protective role for I_{KCa}. [13,14] The contribution of I_{KCa} to *atrial* repolarization is also unclear as some reports demonstrate that I_{KCa} is proarrhythmic while others suggest it is protective. [15,16].

We measured the impact of I_{KCa} block on action potentials in intact myocytes using perforated patch recordings to maintain intrinsic Ca^{2+}cycling. We utilized a well-validated canine model that emulates all key features of human HF including chamber dilatation, impaired contractility, impaired functional capacity, repolarization abnormalities, dysregulated myocyte calcium

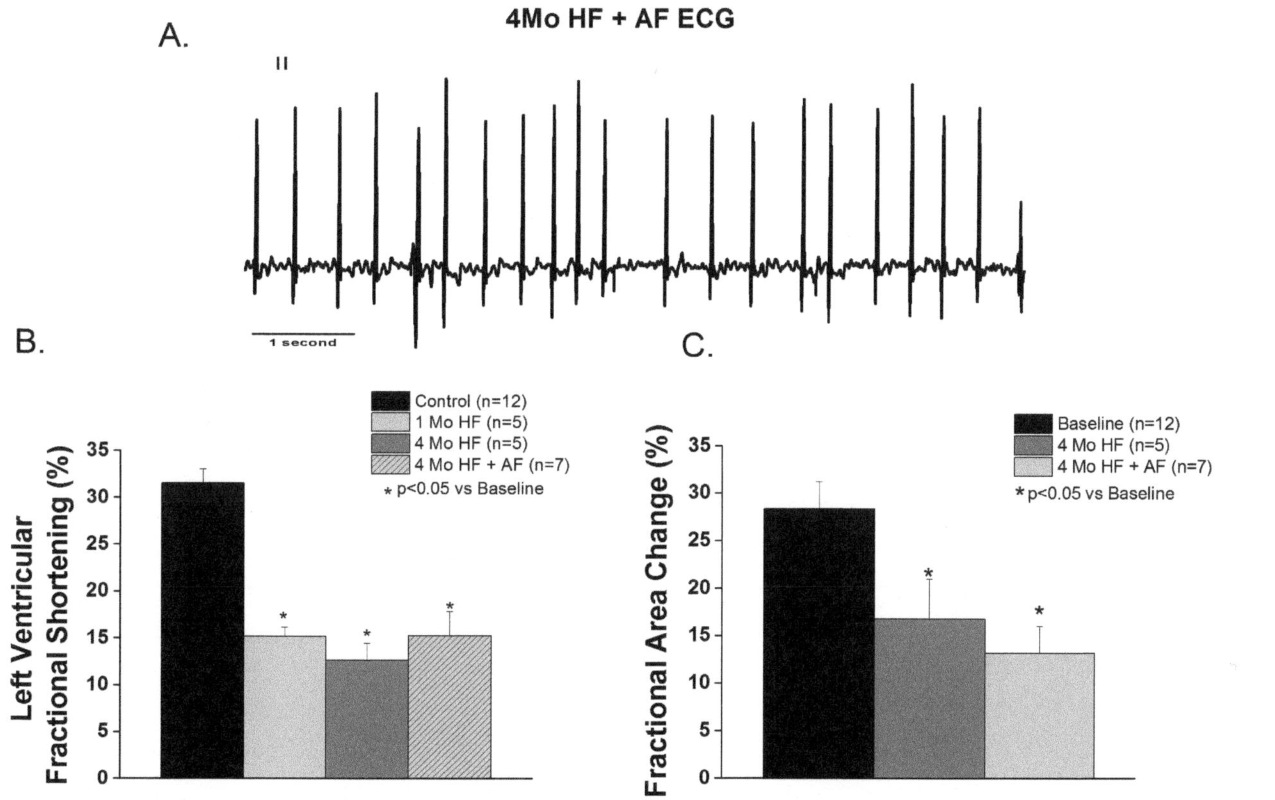

Figure 1. In vivo data from 1 month (1 Mo), 4 month (4 Mo), and 4 month HF with sustained AF (4 Mo HF+AF) canine groups. A. Representative ECG recording from a 4 month HF+AF dog showing the absence of P waves and irregularly irregular QRS complexes characteristic of AF. **B.** LVFS was similarly decreased in the 1 month HF, 4 month HF and the 4 month HF+AF groups compared to baseline. ($p<0.05$ vs baseline). **C.** Atrial contractility was decreased in 4 month HF and 4 month HF+AF groups compared to baseline. ($p<0.05$, N = 5–7 per group).

handling, increased predisposition to AF and increased myocardial fibrosis. [17,18] Complementary experiments were conducted in end-stage human HF. The role of I_{KCa} in AF was evaluated in atrial myocytes from a canine model of chronic HF with sustained AF.

Methods

Heart failure and atrial fibrillation animal models

All animal procedures conformed to the Guide for the Care and Use of Laboratory Animals of the National Institutes of Health, and were approved by the Ohio State University Institutional Animal Care and Use Committee (Protocol: 2010A00000103-R1). Canine heart failure was induced by right ventricular (RV) tachypacing as previously described. [19] Animals were assigned to one or four months of RV tachypacing to induce heart failure.

Atrial fibrillation was induced in dogs with HF using a customized pacemaker (St Jude Medical, Sylmar, CA). One pacing lead was implanted in the right atria (RA) and the second lead was implanted in the RV, with HF induced as previously described. [20] After 10 weeks of RV tachypacing, RA tachypacing was initiated, with the RA stimulated at 10 Hz for 60 seconds, followed by a 10 second pause for automated interrogation of atrial rhythm. This cycle of RA tachypacing was repeated every 70 seconds until AF was detected. Subsequent detection of normal atrial rhythm resulted in resumption of the atrial tachypacing. The total HF duration in the HF+AF group was 4 months. Ventricular pacing was stopped during atrial stimulation, and the ventricular rate was 150–200 BPM during atrial pacing or AF. Serial echocardiograms and ECGs were performed as previously reported. [17,21] Serial pacemaker interrogations were used to monitor cardiac rhythm.

Myocyte Isolation and Tissue Collection

On the day of the terminal procedure, the dogs were anesthetized with pentobarbital sodium (50 mg/kg intravenously; Nembutal, Abbott Laboratories). The heart was rapidly removed and perfused with cold cardioplegia solution containing the following (mM): NaCl 110, $CaCl_2$ 1.2, KCl 16, $MgCl_2$ 16 and $NaHCO_3$ 10. Cannulation of the left circumflex artery was used to perfuse left atria and ventricle following removal of the right atrium and right ventricle, as previously described. [22] Adjacent tissue samples were collected and snap frozen for protein analyses. Tyrode's solution (mM) containing NaCl 130, KCl 5.4, $MgCl_2$ 3.5, NaH_2PO_4 0.5, Glucose 10, HEPES 5 and taurine 20, was used as the initial perfusate. During the cell isolation process the heart was perfused with three different solutions (36°C). The heart was initially perfused for 10 minutes with Tyrode's solution with 0.1 mM EGTA; this was followed by perfusion with Tyrode's solution containing 0.3 mM Calcium, 0.12 mg/ml of Trypsin Inhibitor (NIBCO) and 1.33 mg/ml of collagenase (Type II, Worthington) for a maximum of 45 minutes. Then following enzymatic digestion, the heart was perfused with normal Tyrode's solution for five minutes to remove residual enzyme. Subsequently, left ventricular mid-myocardial and left atrial myocytes were obtained through secondary digestion, as previously described. [22] After secondary digestion the cells were re-suspended in

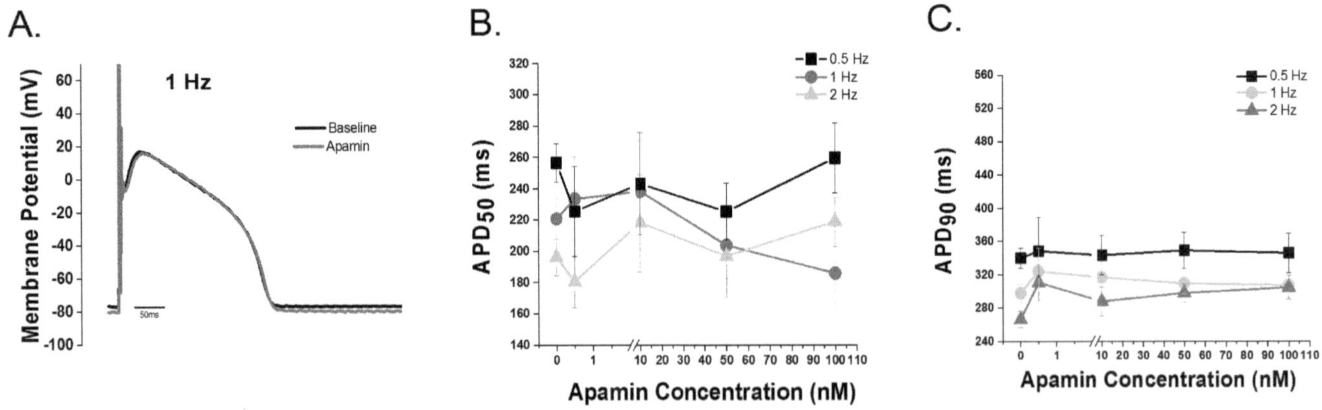

Figure 2. I_{KCa} inhibition does not alter repolarization in control ventricular cells. A. Representative action potential tracing before and after 100 nM apamin recorded at 1 Hz. **B.** APD_{50} and **C.** APD_{90} dose response data (0–100 nM apamin) recorded at stimulation rates of 0.5, 1 and 2 Hz. (p = NS, n = 5–11 cells per group; 8 animals). The Grubb's test for outlier data was applied and one cell was rejected and is not included in the summary data.

incubation buffer. [23] This isolation procedure typically yields 70–90% and 40–60% rod shaped ventricular and atrial myocytes, respectively. All myocyte electrophysiology experiments were conducted within 10 hours of isolation.

In parallel experiments, failing human cardiac tissue was obtained after written informed consent with the documentation of consent securely stored as approved by the Institutional Review Board approval of The Ohio State University (IRB 2008H0113

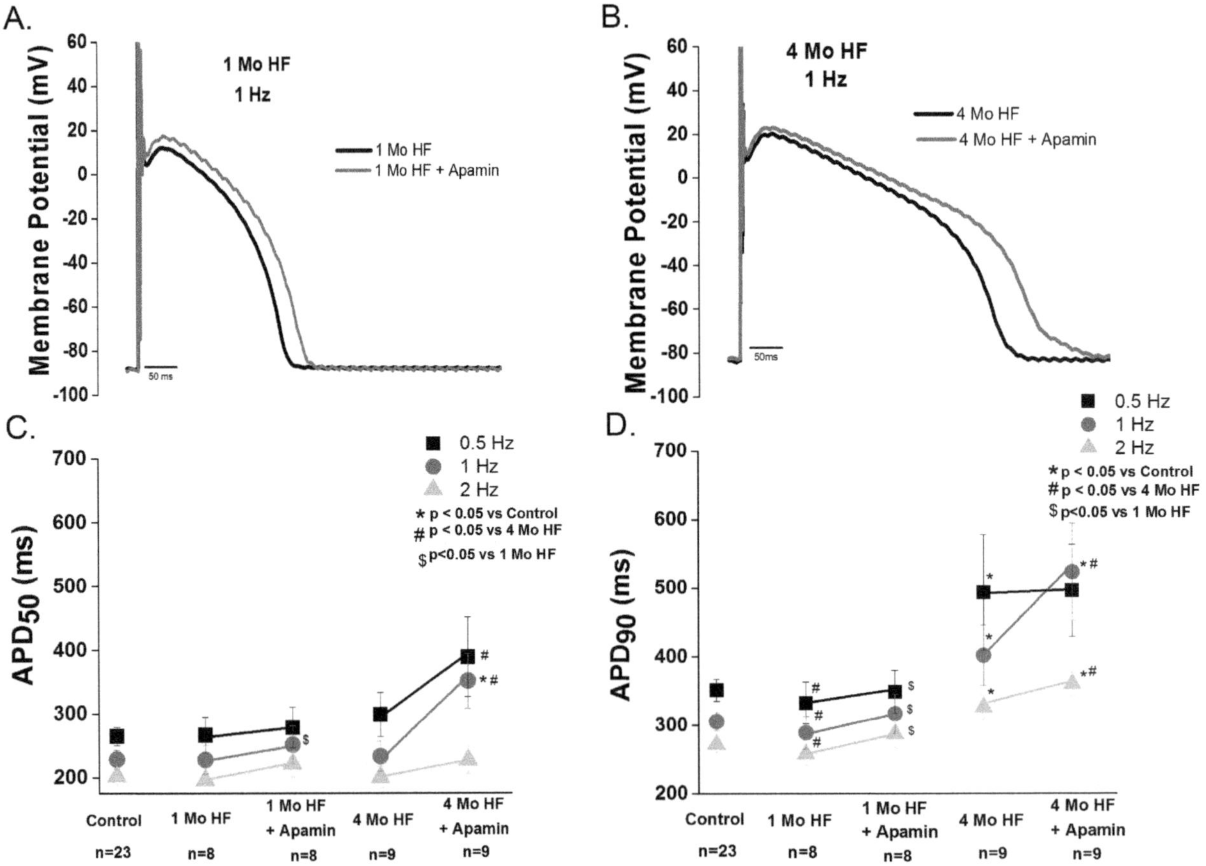

Figure 3. Apamin modulates ventricular repolarization during HF. Representative action potential of a 1 month (**A**) HF and 4 month HF (**B**) ventricular cell before and after apamin superfusion. **C.** Summary data of APD_{50} in control,1 month and 4 month HF before and after apamin treatment. No difference between 1 month HF, 4 month HF and control is observed (2–8 animals per group). Apamin treatment of 1 month HF cells causes a prolongation only at 2 Hz($p<0.05$), likewise apamin treatment of 4 month HF cells causes a prolongation at 0.5 Hz ($p<0.05$) and 1 Hz ($p<0.05$). **D.** Apamin prolongs APD_{90} in both 1 and 4 month HF ($p<0.05$).

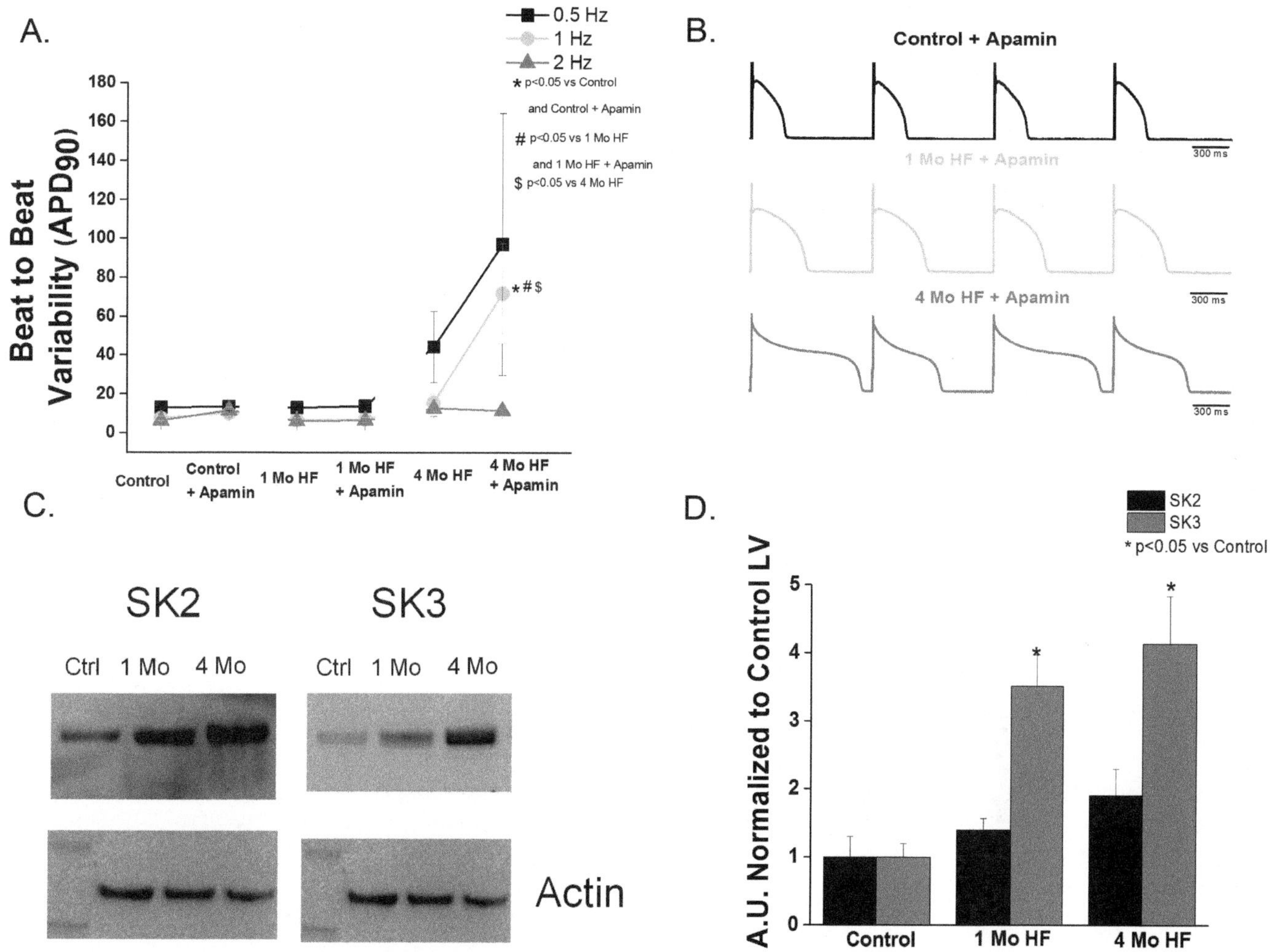

Figure 4. I_{KCa} contributes to ventricular repolarization stability in canine HF, and HF increases SK3 expression. A. Beat to beat variability of APD_{90} (BTBV, ms) is unchanged in both 1 month or 4 month HF vs. controls. I_{KCa} block increases the BTBV in the 4 month, but not the 1 month HF group (p<0.05 vs control, 1 month HF and 4 month HF; 2–8 animals per group). **B.** Representative AP tracings of control, 1 month HF and 4 month HF during superfusion with 100 nm apamin. **C.** Representative blots of SK2 and SK3. **D.** SK3 in the 1 and 4 month HF groups is increased (p<0.05 vs control) while SK2 is unchanged (N = 4–5).

and IRB 2012H0197), in accordance with the 1964 Declaration of Helsinki and its later amendments. Additional human cardiac tissue was obtained from the Lifeline of Ohio Organ Procurement program (http://lifelineofohio.org). For these tissues, the Institutional Review Board waived the need for consent and these tissues were used according to the Ohio State University guidelines regarding the use of data and/or specimens.

Left ventricular mid-myocardial and left atrial appendage myocytes were isolated and adjacent tissues were collected from explanted end-stage failing hearts (n = 6; obtained from the Ohio State University Wexner Medical Center transplant program). After cannulation of a superficial coronary artery to perfuse the left atrium and/or left ventricle, the methods for myocyte isolation were as described for canine samples above. Left ventricular mid myocardium and left atrial appendege tissues were collected from non-failing heart for Western blotting purposes (n = 8 obtained from Lifeline of Ohio). Non-HF status was confirmed in these tissues by lack of CaMKII pS286 hyperphosphorylation.

Action Potential (AP) Measurements

Amphotericin-B perforated patch clamp techniques with a bath temperature of 36±0.5°C were used. The myocytes were placed in a laminin-coated cell chamber (Cell Microcontrols, Norfolk, VA) and superfused (~1 mL/min) with bath solution containing (mM): 135 NaCl, 5 $MgCl_2$, 5 KCl, 10 glucose, 1.8 $CaCl_2$, and 5 HEPES with pH adjusted to 7.40 with NaOH. Borosilicate glass micropipettes with tip resistance of 1.5–3 MΩ, were filled with pipette solution containing the following (mM): 100 K-aspartate, 40 KCl, 5 MgCl, 5 EGTA, 5 HEPES, pH adjusted to 7.2 with KOH.

APs were recorded in a train of 25 traces at 0.5, 1 and 2 Hz at baseline and after apamin perfusion. The average of the last 10 traces (i.e. from trace 16–25) was used to calculate the action potential duration (APD). APD was calculated at 50 and 90 percent of repolarization (APD_{50} and APD_{90}).

To evaluate repolarization instability, beat to beat variability (BTBV) of APD_{90} was assessed as the standard deviation of the APD_{90}, as previously described. [24,25] Early afterdepolarization (EAD) propensity was assessed as the percentage of cells exhibiting

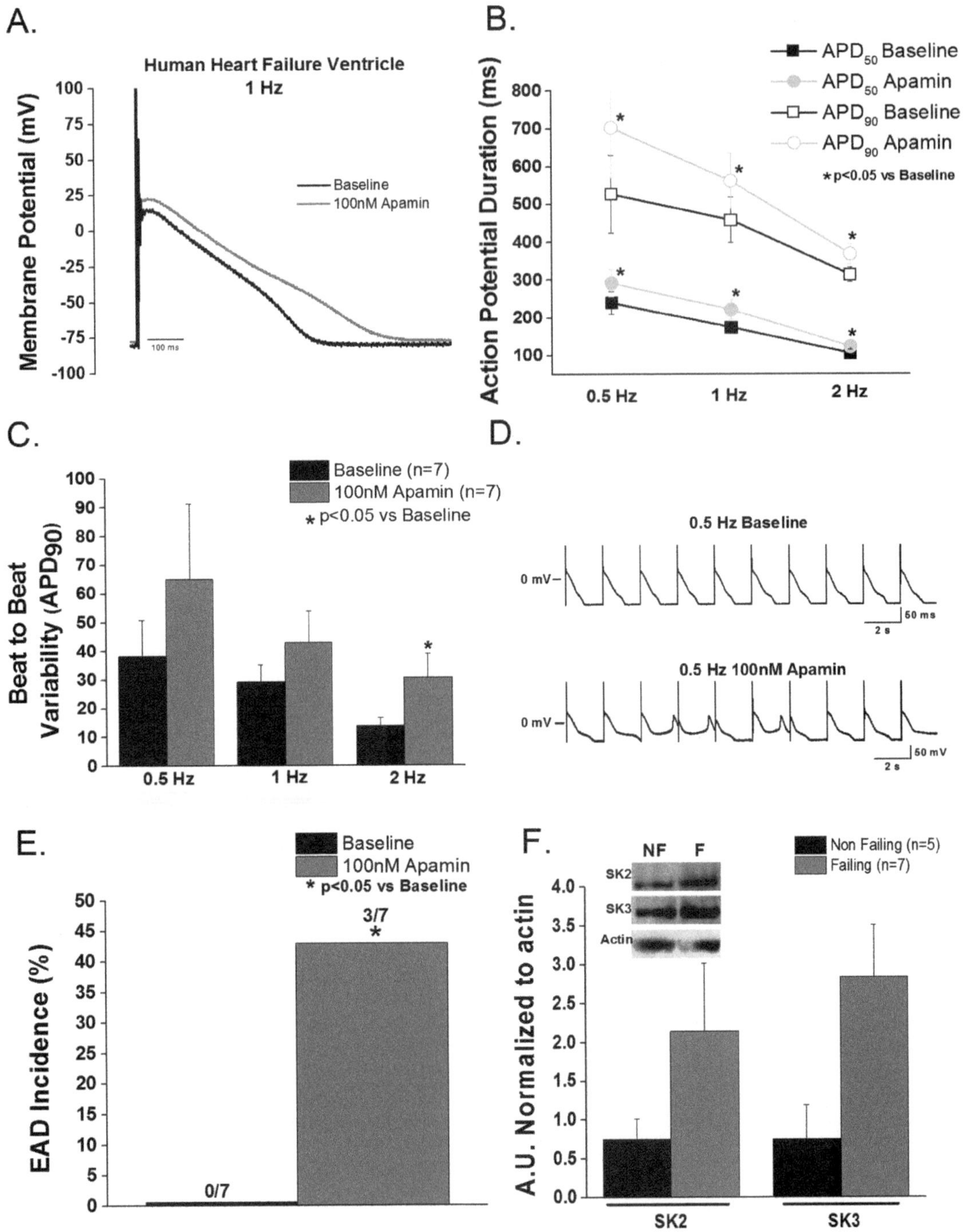

Figure 5. Apamin modulates ventricular repolarization in end-stage human HF. A. Representative action potential recorded at 1 Hz from an end-stage human HF ventricular myocyte before and after apamin. **B.** Apamin superfusion prolongs APD_{50} and APD_{90} in end-stage human HF ventricular myocytes at all rates ($p<0.05$ vs baseline, $n=7$). **C.** Apamin superfusion increases ($p<0.05$ vs baseline) BTBV (ms) at 2 Hz. **D.** Representative action potential showing late phase 3 EADs after apamin superfusion. **E.** Apamin treatment increases EAD incidence in failing human ventricular myocytes. ($p<0.05$ vs baseline) **F.** Representative blots of control and end-stage human HF SK2 and SK3 proteins (SK2 $p=0.556$ and SK3 $p=0.141$ vs. control). HF: N=7 (4 male/3 female); age=52±13 years and LV ejection fraction of 14.5±5.2%; non-failing controls: n=5 (2 male/3 female); age=47±12 years.

EADs. Recordings exhibiting EADs were excluded from APD and BTBV measurements.

Data collection was done at baseline and after superfusion with the I_{KCa} blocker apamin (100 nM), a concentration known to block SK1, SK2 and SK3 encoded-current.[26–28] An Axopatch 200A amplifier with Digidata 1440A (Molecular devices, Sunnyvale, CA) and Clampex 10.2 software was used for data acquisition. At the initiation of each recording the resting potential was examined. For canine cells, atrial cells with a resting membrane potential of ≥ −55 mV were recorded; for ventricular

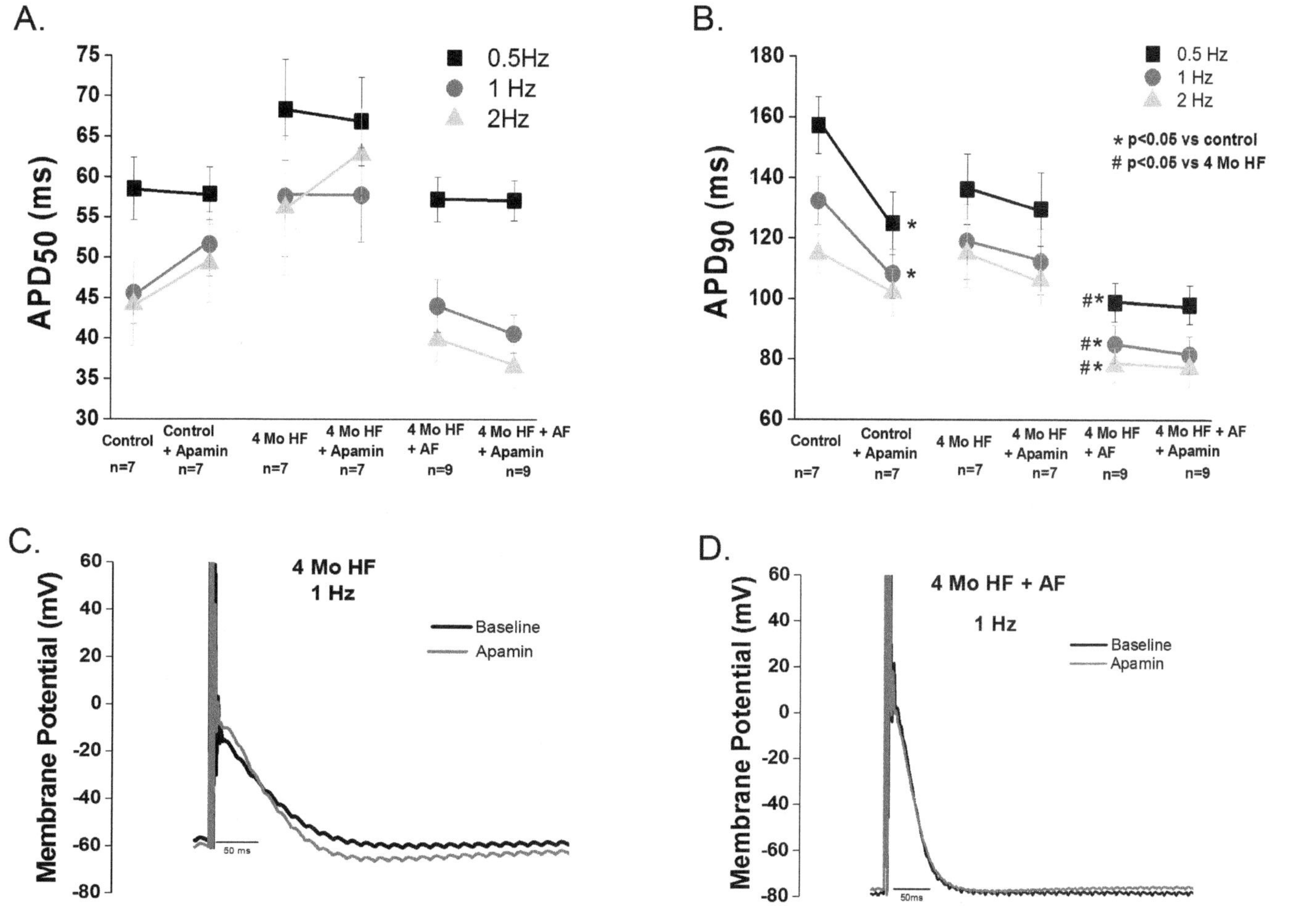

Figure 6. I_{KCa} block does not affect repolarization in normal or diseased atrial myocytes. A. 100 nM apamin does not affect atrial APD_{50} in any of the studied groups (i.e. control, 4 month HF and 4 month HF+AF, n = 7–9 cells per group) **B.** 100 nM apamin shortened the APD_{90} in controls at 0.5 and 1 Hz. ($p<0.05$). HF+AF had a shorter baseline APD_{90} compared to control and HF ($p<0.05$), however no change in APD_{90} was observed after apamin treatment in either 4 month HF or 4 month HF+AF groups. (n = 7–9 cells per groups) **C and D.** Atrial action potential tracings before and after apamin treatment from the 4 month HF group and the 4 month HF+ AF group (2–6 animals per group).

cells those with a resting membrane potential of ≥ −70 mV were recorded. For the human cells, every cell with complete baseline and apamin-treatment data was included. One apamin-treated ventricular canine cell action potential recording was excluded as an outlier.

Calcium transient Measurements

Calcium transients were recorded using Ca^{2+} sensitive dye Fluo-4AM (10 µM) and an Olympus Fluoview 1000 confocal microscope in line scan mode. Myocytes were loaded with dye for 25 minutes at room temperature. Fluo-4 was excited with a 488 nm argon laser and fluorescence collected at wavelength 500–600 nm. Myocytes were paced by extracellular stimulation at 1 Hz with platinum electrodes. External solution contained (mM): 140 NaCl, 5.4 KCl, 2 $CaCl_2$, 0.5 $MgCl_2$, 10 HEPES and 5.6 glucose (pH 7.3).

Immunoblots

Following protein quantification, tissue lysates were analyzed on Mini-PROTEAN tetra cell (BioRad) on a 4–15% precast TGX gel (BioRad) in Tris/Glycine/SDS Buffer (BioRad). Gels were transferred to a nitrocellulose membrane using the Mini-PROTEAN tetra cell (BioRad) in Tris/Glycine buffer with 20% methanol (v/v, BioRad). Membranes were blocked for 1 hour at room temperature using a 3% BSA solution and incubated with primary antibody overnight at 4°C. Antibodies included: SK2 (Alomone, Santa Cruz), SK3 (Alomone, Santa Cruz), GAPDH (Fitzgerald), and actin (Sigma). Secondary antibodies included donkey anti-mouse-HRP and donkey anti-rabbit-HRP (Jackson Laboratories). Densitometry was performed using Image lab software and all data was normalized to GAPDH or actin levels present in each sample.

Data Analysis

Cellular electrophysiology and Ca^{2+} imaging data were analyzed using Clampfit 10.3 software (Axon Instruments) and Origin 9.0 software (OriginLab, Northampton, MA, USA). APD data was examined for outliers by application of the Grubb's test, which rejected one control ventricular myocyte (GraphPad). All APD paired data were compared by paired student t-test. Unpaired data and comparisons between groups were analyzed by one-way ANOVA with post hoc least significant difference testing. Differences in EADs incidence were tested with Pearson's Chi-Square test. For protein experiments, differences were

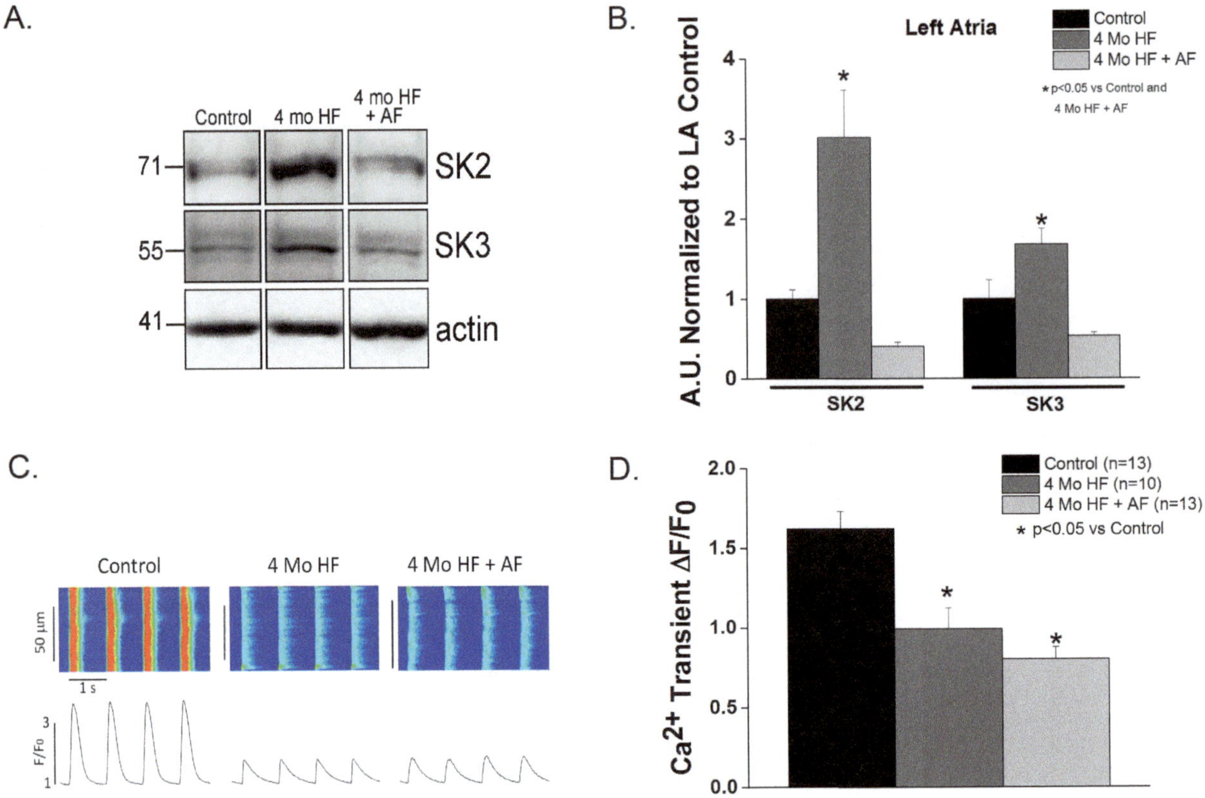

Figure 7. Atrial SK expression and calcium transients in chronic HF with and without AF. A. Representative Western blots of SK2 and SK3. **B.** SK2 and SK3 are increased 3- and 2-fold, respectively in the 4 month HF atria. ($p<0.05$ vs control and 4 month HF+AF) No differences between control and 4 month HF+AF were found in any of the subunits. (N = 3) **C.** Representative calcium transient line scans. **D.** Calcium transient amplitude was decreased in the 4 month HF and 4 month HF+AF groups compared to control ($p<0.05$ vs control; 3–8 animals per group).

assessed with a paired Student's *t* test (2-tailed) or ANOVA, as appropriate, for continuous data. The Bonferroni test was used for post-hoc testing. All data are presented as mean ± SE and $p<0.05$ was the criterion for statistical significance for all comparisons.

Chemicals

All chemicals were purchased from Sigma-Aldrich (St. Louis, MO, USA) and Fisher Scientific (Pittsburg, PA, USA), unless otherwise noted. All buffers and solutions were prepared daily.

Results

In vivo cardiac remodeling

Left ventricular fractional shortening (LVFS) was similarly reduced in the 1 month HF, 4 month HF and 4 month HF+AF groups (Figure 1B), consistent with HF. Electrocardiograms (ECGs) in all canines assigned to the HF+ AF group demonstrated sustained atrial tachyarrhythmias, evident as the absence of P waves and the irregularly irregular ventricular rate characteristic of AF (Figure 1A). Additionally, atrial contractility, measured as left atrial fractional area change (FAC), was significantly reduced in both the 4 month HF and 4 month HF+AF groups compared to baseline ($p<0.05$) as shown in Figure 1C. Notably, the presence of sustained AF did not cause a further decrement in atrial contractility compared to HF alone.

I_{KCa} inhibition in control ventricular myocytes

Action potentials before and after apamin treatment were recorded from control canine ventricular myocytes. Varying apamin concentrations (0.5–100 nM) were tested in order to generate a concentration response curve. Apamin did not alter APD_{50} or APD_{90} in control ventricular myocytes (Figure 2A).

I_{KCa} inhibition and SK expression in failing ventricle

Canine. We observed no HF-induced difference in APD_{50} or APD_{90} in the 1 month HF myocytes compared with control myocytes. However, apamin (100 nM) caused a significant prolongation of the APD_{90} in one month HF ($p<0.05$; Figure 3 A–D). In contrast to 1 month HF, 4 month HF significantly increased APD_{90} relative to control ventricular myocytes ($p<0.05$ vs control). Furthermore, when I_{KCa} was blocked in 4 month HF ventricular myocytes (100 nM apamin), there was a significant prolongation of the APD_{50} at lower rates (i.e. $p<0.05$ vs control at 0.5 and 1 Hz) and a further prolongation in the APD_{90} ($p<0.05$ vs control and baseline 4 month HF).

In order to assess repolarization instability induced by block of I_{KCa}, we measured the beat to beat variability (BTBV) of $APD_{90}\pm$ apamin. HF alone did not increase the BTBV in either HF group compared to controls. Block of I_{KCa} significantly increased BTBV in the 4 month, but not one month, HF group. (Figure 4A,B).

Canine cardiac I_{KCa} encoding proteins SK2 and SK3 were measured in control, 1 month HF and 4 month HF ventricular tissues. No significant change in SK2 protein expression in either HF group ($p>0.05$ vs control) was found. An ~4-fold increase in

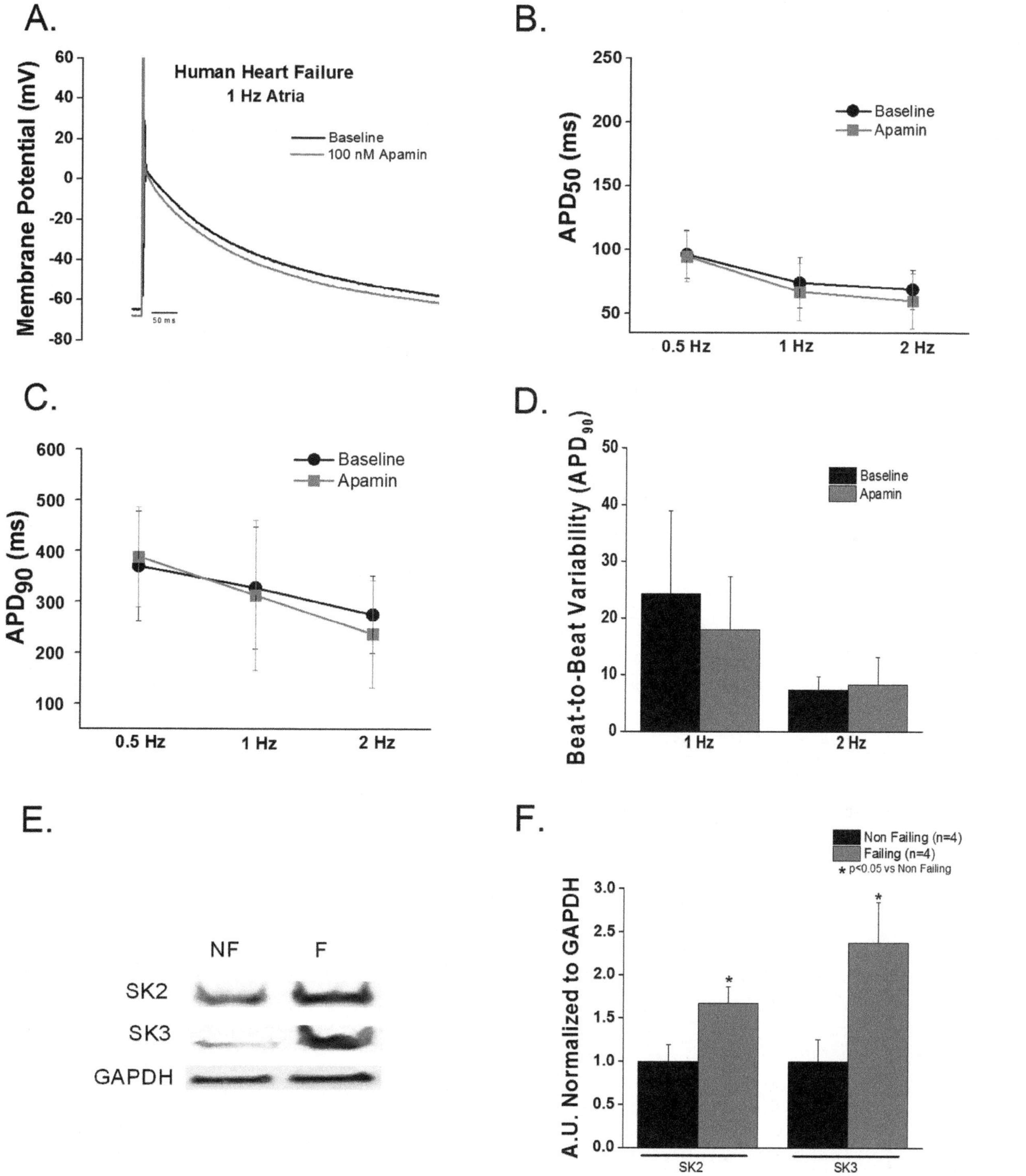

Figure 8. Apamin does not modulate repolarization in end-stage human HF atrial myocytes. A. Representative atrial action potential tracing recorded at 1 Hz. **B and C.** Apamin did not change APD_{50} or APD_{90} in human atrial myocytes. (n = 3) **D.** Apamin superfusion did not increase BTBV (ms). **E.** Representative SK2 and SK3 Western blots. **F.** HF increased SK2 and SK3 expression in left atrial tissue ($p<0.05$ vs non-failing). HF: N = 4 (2 male/2 female); age = 56±4 years and LV ejection fraction of 14.5±1.1%; non-failing controls: n = 4 (2 male/2 female); age = 46±14 years.

SK3 expression was found in both 1 month and 4 month HF groups. ($p<0.05$ vs control) (Figure 4C,D).

End-stage human heart failure. In end-stage human HF, inhibition of I_{KCa} (100 nM apamin) caused a significant prolongation of both APD_{50} and APD_{90} compared to baseline ($p<0.05$, Figure 5 A, B). In addition to AP prolongation, BTBV was significantly increased at 2 Hz in end-stage human HF ventricular cells compared to baseline (Figure 5C). I_{KCa} blockade induced late phase 3 early afterdepolarizations (EADs) in ~40% of myocytes; while no EADs were observed at baseline (Figure 5D,E).

Human cardiac I_{KCa} encoding proteins SK2 and SK3 were measured in control and end-stage human HF ventricular tissue lysate (Figure 5F). While there was a trend toward increased SK2 expression in HF, this did not achieve statistical significance. SK3 protein also showed a tendency to increase in human end-stage HF compared to control ($p = 0.14$).

I_{KCa} inhibition and SK expression in atrial myocytes

Canine. Neither HF nor AF caused any change in APD_{50} compared to control. HF with superimposed AF caused significant APD_{90} shortening compared to control and 4 month HF ($p<0.05$ vs control and 4 Mo HF). I_{KCa} blockade (100 nM apamin) in control atrial myocytes did not change APD_{50} (Figure 6A) but caused an unexpected shortening of the APD_{90} at 0.5 and 1 Hz ($p<0.05$ vs baseline) as shown in Figure 6B. I_{KCa} blockade in the 4 month HF and 4 month HF+AF atrial cells did not cause any change in the APD_{50} or the APD_{90} (Figure 6). In further contrast to what we observed in the ventricle, no change in the BTBV of repolarization was observed in either the control, 4 month HF or the 4 month HF+AF groups after I_{KCa} blockade (data not shown). Thus, contrary to what we observed in the ventricle, I_{KCa} does not modulate repolarization in the atria in our chronic HF model.

The cardiac I_{KCa} encoding proteins SK2 and SK3 were measured in left atrial appendage tissue from the three groups (i.e. Control, 4 month HF and 4 month HF+AF). A 3-fold and 2-fold increase in SK2 and SK3, respectively in the 4 month HF group was observed compared to both control and 4 month HF+AF groups ($p<0.05$, Figure 7A, B); while the 4 month HF+AF group did not differ from control. HF, with or without sustained AF, caused a similar significant decrease in calcium transient amplitude compared to controls ($p<0.05$ vs control, Figure 7C, D).

End-stage human heart failure. Human end-stage HF atrial myocytes showed no significant change in either APD_{50} or APD_{90} when treated with apamin (100 nM). Contrary to what we observed in the ventricular cells no difference was observed in BTBV or afterdepolarizations after apamin treatment in human HF atrial cells (Figure 8). SK2 and SK3 were significantly increased in atrial human HF samples compared with atrial samples from non-failing individuals ($p<0.05$, Figure 8).

Discussion

It is well known that HF is a substrate for AF and these are common co-existing disease states. [1,20] HF patients are at an increased risk for both atrial and ventricular arrhythmias, which contribute to morbidity and mortality. [2] Our main findings were two-fold: first, we did not find any modulation of atrial myocyte repolarization by I_{KCa} in the settings of normal, failing or sustained AF hearts. Secondly, I_{KCa} is activated during HF contributing to stability of ventricular repolarization. Thus, block of I_{KCa} in chronic HF ventricular myocytes prolonged repolarization and increased repolarization instability; these effects have been shown to predict proarrhythmia. [29] Consistent with our findings, I_{KCa} has been previously suggested to play a protective role in the human ventricle during HF. [14].

One interesting question is how I_{KCa} becomes an important modulator of ventricular repolarization during heart failure. Potential explanations for this finding include 1) increased channel expression; 2) altered channel sensitivity to calcium; 3) increased calcium concentrations; or 4) loss of other repolarizing current(s), thereby unmasking the role of I_{KCa}.

In considering these possibilities, we observed an increase in SK3, but not SK2 in our canine HF model. However, we did not observe a statistically significant increase in either SK2 or SK3 in human HF, although there was a trend toward an increase in SK3 ($p = 0.14$); our findings are in contrast to a previous report where SK2 expression was increased in human HF. [14] While the expression was not significantly increased in human HF, the inter-species differences we observed may be explained by the intrinsic enhanced variability in explanted human end-stage heart failure samples resulting from inhomogeneities in etiology, comorbidities and drug treatments.

Other possible explanations for our findings are altered channel sensitivity to calcium, altered calcium cycling, or altered repolarization. Recently it was reported in human end-stage HF that SK channel sensitivity to calcium was increased in ventricular myocytes, [14] which could contribute in part to our findings. Of note, other proteins such as: protein kinase, calmodulin and protein phosphatase A, [7,30] are also known to contribute to the regulation of SK channels, and thus may modulate I_{KCa} during HF.

Since I_{KCa} is a calcium-activated potassium current, HF-induced changes in ventricular calcium handling should directly affect the current. We have previously reported that in our HF model, there is a significant reduction in SR calcium release and calcium transient amplitude, which would reduce rather than augment I_{KCa}. [31] In support of this interpretation, a recent report indicates that SR release is necessary and sufficient for I_{KCa} activation. [32] Considering the HF-induced reduction in calcium cycling, and the lack of apamin effect in control cells where calcium cycling is robust, this suggests that altered calcium cycling is not responsible for the protective role of I_{KCa} in heart failure.

Reduced ventricular repolarization reserve may unmask the role of small currents such as I_{KCa}. [33] Decreased repolarization reserve is well-described in the ventricle during HF and attributed to reductions in repolarizing currents such as I_{K1}, I_{Kr} and I_{Ks}. These changes predispose to repolarization instability and/or arrhythmias.[33–35] Since I_{KCa} blockade prolonged the AP only during HF and not in controls, we suggest that the contribution of I_{KCa} becomes evident only in settings of decreased repolarization reserve. Thus we suggest that increased channel expression, altered calcium sensitivity of SK channels, or altered repolarization reserve may contribute to the stabilizing role of I_{KCa}.

I_{KCa} has been suggested as a therapeutic target for AF. [36] I_{KCa} is defined pharmacologically as apamin-sensitive current, as apamin blocks SK1, SK2 and SK3-encoded channels [9]. One potential problem with this approach is non-selective effects on other ion currents. However, a recent paper surveying apamin effects on human ion channel protein function has demonstrated a high degree of specificity for SK-encoded I_{KCa}, even at a concentration five-fold higher than in the present study. [10] A potential limitation of previous studies evaluating I_{KCa} blockade has been a focus on primarily one cardiac chamber; this is limiting since electrical remodeling during HF is chamber-dependent. Specifically during chronic HF, the atrial action potential is shortened [20,37,38] while the ventricular action potential is prolonged. [39].

Interest in I_{KCa} as a therapeutic target for atrial arrhythmias followed reports of a genetic predisposition to lone AF attributed to a single nucleotide mutation in the gene KCNN3, which encodes for SK3. [40,41] The exact mechanism(s) by which a single mutation affects SK channel function remains unclear. Data supporting both loss of function and gain of function as possible mechanisms for AF have been reported in multiple models. [15,16] Additionally, SK2 and SK3 down regulation have been associated with human AF. [42].

One goal of this study was to elucidate the role of I_{KCa} in atrial electrophysiology during HF and HF with superimposed AF. Considering HF alone, contrary to previous reports, [15,16] I_{KCa} blockade failed to prolong the atrial action potential in either control or HF atrial myocytes, at physiologic rates. Our findings are different from a recent report where I_{KCa} blockade prolonged the atrial action potential in a whole atrial preparation in a reverse rate-dependent fashion; however this only occurred at rates slower than those used in the present study. [16].

The atrial action potential was not prolonged with I_{KCa} block in HF despite increased both SK2 and SK3 expression. Possible explanations include altered protein trafficking, altered channel calcium sensitivity or altered myocyte calcium handling. We previously reported that HF causes a decrease in calcium current in our 4 months HF tachypacing induced canine model, [20,43] and in the present study we report reduced calcium transient amplitude. Surprisingly, even in control myocytes where the calcium transient and current are normal, apamin failed to prolong the action potential.

Since a role for I_{KCa} blockers in the treatment of AF has been suggested [11,36] we also evaluated a HF model with superimposed AF. In a recent report in a canine atrial tachypacing AF model, with preserved LV function, I_{KCa} reduction via a drug which reduced calcium sensitivity of the channel caused a significant prolongation of left atrial action potentials. [15] This contrasts with our AF results in the setting of chronic HF, where I_{KCa} blockade failed to prolong the action potential. Notably, we observed that atrial HF myocytes had similar calcium transient amplitudes whether or not AF was superimposed, suggesting that calcium cycling in HF may be insufficient to activate the current.

In agreement with a previous study of patients with chronic AF who had decreased expression of SK proteins, we found that AF superimposed on HF caused a decrease in the SK2 and SK3 protein expression relative to HF alone. [42] Thus, the lack of apamin effect in the 4 months HF+AF atrial cells may be explained by a decrease in protein expression and/or a decrease in the calcium available for current activation. Since I_{KCa} is a very small current ($\sim$14 pS) [44] and repolarization is accelerated in AF (AP is shortened [45]), it may be less likely that a change in I_{KCa} would affect the overall AP duration. The same logic might apply in chronic HF, where atrial repolarization is also accelerated. [20,37].

While we did not find a beneficial role for I_{KCa} block in HF or AF, I_{KCa} blockade might have utility in disease states where atrial repolarization is prolonged, or if there is spatial dispersion of atrial repolarization. Additionally, a recent study shows that I_{KCa} blockade in pulmonary veins terminates AF suggesting a potential role for I_{KCa} blockers in paroxysmal AF. [15].

Limitations

Several studies have shown a gradient of SK channel expression and I_{KCa} current density across the human ventricular wall. [14] However, our experiments used only mid-myocardial myocytes. A similar limitation occurred in the atria, where we only studied cells from the left atrial appendage, and there may be a difference in I_{KCa} between free wall and appendage. [16] Additionally, we used only single cells which may differ in response compared to coupled cells or intact tissue.

One confounding variable in studying I_{KCa} is that the activity varies during the cardiac cycle in a calcium concentration-dependent manner. [32] To assess the role of I_{KCa} in an integrated system, we used perforated patch action potential recordings to permit maintenance of intrinsic calcium cycling, rather than conducting voltage clamp studies to assess the current.

We relied on a pharmacologic approach to define I_{KCa}. As with any pharmacologic approach there is a concern about non-specific effects. A recent report evaluated apamin selectivity in multiple human cardiac ion channels including L-type calcium channels, and confirmed the selectivity of apamin for I_{KCa} at 500 nM which is 5-fold higher than the concentration in the present study. [10] However, it has also been reported that apamin inhibits calcium current in neonatal chick and fetal cells. [46] These reported differences of apamin on calcium current may reflect maturation-dependent differences in channel subunit expression. [47] We did not directly evaluate the effects of apamin on calcium current, but our experimental system is closest to that in the recent report by Yu et al. [10], suggesting that block of calcium current was unlikely to mediate the observed effects of apamin in the present study.

Conclusions

These experiments highlight the need to evaluate novel therapeutic targets for arrhythmias in both atria and ventricles. In chronic HF, I_{KCa} plays a protective role in the ventricle and currrent block is proarrhythmic. Notably, in early HF (1 month canine HF), I_{KCa} blockade is not proarrhythmic, perhaps reflecting a relatively preserved repolarization reserve with a diminished dependence on I_{KCa} for repolarization stability compared to chronic HF.

We found that I_{KCa} does not play a role in repolarization in the atria as current block does not prolong the action potential in either human or canine HF. Similarly, I_{KCa} does not play a role in repolarization of the atrial AP during sustained AF with concurrent chronic HF, despite increased protein expression.

Collectively, our data do not support a role for I_{KCa} blockers for the treatment of atrial arrhythmias. Rather, our findings suggest that therapeutic strategies to reduce I_{KCa} may be unsafe in the setting of atrial arrhythmias with concurrent HF due to potential proarrhythmic effects in the ventricles.

Acknowledgments

Technical support provided by Jeanne Green and Destiny Allen. Human cardiac tissue was obtained through IRB approved protocols and also through collaboration of the Dorothy Davis Heart and Lung Research Institute of the Ohio State University Wexner Medical Center with the Lifeline of Ohio Organ Procurement program.

Author Contributions

Conceived and designed the experiments: IMB SG PJM CC. Performed the experiments: IMB VPL PVP PW AB QL. Analyzed the data: IMB VPL PVP PW AB JY PJM CC. Contributed reagents/materials/analysis tools: KM PFB PMLJ AK PJM. Contributed to the writing of the manuscript: IMB PVP VVF SG PJM CC.

References

1. Kannel WB, Wolf PA, Benjamin EJ, Levy D (1998) Prevalence, incidence, prognosis, and predisposing conditions for atrial fibrillation: population-based estimates. Am J Cardiol 82: 2N–9N.
2. Wang TJ, Larson MG, Levy D, Vasan RS, Leip EP, et al. (2003) Temporal relations of atrial fibrillation and congestive heart failure and their joint influence on mortality: the Framingham Heart Study. Circulation 107: 2920–2925. doi: 10.1161/01.CIR.0000072767.89944.6E.

3. Xu Y, Tuteja D, Zhang Z, Xu D, Zhang Y, et al. (2003) Molecular identification and functional roles of a Ca(2+)-activated K+ channel in human and mouse hearts. J Biol Chem 278: 49085–49094. doi: 10.1074/jbc.M307508200.
4. Vergara C, Latorre R, Marrion NV, Adelman JP (1998) Calcium-activated potassium channels. Curr Opin Neurobiol 8: 321–329. doi: 10.1016/S0959-4388(98)80056-1.
5. Ro S, Hatton WJ, Koh SD, Horowitz B (2001) Molecular properties of small-conductance Ca2+-activated K+ channels expressed in murine colonic smooth muscle. Am J Physiol Gastrointest Liver Physiol 281: G964–G973.
6. Tuteja D, Xu D, Timofeyev V, Lu L, Sharma D, et al. (2005) Differential expression of small-conductance Ca2+-activated K+ channels SK1, SK2, and SK3 in mouse atrial and ventricular myocytes. Am J Physiol Heart Circ Physiol 289: H2714–H2723. doi: 10.1152/ajpheart.00534.2005.
7. Xia XM, Fakler B, Rivard A, Wayman G, Johnson-Pais T, et al. (1998) Mechanism of calcium gating in small-conductance calcium-activated potassium channels. Nature 395: 503–507. doi: 10.1038/26758.
8. Wei AD, Gutman GA, Aldrich R, Chandy KG, Grissmer S, et al. (2005) International Union of Pharmacology. LII. Nomenclature and molecular relationships of calcium-activated potassium channels. Pharmacol Rev 57: 463–472. doi: 10.1124/pr.57.4.9.
9. Grunnet M, Jensen BS, Olesen SP, Klaerke DA (2001) Apamin interacts with all subtypes of cloned small-conductance Ca2+-activated K+ channels. Pflugers Arch 441: 544–550.
10. Yu CC, Ai T, Weiss JN, Chen PS (2014) Apamin does not inhibit human cardiac Na+ current, L-type Ca2+ current or other major K+ currents. PLoS One 9: e96691. doi: 10.1371/journal.pone.0096691 [doi];PONE-D-14-01991 [pii].
11. Li N, Timofeyev V, Tuteja D, Xu D, Lu L, et al. (2009) Ablation of a Ca2+-activated K+ channel (SK2 channel) results in action potential prolongation in atrial myocytes and atrial fibrillation. J Physiol 587: 1087–1100. doi: 10.1113/jphysiol.2008.167718.
12. Gui L, Bao Z, Jia Y, Qin X, Cheng ZJ, et al. (2013) Ventricular tachyarrhythmias in rats with acute myocardial infarction involves activation of small-conductance Ca2+-activated K+ channels. Am J Physiol Heart Circ Physiol 304: H118–H130. doi: 10.1152/ajpheart.00820.2011.
13. Chua SK, Chang PC, Maruyama M, Turker I, Shinohara T, et al. (2011) Small-conductance calcium-activated potassium channel and recurrent ventricular fibrillation in failing rabbit ventricles. Circ Res 108: 971–979. doi: 10.1161/CIRCRESAHA.110.238386.
14. Chang PC, Turker I, Lopshire JC, Masroor S, Nguyen BL, et al. (2013) Heterogeneous upregulation of apamin-sensitive potassium currents in failing human ventricles. J Am Heart Assoc 2: e004713. doi: 10.1161/JAHA.112.004713.
15. Qi XY, Diness JG, Brundel B, Zhou XB, Naud P, et al. (2013) Role of Small Conductance Calcium-Activated Potassium Channels in Atrial Electrophysiology and Fibrillation in the Dog. Circulation 430–440. doi: 10.1161/CIRCULATIONAHA.113.003019.
16. Hsueh CH, Chang PC, Hsieh YC, Reher T, Chen PS, et al. (2013) Proarrhythmic effect of blocking the small conductance calcium activated potassium channel in isolated canine left atrium. Heart Rhythm 10: 891–898. doi: 10.1016/j.hrthm.2013.01.033.
17. Nishijima Y, Feldman DS, Bonagura JD, Ozkanlar Y, Jenkins PJ, et al. (2005) Canine nonischemic left ventricular dysfunction: a model of chronic human cardiomyopathy. J Card Fail 11: 638–644. doi: 10.1016/j.cardfail.2005.05.006.
18. Terentyev D, Gyorke I, Belevych AE, Terentyeva R, Sridhar A, et al. (2008) Redox modification of ryanodine receptors contributes to sarcoplasmic reticulum Ca2+ leak in chronic heart failure. Circ Res 103: 1466–1472. doi: 10.1161/CIRCRESAHA.108.184457.
19. Nishijima Y, Feldman DS, Bonagura JD, Ozkanlar Y, Jenkins PJ, et al. (2005) Canine nonischemic left ventricular dysfunction: a model of chronic human cardiomyopathy. J Card Fail 11: 638–644.
20. Sridhar A, Nishijima Y, Terentyev D, Khan M, Terentyeva R, et al. (2009) Chronic heart failure and the substrate for atrial fibrillation. Cardiovasc Res 84: 227–236. doi: 10.1093/cvr/cvp216.
21. Nishijima Y, Sridhar A, Viatchenko-Karpinski S, Shaw C, Bonagura JD, et al. (2007) Chronic cardiac resynchronization therapy and reverse ventricular remodeling in a model of nonischemic cardiomyopathy. Life Sci 81: 1152–1159. doi: 10.1016/j.lfs.2007.08.022.
22. Bonilla IM, Sridhar A, Nishijima Y, Gyorke S, Cardounel AJ, et al. (2013) Differential effects of the peroxynitrite donor, SIN-1, on atrial and ventricular myocyte electrophysiology. J Cardiovasc Pharmacol 61: 401–407. doi: 10.1097/FJC.0b013e31828748ca.
23. Bonilla IM, Sridhar A, Gyorke S, Cardounel AJ, Carnes CA (2012) Nitric oxide synthases and atrial fibrillation. Front Physiol 3: 105. doi: 10.3389/fphys.2012.00105.
24. Thomsen MB, Volders PG, Beekman JD, Matz J, Vos MA (2006) Beat-to-Beat variability of repolarization determines proarrhythmic outcome in dogs susceptible to drug-induced torsades de pointes. J Am Coll Cardiol 48: 1268–1276. doi: 10.1016/j.jacc.2006.05.048.
25. Bonilla IM, Vargas-Pinto P, Nishijima Y, Pedraza-Toscano A, Ho HT, et al. (2013) Ibandronate and Ventricular Arrhythmia Risk. J Cardiovasc Electrophysiol. doi: 10.1111/jce.12327.
26. Weatherall KL, Seutin V, Liegeois JF, Marrion NV (2011) Crucial role of a shared extracellular loop in apamin sensitivity and maintenance of pore shape of small-conductance calcium-activated potassium (SK) channels. Proc Natl Acad Sci U S A 108: 18494–18499. doi: 10.1073/pnas.1110724108.
27. Weatherall KL, Goodchild SJ, Jane DE, Marrion NV (2010) Small conductance calcium-activated potassium channels: from structure to function. Prog Neurobiol 91: 242–255. doi: 10.1016/j.pneurobio.2010.03.002.
28. Grunnet M, Jespersen T, Angelo K, Frokjaer-Jensen C, Klaerke DA, et al. (2001) Pharmacological modulation of SK3 channels. Neuropharmacology 40: 879–887. doi: 10.1016/S0028-3908(01)00028-4.
29. Thomsen MB, Oros A, Schoenmakers M, van Opstal JM, Maas JN, et al. (2007) Proarrhythmic electrical remodelling is associated with increased beat-to-beat variability of repolarisation. Cardiovasc Res 73: 521–530. doi: 10.1016/j.cardiores.2006.11.025.
30. Bildl W, Strassmaier T, Thurm H, Andersen J, Eble S, et al. (2004) Protein kinase CK2 is coassembled with small conductance Ca(2+)-activated K+ channels and regulates channel gating. Neuron 43: 847–858. doi: 10.1016/j.neuron.2004.08.033.
31. Belevych AE, Terentyev D, Terentyeva R, Nishijima Y, Sridhar A, et al. (2011) The relationship between arrhythmogenesis and impaired contractility in heart failure: role of altered ryanodine receptor function. Cardiovasc Res 90: 493–502. doi: 10.1093/cvr/cvr025.
32. Terentyev D, Rochira JA, Terentyeva R, Roder K, Koren G, et al. (2013) Sarcoplasmic reticulum Ca2+ release is both necessary and sufficient for SK channel activation in ventricular myocytes. Am J Physiol Heart Circ Physiol In Press. doi: 10.1152/ajpheart.00621.2013.
33. Roden DM (1998) Taking the "idio" out of "idiosyncratic": predicting torsades de pointes. Pacing Clin Electrophysiol 21: 1029–1034.
34. Winslow RL, Rice J, Jafri S, Marban E, O'Rourke B (1999) Mechanisms of altered excitation-contraction coupling in canine tachycardia-induced heart failure, II: model studies. Circ Res 84: 571–586. doi: 10.1161/01.RES.84.5.571.
35. Kaab S, Nuss HB, Chiamvimonvat N, O'Rourke B, Pak PH, et al. (1996) Ionic mechanism of action potential prolongation in ventricular myocytes from dogs with pacing-induced heart failure. Circ Res 78: 262–273. doi: 10.1161/01.RES.78.2.262.
36. Nattel S (2009) Calcium-activated potassium current: a novel ion channel candidate in atrial fibrillation. J Physiol 587: 1385–1386. doi: 10.1113/jphysiol.2009.170621.
37. Workman AJ, Pau D, Redpath CJ, Marshall GE, Russell JA, et al. (2009) Atrial cellular electrophysiological changes in patients with ventricular dysfunction may predispose to AF. Heart Rhythm 6: 445–451. doi: 10.1016/j.hrthm.2008.12.028.
38. Schreieck J, Wang Y, Overbeck M, Schomig A, Schmitt C (2000) Altered transient outward current in human atrial myocytes of patients with reduced left ventricular function. J Cardiovasc Electrophysiol 11: 180–192.
39. Glukhov AV, Fedorov VV, Kalish PW, Ravikumar VK, Lou Q, et al. (2012) Conduction remodeling in human end-stage nonischemic left ventricular cardiomyopathy. Circulation 125: 1835–1847. doi: 10.1161/CIRCULATIONAHA.111.047274.
40. Chang SH, Chang SN, Hwang JJ, Chiang FT, Tseng CD, et al. (2012) Significant association of rs13376333 in KCNN3 on chromosome 1q21 with atrial fibrillation in a Taiwanese population. Circ J 76: 184–188. doi: 10.1253/circj.CJ-11-0525.
41. Ellinor PT, Lunetta KL, Glazer NL, Pfeufer A, Alonso A, et al. (2010) Common variants in KCNN3 are associated with lone atrial fibrillation. Nat Genet 42: 240–244. doi: 10.1038/ng.537.
42. Yu T, Deng C, Wu R, Guo H, Zheng S, et al. (2012) Decreased expression of small-conductance Ca2+-activated K+ channels SK1 and SK2 in human chronic atrial fibrillation. Life Sci 90: 219–227. doi: 10.1016/j.lfs.2011.11.008.
43. Kubalova Z, Terentyev D, Viatchenko-Karpinski S, Nishijima Y, Gyorke I, et al. (2005) Abnormal intrastore calcium signaling in chronic heart failure. Proc Natl Acad Sci U S A 102: 14104–14109. doi: 10.1073/pnas.0504298102.
44. Park YB (1994) Ion selectivity and gating of small conductance Ca(2+)-activated K+ channels in cultured rat adrenal chromaffin cells. J Physiol 481 (Pt 3): 555–570.
45. Van Wagoner DR, Pond AL, Lamorgese M, Rossie SS, McCarthy PM, et al. (1999) Atrial L-type Ca2+ currents and human atrial fibrillation. Circ Res 85: 428–436. doi: 10.1161/01.RES.85.5.428.
46. Bkaily G, Sculptoreanu A, Jacques D, Economos D, Menard D (1992) Apamin, a highly potent fetal L-type Ca2+ current blocker in single heart cells. Am J Physiol 262: H463–H471.
47. Brillantes AM, Bezprozvannaya S, Marks AR (1994) Developmental and tissue-specific regulation of rabbit skeletal and cardiac muscle calcium channels involved in excitation-contraction coupling. Circ Res 75: 503–510.

Permissions

All chapters in this book were first published in PLOS ONE, by The Public Library of Science; hereby published with permission under the Creative Commons Attribution License or equivalent. Every chapter published in this book has been scrutinized by our experts. Their significance has been extensively debated. The topics covered herein carry significant findings which will fuel the growth of the discipline. They may even be implemented as practical applications or may be referred to as a beginning point for another development.

The contributors of this book come from diverse backgrounds, making this book a truly international effort. This book will bring forth new frontiers with its revolutionizing research information and detailed analysis of the nascent developments around the world.

We would like to thank all the contributing authors for lending their expertise to make the book truly unique. They have played a crucial role in the development of this book. Without their invaluable contributions this book wouldn't have been possible. They have made vital efforts to compile up to date information on the varied aspects of this subject to make this book a valuable addition to the collection of many professionals and students.

This book was conceptualized with the vision of imparting up-to-date information and advanced data in this field. To ensure the same, a matchless editorial board was set up. Every individual on the board went through rigorous rounds of assessment to prove their worth. After which they invested a large part of their time researching and compiling the most relevant data for our readers.

The editorial board has been involved in producing this book since its inception. They have spent rigorous hours researching and exploring the diverse topics which have resulted in the successful publishing of this book. They have passed on their knowledge of decades through this book. To expedite this challenging task, the publisher supported the team at every step. A small team of assistant editors was also appointed to further simplify the editing procedure and attain best results for the readers.

Apart from the editorial board, the designing team has also invested a significant amount of their time in understanding the subject and creating the most relevant covers. They scrutinized every image to scout for the most suitable representation of the subject and create an appropriate cover for the book.

The publishing team has been an ardent support to the editorial, designing and production team. Their endless efforts to recruit the best for this project, has resulted in the accomplishment of this book. They are a veteran in the field of academics and their pool of knowledge is as vast as their experience in printing. Their expertise and guidance has proved useful at every step. Their uncompromising quality standards have made this book an exceptional effort. Their encouragement from time to time has been an inspiration for everyone.

The publisher and the editorial board hope that this book will prove to be a valuable piece of knowledge for researchers, students, practitioners and scholars across the globe.

List of Contributors

Victor C. Kok
Public Health and Clinical Informatics Research Group, Department of Biomedical Informatics, Asia University, Wufeng, Taichung, Taiwan
Department of Internal Medicine, Kuang Tien General Hospital, Shalu, Taichung, Taiwan

Jorng-Tzong Horng
Public Health and Clinical Informatics Research Group, Department of Biomedical Informatics, Asia University, Wufeng, Taichung, Taiwan
Department of Computer Science and Information Engineering, National Central University, Jhongli, Taoyuan, Taiwan

Wan-Shan Chang
Department of Computer Science and Information Engineering, National Central University, Jhongli, Taoyuan, Taiwan

Ya-Fang Hong
Institute of Molecular Biology, Academia Sinica, Nankang, Taipei, Taiwan

Tzu-Hao Chang
Graduate Institute of Biomedical Informatics, Taipei Medical University, Taipei, Taiwan

Matthew A. Schechter, Michael K. H. Hsieh, Linda W. Njoroge, Bryan J. Feger, Constantine D. Troupes, Whitney L. Nagel, Gina P. Landinez, Kishan M. Shah, Lucia Santacruz, Carmelo A. Milano, Valentino Piacentino III and Dawn E. Bowles
Department of Surgery, Duke University Medical Center, Durham, North Carolina, United States of America

J. Will Thompson, Erik J. Soderblom and M. Arthur Moseley
Duke Proteomics Core, Duke University Medical Center, Durham, North Carolina, United States of America

Kathleen A. Hershberger and Matthew D. Hirschey
Sarah W. Stedman Nutrition and Metabolism Center, Duke University Medical Center, Durham, North Carolina, United States of America
Department of Medicine, Duke University Medical Center, Durham, North Carolina, United States of America

Olga R. Ilkayeva
Sarah W. Stedman Nutrition and Metabolism Center, Duke University Medical Center, Durham, North Carolina, United States of America

Virginia A. Burns
Duke Translational Research Institute, Duke University Medical Center, Durham, North Carolina, United States of America

Matthew W. Foster
Division of Pulmonary, Allergy and Critical Care, Medicine, Duke University Medical Center, Durham, North Carolina, United States of America

Luciana Mesquita Passamani
School of Physiology & Pharmacology, Bristol Heart Institute, Medical Sciences Building, University of Bristol, Bristol, United Kingdom
Department of Physiological Sciences, Health Sciences Center, Federal University of Espı´rito Santo, Vito´ ria, Espírito Santo, Brazil

Ana Paula Abdala and Julian Francis Richmond Paton
School of Physiology & Pharmacology, Bristol Heart Institute, Medical Sciences Building, University of Bristol, Bristol, United Kingdom

Davi José de Almeida Moraes
Department of Physiology, School of Medicine of Ribeirã o Preto, University of São Paulo, Ribeirão Preto, São Paulo, Brazil

Karla Nívea Sampaio
Department of Pharmaceutical Sciences, Health Sciences Center, Federal University of Espírito Santo, Vitória, Espírito Santo, Brazil

José Geraldo Mill
Department of Physiological Sciences, Health Sciences Center, Federal University of Espírito Santo, Vitória, Espírito Santo, Brazil

Laszlo Deres, Krisztian Eros, Adam Riba and Robert Halmosi
First Department of Medicine, Division of Cardiology, University of Pécs, Pécs, Hungary
Szentagothai Janos Research Center, University of Pécs, Medical School, Pécs, Hungary

Eva Bartha, Anita Palfi and Kalman Toth
First Department of Medicine, Division of Cardiology, University of Pécs, Pécs, Hungary

Janos Lantos
Department of Surgical Research and Techniques, University of Pécs, Pécs, Hungary

Tamas Kalai and Kalman Hideg
Department of Organic and Medicinal Chemistry, University of Pécs, Pécs, Hungary

Balazs Sumegi
Szentagothai Janos Research Center, University of Pécs, Medical School, Pécs, Hungary
Department of Biochemistry and Medical Chemistry, Medical School, University of Pécs, Pécs, Hungary
MTA-PTE Nuclear-Mitochondrial Interactions Research Group, Pécs, Hungary

Ferenc Gallyas
Department of Biochemistry and Medical Chemistry, Medical School, University of Pécs, Pécs, Hungary
MTA-PTE Nuclear-Mitochondrial Interactions Research Group, Pécs, Hungary

Manoraj Navaratnarajah, Urszula Siedlecka, Michael Ibrahim, Carin van Doorn, Gopal Soppa, Ajay Gandhi, Adarsh Shah, Punam Kukadia, Magdi H. Yacoub and Cesare M. Terracciano
Harefield Heart Science Centre, Imperial College London, National Heart and Lung Institute, Laboratory of Cellular Electrophysiology, Harefield Hospital, Harefield, Middlesex, United Kingdom

Brendan N. Putko, Zuocheng Wang, Jennifer Lo, Harald Becher and Gavin Y. Oudit
Division of Cardiology, Department of Medicine, University of Alberta, Edmonton, Alberta, Canada
Mazankowski Alberta Heart Institute, University of Alberta, Edmonton, Alberta, Canada

Todd Anderson
Libin Cardiovascular Institute, University of Calgary, Calgary, Alberta, Canada

Jason R. B. Dyck
Mazankowski Alberta Heart Institute, University of Alberta, Edmonton, Alberta, Canada
Department of Pediatrics, University of Alberta, Edmonton, Alberta, Canada

Zamaneh Kassiri
Mazankowski Alberta Heart Institute, University of Alberta, Edmonton, Alberta, Canada
Department of Physiology, University of Alberta, Edmonton, Alberta, Canada

Chun Li and Xingyun Chai
Modern Research Center for Traditional Chinese Medicine, Beijing University of Chinese Medicine, Beijing, China

Yong Wang, Tianjiao Shi, Yan Wu, Jing Han and Wei Wang
Basic Medical College, Beijing University of Chinese Medicine, Beijing, China

Qi Qiu
Anzhen Hospital of Capital Medical University, Beijing, China

Michal Mor, Wesam Mulla, Sigal Elyagon and Shani Dror
Cardiac Arrhythmia Research Laboratory, Department of Physiology and Cell Biology, Faculty of Health Sciences, Ben-Gurion University of the Negev, Beer-Sheva, Israel

Hovav Gabay
Cardiac Arrhythmia Research Laboratory, Department of Physiology and Cell Biology, Faculty of Health Sciences, Ben-Gurion University of the Negev, Beer-Sheva, Israel
Department of Emergency Medicine, Recanati School for Community Health Professions, Faculty of Health Sciences and PREPARED Center for Emergency Response Research, Ben-Gurion University of the Negev, Beer-Sheva, Israel

Yoram Etzion
Cardiac Arrhythmia Research Laboratory, Department of Physiology and Cell Biology, Faculty of Health Sciences, Ben-Gurion University of the Negev, Beer-Sheva, Israel
Division of Internal Medicine, Soroka University Medical Center, Beer-Sheva, Israel

Noah Liel-Cohen
Cardiology Department, Soroka University Medical Center, Beer-Sheva, Israel

Marina T. Durand, Christiane Becari, Mauro de Oliveira, Carlos Alberto Aguiar Silva, Rubens Fazan Jr, Helio C. Salgado
Department of Physiology, School of Medicine of Ribeirão Preto, University of São Paulo, Ribeirão Preto, São Paulo, Brazil

Jussara M. do Carmo
Department of Physiology and Biophysics, University of Mississippi Medical Center, Jackson, Mississippi, United States of America

Cibele M. Prado
Department of Pathology, School of Medicine of Ribeirão Preto, University of São Paulo, Ribeirão Preto, São Paulo, Brazil

Aline S. Bossa, Jorge Kalil, Edecio Cunha-Neto, Ludmila Rodrigues Pinto Ferreira
Laboratory of Immunology, Heart Institute (InCor), University of São Paulo School of Medicine, São Paulo, Brazil
Division of Clinical Immunology and Allergy, University of São Paulo School of Medicine, São Paulo, Brazil

Vera M. C. Salemi, Suzete C. Ferreira and Charles Mady
Cardiomyopathy Unit, Heart Institute (InCor), University of São Paulo School of Medicine, São Paulo, Brazil

Susan P. Ribeiro
Division of Clinical Immunology and Allergy, University of São Paulo School of Medicine, São Paulo, Brazil

Daniela S. Rosa
Division of Immunology, Department of Microbiology, Immunology and Parasitology-Federal University of São Paulo-UNIFESP, São Paulo, Brazil

Anna Shoko Nishiya
Pró - Sangue Foundation, São Paulo, Brazil; Institute for Investigation in Immunology (iii), INCT, São Paulo, Brazil

Marino DiFranco, Marbella Quiñonez and Julio L. Vergara
Department of Physiology, David Geffen School of Medicine, University of California Los Angeles, Los Angeles, California, United States of America

Perry Shieh
Department of Neurology, David Geffen School of Medicine, University of California Los Angeles, Los Angeles, California, United States of America

Gregg C. Fonarow, Daniel Cruz, Mario C. Deng
Division of Cardiology, Department of Medicine, David Geffen School of Medicine, University of California Los Angeles, Los Angeles, California, United States of America

Holly R. Middlekauff
Department of Physiology, David Geffen School of Medicine, University of California Los Angeles, Los Angeles, California, United States of America
Division of Cardiology, Department of Medicine, David Geffen School of Medicine, University of California Los Angeles, Los Angeles, California, United States of America

Li-hui Zheng, Ling-min Wu, Yan Yao, Wen-sheng Chen, Jing-ru Bao, Wen Huang, Rui Shi, Kui-jun Zhang and Shu Zhang
State Key Laboratory of Cardiovascular Disease, Clinical EP Lab & Arrhythmia Center, Fuwai Hospital, National Center for Cardiovascular Diseases, Chinese Academy of Medical Sciences and Peking Union Medical College, Beijing, China

Charles E. Leonard, Hanieh Razzaghi, Cristin P. Freeman and Jason A. Roy
Center for Clinical Epidemiology & Biostatistics, Department of Biostatistics & Epidemiology, Perelman School of Medicine at the University of Pennsylvania, Philadelphia, Pennsylvania, United States of America
Center for Pharmacoepidemiology Research and Training, Perelman School of Medicine at the University of Pennsylvania, Philadelphia, Pennsylvania, United States of America

Craig W. Newcomb
Center for Clinical Epidemiology & Biostatistics, Department of Biostatistics & Epidemiology, Perelman School of Medicine at the University of Pennsylvania, Philadelphia, Pennsylvania, United States of America,

Sean Hennessy
Center for Clinical Epidemiology & Biostatistics, Department of Biostatistics & Epidemiology, Perelman School of Medicine at the University of Pennsylvania, Philadelphia, Pennsylvania, United States of America
Center for Pharmacoepidemiology Research and Training, Perelman School of Medicine at the University of Pennsylvania, Philadelphia, Pennsylvania, United States of America
Department of Pharmacology, Perelman School of Medicine at the University of Pennsylvania, Philadelphia, Pennsylvania, United States of America

Mariana Gavioli, Aline Lara, Pedro W. M. Almeida, Denis D. Damasceno, Cibele Rocha-Resende, Marina Ladeira
Department of Physiology and Biophysics, Institute of Biological Sciences, Universidade Federal de Minas Gerais, Belo Horizonte, Brazil

Augusto Martins Lima, Marcos Barrouin Melo, Marco Antonio Peliky Fontes, Robson A. Souza Santos and Silvia Guatimosim
Department of Physiology and Biophysics, Institute of Biological Sciences, Universidade Federal de Minas Gerais, Belo Horizonte, Brazil
National Institute of Science and Technology in Nanobiopharmaceutics, Universidade Federal de Minas Gerais, Belo Horizonte, MG, Brazil

Rodrigo R. Resende
Department of Biochemistry, Institute of Biological Sciences, Universidade Federal de Minas Gerais, Belo Horizonte, Brazil

Patricia M. Martinelli
Department of Morphology, Institute of Biological Sciences, Universidade Federal de Minas Gerais, Belo Horizonte, Brazil

Patricia C. Brum
School of Physical Education and Sport, Universidade de São Paulo, São Paulo, Brazil

Marco A. M. Prado
Robarts Research Institute, University of Western Ontario, Department of Physiology and Pharmacology, Department of Anatomy & Cell Biology, Schulich School of Medicine & Dentistry, University of Western Ontario, London, Canada

Juan F. Gomez, Karen Cardona, Laura Martinez, Javier Saiz and Beatriz Trenor
Instituto de Investigación en Ingeniería Biomédica, UniversitatPolitècnica de València, Valencia, Spain

Neeta Adhikari, Marjorie Carlson, Adam Mitchell, Peter Eckman and Jennifer L. Hall
Lillehei Heart Institute, Department of Medicine, University of Minnesota, Minneapolis, Minnesota, United States of America

Weihua Guan
Division of Biostatistics, University of Minnesota, Minneapolis, Minnesota, United States of America

Brian Capaldo and Aaron J. Mackey
Center for Public Health Genomics, University of Virginia, Charlottesville,Virginia, United States of America

Sundaram Ramakrishnan
Department of Pharmacology, University of Minnesota, Minneapolis, Minnesota, United States of America

Dinesha Walek
University of Minnesota Genomics Center, University of Minnesota, Minneapolis, Minnesota, United States of America

Manu Gupta
National Institute of Heart Research, Cardiovascular Biomedical Research Unit, Royal Brompton and Harefield Trust, London, United Kingdom

Ranjit John
Department of Surgery, Cardiothoracic Surgery Division, University of Minnesota, Minneapolis, Minnesota, United States of America

Euan Ashley
Center for Inherited Cardiovascular Disease, Department of Medicine, Stanford University, Stanford, California, United States of America

Paul J. Barton
Heart Science Centre, National Heart and Lung Institute, Imperial College, London, United Kingdom

Yujie Zhu, Mohamed A. Hanafy, Cheryl R. Killingsworth, Gregory P. Walcott, Martin E. Young,
Steven M. Pogwizd
Department of Medicine, University of Alabama at Birmingham, Birmingham, Alabama, United States of America

Kosuke Minai, Takayuki Ogawa, Makoto Kawai, Kimiaki Komukai, Toshikazu Tanaka, Kazuo Ogawa,

Tomohisa Nagoshi, Satoshi Arase, Satoshi Morimoto, Yasunori Inoue, Hiroshi Sekiyama, Akihiro Urabe, Seiichiro Matsuo, Kenichi Hongo and Michihiro Yoshimura
Division of Cardiology, Department of Internal Medicine, The Jikei University School of Medicine, Tokyo, Japan

Gaetano Valenza
Neuroscience Statistics Research Laboratory, Department of Anesthesia, Critical Care & Pain Medicine, Harvard Medical School, Massachusetts General Hospital, Boston, Massachusetts, United States of America; and Department of Brain and Cognitive Science, Massachusetts Institute of Technology, Cambridge, Massachusetts, United States of America
Research Center E. Piaggio and Department of Information Engineering, University of Pisa, Pisa, Italy

Luca Citi
Neuroscience Statistics Research Laboratory, Department of Anesthesia, Critical Care & Pain Medicine, Harvard Medical School, Massachusetts General Hospital, Boston, Massachusetts, United States of America; and Department of Brain and Cognitive Science, Massachusetts Institute of Technology, Cambridge, Massachusetts, United States of America
School of Computer Science and Electronic Engineering, University of Essex, Colchester, United Kingdom

Riccardo Barbieri
Neuroscience Statistics Research Laboratory, Department of Anesthesia, Critical Care & Pain Medicine, Harvard Medical School, Massachusetts General Hospital, Boston, Massachusetts, United States of America; and Department of Brain and Cognitive Science, Massachusetts Institute of Technology, Cambridge, Massachusetts, United States of America

Naoko Matsushita
Department of Molecular and Cellular Pharmacology, Iwate Medical University School of Pharmaceutical Sciences, Shiwa, Iwate, Japan
Department of Pharmacology, Iwate Medical University School of Medicine, Shiwa, Iwate, Japan

Toshihide Kashihara, Tsutomu Nakada and Mitsuhiko Yamada
Department of Molecular Pharmacology, Shinshu University School of Medicine, Matsumoto, Nagano, Japan

Hisashi Shimojo
Department of Pathology, Shinshu University School of Medicine, Matsumoto, Nagano, Japan

Satoshi Suzuki and Yasuchika Takeishi
Department of Cardiology and Hematology, Fukushima Medical University, Fukushima, Fukushima, Japan

Ulrike Mende
Cardiovascular Research Center, Division of Cardiology, Rhode Island Hospital & The Alpert Medical School of Brown University, Providence, Rhode Island, United States of America

Eiichi Taira
Department of Pharmacology, Iwate Medical University School of Medicine, Shiwa, Iwate, Japan

Atsushi Sanbe
Department of Pharmacotherapeutics, Iwate Medical University School of Pharmaceutical Sciences, Shiwa, Iwate, Japan

Masamichi Hirose
Department of Molecular and Cellular Pharmacology, Iwate Medical University School of Pharmaceutical Sciences, Shiwa, Iwate, Japan

Ingrid M. Bonilla and Victor P. Long, III
College of Pharmacy, The Ohio State University, Columbus, Ohio, United States of America

Dorothy M. Davis Heart and Lung Research Institute, The Ohio State University Wexner Medical Center, Columbus, Ohio, United States of America

Pedro Vargas-Pinto
College of Veterinary Medicine, The Ohio State University, Columbus, Ohio, United States of America

Patrick Wright, Andriy Belevych, Qing Lou, Philip F. Binkley, Vadim V. Fedorov, Sandor Györke, Paulus M. L. Janssen, Ahmet Kilic and Peter J. Mohler
Dorothy M. Davis Heart and Lung Research Institute, The Ohio State University Wexner Medical Center, Columbus, Ohio, United States of America

Kent Mowrey,
St Jude Medical, Sylmar, California, United States of America

Jae Yoo,
College of Pharmacy, The Ohio State University, Columbus, Ohio, United States of America,

Cynthia A. Carnes
College of Pharmacy, The Ohio State University, Columbus, Ohio, United States of America,
College of Veterinary Medicine, The Ohio State University, Columbus, Ohio, United States of America

Index